# Medicinal Cannabis and CBD in Mental Healthcare

Kylie O'Brien • Philip Blair

# Medicinal Cannabis and CBD in Mental Healthcare

Springer

Kylie O'Brien
Torrens University Australia
Adelaide, Sth Australia
Australia

Philip Blair
Private Practise
Castle Rock, WA
USA

ISBN 978-3-030-78558-1 ISBN 978-3-030-78559-8 (eBook)
https://doi.org/10.1007/978-3-030-78559-8



This Springer imprint is published by the registered company Springer Nature Switzerland AG
The registered company address is: Gewerbestrasse 11, 6330 Cham, Switzerland

# Foreword

Dr. Kylie O'Brien, PhD, the Chief Scientific Officer at Releaf Group Ltd and Adjunct Professor at Torrens University, and Dr. Philip Blair, a family physician and retired United States Army colonel who has utilized medical cannabis in his practice for a number of years, have written a comprehensive textbook on the relationship between cannabinoids, including cannabis, and mental health. This important book will be a resource for clinicians and patients around the world.

Cannabis remains a polarizing topic around the world. Some say that cannabis is harmless and that it can treat almost any medical condition while others refer to it as the "Devil's Drug" with no place in medical practice. Neither extreme view is true. Unfortunately, though, patients and their doctors are caught in the middle of this battle, and it has become hard to learn the truth about cannabis and cannabinoids and to access doctors comfortable with utilizing cannabinoids in their practices. It is my sincere hope that this book will help address this problematic situation.

The authors, one a well-known educator and the other a noted clinician, work to dispel many misunderstandings about cannabis, primarily known as a recreational drug. The level of detail shows the authors' obvious passion for this topic. More recently, though, evidence has been building to support the use of cannabis and cannabinoids as pharmacotherapies for a host of medical indications.

The book opens with an introduction, followed by a chapter describing the endocannabinoid system as a foundation for understanding the hypothetical rationale for cannabinoids as medications. Chapter 3 discusses the relationship between the endocannabinoid system and stress. Chapter 2 plays a vital role by explaining what medical cannabis is and what it is comprised of. Unfortunately, many people have different understandings of what medical cannabis refers to. The authors explain the roles of delta-9-tetrahydrocannabinol (THC) and cannabidiol (CBD), but they also introduce terpenes and other phytocannabinoids. From there, the book covers specific medical conditions—anxiety, depression, post-traumatic stress disorder (PTSD), insomnia, Alzheimer's Disease, and autism spectrum disorder.

For each medical condition, the authors present key information about each condition before reviewing the state of the evidence—both preclinical and clinical—for cannabinoids as possible treatments for these conditions. The depth in each chapter is considerable as the authors dissect the role of the endocannabinoid system in each condition, why cannabinoids may alleviate symptoms in each condition, and the current state of the evidence for cannabinoids for each. They place a particular focus on THC and CBD as those are the most commonly utilized cannabinoids in most medical practices. Case studies are used to illustrate clinical considerations that are likely to arise. The authors acknowledge that the level of evidence for various cannabinoids for different medical conditions varies widely, but they want to ensure that patients and clinicians have all of the evidence at their disposal so that they can make informed decisions about their health.

The authors should be commended for making an important contribution to the science of cannabinoids by creating an exhaustive resource. Patients and clinicians alike will find this book to be an important resource, especially with misinformation on cannabis being so plentiful these days. We clearly need additional rigorous research on the potential medical benefits of cannabinoids. For several reasons, the rate and scale of the research has not kept pace with the surging public interest. Drs. O'Brien and Blair, however, recognized the need for guidance today for patients and clinicians discussing the possibility of cannabinoid pharmacotherapy for mental health conditions, and they have made an impressive contribution.

Associate Professor of Psychiatry
Harvard Medical School
Boston, MA, USA

Kevin P. Hill

# Disclaimer

This book was written for the purposes of healthcare practitioner education. It is not intended as medical advice for any individual. Individuals interested in the potential use of medicinal cannabis for their own health concerns are advised to consult an appropriate healthcare practitioner knowledgeable in its use.

# Contents

# Introduction

# 1

## Why This Book?

More than 10% of the world's population suffer from some kind of mental illness and in the United States of America (USA), almost one in five have a mental illness with women and young adults/adolescents being the most affected [1, 2]. What extraordinary figures. Mental health issues such as anxiety, depression, and post-traumatic stress disorder (PTSD) consistently come up as some of the main reasons people use cannabis medicinally. Yet, little is really understood by the medical fraternity about how cannabis may be able to alleviate such problems. There is still much unnecessary stigma attached to the smoking of "marijuana," and unfortunately this seems to have spilled over and tarred its medical use somewhat. This is a key reason for writing this book—to demonstrate that while much more needs to be discovered, there is also much scientific evidence already in relation to many medical conditions, including mental health conditions.

Cannabis is not new, but it is to most medical practitioners practicing right now. It has a history of use of thousands of years in many cultures including China, India, and Egypt, to name just a few. Cannabis was used by some of the greats of medicine in the western world in the 1800s including Sir William Osler (USA) and Sir John Russell Reynolds (UK). It was in common medical use in the USA, prescribed by medical practitioners until it was prohibited in 1937 with the passing of the Marijuana Tax Act 1937 over the objections of the American Medical Association. What then has ensued has been an effective smear campaign, overregulation, and politicization, which has effectively denied access to this ancient and medicinal herb to over 100 countries as a result of the United Nations Single Convention on Narcotic Drugs of 1961.

Prescribing medicinal cannabis is somewhat different to prescribing a pharmaceutical, simply because it is an herbal medicine and it does need to be individualized to the patient. The patient needs to take an active role in the titration of dosage. The practice of individualizing herbs is what herbal medicine practitioners do every



K. O'Brien, P. Blair, *Medicinal Cannabis and CBD in Mental Healthcare*,
https://doi.org/10.1007/978-3-030-78559-8_1

day, but it is not what a western medical doctor normally does. To make things more complex, everyone's endocannabinoid system is different, and therefore different people will respond differently.

The concern voiced by many of our medical colleagues is typically around "the evidence" that medicinal cannabis works. As laws and regulations associated with cannabis change and barriers to access and stigma break down, more patients are becoming curious about medicinal cannabis and are wanting to know if it might help them. Some have already taken the decision into their own hands of course, since their personal physician will not discuss cannabinoids intelligently. Few medical practitioners have been educated about the endocannabinoid system or the depth of established evidence for medicinal cannabis in practice. And, since it's not a pharmaceutical drug, they simply do not know how medicinal cannabis might work or how to manage patients with herbal extracts. For this reason we decided to write this book for healthcare practitioners.

There is much research into medicinal cannabis already: as of January 2021, PubMed lists over 32,000 reports on cannabinoids and over 13,000 US National Institutes of Health (NIH) grants. The spectrum of studies is expansive due to the lack of approved model drugs, nonconformity of herbal extracts, and the extraordinary pleotropic mechanisms of cannabinoid action. Preclinical research serves to help us understand how the endocannabinoid system works, how the endocannabinoid system becomes dysfunctional in particular diseases or conditions, what are the mechanisms of action in different conditions, and how effective is cannabinoid therapy in mitigating such illness (typically through the use of animal models of disease, cell cultures, or ex vivo tissue). It is easier to conduct preclinical research, relatively speaking, and knowledge gained there is typically used to provide a rationale for then conducting research in humans. This is the pharmaceutical approach to research.

Human evidence comes in many forms including epidemiological studies, case studies, randomized controlled trials, and systematic reviews. There is comparatively less research in humans simply because it has been so difficult for researchers to be able to conduct research into medicinal cannabis for a variety of reasons. The exception here might be Israel which seems to have adopted a more open approach to research into cannabis. The foremost reason for this difficulty is tied to the manner in which cannabis has been regulated and restricted. Other reasons relate to funding. Government research funding is often difficult to procure. There is also less interest in medicinal cannabis from wealthy pharmaceutical companies as it is difficult to patent plants. The pharmaceutical model requires something to patent.

## The Structure of the Book

This book has been written to pull together some of the scientific evidence for the use of medicinal cannabis in common mental health conditions and insomnia. While insomnia is not a mental health condition per se, it often goes hand in hand with other conditions such as anxiety and poor sleep which can certainly affect our mental health. It begins with a description of the endocannabinoid system in some depth (Chap. 2). Chapter 3 discusses the endocannabinoid system and stress. Chapter 4 examines what medicinal cannabis is and its key constituents (the phytocannabinoids, terpenes, and other plant nutrients) with a focus on cannabidiol (CBD) and tetrahydrocannabinol (THC). The remainder of the book covers the six clinical topics of anxiety, depression, post-traumatic stress disorder (PTSD), sleep disorders (insomnia), Alzheimer's disease, and autism spectrum disorder (ASD). We chose to include a chapter on cannabis routes of delivery, pharmacokinetics and safety at the end of the book, rather than including this information in Chap. 4 (already a long chapter) so as to not interrupt the flow of the book. The final chapter, the Conclusion, completes the book.

The approach we have taken to the topic of mental health and medicinal cannabis is to summarize key information about each condition, including its pathophysiology, and then look at scientific evidence of how the endocannabinoid system is involved in the particular condition. We then examine the evidence that CBD and THC in particular may be able to contribute to its treatment by looking at potential mechanisms of action, preclinical evidence of efficacy, and clinical evidence of efficacy. We include some information on terpenes and other phytocannabinoids in some chapters also. Finally, we end with some dosing guidelines for use of medicinal cannabis products for the treatment of that particular condition, with a focus on treatment with CBD-dominant products, and one or two case studies from Dr. Blair's clinical practice.

We have chosen to focus in particular on CBD and also THC in this book, but recognize that there are other phytocannabinoids and terpenes which are showing promise. It is Dr. Blair's clinical experience and success with prescribing CBD-dominant products that provided the impetus to focus this book including the case studies on CBD. In countries such as Australia, where it is an offense under its driving laws to drive with any amount of THC in your body, the prescribing of products containing THC is somewhat fraught. Many patients prefer not to run the gauntlet and choose to use CBD products. Other patients prefer not to have any of the potential side effects that may be associated with THC, though as you will come to understand, these are dose-dependent. And for many conditions, CBD-dominant products work very well.

## Limitations

There are limitations to what can be covered in a book, and we are aware of our own limitations as academics and clinicians. The heroes are all the scientists whose work we have sought to summarize and bring together, as it is those women and men who have spent much time and effort to produce the scientific evidence that ultimately provides the rationale for the use of medicinal cannabis in the treatment of so many diseases. We have sought to cover the pathophysiology of each condition sufficiently; however, we are aware that in each of these conditions, there is emerging knowledge and theories and it is likely we may have missed information. We seek your forgiveness where we may not have been complete or have missed something.

We understand that by the time this book goes to print, even more studies will have been published. We encourage our healthcare practitioner colleagues to keep up with the literature as it emerges.

## Medicinal Cannabis as Part of a Holistic Therapeutic Approach

Medicinal cannabis is not a magic bullet, and as practitioners we are treating a person who has become out of balance in some way. We must consider all the factors that may have brought about this imbalance: stress, poor nutrition, lack of physical activity, poor sleep, lack of sunshine (vitamin D), and others. Medicinal cannabis should be an important component of a holistic treatment strategy that may also include western pharmaceuticals. We would stress that as practitioners, you need to help the patient address all of those factors that have led to the dis-ease, and if you don't have knowledge in a particular area such as nutrition, for example, expand your network and refer your patient to other practitioners who may have such knowledge. This is integrative medicine. You don't need to be an expert in everything. But you do need to keep an open mind and be aware of other modalities that can help your patients. Remember to empower your patients with knowledge. In the end, it is they who must heal themselves.

## Your Journey

This book has been written for our healthcare practitioner colleagues and lay-scientists who are making a substantial impact on medical knowledge. It seeks to set out the scientific evidence in a logical manner so that you can establish a clinical basis for the use of medicinal cannabis therapy in mental health disorders, based on understanding how the endocannabinoid system and other factors are involved in the pathophysiology of such conditions. Perhaps, you will be better prepared when your next patient, family member, or friend asks you about the use of cannabinoids for one of these conditions. At the very least, we hope that you come away with an appreciation that indeed there is much already known about how medicinal cannabis may be able to help treat several mental health conditions and that it will give you some measure of confidence that the field of cannabinoid medicine is becoming scientifically more robust.

## A Final Note from Dr. Blair

In my 43 years of medical practice in family, combat, and occupational medicine as well as disease management, the last 6 years which has focused predominantly on medicinal cannabis practice have been the most revealing and satisfying of my career. They have been revealing in studying an entirely new and exciting physiological science that finally explains why we get sick and how to stay well. These last 6 years have been extraordinarily satisfying for me in reducing human suffering, restoring productive lives, and resolving many here-to-fore untreatable illnesses. Why else would I be continuing these labors so far beyond retirement? All of this with rare adverse reactions, if any, are associated with medicinal cannabis, but with a plethora of beneficial effects. That final point is an important reason for my participation. I want you to feel comfortable about the safety of quality cannabinoids for your practice.

We hope we are able to inspire you to consider medicinal cannabis first rather than last in your treatment options.

## References

1. de Roon-Cassini T, Stollenwerk RM, Beatka M, Hillard CJ. Meet your stress management professionals: the endocannabinoids. Trends Mol Med. 2020;26(10):953–68.
2. Ritchie H, Roser M. Mental health. Our World in Data, online 2018. https://ourworldindata.org/mental-health.

# 2 Endocannabinoid System

## Introduction

The endocannabinoid system (ECS) is one of the most important neuroregulatory systems in our body. Discovered in the early 1990s, not only is the ECS is a major modulator of synaptic activity within the brain but it also has wide-ranging effects in other parts of the body, including on our immune system [1]. Briefly, it is composed of endogenous ligands or endocannabinoids (endo = within), receptors for these ligands, and proteins (enzymes) involved in the metabolism and degradation of the endocannabinoids.

This ECS is an intelligent system. What often surprises people, particularly those who are critical of cannabis and its potential role as a therapeutic agent, is that we make our own cannabinoids in our bodies: "endocannabinoids." The classic understanding of how endocannabinoids act is that they are synthesized on demand when needed, bind with receptors to effect change and then are quickly degraded when they have served their purpose (though this may not be the whole story since it appears there are intracellular reservoirs of endocannabinoids, discussed later). We have receptors for these endocannabinoids throughout the whole body including the brain, organs, connective tissue, skin, and organs and cells of our immune system. In fact, our ECS is involved in the development of the fetus, so we wouldn't be here without it. This is probably the main reason that the phytocannabinoids, the active constituents of the plant *Cannabis sativa*, actually work—they are tapping into a system that is already present in the body. It is not just humans who possess an ECS. The ECS is present in animals, both vertebrates and invertebrates, too.

**This Chapter**
This chapter will explore the purpose of the ECS, its components, its various mechanisms of action including its role in neuroprotection, the role of the ECS in development, and its role in disease. It will also discuss the role of diet in ensuring a healthy ECS.



K. O'Brien, P. Blair, *Medicinal Cannabis and CBD in Mental Healthcare*,
https://doi.org/10.1007/978-3-030-78559-8_2

## Purpose of the Endocannabinoid System

The ECS is responsible for homeostasis of most systems in the body. The ECS modulates:

- Immune system (innate, adaptive); inflammation
- Pain/analgesia
- Stress response, emotions/moods, cognitive function, memory and memory extinction, relief from dwelling on pain and fear
- Sleep
- GI tract homeostasis including regulation of food intake and satiation, gastroprotection, nausea and emesis, gastric secretion, visceral sensation, GI motility, ion transport, intestinal inflammation, and cell proliferation in the gut
- Energy homeostasis and regulation of lipid and glucose metabolism
- Embryological development
- Cycle of cell life and death, cancer cell control, cyto-protection
- Neurotransmitters, neuroprotection, neural plasticity
- Many others [2–9]

When malfunctioning, the ECS can contribute to pathological states [10]. The ECS plays a key role in the regulation of our mind and emotions. The ECS has a bidirectional involvement in stress modulation: it plays a key role in regulating our reaction to stress and stress can modulate the functioning of the ECS, discussed in the next chapter in detail [11]. So, let us first look in more detail at what makes up the ECS.

## Components of the Endocannabinoid System: Overview

The ECS is generally understood to be composed of three components:

1. Endogenous ligands (endocannabinoids), the two key ones being N-arachidonoylethanolamine (anandamide, abbreviated to AEA) and 2-arachidonoylglycerol (2-AG), with at least three others which may also be endocannabinoids
2. Cannabinoid (CB) receptors, metabotropic receptors coupled to G-proteins, the two key ones being CB1 and CB2 receptors, which bind with the endocannabinoids (however there are several other classes of receptors which appear to bind with endocannabinoids also)
3. Enzymes responsible for their synthesis and metabolism [12, 13]

This is the simplistic view of the ECS. In reality it is much more complex and there are several ECS-related entities. These include other receptors to which endocannabinoids can bind, such as the deorphanized metabotropic G-protein receptors

(GPR18, GPR55, GPR119), the intranuclear peroxisome proliferator-activated receptors (PPARs), and members of the transient receptor potential (TRP) ion channel superfamily. It also includes other potential ligands that are part of the N-acyl ethanolamine family including palmitoylethanolamide (PEA) and oleoylethanolamide [8].

## Endogenous Ligands: Endocannabinoids

**Some Terminology**

**Ligand:** A ligand is a substance that forms complexes with receptors (proteins) to cause a biological action [14]. We have endogenous ligands, e.g., the endocannabinoids, and exogenous ligands (e.g., the phytocannabinoid tetrahydrocannabinol is an exogenous ligand).

**Modulation:** Receptors may be activated at their "regular" binding site to which endogenous ligands bind, and this is called *orthostatic modulation.* Ligands can also bind at a different site, termed *allosteric modulation.* Ligands can be "positive allosteric modulators," which means they enhance the effects of the natural ligand, or they can be "negative allosteric modulators," reversing the effects of the natural ligand.

**Agonists and Antagonists:** Ligands may be full agonists, partial agonists, neutral antagonists, partial inverse agonists, or full inverse agonists. Whether a ligand is a partial or full agonist at a receptor can depend on the type of cell being innervated [14].

### Endocannabinoids in Brief

Endocannabinoids are lipophilic, that is, lipid-loving. The main endocannabinoids are arachidonoylethanolamine (anandamide, abbreviated to AEA) and 2-arachidonoylglycerol (2-AG), with three others identified: 2-Arachidonyl glyceryl ether (2-AGE, noladin ether), O-Arachidonoyl ethanolamine (O-AEA, virodhamine), and N-Arachidonoyl dopamine (NADA) [5]. AEA was first isolated in 1992 from porcine brain [15] and is a partial agonist at the two cannabinoid receptors (called CB1 receptors and CB2 receptors) [1]. 2-AG was isolated in 1995 in canine gut [16] and in the brain [17]. It is a full agonist at CB1 receptors and CB2 receptors [1].

The life cycle of the endocannabinoids involves synthesis, binding to receptors, then rapid degradation, and removal. The metabolic enzymes involved in the synthesis and degradation of the endocannabinoids thus regulate their in vivo availability and are responsible for maintaining what is known as the "endocannabinoid tone" [18].

## Synthesis of AEA and 2-AG

Unlike other neurotransmitters such as serotonin and dopamine which are stored in vesicles, the classic understanding is that both AEA and 2-AG are synthesized postsynaptically on demand in response to an internal signal, through a process of enzymatic cleavage of membrane-bound lipid precursors present in the phospholipid layer [1, 19]. They are not as rapidly acting as typical neurotransmitters for this reason [14]. AEA and 2-AG primarily act presynaptically on CB1 receptors, and their main action in nerves is to reduce neuronal release of other transmitters [1]. Thus, when synthesis is triggered, the endocannabinoids move in a retrograde fashion, from postsynaptic to the presynaptic region.

The precursors and enzymes that synthesize endocannabinoids are present on the cell surface (which supports the idea that endocannabinoids are generated within the plasma membrane). Both AEA and 2-AG are formed from membrane-bound phospholipid arachidonic acid (AA), synthesized in postsynaptic terminals following increased levels of intracellular calcium [20, 21]. The endocannabinoids are then released by diffusion, either passively or facilitated by lipid-binding proteins [22, 23].

**AEA** formation begins with the transfer of arachidonic acid (AA) from the sn-1 position of 1,2-sn-di-arachidonyl-phosphatidylcholine to phosphatidylethanolamine, which generates the AEA precursor N-arachidonoyl phosphatidylethanolamine (NAPE). NAPE is then converted into AEA by the enzyme NAPE-selective phospholipase D [1, 24]. The on-demand synthesis of AEA is not as well understood as for 2-AG [25]. The other N-acylethanolamides, OEA, PEA, and SEA (stearoylethanolamide), also use this pathway.

**2-AG** is an ester formed from membrane phospholipids when the arachidonic acid-containing diacylglycerol (DAG) reacts with glycerol in a process catalyzed by sn-1-selective diacylglycerol lipase α (DAGL α) or by DAGLβ [1, 11, 26, 27]. This pathway appears to dominate in the CNS [28]. However, there are other pathways for synthesis of 2-AG which have not been investigated as extensively:

1. A process involving lysophosphatidic acid (LPA) hydrolysis by an LPA phosphatase.
2. A process involving the conversion of phosphatidyl lipid (e.g., PI) to 2-arachidonoyllyso PI, via the action of a PLA1, and then to 2-AG by the action of lyso-PLC (for more details, see Murataeva et al. [27]).

When the postsynaptic neuron becomes depolarized by a neurotransmitter such as glutamate acting on an excitatory postsynaptic receptor, an increase in intracellular calcium occurs which induces the postsynaptic synthesis of 2-AG and its release into the synaptic cleft. 2-AG is only produced within the regions where this activation occurs [1].

The presence of more than one route for synthesis of 2-AG is thought to possibly reflect its involvement in cellular metabolism as well as its role as a neurotransmitter [21, 22].

## Binding to Receptors (Extracellular and Intracellular)

Both 2-AG and AEA bind to the two main extracellular receptors for cannabinoids, CB1 and CB2 receptors, and are said to be agonists of these receptors (which means that they activate the receptors). 2-AG is a full CB1 receptor agonist and full CB2 receptor agonist, whilst AEA is a partial CB1 receptor agonist and partial CB2 receptor agonist [1, 14].

Endocannabinoids also bind to other non-CB1/CB2 receptors such as GPR55, as well as intracellular binding sites (such as the transient receptor potential vanilloid 1 or TRPV1 channel), and to receptors residing in the nucleus (e.g., peroxisome proliferator-activated receptors, e.g., PPAR-α receptors) [22, 29], described in more detail.

### Transport Across the Plasma Membrane

How AEA is transported in and out of cells (i.e., across the plasma membrane) is not well understood, and several hypotheses exist including passive diffusion (in which AEA may form complexes with cholesterol, in microdomains called "lipid rafts"; b) facilitated transport via an endocannabinoid transporter; and caveolae-related endocytosis [24, 29]. The mechanisms of intracellular trafficking are also not well understood [29].

Once AEA has crossed the plasma membrane, it is transported within the cytoplasm by intracellular transporters (these include fatty acid-binding proteins 5 and 7 and heat shock protein 70) to various targets such as the nucleus and to storage compartments that have been identified, called adiposomes (2-AG is also likely to be transported in a similar manner intracellularly) [24].

### Intracellular Reservoirs Challenge Classic Understanding of Endocannabinoid On-Demand Synthesis

The discovery of intracellular reservoirs of AEA, which are lipid droplets called adiposomes, as well as intracellular transporters, has thus called into question the classic understanding that endocannabinoids are synthesized on demand [24, 29]. Adiposomes then may play a crucial role in accumulating AEA. They may also play a role in connecting plasma membrane to internal organelles [30]. Future research will no doubt unravel more about the internal activities of the endocannabinoids within cells.

## Degradation of Endocannabinoids

Once the endocannabinoids have served their purpose (e.g., activating receptors), a reuptake system terminates their action [22]. The endocannabinoids are internalized into the cell and metabolized or degraded quickly [31]. It is thought that an endocannabinoid cell membrane transporter system is involved in the control of AEA and 2-AG transport and metabolism and the rapid removal of the endocannabinoids from circulation, though this process is not at all well understood at this point [1, 20].

**AEA Degradation**

The AEA degradation enzymes (fatty acid amide hydrolase [FAAH-1 and FAAH-2]) are bound to intracellular membranes [29], and fatty acid-binding proteins (FABP) transport AEA to intracellular FAAH for inactivation and degradation. FAAH hydrolyzes AEA to arachidonic acid and ethanolamine [27]. The AEA-degrading enzyme FAAH is widely expressed in the brain, in postsynaptic structures [32]. There are other enzymes that can cleave AEA, albeit poorly (e.g., N-acylethanolamine-hydrolyzing acid amidase), and these are located within lysosomes [29]. In addition to hydrolysis by FAAH, AEA can also be broken down by several other enzymes, and the:

- Cyclooxygenase-2 (COX-2) (via oxygenation): metabolizes AEA into prostaglandin-ethanolamides (PGs-EA)
- 15-Lipoxygenase: converts AEA to hydroxy-anandamides or hydroxyeicosatetraenoyl-ethanolamides (HETEs-EA)
- Several cytochrome P450 monooxygenases: convert AEA into epoxyeicosatrienoyl-ethanolamides (EETs-EA)

The oxygenated derivatives of AEA have biological actions, though their impact on human health is not yet clear [30].

**2-AG Degradation**

2-AG metabolization has at least eight different enzymes participating. These either degrade 2-AG into its component parts of arachidonic acid and glycerol or transform 2-AG into highly bioactive signal molecules [27]. The enzymes which metabolize 2-AG are located postsynaptically and presynaptically, providing parallel mechanisms for spatial control of endocannabinoid signaling. Monoacylglycerol (MAGL) is considered the main enzyme that degrades 2-AG, responsible for around 85% of its hydrolysis, and MAGL co-localizes with CB1 receptors in axon terminals [20]. However, there are at least three other serine hydrolases that contribute to degradation of 2-AG which are fatty acid amide hydrolase (FAAH), serine hydrolase α-β-hydrolase domain 6 (ABHD6), and serine hydrolase α-β-hydrolase domain (ABHD12). These pathways all lead to two main degradation products: arachidonic acid (AA) and glycerol [27].

**New Signaling Molecules Generated**

In addition to their roles as endocannabinoids, 2-AG and AEA are important intermediates in lipid metabolism—they act as precursor pools for arachidonic acid from which eicosanoids are subsequently produced [20]. 2-AG and AEA are substrates for COX-2 (producing prostamides and prostaglandin glycerol esters) and are also substrates for lipoxygenase (LOX, producing hydroperoxy derivatives) as well as CYP enzymes (producing hydroxy-eicosatetraenoic ethanolamide molecules or epoxy-eicosatrienoic acids) [20]. We have previously pointed out some of the additional metabolic pathways of AEA and resultant metabolites.

Here are some of the other 2-AG metabolism pathways which produce new signaling molecules:

- COX-2 oxidizes 2-AG under certain circumstances to produce prostaglandin glycerol esters ($PGE_2$ glycerol ester). $PGE_2$-G is a multifunctional signaling molecule involved in immune system modulation, hyperalgesia, and enhanced neuronal activity. However, in other circumstances COX-2 converts 2-AG into a pro-nociceptive prostanoid [33].
- Phosphorylation of 2-AG by acyl glycerol kinase(s) creates lysophosphatidic acid (LPA) which activates different signaling pathways.
- Lipoxygenases (LOX) can oxidize 2-AG to produce hydroperoxy derivatives of 2-AG [20].

What is important to note is that these latter 2-AG metabolites often have the opposite bioactivity to that of 2-AG, that is, they are excitatory rather than inhibitory. Thus, inhibiting the metabolic enzymes can have important consequences at the cellular level [27].

Thus, many of the degradation products of endocannabinoids are also biologically active in the ECS and beyond. They also play a significant role in maintaining the homeostatic balance of the ECS as well as additional modulation.

The key synthesis and degradation pathways of AEA and 2-AG are set out in Fig. 2.1.

### A Fine-Tuned Modulation System

Why is it that there are so many degradation pathways involved? Simply, it seems to be all about having a fine-tuned modulation system. If there are large amounts of 2-AG produced in the postsynaptic cell, it may be degraded postsynaptically by ABDH6 into arachidonic acid and glycerol. The remaining 2-AG which has diffused across the synapse has interacted with CB1 receptors on the presynaptic terminal. There, presynaptically, this 2-AG can be degraded by MAGL, COX-2, or ABHD12. As explained elegantly by Murataeva et al. [27], "Depending on the amount of 2-AG produced, and the enzymes involved, the duration and spatial spread of 2-AG can be controlled and additional modulators (eg.$PGE_2$-G and 2A-LPA) produced."

## AEA and 2-AG in More Detail

There are differences between AEA and 2-AG in terms of their binding affinity to the endocannabinoid receptors, expression and concentration in the brain, and their function and agonist effect. Some key differences between AEA and 2-AG are set out in Table 2.1.

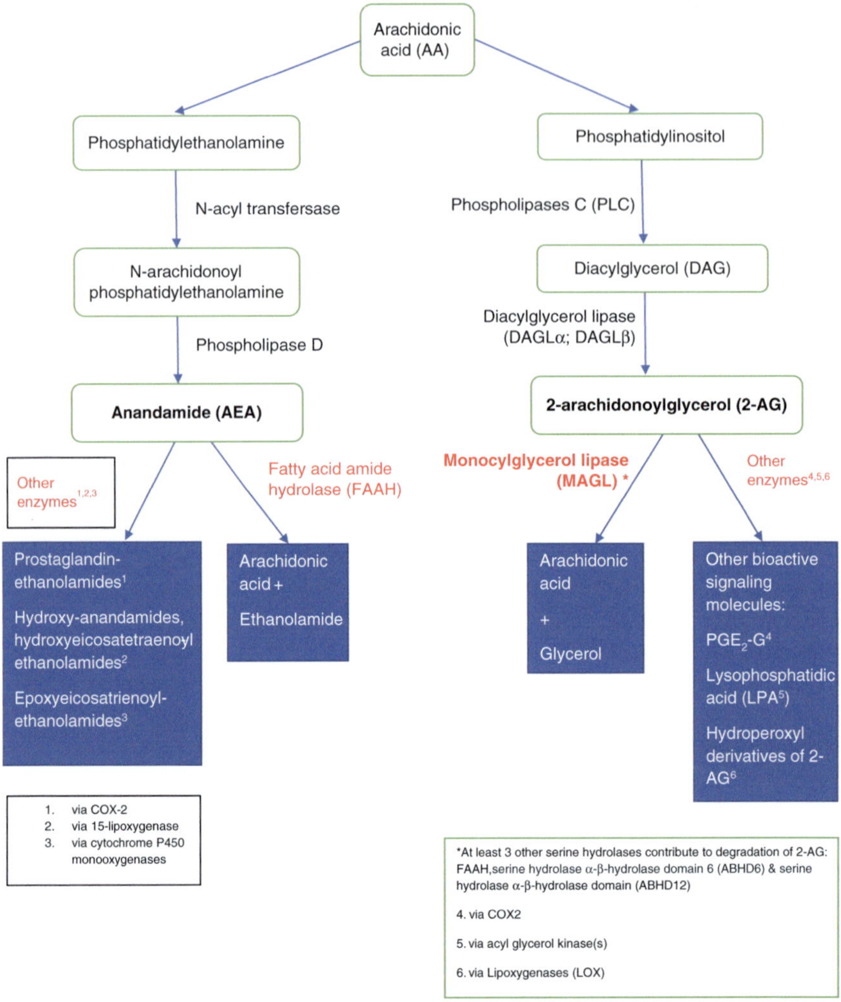


**Fig. 2.1** Endocannabinoid synthesis and degradation pathways: AEA and 2-AG

## Anandamide (AEA)

AEA is a partial agonist at CB1 and CB2 receptors, has a greater affinity for CB1 receptors (than CB2 receptors), and has a lower relative intrinsic activity at CB2 receptors compared with CB1 receptors. AEA's affinity for the CB1 receptor is similar to that of THC, but its affinity for the CB2 receptor is less than that of THC [35].

During development, AEA does not function as a retrograde transmitter. It is tonically active during development and acts as a growth factor: its role is to promote and regulate neuronal development where it is critical in synapse formation

**Table 2.1** Differences between AEA and 2-AG

| Characteristic | AEA | 2-AG |
|---|---|---|
| **Affinity to CB1 and CB2 receptors** | Binds with greater affinity to CB1 receptors (compared with CB2 receptors) | Binds to both CB1 and CB2 receptors |
| **Agonist effect at CB1 receptors** | Partial agonist at CB1 receptors; higher affinity for CB1 receptors compared with CB2 receptors; similar affinity as THC for CB1 receptors | Full agonist at CB1 receptors; slightly higher affinity for CB1 receptors compared with CB2 receptors; has a higher CB1 and CB2 potency than AEA and higher CB1 and CB2 intrinsic activity than AEA |
| **Agonist effect at CB2 receptors** | Partial agonist at CB2 receptors; lower affinity for CB2 receptors compared with CB1 receptors; lower relative intrinsic activity at CB2 receptors compared with CB1 receptors; affinity for CB2 receptors is less than THC's affinity for CB2 receptors | Full agonist, primary binding ligand for CB2 receptors |
| **Concentration in brain** | Lower concentrations in the brain than 2-AG | Greater concentrations in the brain than AEA (1000× greater than AEA) |
| **Breadth of expression in brain** | Less broadly expressed in the brain than 2-AG | More broadly expressed in the brain than AEA |
| **Function** | AEA regulates tonic basal synaptic transmitter release<br>Acts as a growth factor during development. | Main working endocannabinoid in the brain; acts as a phasic signal triggered during sustained neuronal depolarization and mediates forms of synaptic plasticity<br>Acts as a stress modulator in adult life |
| **When more tonically active/ action** | More tonically active during development; acts as a growth factor during development and a stress modulator in adulthood | More tonically active during adulthood; acts as a neuromodulator |

Parker [1], Katona and Freund [34], Atkinson and Abbot [14], Pertwee et al. [35], Chen et al. [36], Zou and Kumar [37]

and axonal pathfinding [14, 38]. In contrast, in adulthood AEA acts as a stress response modulator, and the effects within the brain are very localized. Similar to 2-AG, it acts as a retrograde neurotransmitter and affects cells in the immediate vicinity but not beyond—it doesn't have diffuse action like hormones do, and it doesn't affect the body systemically like phytocannabinoids can [14].

Whilst AEA is not as tonically active as 2-AG in the adult brain, if AEA is induced to be constantly active, the brain downregulates its responsiveness to AEA. This in turn can decrease its neuromodulatory function and disrupt the signaling function mediated by stress-responsive variations in AEA levels [14].

### AEA Binds to Many Non-cannabinoid Receptors

AEA binds to several non-cannabinoid receptors including:

- Transient receptor potential cation channel subfamily V member 1 (TRPV1) receptors
- Peroxisome proliferator-activated (PPAR-α and PPAR-ϒ [alpha and gamma]) receptors (receptors that target genes involved in regulation of metabolism and energy homeostasis, inflammation, and cell differentiation [39])
- G-protein receptor 55 (GPR55) [22]

AEA also reduces conductance of several other receptors including:

- α-7 nicotinic receptors
- Glycine receptors
- 5HT3 serotonergic receptors [22]

### 2-Arachidonylglycerol (2-AG)

2-AG is a full agonist at both CB1 and CB2 receptors with a slightly higher affinity for CB1 receptors compared with CB2 receptors. 2-AG has a higher CB1 and CB2 potency than AEA and higher CB1 receptor relative intrinsic activity than AEA [35].

The basal level of 2-AG in the brain is around 1000 times that of AEA [37]. 2-AG is more tonically active in the adult CNS, acting more as a neuromodulator [14]. It does this through acting as a retrograde neurotransmitter, exerting effects on CB1 receptors located on the presynaptic regulatory neurons which may be excitatory (neurotransmitter = glutamate) or inhibitory (neurotransmitter = GABA receptors). In the brain such CB1 receptors are located in various regions such as the hippocampus, mesolimbic dopamine area (nucleus accumbens, ventral tegmental area), amygdala, cingulate cortex, prefrontal cortex, and cerebellum [14], and as we will see later, many of these areas are involved in the regulation of emotions, cognition, fear, and memory. 2-AG is a particularly fast retrograde synaptic messenger [40].

## Key Difference Between Endocannabinoids and Phytocannabinoids

There is a key point of difference between endocannabinoids and phytocannabinoids or synthetic cannabinoids: the metabolism of the endocannabinoids is rapid, whereas metabolism of phytocannabinoids takes several hours. For example, the half-life $t_{1/2}$ of cannabidiol (CBD) is 20–36 h [41]. The mean urinary excretion $t_{1/2}$ of the THC metabolite, THCCOOH, is 1.3 days for an infrequent user, and the median $t_{1/2}$ is 1.4 days for a frequent user during the first 5 days; but in frequent users, terminal excretion half-lives of up to 10.3 days have been observed. Detection time of the last THCCOOH- and cannabinoid-positive urine specimen and time to first negative specimen are increased in frequent users compared with infrequent users [42].

## Endocannabinoid-Like Compounds: PEA, OEA, and Oleamide

N-palmitoylethanolamide (PEA), oleoylethanolamide (OEA), and oleamide are considered *endocannabinoid-like* compounds and are part of the extended ECS. An N-acylethanolamine (NAE) is a fatty acid amide formed when an acyl group links with a nitrogen atom of ethanolamine. N-palmitoylethanolamide (PEA) and oleoylethanolamide (OEA) as well as the endocannabinoid anandamide (arachidonoylethanolamine) are examples of NAEs.

### N-palmitoylethanolamide (PEA) and Oleoylethanolamide (OEA)

OEA and PEA are structurally similar to AEA, are found in the gastrointestinal tract, and can induce analgesia (PEA) and modulate food intake and body weight (OEA) [22, 43, 44]. FAAH (the enzyme that degrades AEA) also breaks down PEA and OEA, and it has been found that FAAH inhibitors elevate all three [1, 45]. Although PEA and OEA are structurally similar to AEA, current thinking is that neither PEA or OEA bind to CB1 and CB2 receptors, though there is some evidence that PEA can directly or indirectly stimulate as yet unidentified CB2-like receptors [43, 46] and there is some evidence that PEA might bind with CB1 receptors [47] (yet to be confirmed) [48].

PEA acts through PPAR-α (which regulates gene networks which control pain and inflammation), GPR55, and GPR119 receptors and may sensitize TRPV1 channels on sensory neurons [43, 49–51]. PEA may play a role as an antioxidant, analgesic, anti-nociceptive, and anti-inflammatory mediator and might also act as an "entourage" compound for endocannabinoids, by inhibiting the inactivation of endocannabinoids (thereby enhancing their action) [44, 46].

OEA acts through PPAR-α, GPR119, and TRVP1 receptors, with a high affinity for PPAR-α [52, 53]. OEA can modulate the control of food intake, as well as lipid and glucose metabolism, as well as have analgesic effects and potential anti-inflammatory and anti-fibrosis actions [52, 53]. OEA has shown clear effects in the treatment of obesity and obesity-related metabolic conditions and may show promise in the management of risk factors associated with non-alcoholic fatty liver disease [53].

### Oleamide

Oleamide, a derivative of oleoylglycine, has been suggested as another member of the ECS family but appears to be synthesized in a pathway unrelated to other endocannabinoids. Oleamide is generated by the neuropeptide processing enzyme, peptidylglycine alpha-amidating monooxygenase (PAM) [54]. Oleamide is structurally related to AEA and is an endogenous amide of the fatty acid oleic acid (a major monounsaturated fatty acid found in olive oil) [55]. The FDA has approved a health claim for high oleic oils in the prevention of coronary heart disease [56]. It was first isolated in the cerebrospinal fluid of sleep-deprived cats [32]. Oleamide is a full agonist of CB1 receptors, has similar effects to AEA in vivo, and is degraded by FAAH [55]. Animal research indicates that oleamide is produced in brain microsomes of mice [57] as well as in neuroblastoma cells, with levels found to be 78 times greater than AEA [55, 58]. Research has demonstrated that oleamide is able to inhibit gap junction-mediated cell-cell communication as well as modulate other neurotransmitter systems, including modulating some of the serotoninergic receptors and inhibitory ionotropic receptors (e.g., $GABA_A$ receptor) [55]. In mice neuroblastoma cells, oleamide can inhibit or stimulate formation of cAMP following $G_{i/o}$ inactivation and in a manner sensitive to CB1 antagonists and has similar CB1 receptor agonist activity as AEA. This supports the idea that in addition to allosteric modulation and possible entourage effects (due to FAAH inhibition), oleamide is also an endocannabinoid which directly acts at the CB1 receptor [55].

Both AEA and oleamide induce sleep [55] though how it does so is not completely understood. It is likely that it interacts with several neurotransmitter systems, and it seems cannabinergic pathways are involved as cannabinoid agonists can inhibit its hypnotic action [59]. Oleamide can elicit the classic tetrad of behaviors that are used to identify cannabinergic activity and has a similar activity profile to AEA [55]. Could the benefits of diets high in oleic acid oils come from its endocannabinoid effects?

## Cannabinoid Receptors

### Discovery of Cannabinoid Receptors

The structure for the exogenous cannabinoid ligand THC was discovered in 1964 [60], well ahead of the discovery of the endogenous cannabinoids (AEA, 2-AG) or the actual receptors for the cannabinoids (endo- and exo-). It was not until 1990 that an orphan G-protein-coupled receptor (SKR6) derived from a rat cerebral cortex cDNA library was discovered to mediate the pharmacological effects of THC, and it was this discovery that identified the first cannabinoid receptor, referred to as the CB1 receptor [61]. In 1993, a second G-protein-coupled receptor (CX5) expressed in the human promyelocytic leukemic cell line HL60 was discovered and identified as the second cannabinoid receptor, referred to as the CB2 receptor [62]. Receptors for cannabinoid ligands, whether such ligands are endogenous or exogenous (i.e., phytocannabinoids), are thus referred to as "cannabinoid receptors."

CB1 and CB2 receptors are members of the superfamily of G-protein-coupled receptors (GPCRs) [35]. Both are metabotropic receptors coupled through G-proteins to adenylyl cyclase and mitogen-activated protein kinase (MAPK). They inhibit adenylyl cyclase and activate mitogen-activated protein kinase (MAPK) by signaling through $G_{i/o}$ proteins. For the CB1 receptor, this can also impact on potassium and calcium currents [1, 11, 35].

### Location of Cannabinoid Receptors

CB1 and CB2 receptors differ in where they are predominantly located; however, there are several parts of the body where they both appear. Essentially, CB1 receptors are abundant in the central nervous system (CNS) but are also present in periphery, in many other parts of the body, whilst CB2 receptors are abundant in the periphery, being particularly concentrated in cells and organs of the immune system though are also present in other parts of the body. Table 2.2 sets out the anatomical locations of CB1 and CB2 receptors, much of which has been derived from animal research.

**Table 2.2** Anatomical location of CB1 and CB2 receptors

| CB1 receptors | CB2 receptors |
|---|---|
| **Abundant in the central nervous system**<br>Brain (neurons in particular; also in cerebral blood vessels and present to some extent in microglia), spinal cord<br>**Also in periphery:**<br>Peripheral nervous system: sympathetic nerve terminals, trigeminal ganglion, dorsal root ganglion, dermic endings of primary sensory neurons; neurons of parasympathetic nervous system<br>Eye<br>Adipose tissue, connective tissue (e.g., fascia, fibroblasts), skeletal muscle, bone (osteoblasts, osteoclasts), smooth muscle (vascular and visceral)<br>GI tract: myenteric and submucosal plexuses of enteric nervous system (mostly by motor neurons, interneurons, primary afferent neurons but also epithelial cells); non-neuronal cells in intestinal mucosa (enteroendocrine cells, immune cells, enterocytes); endings of vagus nerve; ileum longitudinal smooth muscle; pancreas<br>Liver: hepatocytes, stellate cells, vascular endothelial cells<br>Heart<br>Kidney<br>Bladder<br>Adrenal gland<br>Spleen, tonsils<br>Lung<br>Endocrine glands (e.g., thyroid, adrenals, pituitary gland), exocrine glands<br>Skin (keratinocytes, hair follicle cells, sebaceous glands, sensory neurons, immune cells)<br>Reproductive organs: male (testes) and female (uterus, ovaries); placenta<br>Blood vessels, vascular endothelial cells, blood (leukocytes); smooth muscle cells<br>Immune cells (including macrophages, mast cells) | **Abundant in the periphery; highly concentrated in the tissues and cells of the immune system**<br>Monocytes, macrophages<br>CD4+ and CD8+ T cells, B cells, NK cells, neutrophils, mast cells<br>Spleen, tonsils, thymus<br>**Also in:**<br>CNS (present in lower levels in CNS): cell bodies and dendrrites of central neurons; cortex, brainstem, cerebellum, striatum, hippocampus, amygdala, retina; neuronal, glial (incl astrocytes, microglia) and endothelial cells of the brain<br>Spinal cord and dorsal root ganglia; primary sensory neurons<br>Liver; activated hepatic stellate cells<br>GI tract: predominantly peripheral distribution (highest expression on immune cells but also found on enteric neurons: neurons in myenteric and submucosal plexus of enteric nervous system); colonic epithelial cells; intestinal mucosa-enterocytes<br>Adipocytes<br>Leukocytes<br>Bone marrow; bone (osteoclasts, osteoblasts, osteocytes)<br>Heart: myocardium, cardiomyocytes, cardiomyoblasts<br>Muscle cells<br>Human vascular smooth muscle; endothelial cells<br>Pancreas (exocrine, enterocrine)<br>Lung<br>Skin: including keratinocytes, sebaceous glands, sensory neurons, immune cells<br>Reproductive organs and cells (e.g., ovary); placenta<br>Kidneys<br>Bladder<br>Various human tumors |

Health Canada [63], McGeeney [64], Pacher and Mechoulam [65], Kupczyk et al. [66], McPartland et al. [10], Parker [1], Maccarrone et al. [18], Ellert-Miklaszewska et al. [67], Chua et al. [68], Hedlund [69], Lotersztajn et al. [70], Galiegue et al. [71], Cacciola et al. [72], Rezkalla and Kloner [73]; Matias and Di Marzo [6]; Park et al. [74]; Mackie [75]; Gonzales et al. [76]; Borowska et al. [77]; Rossi et al. [78]; Rajesh et al. [79]; Pacher et al. [80]; Shestra et al. [81]; Caterina [82]; Pucci et al. [83]; Ramot et al. [84]; Pesce et al. [85]; Chen et al. [36]; Onaivi et al. [86]; Anand et al. [87]; El-Talatini et al. [88]; Bermúdez-Silva et al. [89]; Ofek et al. [90]; Pini et al. [91]; Xu et al. [92]; Sharkey & Wiley [93]; Zou & Kumar [37]; Fede et al. [94]; Alfulaij et al. [95]; Mahavadi et al. [96]

- CB1 receptors are particularly concentrated in the CNS, but occur in a many organs of the body also. CB1 receptors inhibit the release of excitatory and inhibitory neurotransmitters including dopamine, GABA, glutamate, noradrenaline, and acetylcholine [97].
- CB2 receptors are found predominantly in peripheral tissues, especially in immune cells where they act as immunomodulators; however, they are also present in the brain and other parts of the body [13].

## Location of CB1 Receptors: Overview

Originally considered mainly a CNS receptor, it is now known that the CB1 receptor is represented in many tissues and organs, though at a lower expression level than in the brain [1]. See Table 2.2 for details. Much of the research into cannabinoid receptors has been conducted in rats [98]. There is significant similarity in the amino acid sequence for CB1 receptors between human and rat, with 97% sequence identity between the two [99].

CB1 receptors are found mainly at the terminals of central and peripheral neurons [35]. Activation of CB1 receptors leads to central and peripheral effects, and specific effects on the nervous, cardiovascular, gastrointestinal, reproductive, and other systems are essential for normal physiological functioning [65]. As discussed previously, binding of endogenous ligands to CB1 receptors typically mediates inhibition of the ongoing release of several different excitatory and inhibitory neurotransmitters [35]. The CB1 is the receptor responsible for the "high" associated with recreational use of cannabis since this is the receptor that tetrahydrocannabinol (THC, the component of *Cannabis sativa* that is potentially intoxicating) binds to in the brain. CB1 receptors in various parts of the brain play a key role in the regulation of our emotions, cognition, and memory and control of motor function and analgesia [35].

CB1 receptors have one or more allosteric sites in addition to orthosteric sites. Ligands which bind at the allosteric sites can enhance or inhibit the activation of the CB1 receptor by direct agonists [35].

### Neuroprotection

In vivo research in mice investigating traumatic brain injury indicates that generation of 2-AG and activation of plasma CB1 receptors mediate neuroprotective responses through several pathways including suppression of reactive oxygen species (ROS) formation, vasodilation, inhibition of proinflammatory mediators, and inhibition of excitotoxicity [92, 100, 101]. CB2 receptors are found on resident inflammatory cells in the CNS and facilitate neuroprotection by reducing the inflammatory response [92].

## CB1 Receptors in the CNS

CB1 receptors are particularly concentrated in the central nervous system (CNS, brain, and spinal cord), as well as many organs of the body. CB1 receptors are found in many regions of the brain, with a high concentration of CB1 receptors in sensory and motor regions of the brain [1]. Human research has confirmed that cannabinoid receptor binding sites are present mainly in the forebrain regions associated with higher cognitive functions; forebrain, midbrain, and hindbrain regions associated with movement control; and hindbrain areas associated with control of motor and sensory functions of the autonomic nervous system [102]. Very high concentrations of cannabinoid receptor binding sites occur in the dentate gyrus, Ammon's horn, and subiculum of the hippocampal formation and high concentrations in the entorhinal cortex and amygdaloid complex [102].

CB1 receptors are expressed in the hippocampus, mesolimbic dopamine areas (ventral tegmental area and nucleus accumbens), cingulate cortex, prefrontal cortex, and cerebellum [14].

Cannabinoid receptor binding sites are present in all regions of the neocortex with the greatest densities in the associational cortical regions of the frontal and limbic lobes, moderate densities in the secondary sensory and motor cortical regions, and lowest densities in the primary sensory and motor regions in human brains. There are relatively high concentrations of cannabinoid receptors in the cortical regions of the left hemisphere, associated with verbal language [102].

There is a low density of CB1 receptors in the brainstem regions controlling cardiovascular and respiratory functions [41]. CB1 receptors are also found in astrocytes, oligodendrocytes, and glia as well as inside of cells [103–105].

### Glutamate and GABAergic Receptors

The expression of CB1 receptors in the brain is very high, with amounts of protein similar to $GABA_A$ and NMDA receptors [103]. CB1 receptors are considered the most abundant metabotropic receptors in brains of mammals [22, 106]. CB1 receptors are present in many types of cells in the brain, but levels of expression vary between locations [103]. In addition, within the same brain region, strength of G protein activation can differ between types of neurons [103]. For example, mice studies indicate that within the hippocampus, the strength of the G protein activation by glutamatergic neurons CB1 receptors is much greater than that induced by GABAergic interneurons [103, 106].

The ECS is particularly well positioned to regulate the activity of neurotransmitters involved in regulation of emotions, since CB1 receptors are present on brain glutaminergic, GABAergic, serotonergic, and noradrenergic axon terminals [108]. In addition, CB1 receptors are present in mitochondria and may exert effects on memory formation [109].

In terms of regional brain expression, CB1 receptors:

- **Are highly expressed** in areas of the brain associated with mood/emotions and cognitive processes (e.g., cingulate cortex, frontal cortex, amygdala, hippocampus) and areas involved with movement control (basal ganglia, cerebellum).
- **Are moderately expressed** in the dorsal root of the spinal cord and the periaqueductal gray matter (PAG), which are areas involved in nociceptive processing (i.e., neural substrates for analgesic effects), and in the hypothalamus (i.e., a neural substrate for neuroendocrine effects).
- **Have a relatively low expression** in brain areas associated with control of essential vegetative functions [22, 103].

Within cortical areas of the brain, there are two major neuronal subpopulations that express CB1 receptors, and these have opposite actions in regulating the brain's excitatory state: cortical GABAergic interneurons (inhibitory action) and cortical glutaminergic neurons (excitatory action) and the relative abundance of CB1 receptors differs between these neuronal subpopulations [103, 110]. In the cortex, there are high levels of CB1 receptors in GABAergic neurons but much lower levels of CB1 receptors in glutamate receptors. Yet in other regions of the brain, for example, the hypothalamus, there is a relatively low level of CB1 receptors overall, but their level of expression is similar in glutamatergic and GABAergic neurons [103, 111]. Other types of neurons including noradrenergic, cholinergic, serotonergic, and perhaps also dopaminergic neurons are also found to contain low-to-moderate levels of CB1 receptor protein; [103, 112]. For example, rodent experiments have also found CB1 receptors in serotonergic neurons (5-HT) of the dorsal raphe nucleus [113] and noradrenergic neurons in the forebrain [114]. To complicate matters a little more, there is not a direct correlation between abundance of expression of CB1 receptors and levels of cannabinoid-dependent signaling. For example, the hypothalamus which contains relatively low CB1 receptor levels has higher levels of cannabinoid-dependent signaling than other brain regions that express much higher levels of CB1 receptors [115]. Other studies suggest that hippocampal glutaminergic CB1 receptors have a much higher efficacy of G protein-dependent signaling compared with neighboring GABAergic interneurons. Why this is so is not yet understood [103]. It seems that G protein-coupling efficacy is not an intrinsic property of CB1 receptors, but is feature which depends on cell type or where the CB1 receptors are expressed [103]. See Busquets-Garcia et al. [103] for a greater discussion.

CB1 receptors are generally found on the *presynaptic terminals* of the axons of neurons (central and peripheral nerves) that release other neurotransmitters, though low levels of CB1 receptors can be found in proximal axonal regions, dendrites, and the cell body [22, 116, 117]. CB1 receptors inhibit the release of excitatory and inhibitory neurotransmitters including glutamate (excitatory neurotransmitter) and GABA (inhibitory neurotransmitter) through coupling to $Ca^{2+}$ and $K^{+}$ channels, but there are other neurotransmitters that they can affect too including acetylcholine, 5-hydroxytryptamine (5-HT, serotonin), and norepinephrine (NE) [1, 97, 118, 119]. The most common effect of CB1 agonists (e.g., AEA, 2-AG, THC in cannabis) at these sites is inhibition of synaptic transmission by inhibiting neurotransmitter release [1]. The effects downstream, then, will depend on whether the neurotransmitter is an excitatory one like glutamate or an inhibitory one, such as GABA.

The ECS is an intelligent system. Glutamate is a key excitatory neurotransmitter, and CB1 receptors are located both presynaptically and postsynaptically at glutamatergic synapses: this allows control of excessive glutamate release and defense against excitotoxicity or overactivation of glutamatergic receptors [100, 120, 121]. This can also limit calcium influx and activation of calcium-dependent pathways which may be destructive in nature. CB1 receptors are also located on GABAergic neurons (which are inhibitory in nature) [121]. Cannabinoids which bind with CB1 receptors may therefore play a role in glutamate homeostasis [121].

#### CB1 Receptors Are More Abundant than Mu-Opioid Receptors

CB1 receptors appear ten times more frequently in the brain than mu-opioid receptors, and cannabinoid receptors can co-localize with opioid receptors, augmenting the pain-relieving effects of opioids [122, 123]. CB1 receptor agonists cause dopamine release in the nucleus accumbens, which may assist in pain disorders, though dopamine release in the mesolimbic dopamine system is seen in drugs of abuse [124]. Activation of CB1 receptors is involved in pain modulation via inhibition of neurotransmitters including GABA, glutamate, noradrenaline, and acetylcholine [34].

#### CB1 Receptors and Cerebromicrovascular Endothelial Cells

CB1 receptors are expressed on the cerebromicrovascular endothelial cells, key cells that make up the blood-brain barrier. These receptors are involved in ECS-mediated vasodilation, astrocytes and microglia, key sources of inflammatory mediators following, for example, a trauma to the brain [92]. Note that CB2 receptors and TRPV1 receptors are also expressed on microvascular endothelial cells [100]. According to Shohani and colleagues [101], the co-localization of CB1 receptors, CB2 receptors, and TRPV1 receptors on brain endothelial cells in humans is suggestive of an ability to affect the functioning of the cerebral microvascular endothelium and a role in regulation of cerebral blood flow and blood-brain barrier permeability [101].

### CB1 Receptors in Peripheral Nervous System and Periphery

CB1 receptors are also found in the periphery, as seen in Table 2.2.

#### CB1 Receptors in the Peripheral Nervous System

CB1 receptors are also plentiful in the peripheral nervous system, mostly in the sympathetic nerve terminals. They have also been found in trigeminal ganglion, in dorsal root ganglion, and on neurons of the parasympathetic nervous system [1, 37]. CB1 receptors are also present on dermic nerve endings of primary sensory neurons, regulating nociception from afferent nerve fibers [37].

### CB1 Receptors in the Gut

CB1 receptors are present in the gut and in the enteric nervous system as well as non-neuronal cells in the intestinal mucosa [37, 93]. Such non-neuronal cells include immune cells, enteroendocrine cells, and enterocytes. CB1 receptors are involved in modulating many different gastrointestinal tract functions including mobility, gastric fluid secretion, and permeability of the intestinal epithelium and neurotransmitters and hormones through both neuronal and non-neuronal mechanisms [37].

### CB1 Receptors in the Skin

CB1 receptors have also been found in the skin, predominantly on cutaneous nerves, for example, on large, myelinated nerve fibers in the papillary dermis as well as on small nerve fibers associated with hair follicles. They have also been found on nerve fibers of the epidermis, though sporadically, and CB1R immunoreactivity has been shown in keratinocytes in the stratum spinosum and stratum granulosum, on differentiated epithelial cells of infundibulum, and in association with hair follicles (the inner hair root sheet). CB1 receptors are also expressed on a portion of CD68-positive macrophages and on dermal mast cells. Normal human epidermal keratinocytes have the biochemical equipment to synthesize, bind, and metabolize AEA [66]. CB1 receptors and TRPV-1 are co-localized on sensory neurons in the skin [125].

### CB1 Receptors in the Liver

CB1 receptors are only expressed in very low levels in the liver under normal circumstances; however, they become upregulated in different types of hepatic cells where they contribute to hepatic insulin resistance, lipogenesis, and fibrosis [18, 37].

### Contrary Actions in the Periphery Compared with CNS: CB1 Receptors in Adipocytes

CB1 receptors have been found in adipocytes, and in a recent study Suarez et al. [126], we see a difference between the actions of CB1 receptors there compared with in the CNS. In a study in obese rats compared with normal rats, genetic knockout of the adipocyte CB1 receptor (mice were bred to not express CB1 receptors) in peripheral adipocytes was associated with improvements in metabolism (including normalization in insulin resistance and glucose intolerance) which were accompanied by normalization of depressive-like behavior, increased adult neurogenesis, and reduced inflammation in the hippocampus and hypothalamus [126]. This study supports the role of adipocyte-brain cross-talk in which adipocyte-specific CB1 receptors are found to be involved in obesity-related depressive-like behavior, adult neurogenesis, and neuroinflammation in the hippocampus and hypothalamus [126]. These results are in contrast with what has been found when CB1 receptors are blocked in the CNS. Rimonabant, a CNS CB1 receptor antagonist marketed as a weight loss drug, was removed from the market as it caused depression and suicide ideation, indicating that functioning CB1 receptors are required for regulation of mood disorders. Yet in this study, blocking peripheral CB1 receptors on adipocytes had the opposite effects, suggesting that activation of CB1 receptors in adipocytes is in some way involved in depression, metabolic defects, and neuroinflammation. More research in the future will no doubt elucidate how such proposed cross-talk is actually mediating such changes.

## Intracellular CB1 Receptors

Although CB1 receptors are mainly localized in the cell plasma membrane, there are also *intra*cellular CB1 receptors in many different types of cells including non-neuronal cells, undifferentiated neuronal cells, and hippocampal cells. Intracellular CB1 receptors located within acid-filled endo/lysosomes have different functionalities than those localized to the plasma membrane. These endo/lysosome localized CB1 receptors don't contribute to the subpopulation of CB1 receptors that are expressed at the cell surface, that is, they don't translocate to the plasma membrane. On activation, CB1 receptors on endo/lysosomes can increase the release of calcium from the endoplasmic reticulum and lysosomes and can increase the permeability of lysosomes [37]. These intracellular CB1 receptors work through a different mechanism of action. When activated, CB1 receptors at the cell surface inhibit cAMP formation and calcium influx, whilst the internal CB1 receptors mediate signaling pathways through β-arrestin [37].

CB1 receptors are also abundant on the outer membranes of mitochondria, the intracellular organelle that plays a key role in regulating cellular aerobic metabolism and apoptosis [92]. Activation of mitochondrial CB1 receptors (mtCB1) influences mitochondrial cyclic adenosine monophosphate (cAMP) accumulation, protein kinase A (PKA) activity, complex I activity, and mitochondrial respiration [92]. The association between mitochondrial CB1 receptors and mitochondrial functioning is important given that mitochondrial dysfunction is implicated in many pathological conditions [37]. We will discuss mitochondrial CB1 receptors again shortly.

## Different Isoforms of CB1 Receptors

To make matters even more interesting, researchers have isolated three different isoforms of the CB1 receptor. These are: CB1, CB1a, and CB1b, and they differ in their ligand binding and downstream signaling [127]. The CB1a and CB1b isoforms are formed due to deletions and alterations in the N-terminal sequence of amino acids and therefore are shorter than the CB1 isoform. These isoforms appear to have different expression in the brain and periphery [127]. In the human brain, the main isoform was found to be the CB1 isoform and there is a relatively low level of CB1a receptors and the CB1b receptors were practically absent. This was the case for various brain regions tested including the nucleus accumbens, hippocampus and cortex. In skeletal muscle, a similar pattern was found in relation to isoform expression. However, in the liver, the CB1b was the main isoform, with 10 times greater expression compared with CB1 receptor expression. The human CB1b isoform was found to be highly expressed in hepatocytes as well as in pancreatic β-cells where it is a stronger modulator of adenylyl cyclase activity than the other isoforms [127].Why might this be important? Much research has been conducted into the action of CB1 receptor agonists, inverse agonists and antagonists in the past. The ECS is overactivated in obesity and reflected in the higher levels of CB1 isoforms present in the liver and pancreas. The following research determined that the activity of CB1 receptor inverse agonists depends on the specific isoform. In this study, researchers tested whether the two main isoforms found in pancreatic β-cells and hepatocytes (the CB1 and CB1b isoforms) responded differently to a global CB1 receptor inverse agonist (rimonabant) compared with a peripherally-restricted CB1 receptor inverse agonist (called JD-5037). They found that the binding affinity of rimonabant was slightly stronger for the CB1 receptor (around 3 times) but the binding affinity of (peripherally acting) JD-5037 affinity was much stronger for the CB1b receptor (around 30 times) [127]. They also found that the peripherally acting JD-5037 strongly enhanced insulin secretion from isolated human islets in a concentration-dependent way, and that rimonabant (centrally acting) stimulated insulin secretion to a lesser extent than JD-5037.This is relevant when we start to look at diseases like diabetes. The CB1b isoform influences metabolically active tissues and blocking it enhances insulin secretion in a glucose-dependent way. The peripheral CB1b receptor isoform was shown to have stronger inhibitory action on adenylyl cyclase than CB1 or CB1a isoforms, and the researchers postulate that its presence in β-cells probably modulates the intensity of cAMP/PKA downstream signaling. Peripheral blockade of CB1 receptors might result in positive effects on glucose homeostasis, something that has been observed in globally-acting inverse agonists previously [127]. Importantly, rimonabant's critical drawback, being a globally-acting CB1 receptor inverse agonist, was that when it was used in humans, it caused significant, serious psychological effects which saw it withdrawn from the market as a drug. Therapeutic agents that are able to act peripherally might avoid some of these issues. Future research will no doubt ascertain whether this is the case or not.

**CB1 Receptors in Brainstem: Has Anyone Died of a Cannabis Overdose?**
According to the World Health Organization, the absence of mortality due to THC may reflect the low density of cannabinoid CB1 receptors in brainstem regions that control vital cardiovascular or respiratory functions [41]. Whilst this anatomical finding is often used to claim that no one has ever died of a cannabis overdose (and indeed this is what is implied by the WHO report on THC) [41], this purported lack of deaths associated with cannabis may not, in fact, be the case. Deaths due to acute myocardial infarction associated with cannabis use have been reported [128]. We explore this topic in the chapter on Routes of Delivery, Pharmacokinetics and Safety.

## Functions of CB1 Receptors

CB1 receptors maintain the intricate balance between neuronal inhibition and excitation, in particular in GABAergic, glutamatergic, and dopaminergic transmission [14]. In the brain, the action of CB1 receptors in presynaptic neurons largely decreases GABA release (remember GABA is an inhibitory neurotransmitter). In the ventral tegmental area, this has the overall effect of facilitating dopamine release, where a decrease in the (inhibitory) GABAergic tone facilitates phasic, burst firing of dopamine [129]. However, in other areas of the brain like the hippocampus, the CB1 receptor behaves as an excitatory receptor, increasing the excitatory neurotransmitter glutamate [14]. As mentioned previously, CB1 receptors are located both pre- and postsynaptically on glutamatergic neurons, and this co-location may serve to regulate or control excitotoxicity or overactivation of glutamatergic receptors [121].

As explained by Pamploma and Takahashi [22], research suggests that CB1 receptors have "functional selectivity" which means they can mediate quantitatively and qualitatively different actions for different ligands; this is mediated by induction of conformational changes in the CB1 receptor's structure or selection of specific conformations from a pool of heterogeneous receptors. In this way, different endocannabinoids may potentially activate distinct signaling pathways depending on their affinity for different CB1 receptor conformational states. Such functional selectivity is partly explained by the fact that there are different binding sites on cannabinoid receptors [22]. CB1 receptors may be allosterically modulated by receptor dimerization and can form homodimers with up to four subunits of other CB1 receptors as well as heterodimers with D2 dopamine receptors, mu-opioid receptors, A2A adenosine receptors, β2 adrenergic receptors, and OX1 orexin receptors which can interfere with CB1 receptor signaling [22].

Cannabinoid receptors are also mobile, not static—they move in and out of the synaptic region dynamically, and this can occur via endocytosis, desensitization, or receptor internalization. According to Pamploma and Takahashi [22], receptor mobility may mediate the plasticity of this receptor system and may have important implications for pharmacodynamic tolerance, with changes in CB1 receptors the key mediators of tolerance to cannabinoids. It is known that cannabinoid receptors desensitize quickly following high or repeated doses of agonists, and chronic treatment has been associated with rapid reduction in CB1 receptor functionality, binding sites, or both [22]. This has implications for disease states with endocannabinoid dysfunction and potential modulation of the ECS.

CB1 receptors play an important role in neuronal protection. Neuronal CB1 receptors are abundant on the plasma membranes of neurons. Recent research also indicates a substantial presence on neuronal mitochondrial outer membranes [92], discussed in the next section. The neuroprotective effects of cannabinoids have traditionally been assigned to alterations in membranes induced by these plasma membrane CB1 receptors; however, a recent study using a model of traumatic brain injury found a relatively small upregulation of plasma membrane CB1 receptors and a strong upregulation of mitochondrial CB1 receptors instead in the first 24 h following TBI [92].

## Functions of Mitochondrial CB1 Receptors

The role of mitochondrial CB1 receptors (mtCB1) in traumatic brain injury (TBI) has been investigated using various models [92, 100, 101]. The sequelae of TBI include metabolic defects and neuronal apoptosis which lead to neurodegenerative processes, with subsequent brain atrophy and impairment of cognition. In cultured neurons and mice experiments, mtCB1 were rapidly upregulated after TBI, and activation of mtCB1 promoted metabolic defects accompanied with a deficit in ATP but paradoxically protected neurons from apoptosis. On the one hand, upregulation of mtCB1 inhibited the mitochondrial cAMP/PKA/complex I which exacerbated metabolic defects, energy insufficiency, and neuronal apoptosis, but on the other hand, activation of mtCB1 upregulated mitochondrial AKT/complex V activity which alleviated the ATP shortage in metabolic defects and had anti-apoptosis effects [92]. Clearly what is happening at the level of the mitochondria as a result of TBI is complex, and future research may elucidate whether phytocannabinoids are able to directly impact on mtCB1 activity in a positive way.

## CB2 Receptors

CB2 receptors are found predominantly in peripheral tissues, especially in immune cells and organs where they act as immunomodulators; however, they are also present in the brain and other parts of the body including cardiovascular, gastrointestinal, bone, neuronal, and liver cells and tissue [13, 65, 73]. There is around 81% amino acid sequence identity between rat and human CB2 receptors [130].

### CB2 Receptors and the Immune System

CB2Rs are expressed particularly in cells and organs of the immune system and, when activated, can modulate immune cell migration and cytokine release within and outside the brain [35]. They are expressed in:

- The immune tissues: including the marginal zone of the spleen, thymus, tonsils, gastrointestinal tract
- Nearly all human peripheral blood immune cells (CD4+ and CD8+ T cells, B cells, macrophages, monocytes, natural killer cells, and neutrophils) [64], with the following rank order of mRNA levels: B cells > NK cells > monocytes > PMNs > T cells [65]

CB2 receptors are predominant in leukocytes and are key mediators of cannabinoid regulation of the immune and inflammatory systems. For example, stimulation of macrophage CB2 receptors inhibits proliferation and release of proinflammatory factors and decreased phagocytosis [5].

Endocannabinoid receptor expression in immune cells is influenced by various inflammatory and other triggers (e.g., bacterial lipopolysaccharide, LPS). Other mechanisms by which inflammatory stimuli can trigger increased endocannabinoids in immune cells are through activation of biosynthetic pathways and/or reducing the expression of the metabolic enzyme(s) which degrade(s) the endocannabinoid(s) [65].

Stimulation of CB2 receptors in cells and tissues of the immune system generally leads to protective mechanisms: inflammation or tissue injury triggers rapid increases in local endocannabinoid levels, which regulate rapid signaling responses in immune cells and other cells, modulating their functions [65]. CB2 activation in immune cells usually mediates immunosuppressive effects, attenuating the autoimmune inflammatory response, thereby limiting tissue injury, i.e., inhibition of proliferation, apoptosis induction, suppression of cytokine and chemokine production and migration of stimulated immune cells, and induction of T regulatory cells [65].

### CB2 Receptors in the Brain

Contrary to what was originally thought, CB2 receptors are expressed in the brain and are an important component of the nervous system. CB2 receptors are implicated in controlling proliferation, differentiation, and survival in neural (as well as non-neural cells) [131].

CB2 receptor proteins and/or mRNA have been found in many areas of the CNS, including the brainstem, pons, cerebellum, cerebral cortex, hippocampus, amygdala, striatum, substantia nigra, thalamus, hypothalamus and olfactory bulb [14, 132–134]. In addition, new evidence is emerging from animal research that CB2 receptors may be involved in brain regions that regulate drug addiction. Functional CB2 receptors have been found in mouse ventral tegmental area dopamine neurons, and activation of these reduces neuronal excitability and reduces cocaine-seeking behavior [36].

CB2 receptors are involved in CNS inflammation, part of the pathophysiology of several conditions such as schizophrenia [135] and other mental health conditions we will examine in later chapters. Incidentally, variations in the CB2 receptor gene have also been correlated with risk for psychosis [136].

CB2 receptors are found in microglia and astrocytes [131]. During neuroinflammation, microglia become activated and CB2 receptor levels increased [65]. CB2 receptor signaling mechanisms include inhibition of adenylyl cyclase, activation of MAPK cascades, and activation of the PI3K-Akt pathway [131]. The upregulation of CB2 receptors in reactive microglia and astrocytes in response to stimuli that provoke local inflammatory processes is thought to be a neuroprotective response to control the production of neurotoxic factors by these reactive cells (e.g., nitric oxide, proinflammatory cytokines, ROS) [131]. In vitro and animal models of acute and chronic neurodegenerative diseases have demonstrated a beneficial effect of CB2 receptor activation [131]. Animal research also indicates that stimulation of CB2 receptors is involved in cannabinoid antitumor activity. For example, stimulation of CB2 receptors on glioma and/or astrocytoma cells induced apoptosis, and CB2 receptors may mediate inhibition of angiogenesis and invasiveness of glioma through several different pathways [131].

### Unique Features of CB2 Receptors Compared with CB1 Receptors

In the brain, CB2 receptors exhibit several unique features in comparison with CB1 receptors:

- Brain CB2Rs have a lower level of expression than CB1Rs.
- Brain CB2Rs are highly inducible. Under certain pathological conditions (e.g., anxiety, addiction, inflammation), CB2 expression is rapidly enhanced in the brain, suggesting a close relationship between changes in CB2 receptor expression and various psychiatric as well as neurological disorders.
- Brain CB2 receptors have a specific distribution. Brain CB2 receptors are mainly expressed in neuronal somatodendritic areas (postsynaptic); therefore, the activation of CB2 receptors may lead to opposite effects compared to CB1 receptors. For example, CB1 receptors are predominantly expressed on neuronal terminals, in particular on presynaptic GABAergic terminals in ventral tegmental area (VTA) dopamine (DA) neurons, and their activation reduces GABA release onto DA neurons. Since GABA is an inhibitory neuron, this leads to an increase in DA neuronal firing through a disinhibition mechanism. In contrast, CB2Rs are mainly located on postsynaptic somatodendritic areas, and their activation decreases VTA DA neuron firing and excitability [36].

CB2 receptors appear to play an important neuroprotective function. Thus, therapies targeting the CB2 receptor hold promise for the treatment of neuropsychiatric and neurological diseases and, as a bonus, avoid the CB1R-mediated side effects [36].

### CB2 Receptors in Other Organs and Tissues

CB2 receptors, endocannabinoids, and their enzymes are present in low levels in cardiovascular, gastrointestinal, bone, neuronal, and liver cells and tissue (see Table 2.2) and appear to play a limited (if any) role in normal physiological functioning of these organs. However, under pathological states, CB2 expression can be markedly upregulated (with increased endocannabinoid levels) as part of an inflammatory response [65].

CB2 receptors have been found in cardiomyocytes and in smooth muscle of blood vessels. There have been reports linking smoking of cannabis to cardiovascular events including atrial fibrillation, ventricular arrhythmias, and acute myocardial ischemia, though the exact mechanism of the vascular effect of cannabis is presently unknown [128].

### CB2 Receptors in Skin

CB2 receptors are also present in our skin, in the following structures:

- Large myelinated nerve fiber bundles of the superficial and deep reticular dermis.
- Small unmyelinated nerves of the papillary dermis.
- Epidermal nerves (sometimes).
- Epidermis: CB2 receptor immunoreactivity has mostly been found in the basal layer.
- Undifferentiated cells of the infundibulum.
- Outer hair root sheet.
- Hair follicle bulb [66].

## Mechanisms of Action of the Endocannabinoid System (ECS)

There are several mechanisms of action by which the endocannabinoids exert their effects. The classic understanding that is well documented is what happens within the nervous system, and the simplistic understanding there has given way to a much more complex picture, as we will see. However, the ECS is involved in just about every cell in the body. We will now take a look at some of the ways in which the ECS works.

### Classic Understanding of How the ECS Works in the Nervous System

In the nervous system, the classic understanding of how the ECS promotes homeostasis, centrally and also peripherally (e.g., enteric nerves), is by reducing the rate of neuronal firing or transmission by limiting the release of other neurotransmitters. Under normal homeostatic conditions, the endocannabinoids are at low levels; however, they become synthesized in the postsynaptic neurons in large quantities when stimulated in response to, for example, painful stimuli, bacterial or viral infection, stress, inflammation, and exercise [5, 137]. To be more specific, endocannabinoids are synthesized on demand in the postsynaptic neuron from plasma membrane phospholipids in response to increased intracellular calcium concentration and/or activated G-coupled receptors [22, 37].

The basal level of 2-AG is much higher (1000 times) than AEA in the brain, and thus it is thought that 2-AG is the primary endogenous ligand for cannabinoid receptors throughout the CNS. AEA, however, still plays a role in synaptic transmission as it can activate TPPV1 and inhibit L-type calcium channels, and it can negatively regulate the biosynthesis of 2-AG and physiological effects in the striatum [37].

In the nervous system, the endocannabinoids travel in a retrograde manner and bind with cannabinoid receptors on presynaptic terminals, acting as "retrograde messengers" (in the brain, these cannabinoid receptors are predominantly CB1 receptors which are in greater abundance). Whilst it is thought that this endocannabinoid retrograde signaling is mainly mediated by 2-AG, AEA produced in postsynaptic terminals can also activate presynaptic CB1 receptors as well as other non-cannabinoid receptors [37]. The endocannabinoids, mainly 2-AG, easily cross the membrane of the postsynaptic terminal into the synaptic cleft (where cells other than neuronal cells are involved elsewhere, this would be the intracellular space). However, since they are derived from lipid precursors and are uncharged and hydrophobic, they cannot diffuse freely, and it is believed they either diffuse via concentration gradients generated or via endocytosis involving caveolae/lipid rafts via carrier proteins (e.g., fatty acid-binding proteins and heat shock protein) [37]. More research is needed to elucidate the exact mechanisms.

CB1 and CB2 receptors are coupled to $G_{i/o}$ proteins. Binding of endocannabinoids to the cannabinoid receptors suppresses the release of neurotransmitters by inhibiting voltage-gated calcium channels (L, N, P, Q types) (which then reduce presynaptic calcium influx) as well as activating K+ channels and by inhibiting adenylate cyclase and the cAMP/PKA pathway levels [22, 37]. Binding of the endocannabinoids to the cannabinoid receptors essentially causes suppression of neuronal excitation and inhibition of depolarization-induced neurotransmitter release, including monoamines, amino acids, and neuropeptides [22]. What happens downstream depends on whether the neurotransmitter is excitatory (e.g., glutamate) or inhibitory (e.g., ϒ-aminobutyric acid, GABA) [1, 22].

The additional 2-AG in the synaptic cleft is taken up into the presynaptic terminals, though exactly how this is done is not clear, and is then (predominantly) degraded by monoacylglycerol (MAGL) into arachidonic acid and glycerol (as discussed earlier, it is also degraded by other pathways). AEA is degraded by fatty acid amide hydrolase (FAAH) within the presynaptic terminal (or within cells in the case of non-neuronal signaling) into arachidonic acid and ethanolamine [37].

## Complexity of the ECS: Multiple Signaling Pathway Involvement

Now that we have explored the mechanism by which the ECS works in the previous section, we now want to explain that this traditional view (i.e., that CB1 receptors are presynaptic inhibitory receptors acting through $G_{i/o}$ proteins to inhibit neurotransmitter release) is likely to be an oversimplification [22].

Typically, CB1 and CB2 receptors mostly couple to G-protein type Gi/o, inhibiting the activity of adenylate cyclase, formation of cAMP, and activity of protein kinase A (PKA). This can suppress calcium influx via voltage-gated calcium channel (VGCC). However, under certain circumstances, and in a cell type and ligand-dependent way, CB1 receptors can switch its coupling from $G_{i/o}$ to $G_s$ or $G_q$ [37].

CB1 and CB2 receptors can activate multiple intracellular signal transduction pathways. These can include (depending on cell type) protein kinase A, protein kinase C, Raf-1, JNK, mitogen-activated protein kinases (MAPKs), p38 MAPKs, extracellular signal-regulated kinase (ERK 1, 2), c-fos, c-jun, phosphoinositide 3-kinase (PI3K)/protein kinase B (Akt) pathways, mammalian target of rapamycin (mTOR), and many others [37, 138, 139]. Adenylate cyclase and cyclic AMP-protein kinase A (PKA signaling) can also be inhibited [139].

These cellular pathways induce a corresponding change in the function of the cell, tissue, or organ involved [139], and depending on the ligand and subcellular environment, the outcome of this could be promotion of cell survival or cell death [37].

There is increasing evidence of the sophistication of the ECS's ability to fine-tune its actions. For example, the ability of CB1 receptors to signal other unrelated G-proteins (CB1 receptors can also signal via excitatory $G_s$ proteins and stimulate adenylate cyclase and increase formation of cAMP) might be the way in which the body mediates fine-tuning of synaptic activity induced by CB1 activation [22, 140].

Another example of the fine-tuning involved in the ECS is in the enteric nervous system. Whilst endocannabinoids, in particular 2-AG, are retrograde transmitters in the brain, in the enteric nervous system, they are also involved in synaptic control that uses two retrograde messengers working in the opposite direction to control synaptic strength—these are the endocannabinoids themselves plus a purine nucleotide [18].

We can also see that there are widespread cannabinoid receptor-independent effects of endocannabinoids. Endocannabinoids have effects on voltage-gated ion channels including L-type Ca2+, Na+, and K+ channels, and they can interact with ligand-gated ion channels including $5HT_3$ receptors, nicotinic acetylcholine receptors, glycine receptors, ionotropic glutamate receptors, and TRP channels [119].

The view of metabotropic receptors as simple on/off switches of a single transduction system has been superseded by the view that G-protein coupled receptors are functionally diverse and adapt to ligands rather than being statically selected by them and with the cellular environment playing a critical role in receptor pharmacology. As further explained by Pamploma and Takahashi [22], there may be "microdomains" in the cell membrane with specialized lipid compositions (called caveolae and lipid rafts) which may play roles in endocannabinoid signaling processes, like modulating cellular uptake of endocannabinoids, regulating the CB1 receptors' affinity for endocannabinoids, and affecting the activity of enzymes responsible for endocannabinoid synthesis.

In addition, the complexity of cannabinoid signaling is increased by two factors: biased agonism of the cannabinoid receptors and their potential of forming heteromers (with each other or with other G-protein-coupled receptors).

## Biased Agonism

Biased agonism is where the same receptor demonstrates signaling preference among the possible second messenger pathways, and this depends on the ligand. For example, the CB1 receptor usually signals through the Gαi protein leading to decreased cAMP and activation of the β-arrestin 1 and β-arrestin 2 pathways; however, signaling bias is where the ligand prefers (and activates with higher relative efficiency) the β-arrestin pathways over the G-protein-coupled pathway (or vice versa). In other cases, coupling to $G\alpha_s$, $G\alpha_q$, or $G\alpha_{12/13}$ proteins has been demonstrated (with consequent increased cAMP levels, activation of phospholipase C, or Rho pathway, respectively) [8].

## Heteromers

G-protein-coupled receptors are generally made up of several alpha-helical segments linked together in a single-folded chain to form the receptor complex. However, several G-protein-coupled receptors can form heteromers from a combination of two or more individual G-protein coupled receptor subunits, especially if these are densely expressed in the same neuron. Heteromers can form between receptors from the same family, e.g., dopamine $D_1/D_2$ heteromers, or they can form between unrelated receptors, and homo- or heteromerization of receptors leads to intramembrane interactions [8, 141]. Essentially, the pharmacology for agonists and/or antagonists of a particular receptor typically changes when it forms a heteromer with another receptor or when the partner receptor in the heteromer is activated, as a result of the conformational changes in the receptors that occur in the receptor-receptor interface [141]. The CB1 receptor can form functional heteromers with several different types of receptors including δ opioid receptor, $A_{2A}$ receptor, $D_2$ receptor, orexin-1 receptor, and others, whilst CB2 receptors have been shown to be able to form heteromers with CXCR4 chemokine receptors or GPR55 [8].

## The ECS in Non-neural Cells

In non-neural cells, there are other mechanisms of action by which the ECS works. For example, CB1 and CB2 receptors located on enteroendocrine cells, immune cells, and the intestinal epithelium mediate the actions of the endocannabinoids through several mechanisms. These include inhibiting release of enteroendocrine hormones (enteroendocrine cells), suppressing immune activation (immune cells), and regulating tight junctions (intestinal epithelial cells) [18].

Another example of non-neural locations of the ECS is human primary leukocytes, where CB2 receptors demonstrate complex signaling, activating adenylate cyclase via stimulatory Gαs along with the classical Gαi signaling, and induce ERK, p38, and pCREB pathways [142].

In the immune system, there is cross-talk between different types of immune cells involving bioactive lipid molecules, including endocannabinoids. Endocannabinoids can bind to cannabinoid receptors and cooperate with other signaling molecules, thereby modulating the functions of the immune cells—this is particularly true in relation to the adaptive immune response [18]. 2-AG, for example, has been found to act via CB2 receptors, to inhibit the migratory activities of many immune cell types. 2-AG has been found to induce a rapid and transient increase in levels of intracellular free calcium in human HL-60 macrophage-like cells, whilst AEA has been found to inhibit immune function activities such as the production of proinflammatory cytokines [18].

## ECS Signal Transmission Via Microvesicles

Another mechanism of action of ECS signaling involves microvesicles. Extracellular vesicles play a fundamental role in signal transmission in the CNS, but many other different cell types can also release microvesicles, and these mediate intercellular communication [143]. The involvement of microvesicles in the mechanism of action of the ECS has been demonstrated in fascial cells and myofascial pain.

For years, myofascial pain, something that affects up to 85% of people at least once in their lives [144], was thought to only involve muscle. Fascia is now believed to be important in myofascial pain. The ECS is active in myofascial tissue, and human fasciae express both CB1 and CB2 receptors [94]. A recent study found that a synthetic CB2 agonist led to the production of hyaluronan and hyaluronic acid-rich vesicles within a few hours in an in vitro culture of fascial fibroblasts and that after 4 h, these vesicles rich in hyaluronan were visible in both the cytoplasm and extracellular space, demonstrating rapid release into the extracellular environment

[143]. Blockade with a CB2 antagonist blocked the vesicle production, confirming that the release of hyaluronan is a cannabinoid-mediated effect (mediated by the CB2 receptor) [143].

This research demonstrated that fascial cells respond to the ECS, regulating and remodeling the extracellular matrix. Hyaluronan is a key component of the extracellular matrix and is critical in remodeling [145], as well as playing a crucial role in tissue regeneration [146]. An increase in hyaluronan secreted leads to greater fluidity of tissue by facilitating gliding between fascial layers in and beneath the deep fascia during movement [147]. The exciting outcome of this research is that it demonstrates that the mechanism of action by which cannabinoids affect pain perception is not just via the CNS but also via direct peripheral effects which result in structural modification of fascial tissue [143].

The abovementioned examples are some of the ways in which the ECS works within the body. As you can see, it is incredibly complex.

## Other Receptor Targets for Endocannabinoids

The ECS is often modeled as a key-in-a-lock simile, but this is overly simplified because most of the half dozen endocannabinoids and phytocannabinoids have multiple receptor targets with both direct and indirect effects. Other receptors for endogenous and exogenous cannabinoids outside the ECS have also been found, such as the transient receptor potential cation channel subfamily V member 1 (TRPV1), G Protein-coupled Receptor (e.g., GPR55, GPR119), and peroxisome proliferator-activated receptors (e.g., PPAR-α, PPAR-γ) [1]. PPAR-α and PPAR-γ, for example, are found in the cell nucleus, and they move backward and forward to the cytosol in a "ligand-dependent" manner [18].

Some researchers have found that endocannabinoids can simultaneously activate several receptors on the same cell, for example, CB1 receptors and TRPV1 or CB1 receptors plus TRPV1 and PPAR-γ receptors. What is very interesting is that only the interaction with all these receptors produced the complete action of the endocannabinoids [66, 148]. This then provides food for thought in relation to the action of phytocannabinoids and the other plant nutrients found in *Cannabis sativa*, which we explore in a subsequent chapter.

As mentioned previously, there are also many non-receptor targets for the endocannabinoids including ion channels and other important membrane proteins which the endocannabinoids can alter directly [119].

### TRPV1 Receptors

It is important to remember, as we examine the role of the endocannabinoids, the fact that they bind with many other non-cannabinoid receptors. The ECS extends beyond the simplistic idea of endocannabinoids, CB1 and CB2 receptors, and their synthesizing and degrading enzymes. As mentioned previously, AEA binds with transient receptor potential vanilloid 1 (TRPV1) receptors, and under some circumstances, AEA may have a higher affinity at TRPV1 receptors rather than CB1 receptors [22, 149]. When we examine the components of *Cannabis sativa* in a later chapter, we also find that some of the active constituents there bind with TRPV receptors too.

The transient receptor potential (TRP) cation channel family has seven subfamilies that are widely expressed in mammalian tissues: TRPV (vanilloid), TRPC (canonical), TRPN (no mechanoreceptor potential C), TRPM (melastatin), TRPML (mucolipin), TRPP (polycystin), and TRPA (ankyrin) [150, 151]. TRP channels mediate the flux of calcium, sodium, and other cations across cell membranes and also mediate nonionic signaling mechanisms [150]. Abnormalities in TRP channel functions have been implicated in many diseases including chronic pain, cardiovascular disease, cancer, and others [150].

Within the TRPV subfamily, there are six members, 1–6, with only TRPV1 actually activated by vanilloids such as capsaicin (the active constituent of chilli) [151]. TRPV1 receptors are Ca2+-permeable, nonselective ion channels, primarily expressed in sensory neurons of the dorsal root of the spinal cord and the trigeminal ganglion; however, they are also found in brain neurons (e.g., hippocampus and periaqueductal gray matter) and non-neural cells and tissue [1, 22, 151, 152]. Examples of non-neural sites include epithelial cells (keratinocytes, urothelium, gastric epithelial cells, enterocytes, pneumocytes), vascular endothelium, immune cells (mast cells, T cells), smooth muscle, fibroblasts, and hepatocytes [151, 153]. The presence of TRPV1 in areas of the brain such as the CA1 area and dentate gyrus of the hippocampus suggests a role in CNS modulation [152].

TRPV1 is a polymodal sensory signal detector, activated by both physical and chemical stimuli including heat, low pH/acidosis (pH $< 6$), reactive nitrogen species, and oxidative stress, plus several chemicals, in particular capsaicin [152, 154]. For this reason, it is also known as the capsaicin receptor. It serves as the primary heat and capsaicin sensor in humans [155]. TRPV1 is found within the somatosensory system, and is expressed in particular by sensory ganglion neurons or primary afferent neurons that respond to damaging or potentially damaging stimuli (nociceptors), key components at the beginning of the pain pathway [156, 157]. Stimulation of TRPV1 causes a burning sensation, reflective of its role in pain pathways [157]. TRPV1 appears to be upregulated in several diseases including inflammatory bowel disease, irritable bowel syndrome, mastalgia, and others [154].

TRPV1 receptors are understood to play a role in pathogenesis of seizures, with calcium ion accumulation in neurons in the hippocampus contributing to the etiology of epilepsy [152, 158]. TRPV1 is expressed in those areas of the brain associated with epilepsy including the CA1 area and dentate gyrus of the hippocampus [152]. Research indicates that TRPV1 can regulate the dynamics of dopaminergic neuronal function and neurotransmission at several levels and, thus, might be a promising pharmacologic target for conditions associated with hyper-dopaminergic states like schizophrenia and ADHD [159].

AEA has been found to be a full agonist at TRPV1. AEA and capsaicin have similar binding affinities at TRPV1, and it has been posited that AEA may bind in the same location [160, 161]. This may have implications for suppression of pain sensitivity.

Another dimension of effect is added, in that TRPV1 co-localizes and interacts with CB1 receptors in sensory and brain neurons and with CB2 receptors in sensory neurons, which allows intracellular cross-talk between ligands that activate both types of receptors [1].

### Peroxisome Proliferator-Activated Receptors (PPARs)

Peroxisome proliferator-activated receptors (PPARs) are ligand-activated transcription factors, part of the nuclear receptor superfamily [35]. There are three isoforms: PPAR-α, PPAR-β, and PPAR-ϒ. PPARs are believed to be generalized lipid sensors which monitor local changes in metabolism and energy homeostasis, inflammation, and cell differentiation [1, 22]. Whilst much of the research has focused on their role as transcriptional regulators of lipid and glucose metabolism, there is also evidence of their role in regulation of other systems. For example, PPARs are involved in skin homeostasis (all three isoforms are found in skin) [162]. PPARs are involved in inflammation, and PPAR-α and PPAR-ϒ agonists have been found to have anti-inflammatory actions [163]. The different PPAR subtypes are involved in many diseases including diabetes, atherosclerosis, cancer, and fertility [163].

AEA binds to PPAR receptors [22], and two of the other N-acyl ethanolamines, oleoylethanolamide (OEA) and palmitoylethanolamide (PEA), are strong agonists of PPAR-α. Fatty acids and their derivatives (e.g., oleic acid, arachidonic acid, leukotriene β, prostaglandin J2) are also PPAR agonists [1].

### GPR55 Receptors

G-Protein-coupled Receptor 55 (GPR55), highly expressed in the brain, was posited as another endocannabinoid receptor because some effects of compounds thought to be specific for CB1 or CB2 receptors appeared to act independently of them [1]. GPR55 is now considered a de-orphanised receptor that may be involved in developmental processes. For example, it has been shown to regulate growth of cones and axons in the retina [164]. GPR55 is also involved in seizures [158]. AEA and 2-AG are both agonists of GPR55 [165, 166]. Cannabidiol (CBD), one of the key active constituents of *Cannabis sativa*, may be an allosteric modulator of GPR-55 [14] or an antagonist [1]. THC does not act directly on this receptor [14].

When activated, GPR55 triggers many different effects in cells, depending on cell type [167]. Increased GPR55 receptor levels have been implicated in inflammatory bowel disease, cancer, and inflammatory and neuropathic pain [167–171]. Mice bred to have no GPR55 receptors have been found to have lower levels of inflammation and inflammatory and neuropathic pain [170]. Animal research suggests that blockage of GPR55 by cannabidiol (CBD, one of the key active constituents of *Cannabis sativa*) may underlie the mechanism by which it can reduce bowel inflammation [167, 169] and symptoms associated with Dravet syndrome, a severe form of epilepsy [172]. On excitatory axon terminals, GPR55 facilitates the release of the excitatory neurotransmitter glutamate. The mechanism by which CBD may reduce seizures is through blocking GPR55 activation, thereby reducing excess presynaptic glutamate release from hyperactive excitatory neurons [1].

## The Endocannabinoid System in Neuroprotection

Before we delve into later chapters on mental health conditions where we are examine the pathophysiology involved within various brain structures, we will briefly discuss the role of ECS in neuronal homeostasis and neuroprotection in more general terms. Neuroprotection is, of course, particularly relevant in relation to neurodegenerative conditions such as Huntington's disease or Parkinson's disease or conditions such as traumatic brain injury, each of which may be associated with dementia.

As set out well in Sagredo and colleague's paper [121], described here briefly, the ECS plays a key role in neuronal homeostasis and survival. Scientific research evidence indicates that when brain damage occurs, our bodies generate endocannabinoids in response, accompanied by an upregulation of receptors (including CB2 receptors), as well as modifications to intracellular signaling pathways involved in cell repair, homeostasis, and survival. In this way, neurons and glial cells limit the extent of potential damage due to cytotoxic processes including inflammation, oxidative stress, and excitotoxicity which may occur in, for example, neurodegenerative conditions. The ECS is intelligently designed to effect homeostasis and neuroprotection, with key components of cannabinoid signaling located in cellular and molecular substrates critical for neuronal survival. As mentioned earlier, it has been found that CB1 receptors are located both pre- and postsynaptically at glutaminergic synapses, a mechanism to control excess excitation and limit activation of damaging calcium-dependent pathways. Meanwhile, other studies indicate that activation of CB2 receptors located in microglia and astrocytes may play a neuroprotective role to limit neuronal damage by decreasing release of proinflammatory cytokines, nitric oxide, and reactive oxygen species by activated microglia and increasing anti-inflammatory cytokines and pro-survival molecules (e.g., neurotropic factors) [121]. For the details of individual studies demonstrating these findings, see Sagredo et al. [121].

## Development and the Endocannabinoid System

There are critical time points in the development of the brain where neural plasticity is high, and evidence indicates that the ECS is critically involved in brain development. This is important to understand, since exposure to environmental stress including the smoking of cannabis at critical times can lead to dysfunctional regulation of emotions. To understand how this might occur, we need to understand something of how the brain and the ECS develop.

## The ECS in Early Life

Human reproduction is under the control of endocannabinoid signaling. The ECS regulates the functionality of the hypothalamus-hypophysis-gonads axis, as well as regulate the reproductive system locally in males and females [72]. The ECS is widely distributed in the reproductive tract, being present from early embryonal stages and throughout prenatal and postnatal development [173]. The ECS is essential for life: it is involved in gametogenesis, successful embryonal passage through the oviduct and implantation in the uterus, as well as development of the fetus [173, 174]. AEA appears to be involved in synchronization of the embryo-endometrial development for planned implantation, development of the embryo into the blastocyst, as well as embryo transport across the fallopian tubes, though the mechanisms by which AEA does this are unclear [174]. In males, the ECS is involved in regulation of spermatogenic output, sperm viability, and motility [72]. Clearly, in order for successful fertilization of an egg to take place, the ECS of both parties needs to be functioning.

During the fetal stage and postnatal life, the ECS plays an important role in neurodevelopment, as well as neuroprotection, and brain plasticity and repair [11, 173, 175, 176]. In the fetus, the endocannabinoids and especially the CB1 receptors are important for brain development [173]. In mice, CB1 receptors are highly expressed in early fetal stages, starting as early as the first day of embryonic life [177]. Expression of CB1 receptors varies with brain region and may continue to increase after birth into adulthood in some areas and decrease in others [176].

In the developing cerebral cortex, establishment of functional structure and connectivity depends on three main developmental events: (1) proliferation and differentiation of neural progenitors, leading to development of neuronal subtypes; (2) migration of neurons to specific locations; and (3) establishment of synaptic connections between neurons following neuronal differentiation [176]. The ECS regulates neural progenitor differentiation and guides neuronal and glial migration, elongation of axons, and synaptogenesis [173, 176, 178]. After birth, the ECS continues to be involved in neurodevelopment and brain maturation. Activation of CB1 receptors by AEA and 2-AG stimulates pruning of synapses, refining the neuronal phenotype [1].

Endocannabinoids, in particular 2-AG, are present in maternal milk [173]. CB1 receptor activation by 2-AG is understood to play a critical role in initiation of milk suckling in mouse pups, which may be by enabling innervation and/or activation of tongue muscles [173].

In studies, perinatal manipulation of the ECS through cannabis use has been found to alter neurotransmitter and behavioral functions in offspring, and that these sequelae are similar to effects of prenatal stress. This, then, suggests that cannabinoid exposure may interfere with the ability of the fetus to cope with stress [173]. Studies of the offspring of mothers who used cannabis during pregnancy have found detrimental effects including increased risk of sleep disorders [179, 180] and autism [181], though an observational study found no detrimental effects on development of Jamaican children born of mothers who smoked cannabis during pregnancy [182].

We discuss the potential negative effects in more detail in the overview chapter on medicinal cannabis.

## The Adolescent Brain and the ECS

Adolescence is a period of much change within the brain's nervous system, with experience-dependent synaptic pruning occurring, and at this time, the adolescent brain is particularly vulnerable to environmental influences and stresses [175]. Endocannabinoids within different brain areas undergo specific patterns of development, and these appear gender-dependent [175]. For example, CB1 receptors in the prefrontal cortex are at a maximum during early adolescence and then gradually decrease to adult levels, whilst in the limbic areas, declines in CB1 receptors occur gradually in adolescence, and in sensorimotor areas, the changes don't occur until mid-late adolescence [175, 183]. The prefrontal cortex matures last in the adolescent brain. This area is vital for many cognitive functions including executive functioning and mental health, including managing stress responses and anxiety [175].

The brain of the adolescent undergoes extensive maturation, associated with significant reorganization and maturation of the ECS. Cortical development involving synaptic pruning requires normal endocannabinoid function; in fact, endocannabinoids regulate cortical activity right throughout life [184]. At this time of change in the adolescent brain, synchronized neural network activity (termed "cortical oscillations," which underpin cognitive and sensory processing) matures, and the anatomical and physiological functions of neural networks develop. It is believed that endocannabinoids are involved in the regulation of these network activity patterns [175].

Research indicates that CB1R mRNA peaks between the time of neonate and toddler and then decreases until adulthood. DAGLα mRNA expression is lowest in early life and adulthood and peaks between school age and young adulthood [184]. MAGL (enzyme that degrades 2-AG) expression peaks in infancy and then declines thereafter, whilst FAAH (enzyme that degrades AEA) increases after infancy and peaks in adulthood [184]. The higher mRNA levels of FAAH that occur after adolescence suggest that a late developmental switch occurs, where AEA is more strongly regulated after adolescence than in earlier life stages. Expression of key genes in the ECS alters with maturation of cortical function [184].

An important point to understand is that in early life, the brain is particularly impressionable and vulnerable due to this high level of neural plasticity. Stress in early life can alter the development of the ECS and cause sustained deficits in function, in particular in areas such as the hippocampus which are involved with regulation of stress and emotions [11].

## Endocannabinoid System Dysfunction and Disease

### The Concepts of Endocannabinoid Tone and Endocannabinoid Deficiency

Ethan Russo first coined the term "endocannabinoid deficiency syndrome" in 2001 [185, 186]. This theory is founded on the idea that we have an inherent "endocannabinoid tone" which refers to the levels of endocannabinoids; their production, metabolism, and relative abundance; and state of our endocannabinoid receptors. Under certain conditions, endocannabinoid tone becomes deficient and leads to a host of clinical conditions. These deficiencies can be due to genetic causes or may be acquired due to intercurrent injury or disease Russo [186]. The basis for this theory is that many brain disorders are associated with neurotransmitter deficiencies (e.g., acetylcholine in Alzheimer's disease, serotonin and norepinephrine in depression) and that a similar deficiency in endocannabinoid levels might be present in particular disorders that display predictable clinical features as a consequence [186]. As explained by Russo [186], when he first proposed this theory, it was based on a few factors: genetic overlap and comorbidity, symptomatology patterns that were able to be mediated by the ECS, and findings that phytocannabinoids often remedied symptoms. However, since then more objective data lends credence to his theory, including findings of significant differences in levels of AEA in cerebrospinal fluid in migraine sufferers and imaging studies demonstrating a hypofunctioning of the ECS in post-traumatic stress disorder [186].

However, there are diseases in which the ECS is hyperactive, including particular cardiovascular diseases [187]. Therefore, it might be better to describe pathology involving the ECS as "ECS dysfunction," which encompasses ECS deficiency.

## Diseases in Which ECS Dysfunction Is Implicated

Deficiency or dysfunction/dysregulation of the ECS has been implicated in many acute and chronic conditions including (but not limited to) the following conditions, set out below. This list is simply illustrative of the wide variety of clinical conditions in which the ECS is involved and is by no means exhaustive.

| | |
|---|---|
| Depression, anxiety, bipolar, PTSD | Brachial plexopathy |
| Alzheimer's disease | Glaucoma, uveitis |
| Schizophrenia | Seizure disorders |
| Traumatic brain injury | Causalgia |
| Migraine | Neonatal failure to thrive syndrome |
| Multiple sclerosis | Repetitive miscarriages |
| Huntington's disease | Infantile colic |
| Parkinson's disease | Autoimmune disease, e.g., rheumatoid arthritis |
| Amyotrophic lateral sclerosis | Allergic asthma |
| HIV-associated dementia | Allergic dermatitis |
| Irritable bowel syndrome | Insulin resistance, diabetes, obesity |
| Chronic motion sickness | Osteoporosis |
| Fibromyalgia | Cardiovascular disease |
| Anorexia | Nephropathy |
| Dysmenorrhea | Pancreatitis |
| Hyperemesis gravidarum | Psoriasis |
| Phantom limb pain | Autism spectrum disorder, ADHD |

Russo [186, 188]; McPartland et al. [10]; Pacher and Mechoulam [65]; Del Rio et al. [189]; Di Marzo et al. [190]; Aran et al. [225]; Cooper et al. [191])

Dysregulation of endocannabinoid-CB2 signaling more specifically has been implicated in many pathological conditions including cardiovascular, gastrointestinal, liver, kidney, lung, neurodegenerative, pain, psychiatric, cancer, bone, reproductive system, and skin pathologies [65]. Polymorphisms (genetic variability) in the ECS including in CB1 and CB2 receptors and FAAH, the enzyme that degrades AEA, have been linked to several diseases in humans including drug and alcohol abuse, schizophrenia, obesity, and anorexia nervosa [192].

Inflammation, which underpins most chronic illness in some way, is a constant balance between proinflammatory and anti-inflammatory substances, and endocannabinoid and eicosanoid signaling are involved in its homeostatic regulation [193]. Thus, it is not surprising to find the extensive list of diseases in which ECS dysregulation is implicated. This includes depression which is associated with a hypoactivity of the ECS and increased inflammatory markers [193].

Polymorphisms in the genes for CB1 receptors (CNR1) have been linked to different diseases including schizophrenia and depression in Parkinson's disease, and polymorphisms in the gene for CB2 receptors (CNR2) have been linked to postmenopausal osteoporosis [35].

## Endocannabinoid System Dysfunction and Mental Health

Russo speaks of the role of an endocannabinoid system (ECS) deficiency in relation to mental health problems. For example, major depression is now thought of less as a failure of monoamine neurotransmission and more as disorder of CNS plasticity, a condition associated with inflammation, or even a degenerative disease, directly linked to hypo-functioning of the ECS [186, 193, 194]. Animal experiments have found that stress-induced anxiety is significantly negatively correlated with AEA levels and that application of a FAAH inhibitor (remember FAAH degrades AEA) reverses the expression of anxiety-like behaviors [195].

A dysregulation of the ECS has been implicated in several mental health conditions including depression, anxiety, PTSD, Alzheimer's disease, and schizophrenia. For example, the association between endocannabinoid signaling dysfunction and schizophrenia is supported by several studies indicating abnormal endocannabinoid levels in cerebrospinal fluid (CSF) and plasma and CB1 receptor expression [196]. In one study, CSF AEA levels were found to be eight times higher in anti-psychotic-naïve, first episode paranoid schizophrenics than in controls or those with dementia or affective disorder. This elevation of AEA was absent in schizophrenics treated with typical antipsychotics (which antagonize dopamine D2-like receptors), but it remained in schizophrenics treated with atypical antipsychotics (which antagonize $5HT_{2A}$ receptors). Level of AEA in the CSF was found to be inversely correlated with psychotic symptoms ($p = 0.001$), suggesting the increased AEA levels in acute paranoid schizophrenia may reflect a compensatory adaptation [196].

The ECS is involved in regulation of stress and emotions, in particular via its actions in regulating the corticolimbic system and HPA axis, discussed in the next chapter. We will examine the role of the ECS and ECS dysfunction in relation to several mental health disorders in the chapters devoted to those conditions.

## Omega 3 and 6 PUFAs in the Brain Health

After adipose tissue, the highest concentration of lipids is found in the central nervous system (CNS). Omega 3 and Omega 6 polyunsaturated fatty acids (PUFAs) are particularly represented in the brain, with lipids constituting 50–60% of the dry weight of the brain. There is a short chain form of Omega 3 PUFA (α-linolenic acid, ALA) and long-chain forms: docosahexaenoic acid (DHA) and eicosapentaenoic acid (EPA). Omega 6 PUFAs are divided into a short chain form (linoleic acid, LA) and a long-chain form, arachidonic acid (AA). DHA accounts for 10–15% of the total fatty acids in both male and female human brains [197]. Thus, PUFAs are essential to normal development and functioning of the CNS [198].

### Diet and Importance of Omega 3 Fatty Acids for a Healthy ECS

There is a growing evidence base of the importance of polyunsaturated fatty acids (PUFAs) in the pathogenesis of many mental health conditions including anxiety and depression [198]. Omega 3 PUFAs modulate neurobiological processes involved in these two conditions. Potential pathomechanisms include the activity of the (PUFA-derived) ECS and the HPA axis [198].

It is known that low dietary levels of DHA (Omega 3 PUFA) have been found to be associated with increased risk of developing neuropsychiatric diseases, though until recently, the mechanisms of action were largely not well understood [199]. A deficiency in Omega 3 PUFAs to the brain has been associated with mental health conditions such as anxiety and depression [135].

### Studies Linking Omega 3 Deficiency and Mental Health Conditions

Both epidemiological studies [200] and clinical studies link depression, anxiety, and schizophrenia with significantly lower levels of Omega 3 PUFAs and a higher ratio of Omega 6/Omega 3 in the blood and brain [201–203]. For example:

- Lower erythrocyte membrane levels of Omega 3 PUFAs and higher Omega 6/Omega 3 ratios were found in non-depressed patients with social anxiety disorder compared with controls, with a negative correlation found between Omega 3 PUFA levels and anxiety scores [201].
- Current comorbid depressive and anxiety disorder patients and pure depressive disorder patients were found to have lower Omega 3 PUFAs than controls, though Omega 6 levels were no different. Changes in PUFA levels were not associated with pure anxiety. Interestingly there was no difference in PUFAs between patients in remission and controls [204].
- A meta-analysis found significantly lower levels of EPA, DHA, and total Omega 3 PUFAs in 3318 depressed patients [205].

Postmortems in brains of patients who had suffered from major depressive disorder [197] and bipolar disorders [206] and depressed suicide victims [207] have revealed lower levels of DHA in the orbitofrontal cortex (major depressive and bipolar disorders) or prefrontal cortex (suicide victims). Reduced expression of fatty acid biosynthesis genes has been found in the prefrontal cortex of patients with major depressive disorder [202].

Animal studies have also demonstrated diets deficient in Omega 3 PUFAs induce depressive- and anxiety-like symptoms and abnormal social behavior in adult offspring [199, 208–211]. In rats, a disproportionately high Omega 6/Omega 3 ratio diet has been found to alter biochemistry, affect monoaminergic neurotransmitter and glutamate receptors, and impair rodent behavior [209, 212].

### Link Between ECS, Omega 3, and Omega 6

Arachidonic acid (Omega 6) and DHA (Omega 3) are the main forms of PUFA within the brain, and DHA is a key component of neuronal membranes [20, 210]. Since mammals cannot synthesize Omega 3 PUFAs, these need to be provided through diet [210]. To recap, endocannabinoids and endocannabinoid-like compounds are signaling lipids produced from long-chain fatty acids:

- AEA and 2-AG are derived from arachidonic acid (AA, an Omega 6 PUFA)
- Oleylethanolamide (OEA) and palmitoylethanolamide (PEA) are derived from EPA (Omega 3 PUFA)
- DHEA is derived from DHA (Omega 3 PUFA) [198]

### Why Are Omega 3 PUFAs Important for Functioning of the ECS?

As AEA and 2-AG are synthesized from phospholipid-bound arachidonic acid (AA), one might wonder why Omega 3 PUFAs are important in relation to the ECS when AEA and 2-AG are derived from AA, an Omega 6 PUFA? This is perhaps better understood when we consider that there is growing evidence to indicate that there is a complex interaction between Omega 3 and Omega-6 long-chain PUFAs and the ECS and that the ratio of Omega 3/Omega 6 appears to be very important for ECS functioning [20].

Since endocannabinoids (and endocannabinoid-like compounds) are derived from Omega 6 and Omega 3 PUFAs, the effects of PUFAs on mood-related behavior may be mediated through the ECS, at least partly [198]. Animal research now provides evidence that an imbalanced ratio of Omega 6/Omega 3 ratio can have detrimental effects on endocannabinoid signaling and thereby mood/emotions [20, 198].

Several animal studies support the idea that nutritional PUFA intake is tightly linked to brain endocannabinoid levels and have explored potential mechanisms. Through regulating brain endocannabinoids, PUFAs have been shown to impact synaptic plasticity in the hippocampus and endocannabinoid-dependent plasticity and CB1-associated signaling pathways in the prefrontal cortex and the nucleus accumbens. Omega 3 PUFA deficiency may also impact on HPA axis function, though the mechanisms by which it does are not well understood [198]. According to Lafourcade et al. [209], a dietary deficiency of Omega 3 modifies CB1 receptor functions in a way akin to classical agonist desensitization. A result of CB1 receptor desensitization is to eliminate endocannabinoid-mediated synaptic plasticity in those brain areas implicated in regulation of emotions and mood disorders, that is, the prelimbic area of the PFC and the nucleus accumbens [209]. For a detailed discussion, see Larrieu and Laye [198] and Dyall [20].

There are several studies that support the close relationship between the ECS and Omega 3 and Omega 6 PUFAs. For example, long-term supplementation with DHA and EPA has been found to increase endocannabinoid-like DHA and EPA-derived molecules (though their functions are as yet unknown) and decrease levels of AEA and 2-AG [20]. A mice study found that lifelong dietary insufficiency of Omega 3 PUFAs specifically ablated long-term synaptic depression mediated by endocannabinoids in the prelimbic prefrontal cortex and nucleus accumbens. In mice experimentally induced to be Omega 3 deficient, presynaptic CB1 receptors were uncoupled from their effector Gi/o proteins, markedly reducing the CB1 receptor function, and the reduction in CB1 receptor function in mood-controlling structures (induced by the dietary insufficiency) was associated with impaired emotional behavior. This suggests a possible pathogenetic mechanism for behavioral changes caused by Omega 3 PUFA deficiencies and may help explain the link between dietary Omega 3 insufficiency and neuropsychiatric diseases [209].

In another mice study, long-term dietary deficiency of Omega 3 PUFA was found to decrease DHA levels in the brain and impair cannabinoid receptor signaling pathways in mood-controlling parts of the brain such as the prefrontal cortex and hypothalamus [210]. The effect of a synthetic cannabinoid agonist in an anxiety-like behavior test was abolished in Omega 3-deficient mice, supporting the idea that the behavioral changes linked to the dietary Omega 3 deficiency are caused by changes in the ECS in specific regions of the brain [210]. In another study, this time in mice pups, deficiency of Omega 3 PUFAs was found to impair endocannabinoid gating of synaptic activity in the hippocampus [213].

Other studies have explored how Omega 3 PUFAs may positively impact on mood. For example, fat-1 transgenic mice which have enriched DHA levels in the brain (they can convert Omega 6 to Omega 3 fatty acids) show increased hippocampal neurogenesis, which is a mechanism by which Omega 3 PUFAs may influence mood and depression [214].

Thus, there is support for the idea that the ECS is impacted by changes in the dietary Omega 6/Omega 3 ratio.

Further evidence of the intimate relationship between the ECS and Omega 6 PUFAs is found at the opposite end of the life cycle of the two main endocannabinoids. Not only do both AEA and 2-AG require AA for their synthesis, but the breakdown products of AEA and 2-AG include AA, and so these endocannabinoids act as precursor pools for production of eicosanoids and are also converted to other classes of bioactive mediators [20].

### Why Are Dietary Sources of Long-Chain PUFAs Important?

As explained by Dyall [20], endogenous synthesis of long-chain PUFAs (DHA, AA) is low, and brain levels appear to be maintained predominantly by dietary sources and/or liver sources in blood (the liver can synthesize long-chain PUFAs from their shorter chain precursors, LA and ALA, though this is a very inefficient mechanism since these biosynthetic pathways compete with each other due to shared enzymes). Long-chain PUFA levels in the brain respond to dietary intake, demonstrated by the fact that a diet with a ratio of LA (Omega-6)/ALA (Omega 3) of around 1:1 leads to higher brain DHA levels, whilst a ratio of 10:1 (Omega 6/ Omega 3) decreases DHA levels in the brain and increases other products of the LA metabolism pathway (such as docosapentaenoic acid and adrenic acid) [20].

### The Problem with the Western Diet

Originally humans evolved living on a diet in which the ratio of Omega 6/Omega 3 was 1:1 [215]. Whilst the body needs both Omega 6 and Omega 3 essential fatty acids, it needs them in the optimal ratio. Unfortunately, in our modern world, the typical western diet is very skewed towards a high ratio of linoleic acid (LA, Omega 6 PUFA)/α-linolenic acid (ALA, Omega 3 PUFA) of somewhere between 10: 1 and 25:1 [215–217]. A shift away from animal fats towards plant-based oils (e.g., sunflower, canola oil) which are mostly high in LA (the precursor of arachidonic acid, AA) and low in ALA (the precursor of DHA) may have led to this marked increase in LA (Omega 6) intake [217].

Mammals cannot synthesize their own LA and ALA, and so these need to be acquired through diet [218]. LA and ALA are metabolized into long-chain fatty acids, AA and DHA, respectively, using the same enzymatic pathway and are therefore in competition with each other for conversion to their respective long-chain fatty acids and also for their entry into the brain [219]. A greater LA:ALA ratio shifts the balance to a proinflammatory state, with increased prostaglandins, increased platelet aggregation, and increased inflammation [220]. A high level of Omega 6 compared to Omega 3 leaves us relatively deficient in Omega 3 PUFAs.

High levels of Omega 6 or a high Omega 6/Omega 3 ratio promotes chronic inflammatory conditions and has been linked to cardiovascular disease, cancer, hypertension, diabetes, arthritis, osteoporosis, and inflammatory and autoimmune disorders, whereas a low Omega 6/Omega 3 ratio is suppressive of such conditions [215, 221]. Inflammation has also been found to be implicated in the pathogenesis of many mental health conditions including anxiety and depression, as we will see in later chapters.

### Hemp Seeds Have a Very Good Ratio of Omega 6/Omega 3 PUFAs

Interestingly, hemp seeds derived from the cannabis plant (hemp seeds do not contain phytocannabinoids) are probably one of the best foods in terms of the optimal balance of linoleic acid (LA, Omega 6) to α-linolenic acid (ALA, Omega 3) of between 2:1 and 3:1 (similar to the Mediterranean and Japanese diets) [222]. Supplementing the diet with hemp seed oil may counterbalance the increased Omega 6/Omega 3 ratio of western diets [223]. One cautionary note is the limited ability of humans to convert ALA to DHA. Between 8% and 20% of ALA is converted to EPA in humans and between 0.5% and 9% of ALA is converted to DHA. However, one study which compared fish-eaters, non-fish-eating meat-eaters, vegetarians, and vegans found very similar levels of circulating plasma EPA in the fish-eaters, vegetarian, and vegan groups (fish-eaters, 57.5 +/− 43.2μmol/L; meat-eaters; 47.4 +/− 30.3μmol/L; vegetarian, 55.9 +/− 45.3μmol/L; and vegan, 65.1 +/− 45.5μmol/L) and slightly higher DHA in vegetarians compared with meat-eaters (fish-eaters, 239.7 +/− 106.2μmol/L; meat-eaters, 215.6 +/− 96.4μmol/L; vegetarian, 222.2 +/− 138.4μmol/L; and vegan, 195.0 +/− 58.8μmol/L) [224].

Suffice to say, diet remains a very important factor in general health and mental health. Use of medicinal cannabis and other forms of natural medicine should be seen as part of a more holistic approach to health, in particular one in which dietary factors are seen as playing a critical role.

## Conclusion

This chapter has provided an overview of the ECS, a critical neuroregulatory system within the bodies of humans and animals. It is important to understand the ECS, since this provides a foundation for understanding how medicinal cannabis works within our bodies to help alleviate many different and varied conditions, including mental health conditions. The ECS is involved in the homeostasis of nearly all of our bodily systems, and dysregulation of the ECS is implicated in many different human diseases and disorders, including mental health conditions. It is important to recognize the precursors of our endocannabinoids come from what we eat. Attention to diet and nutrition likely plays a key role in maintaining health, avoiding disease, and modulating the ECS.

Let's now look at how the endocannabinoid system is involved in the stress response, given that stress can contribute to many illnesses including mental health illnesses.

## References


1. Parker LA. Cannabinoids & emotional regulation. In: Cannabinoids and the brain. Cambridge: MIT Press; 2017.
2. Ahmet W, Katz S. Therapeutic use of cannabis in inflammatory bowel disease. Gastroenterol Hepatol. 2016;12(11):668–79.
3. Fride E, Feigin C, Ponde DE, et al. (+)-Cannabidiol analogues which bind cannabinoid receptors but exert peripheral activity only. Eur J Pharmacol. 2004;506(2):179–88.
4. Grill M, Hogenauer C, Blesi A, et al. Members of the endocannabinoid system are distinctly regulated in inflammatory bowel disease and colorectal cancer. Sci Rep. 2019;9:2358.
5. Jarvis S, Rassmussen S, Winters B. Role of the endocannabinoid system and medical cannabis. JNP. 2017;13(8):525–31.
6. Matias I, Di Marzo V. Endocannabinoids and the control of energy balance. Trends Endocrinol Metab. 2007;8:27–37.
7. McPartland JM, Duncan M, Di Marzo V, Pertwee RG. Are cannabidiol and $\Delta^9$-tetrahydrocannabivarin negative modulators of the endocannabinoid system? A systematic review. Br J Pharmacol. 2015;172:737–53.
8. Olah A, Szekanecz Z, Biro T. Targeting cannabinoid signaling in the immune system: "high"-ly exciting questions, possibilities, and challenges. Front Immunol. 2017;8:1487. https://doi.org/10.3389/fimmu.2017.01487.
9. Izzo AA, Sharkey KA. Cannabinoids and the gut: New developments and emerging concepts. Pharmacol Ther. 2010;126(1):21–38.
10. McPartland JM, Guy GQ, Di Marzo V. Care and feeding of the endocannabinoid system: a systematic review of potential clinical interventions that upregulate the endocannabinoid system. PLoS One. 2014;9(3):e89566.
11. Goldstein Ferber S, Trezza V, Weller A. Early life stress and development of the endocannabinoid system: a bidirectional process in programming future coping. Dev Psychobiol. 2019;00:1–10.
12. Pertwee RG. The diverse CB1 and CB2 receptor pharmacology of three plant cannabinoids: delta9-tetrahydrocannabinol, cannabidiol and delta9-tetrahydrocannabivarin. Br J Pharmacol. 2008;153:199–215.
13. Schubart CD, Sommer IEC, Fusar-Poli P, et al. Cannabidiol as a potential treatment for psychosis. Eur J Neuropsychopharmacol. 2014;24:51–64.

14. Atkinson DL, Abbot JK. Cannabinoids and the brain: the effects of endogenous and exogenous cannabinoids on brain systems and function. In: Compton MT, Manseau MW, editors. The complex connection between cannabis and schizophrenia. Elsevier Science and Technology; 2017.
15. Devane WA, Hanus L, Breuer A, et al. Isolation and structure of a brain constituent that binds to the cannabinoid receptor. Science. 1992;258(5090):1946–9.
16. Mechoulam R, Ben-Shabat S, Hanus L, et al. Identification of an endogenous 2-monoglyceride, present in canine gut, that binds to cannabinoid receptors. Biochem Pharmacol. 1995;50(1):83–90.
17. Sugiura T, Kondo S, Sukagawa A, et al. 2-Arachidonoylglycerol: a possible endogenous cannabinoid receptor ligand in brain. Biochem Biophys Res Commun. 1995;215(1):89–97.
18. Maccarrone M, Bab I, Biro T, et al. Endocannabinoid signalling at the periphery: 50 years after THC. Trends Pharmacol Sci. 2015;36(5):277–96.
19. Barrie N, Kuruppu V, Manolios E, et al. Endocannabinoids in arthritis: current views and perspective. Int J Rheum Dis. 2017;20(7):789–97.
20. Dyall SC. Interplay between n-3 and n-6 long-chain polyunsaturated fatty acids and the endocannabinoid system in brain protection and repair. Lipids. 2017;52(11):885–900.
21. Stella N, Schweitzer P, Piomelli D. A second endogenous cannabinoids that modulates long-term potentiation. Nature. 1997;388:773–8.
22. Pamplona FA, Takahashi RN. Psychopharmacology of the endocannabinoids: far beyond anandamide. Psychopharm. 2012;26(1):7–22.
23. Piomelli D. The molecular basis logic of endocannabinoid signalling. Nat Rev Neurosci. 2003;4:873–84.
24. Chakrabarti B, Persico A, Battistia N, Maccarrone M. Endocannabinoid signaling in autism. Neurotherapeutics. 2015;12:837–47.
25. Mechoulam R, Hanus LO, Pertwee R, Howlette AC. Early phytocannabinoid chemistry to endocannabinoids and beyond. Nat Rev Neurosci. 2014;15(11):757–64.
26. Bisogno T, Howell F, Williams G, Minassi A, Cascio MG, Ligresti A, et al. Cloning of the first sn1-DAG lipases points to the spatial and temporal regulation of endocannabinoid signaling in the brain. J Cell Biol. 2003;163:463–8.
27. Murataeva N, Straiker A, Mackie K. Parsing the players: 2-arachidonoylglycerol synthesis and degradation in the CNS. Br J Pharmacol. 2014;171(6):1379–91.
28. Kano M, Ohno-Shosaku T, Hashimotodani Y, Uchigashima M, Watanabe M. Endocannabinoid-mediated control of synaptic transmission. Physiol Rev. 2009;89:309–80.
29. Maccarrone M, Dainese E, Oddi S. Intracellular trafficking of anandamide: new concepts for signaling. Trends Biochem Sci. 2010;35(11):601–8.
30. Maccarrone M. Metabolism of the endocannabinoid anandamide: open questions after 25 years. Front Mol Neurosci. 2017;10:166. http://dx.doi.org.ezproxy.uws.edu.au/10.3389/fnmol.2017.00166.
31. Van der Stelt M, Hansen HH, Veldhuis WB, et al. Biosynthesis of endocannabinoids and their modes of action in neurodegenerative diseases. Neurotox Res. 2003;5(3):183–200.
32. Cravatt BF, Giang DK, Mayfield SP, et al. Molecular characterization of an enzyme that degrades neuromodulatory fatty-acid amides. Nature. 1996;384:83–7.
33. Hu SS, Bradshaw HB, Chen JS, Tan B, Walker JM. Prostaglandin E2 glycerol ester, an endogenous COX-2 metabolite of 2-arachidonoylglycerol, induces hyperalgesia and modulates NFkappaB activity. Br J Pharmacol. 2008;153(7):1538–49.
34. Katona I, Freund TF. Multiple functions of endocannabinoid signaling in the brain. Ann Rev Neurosci. 2012;35:529–58.
35. Pertwee RG, Howlett AC, Abood ME, et al. Cannabinoid receptors and their ligands: beyond CB1 and CB2. Pharmacol Rev. 2010;62:588–631.
36. Chen D, et al. Brain cannabinoid 2 receptor: expression, function and modulation. Acta Pharmacol Sin. 2017;38:312–6.
37. Zou S, Kumar U. Cannabinoid receptors and the endocannabinoid system: signaling and function in the central nervous system. Int J Mol Sci. 2018;19(3):833.
38. Rivera P, Bindila L, Pastor A et al. Pharmacological blockade of the fatty acid amide hydrolase (FAAH) alters neural proliferation, apoptosis and gliosis in the rat hippocampus,

hypothalamus and striatum in a negative energy context. Front Cell Neurosci, 27 March 2015; https://doi.org/10.3389/fncel.2015.00098.
39. O'Sullivan SE. An update on PPAR activation by cannabinoids. Br J Pharmacol. 2016;173(12):1899–910.
40. Wilson RI, Nichol RA. Endogenous cannabinoids mediate retrograde signalling at hippocampal synapses. Nature. 2001;410:588–92.
41. World Health Organization (WHO). World Health Organization Expert Committee on Drug Dependence. Cannabidiol (CBD) Critical Review Report. Expert Committee on Drug Dependence Fortieth Meeting Geneva, 4–7 June 2018. World Health Organization (WHO), 2018. Available at: https://www.who.int/medicines/access/controlledsubstances/CannabidiolCriticalReview.pdf.
42. Smith-Kielland A, Skuterud B, Morland J. Urinary excretion of 11-nor-9-carboxy-delta9- tetrahydrocannabinol and cannabinoids in frequent and infrequent drug users. J Anal Toxicol. 1999;23:323–32.
43. Ho W-SV, Barrett DA, Randall MD. Entourage effects of *N*-palmitoylethanolamide and *N*-oleoylethanolamide on vasorelaxation to anandamide occur through TRPV1 receptors. Br J Pharmacol. 2008;155(6):837–46.
44. Lambert DM, Di Marzo V. The palmitoylethanolamide and oleamide enigmas: are the two fatty acid amides cannabimimetic? Curr Med Chem. 1999;6:757–73.
45. De Petrocellis L, Ligresti A, Schiano Moriello A, et al. Effects of cannabinoids and cannabinoid-enriched Cannabis extracts on TRP channels and endocannabinoid metabolic enzymes. Br J Pharmacol. 2011;163:1479–94.
46. Re G, Barbero R, Miolo A, Di Marzo V. Palmitoylethanolamide, endocannabinoids and related cannabimimetic compounds in protection against tissue inflammation and pain: potential use in companion animals. Vet J. 2007;173:21–30.
47. Lin T, Lu C, Wu C, et al. Palmitoylethanolamide inhibits glutamate release in rat cerebrocortical nerve terminals. Int J Mol Sci. 2015;16(3):555–5571.
48. Trautmann SM, Sharkey KA. Chapter three - the endocannabinoid system and its role in regulating the intrinsic neural circuitry of the gastrointestinal tract. In chapter three - the endocannabinoid system and its role in regulating the intrinsic neural circuitry of the gastrointestinal tract. Int Rev Neurobiol. 2015;125:85–126.
49. Appendino G, Ligresti A, Minassi A, et al. Conformationally constrained fatty acid ethanolamides as cannabinoid and vanilloid receptor probes. J Med Chem. 2009;52:3001–9.
50. Godlewski G, Offertaler L, Wagner JA, Kunos G. Receptors for acylethanolamides—GPR55 and GPR119. Prostaglandins Other Lipid Mediat. 2009;89(3–4):105–11.
51. Hansen HS, Artmann A. Endocannabinoids and nutrition. J Neuroendocrinol. 2008;20(1):94–9.
52. Thabuis C, Tissot-Favre D, Bezelgues J-B, et al. Biological functions and metabolism of oleoylethanolamide. Lipids. 2008;43(10):887–94.
53. Tutunchi H, Ostadrahimi A, Saghafi-Asl M, Maleki V. The effects of oleoylethanolamide, an endogenous PPAR-α agonist, on risk factors for NAFLD: a systematic review. Obes Rev. 2019;20(7):1057–69.
54. Mueller P, Driscoll WJ. Biosynthesis of oleamide. Vitam Horm. 2009;81:55–78.
55. Leggett JD, Beckett SRG, D'Antona AM, et al. Oleamide is a selective endogenous agonist of rat and human $CB_1$ cannabinoid receptors. Br J Pharmacol. 2004;141(2):253–62.
56. Federal Drug Administration. FDA completes review of qualified health claim petition for oleic acid and the risk of coronary heart disease. November 19, 2018. Available at: https://www.fda.gov/food/cfsan-constituent-updates/fda-completes-review-qualified-health-claim-petition-oleic-acid-and-risk-coronary-heart-disease. Accessed 10 Jan 2021.
57. Sugiura T, Kondo S, Kodaka T, et al. Enzymatic synthesis of oleamide (*cis*-9, 10-octadecenoamide), sleep-inducing lipid, by rat brain microsomes. Biochem Mol Biol Int. 1996;40:931–8.
58. Bisogno T, Sepe N, De Petrocellis L, et al. The sleep inducing factor oleamide is produced by mouse neuroblastoma cells. Biochem Biophys Res Commun. 1997;239:473–9.
59. Mendelson W, Basile A. The hypnotic actions of the fatty acid amide, oleamide. Neuropsychopharmacology. 2001;25:S36–9.
60. Gaoni Y, Mechoulam R. Isolation, structure, and partial synthesis of an active constituent of hashish. J Am Chem Soc. 1964;86(8):1646–7.

61. Matsuda LA, Lolait SJ, Brownstein MJ, et al. Structure of a cannabinoid receptor and functional expression of the cloned cDNA. Nature. 1990;346:561–4.
62. Munro S, Thomas KL, Abu-Shaar M. Molecular characterization of a peripheral receptor for cannabinoids. Nature. 1993;365:61–5.
63. Health Canada. Information for Health Care Professionals: Cannabis (marihuana, marijuana) and the cannabinoids [Health Canada 2013]. Government of Canada. 2013. Available at: https://www.canada.ca/en/health-canada/services/drugs-medication/cannabis/information-medical-practitioners/information-health-care-professionals-cannabis-cannabinoids.html#chp62. Accessed 30 July 2018.
64. McGeeney BE. Cannabinoids and hallucinogens for headache. Headache. 2013;53(3):447–58.
65. Pacher P, Mechoulam R. Is lipid signaling through cannabinoid 2 receptors part of a protective system? Prog Lipid Res. 2011;50(2):193–211.
66. Kupczyk P, Reich A, Szepietowski JC. Cannabinoid system in the skin – a possible target for future therapies in dermatology. Exp Dermatol. 2009;18:669–79.
67. Ellert-Miklaszewska A, Grajkowska W, Gabrusiewicz K, et al. Distinctive pattern of cannabinoid receptor type II (CB2) expression in adult and pediatric brain tumors. Brain Res. 2007;1137(1):161–9.
68. Chua JT, Argueta DA, DiPatrizio NV, et al. Endocannabinoid system and the kidneys: from renal physiology to injury and disease. Cannabis Cannabinoid Res. 2019;4(1):10–20. https://doi.org/10.1089/can.2018.0060.
69. Hedlund P. Cannabinoids and the endocannabinoid system in lower urinary tract function and dysfunction. Neurourol Urodyn. 2013;33(1):46–53.
70. Lotersztajn S, Teixeira-Clerc F, Julien B, et al. CB2 receptors as new therapeutic targets for liver diseases. Br J Pharmacol. 2008;153(2):286–9.
71. Galiègue S, Mary S, Marchand J, Dussossoy D, et al. Expression of central and peripheral cannabinoid receptors in human immune tissues and leukocyte subpopulations. Eur J Biochem. 1995;232(1):54–61.
72. Cacciola G, Chianese R, Chioccarelli T, et al. Cannabinoids and reproduction: a lasting and intriguing history. Pharmaceuticals (Basel). 2010;3:3275–323.
73. Rezkalla S, Kloner RA. Cardiovascular effects of marijuana. Trends Cardiovasc Med. 2019;29(7):403–7.
74. Park B, Gibbons HM, Mitchell MD, et al. Identification of the CB1 cannabinoid receptor and fatty acid amide hydrolase (FAAH) in the human placenta. Placenta. 2003;24(5):473–8.
75. Mackie K. Cannabinoid receptors: where they are and what they do. J Neuroendocrinol. 2008;20(S1):10–4.
76. Gonzales S, Manzanares J, Berrendero F, et al. Identification of endocannabinoids and cannnaboid receptor mRNA in the pituitary gland. Neuroendocrin. 1999;70(2):137–45.
77. Borowska M, Czarnywojtek A, Sawicka-Gutaj N, et al. The effects of cannabinoids on the endocrine system. Endokrynologia Polska. 2018;69(6):705–19.
78. Rossi F, Bellini G, Luongo L, et al. Cannabinoid Receptor 2 as Antiobesity Target: Inflammation, Fat Storage, and Browning Modulation. J Clin Endocrinol Metab. 2016;101(9):3469–78.
79. Rajesh M, Mukhopadhyay P, Batkai S et al. CB2-receptor stimulation attenuates TNF-α-induced human endothelial cell activation, transendothelial migration of monocytes, and monocyte-endothelial adhesion. Am J Physiolo Heart Circul Physiol. 2007; 293(4): https://doi.org/10.1152/ajpheart.00688.2007.
80. Pacher P, Batkai S, Kunos G. The Endocannabinoid System as an Emerging Target of Pharmacotherapy. Pharmacol Rev. 2006 Sep;58(3):389–462.
81. Shrestra N, Cuffe JSM, Hutchinson DS, et al. Peripheral modulation of the endocannabinoid system in metabolic disease. Drug Discov Today. 2018;23(3):592–604.
82. Caterina M. TRP channel cannabinoid receptors in skin sensation, homeostasis, and inflammation. ACS Chem Neurosci. 2014;5(11):1107–16.
83. Pucci M, Rapino C, Di Francesco A, et al. Epigenetic control of skin differentiation genes by phytocannabinoids. Br J Pharmacol. 2013;170:581–91.
84. Ramot Y, Sugawara K, Zakany N, et al. A novel control of human keratin expression: cannabinoid receptor 1-mediated signaling down-regulates the expression of keratins K6 and K16 in human keratinocytes in vitro and in situ. Peer J. 2013;1:e40.

85. Pesce M, d'Allessadro, Borelli O, et al. A Endocannabinoid-related compounds in gastrointestinal diseases. J Cellular Mol med. 2018;22(2):706–15.
86. Onaivi ES, Ishiguro H, Gu S, Liu Q-R. CNS effects of CB2 cannabinoid receptors: beyond neuro-immuno-cannabinoid activity. J Psychopharmacol. 2012;26(1):92–103.
87. Anand U, Otto WR, Sanchez-Herrera D, et al. Cannabinoid receptor CB2 localisation and agonist-mediated inhibition of capsaicin responses in human sensory neurons. Pain. 2008;138(3):667–80.
88. El-Talatini MR, Taylor AH, Elson JC, et al. Localisation and function of the endocannabinoid system in the human ovary. PLoS One. 2009;4(2):e4579.
89. Bermúdez-Silva FJ, Suárez J, Baixeras E, et al. Presence of functional cannabinoid receptors in human endocrine pancreas. Diabetologia. 2008;51(3):476–87.
90. Ofek O, Karsak M, Leclerc N, et al. Peripheral cannabinoid receptor, CB2, regulates bone mass. PNAS. 2006;103(3):696–701.
91. Pini A, Mannaioni G, Pellegrini-Giampietro D, et al. The role of cannabinoids in inflammatory modulation of allergic respiratory disorders, inflammatory pain and ischemic stroke. Curr Drug Targets. 2012;13(7):984–93.
92. Xu Z, Lu XA, Dai Q, et al. Acute upregulation of neuronal mitochondrial type-1 cannabinoid receptor and its role in metabolic defects and neuronal apoptosis after TBI. Mol Brain. 2016;9(1):75.
93. Sharkey KA, Wiley JW. The role of the endocannabinoid system in the brain-gut axis. Gastroenterology. 2016;151(2):252–66.
94. Fede C, Albertin G, Petrelli L, et al. Expression of the endocannabinoid receptors in human fascial tissue. Eur J Histochem. 2016;60:2643.
95. Alfulaij N, Meiners F, Michalek, J et al. Cannabinoids, the heart of the matter. J Am Heart Assoc. 2018;7:e009099.
96. Mahavadi S, Sriwai W, Huang J, et al. Inhibitory signaling by CB1 receptors in smooth muscle mediated by GRK5/ -arrestin activation of ERK1/2 and Src kinase. Am J Physiol Gastrointest Liver Physiol. 2014;306:G535–45.
97. Freund TF, Katona I, Piomelli D. Role of endogenous cannabinoids in synaptic signalling. Physiol Rev. 2003;83:1017–66.
98. Brownjohn PW, Ashton AC. Cannabinoids and neuropathic pain. Mini Rev Med Chem. 2003. Available at: https://www.academia.edu/10078769/Cannabinoids_and_Neuropathic_Pain?email_work_card=view-paper.
99. Gerard CM, Mollereau C, Vassart G, Parmentier M. Molecular cloning of a human cannabinoid receptor which is also expressed in testis. Biochem J. 1991;279(1):129–34.
100. Mechoulam R, Shohami E. Endocannabinoids and traumatic brain injury. Mol Neurobiol. 2007;36:68–74.
101. Shohami E, Cohen-Yeshurun A, Magid L, et al. Endocannabinoids and traumatic brain injury. Br J Pharmacol. 2011;163(7):1402–10.
102. Glass M, Dragunow M, Faull RL. Cannabinoid receptors in the human brain: a detailed anatomical and quantitative autoradiographic study in the fetal, neonatal and adult human brain. Neuroscience. 1997;77(2):299–318.
103. Busquets-Garcia A, Bains J, Marsicano G. $CB_1$ receptor signaling in the brain: extracting specificity from ubiquity. Neuropsychopharmacology. 2018;43(1):4–20.
104. Han J, Kesner P, Metna-Laurant M, et al. Acute cannabinoids impair working memory through astroglial CB(1) receptor modulation of hippocampal LTC. Cell. 2012;148:1039–50.
105. Mackie K. Distribution of cannabinoid receptors in the central and peripheral nervous system. Handb Exp Pharmacol. 2005;168:299–325.
106. Herkenham M, Lynn AB, Little MD, et al. Cannabinoid receptor localization in brain. Proc Natl Acad Sci U S A. 1990;87:1932–6.
107. Steindel F, Lerner R, Haring M, et al. Neuron-type specific cannabinoid-mediated G protein signalling in mouse hippocampus. J Neurochem. 2013;124:795–807.
108. Hillard CJ, Liu QS. Endocannabinoid signaling in the etiology and treatment of major depressive illness. Curr Pharm Des. 2014;20:3795–811.
109. Hebert-Chatelain E, Desprez T, Serrat R, et al. A cannabinoid link between mitochondria and memory. Nature. 2016;539:555–9.

110. Marsicano G, Lutz B. Expression of the cannabinoid receptor CB1 in distinct neuronal subpopulations in the adult mouse forebrain. Eur J Neurosci. 1999;11(12):4213–25.
111. Wamsteeker JI, Bains JS. A synaptocentric view of the neuroendocrine response to stress. Eur J Neurosci. 2010;32:2011–21.
112. Marsicano G, Kuner R. Anatomical distribution of receptors, ligands and enzymes in the brain and in the spinal cord: circuitries and neurochemistry. In: Kofalvi A (ed). Cannabinoids and the Brain. Springer: New York, NY, 2008;161–201.
113. Haring M, Mariscano G, Lutz B, Monory K. Identification of the cannabinoid receptor type 1 in serotonergic cells of raphe nuclei in mice. Neuroscience. 2007;146:1212–9.
114. Oropeza VC, Mackie K, Bockstaele EJ. Cannabinoid receptors are localised to noradrenergic axon terminals in rat frontal cortex. Brain Res. 2007;1127:36–44.
115. Breivogel CS, Sim LJ, Childers SR. Regional differences in cannabinoid receptor/G-protein coupling in rat brain. J Pharmacol Exp Ther. 1997;282:1632–42.
116. Leterrier C, Laine J, Darmon M, et al. Constitutive activation drives compartment-selective endocytosis and axonal targeting of type 1 cannabinoid receptors. J Neurosci. 2006;26:3141–53.
117. Nyiri G, Cserep C, Szabadits E, et al. CB1 cannabinoid receptors are enriched in the perisynaptic annulus and on preterminal segments of hippocampal GABAergic axons. Neuroscience. 2005;136:811–22.
118. Howlett AC. The cannabinoid receptors. Prostaglandins Other Lipid Mediat. 2002;68-69:619–31.
119. Oz M. Receptor-independent actions of cannabinoids on cell membranes: focus on endocannabinoids. Pharmacol Ther. 2006;111:114–44.
120. Marsicano G, Goodenough S, Monory K, et al. CB1 cannabinoid receptors and on-demand defense against excitotoxicity. Science. 2003;302:84–8.
121. Sagredo O, Pazos RM, Valdeolivas S, Fernández-Ruiz J. Cannabinoids: Novel medicines for the treatment of Huntington's disease. Recent Pat CNS Drug Discov. 2012;7(1):1–8.
122. Joy JE, Watson SJ, Benson JA (eds). Marijuana and medicine: assessing the science base. Washington (DC): National Academies Press (US); 1999.
123. Sim LJ, Xiao R, Selley DE, Childers SR. Differences in G-protein activation by mu- and delta-opioid, and cannabinoid, receptors in rat striatum. European Journal of Pharmacology. 1996;307:97–105.
124. McGeeney BE. Hallucinogens and cannabinoids for headache. Headache. 2012;52(s2):94–7.
125. Akerman S, Kaube H, Goadsby PJ. Anandamide acts as a vasodilator of dural blood vessels in vivo by activating TRPV1 receptors. Br J Pharmacol. 2004;142:1354–60.
126. Suarez J, Rivera P, Rey AA, et al. Adipocyte cannabinoid CB1 receptor deficiency alleviates high fat diet-induced memory deficit, depressive-like behavior, neuroinflammation and impairment in adult neurogenesis. Psychoneuroendocrinology. 2019;110:104418.
127. González-Mariscal I, Krzysik-Walker S, Doyle M, et al. Human CB1 receptor isoforms, present in hepatocytes and β-cells, are involved in regulating metabolism. Sci Rep. 2016;6:33302.
128. Patel RS, Kamil SH, Bachu R, et al. Marijuana use and acute myocardial infarction: a systematic review of published cases in the literature. Trends Cardiovasc Med. 2019;S1050-1738(19):30112–4.
129. Laricchiuta D, Musella A, Rossi S, Centonze D. Behavioural and electrophysiological effects of endocannabinoid and dopaminergic systems on salient stimuli. Front Behav Neurosci. 2014;8:183.
130. Griffin G, Tao Q, Abood ME. Cloning and pharmacological characterization of the rat CB2 cannabinoid receptor. J Pharmacol Exp Ther. 2000;292(3):886–94.
131. Fernandez-Ruiz J, Romero J, Velasco G, et al. Cannabinoid CB2 receptor: a new target for controlling neural cell survival? Trends Pharmacol Sci. 2006;28(1):39–45.
132. Brusco A, Tagliaferro P, Saez T, Onaivi ES. Postsynaptic localization of CB2 cannabinoid receptors in the rat hippocampus. Synapse. 2008;62(12):944–9.
133. Atwood BK, Mackie K. CB2: a cannabinoid receptor with an identity crisis. Br J Pharmacol. 2010;160:467–79.
134. Svízenská I, Dubový P, Sulcová A. Cannabinoid receptors 1 and 2 (CB1 and CB2), their distribution, ligands and functional involvement in nervous system structures-a short review. Pharmacol Biochem Behav. 2008;90(4):501–11.

135. Muller N, Weidinger E, Leitner B, Schwartz MJ. The role of inflammation in schizophrenia. Front Neurosci. 2015;9:372.
136. Ishiguro H, Horiuchi Y, Ishikawa M, et al. Brain cannabinoid CB2 receptor in schizophrenia. Biol Psychiatry. 2010;67(10):974–82.
137. Dietrich A, McDaniel WF. Endocannabinoids and exercise. Br J Sports Med. 2004;38(5):536–41.
138. Demuth DG, Molleman A. Cannabinoid signalling. Life Sci. 2006;78(6):549–63.
139. Wang J, Wang Y, Tong M, et al. New prospect for cancer cachexia: medical cannabinoid. J Cancer. 2019;10(3):716–20.
140. Bosier B, Muccioli GG, Hermans E, et al. Functionally selective cannabinoid receptor signalling: therapeutic implications and opportunities. Biochem Pharmacol. 2010;80:1–12.
141. Franco R, Casado V, Cortes A, et al. G-protein coupled receptor heteromers: function and ligand pharmacology. Br J Pharmacol. 2008;153 Suppl 1(Suppl 1):S90–8.
142. Saroz Y, Kho DT, Glass M, et al. Cannabinoid receptor 2 (CB2) signals via G-alpha-s and induces IL-6 and IL-10 cytokine secretion in human primary leukocytes. ACS Pharmacol Transl Sci. 2019;2:acsptsci.9b00049.
143. Fede C, Pirri C, Petrelli L, et al. Sensitivity of the fasciae to the endocannabinoid system: production of hyaluronan-rich vesicles and potential peripheral effects of cannabinoids in fascial tissue. Int J Mol Sci. 2020;21:2936.
144. Pal US, Kumar L, Mehta G, et al. Trends in management of myofascial pain. Natl J Maxillofac Surg. 2014;5:109–16.
145. Garantziotis S, Savani RC. Hyaluronan biology: a complex balancing act of structure, function, location and context. Matrix Biol. 2019;78-79:1–10.
146. Litwiniuk M, Krejner A, Speyrer MS, et al. Hyaluronic acid in inflammation and tissue regeneration. Wounds. 2016;28:78–88.
147. Cowman MK, Schmidt TA, Raghavan P, Stecco A. Viscoelastic properties of hyaluronan in physiological conditions. F1000Research. 2015;4:622.
148. Costa B, Comelli F, Bettoni I, et al. The endogenous fatty acid amide, palmitoylethanolamide, has anti-allodynic and anti-hyperalgesic effects in a murine model of neuropathic pain: involvement of CB1, TRPV1 and PPARc receptors and neurotrophic factors. Pain. 2008;139:541–50.
149. Di Marzo V, Bisogno T, De Petrocellis L. Anandamide: some like it hot. Trends Pharmacol Sci. 2001;22:346–9.
150. Caterina MJ. An introduction to transient receptor potential ion channels and their roles in disease. In: Szallasi A, editor. TRP channels as therapeutic targets. Academic Press; 2015. p. 1–12.
151. Fernandes ES, Fernandes MA, Keeble JA. The functions of TRPA1 and TRPV1: moving away from sensory nerves. Br J Pharmacol. 2012;166(2):510–21.
152. Iu MN. TRPV1 channel: a potential drug target for treating epilepsy. Curr Neuropharmacol. 2015;13(2):239–47.
153. Szallasi A, Gunthorpe M. Peripheral TRPV1 receptors as targets for drug development: new molecules and mechanisms. Curr Pharm Des. 2008;14(1):32–41.
154. Szallasi A, Cortright DN, Blum CA, Eid SR. The vanilloid receptor TRPV1: 10 years from channel cloning to antagonist proof-of-concept. Nat Rev Drug Discov. 2007;6:357–72.
155. Kwon DH, Zhang F, Suo Y, et al. Heat-dependent opening of TRPV1 in the presence of capsaicin. Nat Struct Mol Biol. 2021;28(7):554–63.
156. Cimino Brown D, Iadarola MJ. TRPV1 agonist cytotoxicity for chronic pain relief. In: Szallasi A, editor. TRP channels as therapeutic targets. Academic Press; 2015.
157. Iftinca M, Defaye M, Altier C. TRPV1-targeted drugs in development for human pain conditions. Drugs. 2021;81(1):7–27.
158. Devinsky O, Cilio MR, Cross H, et al. Cannabidiol: pharmacology and potential therapeutic role in epilepsy and other neuropsychiatric disorders. Epilepsia. 2014;55(6):791–802.
159. Tzavara ET, Li DL, Moutsinelli L, et al. Endocannabinoids activate transient receptor potential vanilloid 1 receptors to reduce hyperdopaminergic-related hyperactivity: therapeutic indications. Biol Psychiatry. 2006;59(6):508–15.

160. Muller C, Lynch DL, Hurst DP, Reggio PH. A closer look at anandamide interaction with TRPV1. Front Mol Biosci. 2020;7:144. https://doi.org/10.3389/fmolb.2020.00144.
161. Ross RA. Anandamide and vanilloid TRPV1 receptors. Br J Pharmacol. 2003;140:790–801.
162. Michalik L, Wahli W. Peroxisome proliferator-activated receptors (PPARs) in skin health, repair and disease. Biochim Biophys Acta. 2007;1771(8):991–8.
163. Youssef J, Badr M. Role of peroxisome proliferator-activated receptors in inflammation control. J Biomed Biotechnol. 2004;2004(3):156–66.
164. Cherif H, Argaw A, Cecyre B, et al. Role of GPR55 during axon growth and target innervation. eNeuro. 2015;2(5):ENEURO.0011-15.2015.
165. Ryberg E, Larsson N, Sjögren S, et al. The orphan receptor GPR55 is a novel cannabinoid receptor. Br J Pharmacol. 2007;152:1092–101.
166. Cheung KAA, Peiris H, Wallace G, et al. The Interplay between the Endocannabinoid System. Epilepsy and Cannabinoids. Int J Mol Sci. 2019;20:6079.
167. Kaplan JS. What is the GPR55 receptor and why is it so important in CBD's benefits? Leafly, April 2018. Available at: https://www.leafly.com/news/science-tech/health-benefits-cbd-on-g-protein-coupled-receptor-55. Accessed 14 Jan 2020.
168. Hasenoehrl C, Feuersinger D, Sturm EM, et al. G protein-coupled receptor GPR55 promotes colorectal cancer and has opposing effects to cannabinoid receptor 1. Int J Cancer. 2018;142(1):121–32.
169. Stancic A, Jandl K, Hasenohrl E, et al. The GPR55 antagonist CID16020046 protects against intestinal inflammation. Neurogastroenterol Motil. 2015;27(10):1432–45.
170. Staton PC, Hatcher JP, Walker DJ, et al. The putative cannabinoid receptor GPR55 plays a role in mechanical hyperalgesia associated with inflammatory and neuropathic pain. Pain. 2008;139(1):225–36.
171. Zhou Y, Wang S, Lou H, Fan P. Chemical constituents of hemp (Cannabis sativa L.) seed with potential anti-neuroinflammatory activity. Phytochem Lett. 2018;23:57–61.
172. Kaplan JS, Stella N, Catterall WA, Westenbroek RE. Cannabidiol attenuates seizures and social deficits in a mouse model of Dravet syndrome. PNAS. 2017;114(42):11229–34.
173. Fride E, Gobshtis N, Dahan N, et al. The endocannabinoid system during development: emphasis on perinatal events and delayed effects. Vitam Horm. 2009;81:139–58.
174. Taylor AH, Ang C, Bell SC, Konje JC. The role of the endocannabinoid system in gametogenesis, implantation and early pregnancy. Hum Reprod Update. 2007;13(5):501–13.
175. Dow-Edwards D, Silva L. Endocannabinoids in brain plasticity: cortical maturation, HPA axis function and behaviour. Brain Res. 2017;1654:157–64.
176. Gaffuri AL, Ladarre D, Lenkei Z. Type-1 cannabinoid receptor signaling in neuronal development. Pharmacology. 2012;90:19–39.
177. Vitalis T, Laine J, Simon A, et al. The type 1 cannabinoid receptor is highly expressed in embryonic cortical projection neurons and negatively regulates neurite growth in vitro. Eur J Neurosci. 2008;28:1705–18.
178. Guy AT, Nagatsuka Y, Ooashi N, et al. Glycerophospholipid regulation of modality-specific sensory axon guidance I the spinal cord. Science. 2015;349(6251):974–7.
179. Dahl RE, Scher MS, Williamson DE, et al. A longitudinal study of prenatal marijuana use: effects on sleep and arousal at age 3 years. Arch Pediatr Adolesc Med. 1995;149(2):145–50. https://doi.org/10.1001/archpedi.1995.02170140027004.
180. Winiger EA, Hewitt JK. Prenatal cannabis exposure and sleep outcomes in children 9-10 years of age in the adolescent brain cognitive development SM study. Sleep Health. 2020;6(6):787–9. https://doi.org/10.1016/j.sleh.2020.05.006.
181. Corsi DJ, Donelle J, Sucha E, et al. Maternal cannabis use in pregnancy and child neurodevelopmental outcomes. Nat Med. 2020;26(10):1536–40. https://doi.org/10.1038/s41591-020-1002-5.
182. Hayes JS, Lampart R, Dreher MC, Morgan L. Five year follow up of rural Jamaican children whose mothers used marijuana during pregnancy. West Indian Med J. 1991;40(3):120–3.
183. Heng L, Beverley JA, Steiner H, Tseng KY. Differential development trajectories for CB1 cannabinoid receptor expression in limbic/associative and sensorimotor cortical areas. Synapse. 2011;65:278–86.

184. Long LE, Lind J, Webster M, Weickert CS. Developmental trajectory of the endocannabinoid system in human dorsolateral prefrontal cortex. BMC Neurosci. 2012;13:87.
185. Russo EB. Clinical endocannabinoid deficiency (CECD): can this concept explain therapeutic benefits of cannabis in migraine, fibromyalgia, irritable bowel syndrome and other treatment-resistant conditions? Neuro Endocrinol Lett. 2004;25(1–2):31–9.
186. Russo E. Clinical endocannabinoid deficiency reconsidered: current research supports the theory in migraine, fibromyalgia, irritable bowel, and other treatment-resistant syndromes. Cannabis Cannabinoid Res. 2016;1(1):154.
187. Sierra S, Luquin N, Navarro-Otan J. The endocannabinoid system in cardiovascular function: novel insights and clinical implications. Clin Auton Res. 2018;28:35–52.
188. Russo E. Clinical endocannabinoid deficiency (CECD): can this concept explain therapeutic benefits of cannabis in migraine, fibromyalgia, irritable bowel syndrome and other treatment-resistant conditions? Neuro Endocrinol Lett. 2008;29(2):192–200.
189. Del Rio C, Milland E, Garccia V, et al. Endocannabinoid system of the skin. A potential approach for the treatment of skin disorders. Biochem Pharmacol. 2018;157:122–33.
190. Di Marzo V, Piscitelli F, Mechoulam R. Cannabinoids and endocannabinoids in metabolic disorders with focus on diabetes. Handb Exp Pharmacol. 2011;203:75–104.
191. Cooper RE, Williams E, Seegobin S, et al. Cannabinoids in attention-deficit/hyperactivity disorder: A randomised-controlled trial. Eur Neuropsychopharmacol. 2017;27(8):795–808.
192. Norrod AG, Puffernbarger RA. Genetic polymorphisms of the endocannabinoid system. Chem Biodivers. 2007;4:1926–32.
193. Boorman E, Zajkowska Z, Ahmed R, et al. Crosstalk between endocannabinoid and immune systems: a potential dysregulation in depression? Psychopharmacology. 2016;233(9):1591–604.
194. Hill MN, Gorzalka BB. Is there a role for the endocannabinoid system in the etiology and treatment of melancholic depression? Behav Pharmacol. 2005;16(5–6):333–52.
195. Bluett RJ, Gamble-George JC, Hermanson DJ, et al. Central anandamide deficiency predicts stress-induced anxiety: behavioral reversal through endocannabinoid augmentation. Transl Psychiatry. 2014;4:e408.
196. Giuffrida A, Leweke F, Gerth C, et al. Cerebrospinal anandamide levels are elevated in acute schizophrenia and are inversely correlated with psychotic symptoms. Neuropsychopharmacology. 2004;29:2108–14.
197. McNamara RK, Hahn C-G, Jandacek R, et al. Selective deficits in the omega-3 fatty acid docosahexaenoic acid in the postmortem orbitofrontal cortex of patients with major depressive disorder. Biol Psychiatry. 2007;62:17–24.
198. Larrieu T, Laye S. Food for mood: relevance of nutritional omega-3 fatty acids for depression and anxiety. Front Physiol. 2018;9:1047.
199. Larrieu T, Hilal ML, Fourrier C, et al. Nutritional omega-3 modulates neuronal morphology in the prefrontal cortex along with depression-related behaviour through corticosterone secretion. Transl Psychiatry. 2014;4:e437.
200. Hibbeln JR. Fish consumption and major depression. Lancet. 1998;351:1213.
201. Green P, Hermesh H, Monselise A, et al. Red cell membrane omega-3 fatty acids are decreased in nondepressed patients with social anxiety disorder. Eur Neuropsychopharmacol. 2006;16:107–13.
202. McNamara RK, Liu Y. Reduced expression of fatty acid biosynthesis genes in the prefrontal cortex of patients with major depressive disorder. J Affect Disord. 2011;129:359–63.
203. Parletta N, Zarnowiecki D, Cho J, et al. People with schizophrenia and depression have a low omega-3 index. Prostaglandins Leukot Essent Fatty Acids. 2016;110:42–7.
204. Thesing CS, Bota M, Milaneschia Y, et al. Omega-3 and omega-6 fatty acid levels in depressive and anxiety disorders. Psychoneuroendocrinology. 2018;87:53–62.
205. Lin P-Y, Huang S-Y, Su K-P. A meta-analytic review of polyunsaturated fatty acid compositions in patients with depression. Biol Psychiatry. 2010;68:140–7.
206. McNamara R, Jandacek R, Rider T, et al. Deficits in docosahexaenoic acid and associated elevations in the metabolism of arachidonic acid and saturated fatty acids in the postmortem orbitofrontal cortex of patients with bipolar disorder. Psychiatry Res. 2008;160:285–99.

207. McNamara RK, Jandacek R, Tso P, et al. Lower docosahexaenoic acid concentrations in the postmortem prefrontal cortex of adult depressed suicide victims compared with controls without cardiovascular disease. J Psychiatr Res. 2013;47:1187–91.
208. Bondi CO, Taha AY, Tock JL, et al. Adolescent behavior and dopamine availability are uniquely sensitive to dietary omega-3 fatty acid deficiency. Biol Psychiatry. 2014;75:38–46.
209. Lafourcade M, Larrieu T, Mato S, et al. Nutritional omega-3 deficiency abolishes endocannabinoid-mediated neuronal functions. Nat Neurosci. 2011;14(3):345–50.
210. Larrieu T, Madore C, Joffre C, Lay S. Nutritional n-3 polyunsaturated fatty acids deficiency alters cannabinoid receptor signaling pathway in the brain and associated anxiety-like behavior in mice. J Physiol Biochem. 2012;68:671–81.
211. Larrieu T, Hilal ML, Desmedt-peyrusse V, et al. Nutritional omega-3 deficiency alters glucocorticoid receptor-signaling pathway and neuronal morphology in regionally distinct brain structures associated with emotional deficits. Neural Plast. 2016;2016:8574830.
212. Bourre JM. Dietary omega-3 fatty acids and psychiatry: mood, behaviour, stress, depression, dementia and aging. J Nutr Health Aging. 2005;9:31–8.
213. Thomazeua A, Bosch-Bouju C, Manzoni O, Laye S. Nutritional n-3 PUFA deficiency abolishes endocannabinoid gating of hippocampal long-term potentiation. Cereb Cortex. 2016;27(4):2571–9.
214. Kang JX, Gleason ED. Omega-3 fatty acids and hippocampal neurogenesis in depression. CNS Neurol Disord Drug Targets. 2013;12(4):460–5.
215. Simopoulos AP. The importance of the ratio of omega 6/omega 3 essential fatty acids. Biomed Pharmacother. 2002;56(8):365–79.
216. Simopoulos AP. Evolutionary aspects of diet: the omega 6/omega 3 ratio and the brain. Mol Neurobiol. 2011;44:203.
217. Wilkinson D. Can food be medicine against cancer? A healthy handbook that combines science, medicine and not-so-common sense. Australia: Inspiring Publishers; 2015.
218. Simopoulos AP. Omega-3 fatty acids in health and disease and in growth and development. Am J Clin Nutr. 1991;54:438–63.
219. Bazinet RP, Layé S. Polyunsaturated fatty acids and their metabolites in brain function and disease. Nat Rev Neurosci. 2014;15:771–85.
220. Leizer C, Ribnicky D, Poulev A, et al. The composition of hemp seed oil and its potential as an important source of nutrition. J Nutraceuticals Funct Med Foods. 2000;2:35–53.
221. Rodriguez-Leyva D, Pierce GN. The cardiac and haemostatic effects of dietary hempseed. Nutr Metab. 2010;7:32.
222. Russo R, Reggiani R. Variability in anti-nutritional compounds in hempseed meal of Italian and French varieties. Plant. 2013;1:25–9.
223. Crescente G, Piccolella S, Esposito A, et al. Chemical composition and nutraceutical properties of hempseed: an ancient food with actual functional value. Phytochem Rev. 2018;17:733–49.
224. Welch AA, Shakya-Shrestha S, Lentjes MAH, et al. 2010. Dietary intake and status of n-3 polyunsaturated fatty acids in a population of fish-eating and non-fish-eating meat-eaters, vegetarians, and vegans and the product-precursor ratio [corrected] of α-linolenic acid to long-chain n-3 polyunsaturated fatty acids: results from the EPIC-Norfolk cohort. Am J Clin Nutr. 2010;92(5):1040–51.
225. Aran A, Eylon M, Harel M et al. Lower circulating endocannabinoid levels in children with autism spectrum disorder. Molecular Autism 2019a;10:2.

# The Endocannabinoid System, Stress, and Mental Health

# 3

## Introduction

The term "stress" and its meaning has evolved over time since Selye first popularized it in a paper in *Nature* in 1936 where he defined stress as "non-specific responses of the body to any demand upon it" [1, 2]. The definition of stress has evolved from one primarily related to an effect to include the concept of stress as a cause of illness [2], including stress in the psychosocial sense.

Hill et al. [3] define stress as anything that presents as a challenge to homeostasis and is typically something that threatens our well-being. It may be a real threat, or a perceived one, but people exposed to the same stress are not necessarily affected in the same manner [4]. Emotions cannot be divorced from stress since they drive the creation and interpretation of factors or events that are causes of stress, and the physiological responses that occur while experiencing stress become encoded as part of the interpreted emotion [2].

Stress is one of the most important and often overlooked etiological and pathological factors in many illnesses, particularly those of chronic nature. While stress is difficult to quantify and sometimes to even describe, it has become a feature of modern, westernized life, and as humans, we are becoming sicker. The element of stress, as a cause, an effect, an exacerbating factor, and/or an enabling factor, is likely to be involved in many illnesses, including mental health conditions. In particular, stress in the sense of a psychosocial stressor appears a feature of modern life.

While some level of stress in our lives may be useful, and indeed serves an important function in survival, it is when stress becomes chronic, unrelenting, prolonged, overwhelming, or extreme that it can start to become unhealthy and affect our mental and physical health. Inadequate control of stress responses contributes to the risk of mental health disorders and increases mortality [5, 6].

Stress can increase the risk of many illnesses including cancer, hypertension, cardiovascular disease, stroke, gastrointestinal problems (including inflammatory bowel disease), a weakened immune system, and others [7, 8]. Long-term stress increases the risk of mental health problems including anxiety and depression, sleep



K. O'Brien, P. Blair, *Medicinal Cannabis and CBD in Mental Healthcare*,
https://doi.org/10.1007/978-3-030-78559-8_3

problems, substance abuse, and pain [7]. Psychosocial stress plays a clear role in the development and continuance of symptoms of major mental health illnesses including depression and schizophrenia [9]. Stress also alters our responses to emotional stimuli [10].

Chronic stress is a risk factor for development and exacerbation of mental illnesses including depression, anxiety, and post-traumatic stress disorder (PTSD) [11–13]. Thus, by understanding the biochemical adaptations that occur with chronic stress, it might be possible to discover targets and treatments for many different mental health conditions [14].

There is evidence that the endocannabinoid system (ECS) is involved in our stress response (both acute and chronic) and in stress regulation. It is altered when stress is chronic and when there is early life stress. The gut microbiome also has a role to play in stress regulation, and the two (ECS and gut microbiome) form a close relationship.

**This Chapter**

In this chapter, we will examine the brain regions involved in stress regulation, what happens to the autonomic nervous system stress response and the neuroendocrine stress response, how inflammation is involved in stress, and how stress impacts on the ECS as well as how the ECS is involved in stress regulation. We will also look at the impact of early life stress on mental health and the ECS functioning, the gut microbiome's involvement in stress, and how the "endocannabinoidome," a term referring to the extended ECS, is involved in mental health.

## Key Brain Structures Involved in the Regulation of Stress

There are several key brain regions involved in the processing and regulation of stress. Sensory information is processed by the thalamus and primary sensory cortical centers and then transmitted to the amygdala via corticothalamic afferent nerves. Two important structures associated with the regulation of stress and emotions are the corticolimbic system (prefrontal cortex, amygdala, hippocampus) and the hypothalamic-pituitary-adrenal (HPA) axis [15].

### Corticolimbic System

The corticolimbic system is made up of:

- Prefrontal cortex (PFC)
- Amygdala (especially the basolateral amygdala, BLA)
- Hippocampus

The corticolimbic system processes a wide range of cognitive and behavioral responses including emotional regulation, decision-making, mnemonic function, and motor programming and control [16]. The corticolimbic system integrates emotion with cognition and also is involved in pain modulation [17]. As clinicians know, pain is known to have a strong emotional component. Chronic pain is a disorder with anxio-depressive symptoms as well as cognitive deficits, and the corticolimbic system is implicated in pathophysiology of maladaptive pain [17, 18].

The brain areas that make up the corticolimbic system are all involved in the stress response, as well as in processing and regulation of emotions, fear, reward, emotional memory, anxiety-related behaviors, and drug abuse, and the ECS is widely distributed throughout these regions [3, 19, 20]. These brain regions regulate normal emotional and cognitive development and behavior [21].

The structures of the corticolimbic system are all connected to each other with both feedforward and feedback processes occurring, where stimulation of the ventral hippocampus and mPFC activates principal cells and interneurons in the basal amygdala and innervated principal cells project back from the basal amygdala to the mPFC [22]. There are also connections between the corticolimbic system and other parts of the brain, and some of these will be explored throughout various chapters. For example, the medial PFC (mPFC) projects to several brain regions involved in control of motivated behavior, anxiety, and depression [22].

## Roles of the Components of the Corticolimbic System

The roles of the basolateral amygdala (BLA) are believed to include modulating learning after stress, memory consolidation, and hippocampus activity during learning and stress [23]. Activation of the BLA involved several aspects of the stress response including pain and anxiety, HPA axis activation, and alterations in cognitive processes through connections with other parts of the amygdala and hypothalamus [24]. It is understood that stress-induced release of corticotropin-releasing hormone in the amygdala contributes to emotional responses to exposure to stress (e.g., anxiety) [6]. Reference to past experience and retrieval of spatial memory are mediated via cross-talk between the mPFC and the hippocampus, and the amygdala is also involved in retrieval of fear associations, something clearly relevant in post-traumatic stress disorder [22]. There is also thalamic input to the mPFC that projects information in relation to affective-motivational behaviors [22].

The amygdaloid complex regulates anxiety and fear, providing valence to memories via its connections to the hippocampus which is where memory consolidation occurs. The hippocampus is involved in feedback regulation of the HPA axis [6].

The prefrontal cortex regulates activity of the amygdala and hippocampus, controlling emotional stress responses and facilitating active coping, and contributes to resilience to stress [6], meanwhile excitatory outputs from the medial PFC and the hippocampus control activity and output of the amygdala [22].

## Hypothalamic-Pituitary-Adrenal (HPA) Axis

The hypothalamic-pituitary-adrenal (HPA) axis, believed to be responsible for our main endocrine response to stress, is made up of:

- Hypothalamus (including the paraventricular nucleus, PVN)
- Pituitary
- Adrenal glands

Anxiety and mood disorders have been found to be associated with a dysfunctional stress response by the HPA axis [25]. Physiological stressors (which disturb internal homeostasis) utilize a bottom-up circuit to activate the HPA axis, via direct recruitment of the HPA axis by brainstem nuclei, while in contrast, psychological stressors utilize top-down processes to activate the HPA axis and produce a neuroendocrine response [26–28]. The hypothalamus, involved in the HPA axis stress response, integrates input from limbic and sensory brain areas to regulate HPA axis activation [6].

The paraventricular nucleus (PVN) of the hypothalamus is a key structure in the physiological stress response and integrates pre-autonomic and neuroendocrine control of energy homeostasis, fluid balance, and our stress response [29].

## Other Areas

There are other brain regions that connect with these regions that are involved in emotional processing, regulation, and responses. For example, here are some of them:

**Nucleus Accumbens** It is located in the rostral and ventral forebrain; receives input from the amygdala, hippocampus, and from cells of the stria terminalis; is believed to be the primary site mediating reward behavior and and to play a role in addictive behaviors associated with drug use [15].

**Anterior Cingulate Cortex (ACC)** It has extensive connections to brain areas involved in emotional processing (including the amygdala), autonomic functions (e.g., lateral hypothalamus, brainstem centers), memory (e.g., hippocampus), and reward (e.g., orbitofrontal cortex, ventral striatum) [30]; integrates neuronal circuitry for "affect regulation" (ability to manage uncomfortable emotions) via connections to both the "emotional" limbic system and the "cognitive" prefrontal cortex [30]; and is involved in assessing emotions, emotional learning, and autonomic regulation, with the posterior portion involved in emotional regulation, autonomic regulation, and pain-related affect [30].

**Medial Cingulate Cortex** It is "cognitive" in nature and is involved in several functions such as emotional appraisal, monitoring of conflict, selection and execution of responses, and others [30].

## The Stress Response

Several stress response systems come into play following exposure to stress including the autonomic nervous system (in particular the sympathetic nervous system), the HPA axis, increased negative emotions and behavioral responses such as increased vigilance that help us avoid a threat [6].

Our central nervous system (CNS) is in communication with all other vital organ systems in our body in two ways: direct transmission of neural signals through the autonomic nervous system and via the neuroendocrine system through hormone release into the circulation affecting downstream organs [31]. The stress response thus has two components: an autonomic response and a neuroendocrine response [24].

The stress response to acute stressors or agents is considered adaptive; it mobilizes necessary resources in response to a threat, real or perceived. However, chronic activation of the stress pathways can be etiological factors in illness and/or exacerbate existing pathologies through alterations in metabolic processes, immune dysregulation, and prolonged systemic drive [2].

### The Autonomic Stress Response

In the autonomic stress response, there is stimulation of sympathetic motor and hormonal outputs via descending neural circuits originating in hypothalamic pre-autonomic control centers. This leads to release of catecholamines in the brain and in the circulation [24].

The central nervous system (CNS) involves the brain and spinal cord, and the peripheral nervous system involves the autonomic nervous system and somatic nervous systems. There are two divisions of the autonomic nervous system (ANS):

- The sympathetic nervous system (SNS)
- The parasympathetic nervous system (PNS)

In terms of evolution, the SNS has evolved to keep us safe from predators in the past. In more recent times, our threats are not wild animals (unless you work in a game reserve possibly) but have become other immediate environmental threats. Think about what happens if you step out onto a busy road and suddenly there's a car you didn't see bearing down on you. It's an immediate threat, and you want your SNS response to become activated fast—it is an appropriate response to an immediate threat to existence. However, we also know that there are other forms of existential threat, perhaps not as immediate but more insidious, psychosocial in nature, that we might experience under more chronic conditions. It is when our physiological stress responses become disproportionate and chronic that is dangerous to our well-being.

Under a threat, perceived or real, the SNS response (also called the "fight or flight" response) mobilizes the body's energy resources such as glucose and oxygen and reallocates these quickly to those systems which must be activated (fast) to help us fight or get away (e.g., our skeletal muscles, heart, and vasculature). Our heart rate, blood pressure, and respiration rate and skin conductance all increase in response to a threat, and meanwhile, energy is diverted away from those areas of the body that are not important at that point in time for our survival (e.g., digestive system, reproductive system) [31]. The SNS is paired with the PNS, much like an accelerator (SNS) and a brake (PNS) on the car [32]: once the threat has passed, the PNS reduces the activation of the SNS and energy and blood flow once more resumes being supplied to areas requiring it for normal physiological functioning [31].

### Sympathetic Nervous System Mechanisms of Action

The SNS is linked neuroanatomically to the limbic system and brainstem and reaches various areas of the body peripherally through the sympathetic ganglia (located bilateral to the spinal cord, extending from the neck to coccyx). There are two neural networks that constitute the SNS and use norepinephrine as a neurotransmitter:

- Alpha-adrenergic fibers: in the cardiovascular system, these constrict blood vessels.
- Beta-adrenergic fibers: in the cardiovascular system, these dilate blood vessels, and importantly, these fibers alone innervate the heart and cause increased heart rate and contractility [31]

### Parasympathetic Nervous System Neuroanatomical Connections

In contrast, the PNS connects directly to peripheral organs via several of the cranial nerves, including the vagal nerve (ninth cranial nerve) and the pelvic splanchnic nerves that provide afferent as well as efferent channels. The PNS uses acetylcholine in particular as its neurotransmitter. The vagal nerve transmits signals to the heart which leads to reduced heart rate and reduced cardiac contractility, but it does not have any direct influence on arterial vasoconstriction or vasodilation (unlike the SNS). Thus, in terms of heart functioning, both heart rate and blood pressure are influenced by the SNS and PNS (since both innervate the heart) [31].

### Measurement of ANS Activity

Popular outcome variables for measuring ANS functioning include heart rate, blood pressure, and heart rate variability (HRV) [31].

## Neuroendocrine Stress Response

In contrast to the fast action of the ANS which utilizes nerve impulses, the neuroendocrine response to stress utilizes hormones traveling via the bloodstream, and for this reason, the neuroendocrine response is slower than the ANS responses to stressors [31].

The adrenal glands release two key stress hormones which impact on cardiovascular and other systems' functions: cortisol from the adrenal cortex and adrenalin (epinephrine) from the adrenal medulla. The CNS constantly monitors the levels of these stress-responsive hormones, and there are negative feedback loops in operation to adjust their levels [31].

Both cortisol and epinephrine influence the SNS:

- Cortisol: influences the sensitivity of the SNS beta-adrenergic receptors; enhances the sensitivity of SNS alpha-adrenergic receptors, catecholamine synthesis, and glucose production; **release** is mediated by the HPA axis.
- Epinephrine: influences the sensitivity of the SNS beta-adrenergic receptors; release is mediated by the sympathoadrenomedullary axis (epinephrine is released from the adrenal medulla into the circulation following direct SNS transmission from the brainstem) [2, 31].

Herman et al. [2] argue in that the case of the two "stress systems," the sympathoadrenomedullary axis and the HPA axis, their relationship with stressors is only one of their functions and in fact, both systems are mainly concerned with metabolism on a day-to-day basis, in that both mobilize energy in the liver to provide resources needed to respond to a challenge (glucocorticoids involved in gluconeogenesis, proteolysis, and lipolysis and epinephrine involved in glycogenolysis and glycolysis).

### The HPA Axis in Stress

Continuing from above, Herman et al. [2] make an important point that the HPA axis is not a "stress system" per se, but rather a normal metabolic system that gets co-opted or recruited by stressors (causal agents of stress). There are several areas of the brain which are involved in its regulation and which play a role when there is a perceived or real threat. The functioning of the HPA axis in stress is described well by Herman et al. [2], and the following summary draws heavily from them.

#### The HPA Axis as a Metabolic System

The control of the functioning of the HPA axis is complex. The HPA axis is under circadian control, and peak activity corresponds to when we wake up, logical as we need to mobilize energy necessary for the activities of our day. The processes which result in the release of glucocorticoids are simply part of the normal metabolic role of the HPA axis which includes facilitation of glyconeogenesis, lipolysis, and proteolysis [2]. It is not just on waking that our glucocorticoid levels increase—levels of glucocorticoids also increase when we anticipate a meal. However, as Herman et al. [2] explain, under a condition of stress, this process essentially gets diverted to produce the glucocorticoids needed to deal with a stressor, some kind of threat to homeostasis (and of course, this could be psychosocial in nature). They make an important point relevant to research and the clinic: in attempting to quantify HPA axis activation in the context of investigating the body's response to stress and/or in illness (i.e., by measuring changes in baseline glucocorticoid levels), one needs to take into account both stressor-elicited secretion and endogenous release patterns (e.g., circadian rhythms) [2].

**Regulation of the HPA Axis**

There are many factors that can activate the HPA axis which might be consistent with the need to provide energy quickly, and this includes disruptions to metabolism, thermoregulation, and fluid balance which are under the homeostatic control of the hypothalamus [2].

The paraventricular nucleus (PVN) of the hypothalamus is a central player in the HPA axis response. The classic understanding of the chain of events occurring in HPA axis activation is that PVN releases corticotropin-releasing hormone (CRH) into the portal vessels. The CRH travels to the anterior pituitary gland and binds with CRH receptors, and this stimulates the anterior pituitary to produce adrenocorticotropic hormone (ACTH) which is released into the systemic circulation. ACTH stimulates the release of glucocorticoid hormones (in humans this is mainly cortisol) from the adrenal cortex [3]. The glucocorticoids mobilize energy stores and produce several different effects on the cardiovascular, immune, metabolic, and neural systems [3]. There is then feedback mechanisms which serve to shut off the HPA axis response and restore homeostasis (discussed later).

As with anything in the body, there is a great deal more complexity involved. A key role of the PVN is integration of pre-autonomic and neuroendocrine control of energy homeostasis, fluid balance, and our stress response [29]. If a stressor that could pose a threat to homeostasis is encountered, information from the stressor is integrated across various different brain circuits prior to reaching the PVN. For example, the PVN is stimulated by afferents from the brainstem and hypothalamus which transmit information. The bed nucleus of the stria terminalis (BST) may be involved in the relay of contextual information [2]. Meanwhile, the subnuclei of the amygdala indirectly drive the HPA axis response via disinhibition mediated by GABAergic connections to PVN-projecting neurons in the hypothalamus and BST [2].

Very importantly, emotions must be considered within the context of stressors and HPA axis activation, since emotions can drive generation and interpretation of stressors [2]. When we look at post-traumatic stress disorder (PTSD) in a later chapter, we can also see how memory (in particular fear memories or memories of a traumatic event) can feed into the HPA axis and how the HPA axis "stress response" becomes dysfunctional [33].

Herman et al. [2] point out that there is a three-step amplification process that occurs as we move from the CRH to ACTH to glucocorticoids, i.e., fg/ml for CRH, pg/ml for ACTH, and then ng/ml for glucocorticoids, and this amplification process can be altered by the anterior pituitary and adrenals via various mechanisms. For example, sympathetic activation can increase glucocorticoid production by the adrenals, and negative glucocorticoid feedback can block release of ACTH from the pituitary [2].

Glucocorticoid signaling affects many systems. Glucocorticoids bind with glucocorticoid receptors and the mineralocorticoid receptors, and these act via many different mechanisms including acting as membrane receptors or transcription factors to effect changes in genes, and their effects on their targets can be fast (minutes) or can last weeks [2]. Glucocorticoid receptors are widely distributed in the CNS, and mineralocorticoid receptors are also present in several brain regions, including some areas such as the hippocampus where they co-localize with glucocorticoid receptors [2, 34].

### Turning Off the HPA Axis

Under normal circumstances, the body tries to restore homeostasis since elevated glucocorticoids, if sustained, cause detrimental effects on health. There are complex and distributed negative feedback processes in the brain and periphery that serve to inhibit the PVN neurons and thereby turn off the HPA axis response [2, 3]. Glucocorticoid receptors in various brain regions including the hippocampus and PFC inhibit the HPA axis through glucocorticoid-mediated negative feedback [2, 3]. The corticolimbic system (i.e., PFC, amygdala, hippocampus) which communicates with the PVN and is involved in positive regulation of the HPA axis is also involved in its inhibition [35]. For example, neurons in the PFC and hippocampus inhibit the HPA axis via hypothalamic and BST GABAergic relays to the PVN [2]. There are also peripheral mechanisms of feedback, for example, from adipocytes [2].

Under normal circumstances, all works well, and following a stressful situation and activation of the HPA axis, negative feedback processes occur, and homeostasis is restored. However, under chronic stress conditions, HPA axis dysregulation can occur, and at the neurological level, this is probably due to inappropriate balance between the excitatory and inhibitory inputs impacting on the output of the PVN [2]. In early stages, this HPA axis dysfunction may be characterized by oversecretion of cortisol, but as time goes by, this can turn into what has been termed "adrenal exhaustion" where not enough cortisol is produced (with consequent low energy levels experienced by the patient) [36].

As you can see, the regulation of the stress response is quite complex. To take a deep dive, please read Herman et al.'s [2] paper.

## Measurement of Neuroendocrine Activity

Commonly, measurements of neuroendocrine activity involve analysis of urine, blood, or saliva samples. Cortisol measurements need to take into account its normal diurnal fluctuations in secretion when investigating neuroendocrine responses to stress [31].

### Sex Differences in the Stress Response System Along the HPA Axis

Substantial research has shown that there are sex differences in the stress response, in numerous components of the HPA axis, and these might explain at least partly why certain diseases are more prevalent in males and females [37]. This includes sex differences in basal cortisol levels, stress responsivity, and glucocorticoid receptors [37].

There are some differences in what has been found with animal data in comparison to human data. Animal data has demonstrated that the glucocorticoid levels generated are higher in females than males after HPA axis stimulation, but human research data has not been quite as clear-cut. Some studies have found no difference for HPA axis response to physical activity, and others have found either no difference in cortisol or higher cortisol in young men compared with young women under various psychological stress situations (real-life stress or laboratory stress tests) [37].

In general, it seems that adult men generate greater increases in cortisol in response to psychological stress than women [37]. This lower cortisol response found in women may be related to hypoactivity of the HPA axis, and it possibly might explain the greater prevalence of autoimmune conditions in women, while the greater stress reactivity and higher cortisol levels might possibly explain the higher prevalence of cardiovascular disease in men [37]. It is not clear yet if such differences between male and female humans in adrenocortical responses to stress are present at birth—there are some studies that suggest there is no difference and at least one study that suggests there may be [37, 38].

## When the Stress Response Becomes Pathological

Allostasis is the body's attempt to stabilize physiological functioning by modifying energy distribution to our vital organs, and the size and duration of the response will vary depending on the threat and the health status of the individual [31]. Allostatic load was defined as "the cost of chronic exposure to fluctuating or heightened neural or neuroendocrine response resulting from repeated or chronic environmental challenge" [39]. Another way of thinking about allostatic load is that it represents the "wear and tear" on the brain and body due to persistent and sustained activations of the stress response systems and the loss of the systems that normally buffer stress responses [6].

The ANS and neuroendocrine stress responses function to help us survive, as we have seen, but the activation of these systems is not always proportional to the nature of the threat. Stress responses can become dysfunctional and consequently negatively impact on health. Larkin et al. [31] explain that failure to maintain allostasis (dynamic homeostasis) in response to an acute environmental stress can lead to patterns of dysfunction of the ANS and/or neuroendocrine responses during chronic stress, and these can be quite different to what is seen in acute stress (e.g., hyperarousal in acute stress may lead to hypo-arousal in chronic stress).

As explained by Larkin et al. [31], dysfunctional ANS and neuroendocrine stress responses include (1) exaggerated reactivity to stress (characterized by increased heart rate, blood pressure, and levels of stress hormones such as cortisol), (2) blunted reactivity to stress, and (3) prolonged recovery from stress (e.g., prolonged recovery of blood pressure and heart rate associated with mental stress), which represent three patterns of "allostatic load," and all of which can place a cumulative burden on body functioning that leads to increased disease risk (including CVD) [31, 40, 41]. Meanwhile, low stress reactivity (blunted reactivity) has been found to be associated with lower immune function, obesity, depression, and addictive behaviors including smoking and alcoholism (but not CVD) [31, 42].

There has been some interesting research investigating stress reactivity and cardiovascular disease (described in Larkin et al. [31]). Exaggerated cardiovascular reactivity to laboratory challenge can predict future cardiovascular morbidity and mortality [41]. Increased ANS reactivity, demonstrated, for example, by magnitude of heart rate and blood pressure reactivity, has been found to be associated with various stressful life situations such as being employed in stressful occupations or being a caregiver for a dementia sufferer [31, 43, 44]. In one study, chronic and momentary work stress (significantly) independently predicted greater heart rate reactivity after adjusting for heart rate, age, smoking, caffeine, and momentary physical activity levels [43].

In another study, caregivers with high levels of social support showed a typical age-related decrease in heart rate reactivity, but those with low levels of social support showed an age-related increase in heart rate reactivity [44] which underscores not only the stressful nature of being a caregiver but also the power of social support. Human beings are social beings, and research shows clearly that social connections and social therapy can have tremendous benefits on reducing mortality and morbidity, including in relation to serious illnesses such as cancer [8].

## Stress and Inflammation

The relationship between stress and inflammation is well-known: stress can be proinflammatory [45]. There is increasing evidence that excessive inflammation plays a key role in the pathophysiology of stress-related diseases and that chronic, mild inflammation provides a common pathway of stress-related diseases [46]. In fact, it has been estimated that 75–90% of diseases are related to activation of the stress system. Common stress-related diseases include cardiovascular disease, metabolic disease (e.g., diabetes), mental health conditions (depression, Alzheimer's disease), neurodegenerative diseases, and cancer [46].

Stressful events trigger multiple neurochemical, neurotransmitter, and hormonal changes mainly through activation of the sympathetic nervous system (SNS) and the HPA axis. While traditionally, the link between stress and disease focused on the SNS and HPA axis, inflammation has more recently emerged as a promising biological mechanism linking stress and disease [46]. Chronic stress can lead to inflammation through production of proinflammatory cytokines such as IFN$\gamma$ and TNF$\alpha$ [47–51]. Increased levels of inflammatory cytokines have been found in people with major depression [50, 52] , and we will look at that in more detail in a later chapter.

While inflammation can induce changes in the brain and body functioning which can contribute to a range of psychiatric conditions [45], it has been argued by several authors that even though for an individual patient, inflammation may be *a* or even *the* cause of depression, depression and other psychiatric conditions are not inflammatory conditions *per se* [45, 53]. The argument is that not every patient with depression has increased inflammation [53] and that inflammation may be one of several causes [45]. Psychological stress and inflammation can also underpin other conditions in the body such as coronary heart disease (CHD) [54] and cancer [8].

## How Does Stress Activate Inflammatory Changes?

Stress can activate an inflammatory response both centrally and peripherally. When the HPA axis is activated, glucocorticoids are released, and these are immunosuppressive and anti-inflammatory, and indeed research indicates that glucocorticoids can reduce many types of proinflammatory cytokines including IL-6 and TNF-α as well as increasingly anti-inflammatory cytokines (e.g., IL-10, TNF-β). However, despite this, glucocorticoids have also been found to have a proinflammatory effect on the immune system. Pro- and anti- inflammatory mechanisms depend on both the type and intensity of the stressor involved. For example, acute stressors tend to enhance immune function, chronic stressors suppress immune function, and intense stressors overactivate the immune system, resulting in an imbalance between pro- and anti-inflammation effects [46]. To bring things back to the basics, there is a lack of balance and illness. We see this departure from balance in many different ways in the body when there is illness, something that ancient medical systems such as Chinese medicine recognized and sought then and seek now to identify and address as part of its fundamental approach to both diagnosis and treatment.

Centrally, neuroinflammation can occur under conditions of stress, with increased microglia activation, increased proinflammatory cytokines, and increased peripherally derived monocytes and macrophages occurring. It is thought that a triad of an overactivated immune system, increased activity via sympathetic nervous system pathways, and reduced glucocorticoid responsiveness may jointly activate the inflammatory responses associated with stress and that glucocorticoids, catecholamines, cytokines, and other chemicals released as a result of stress, in the main, mediate the proinflammatory effect induced by stress [46].

As we will see in later chapters, the theme of inflammation appears again and again in the pathophysiology of various mental health conditions, and while it is not the only pathological factor involved in such conditions, it appears to be a relatively consistent one. When we discuss the therapeutic attributes of medicinal cannabis, one of the key ones is its effect on inflammation.

## Endocannabinoid System and Stress Regulation

The endocannabinoid system (ECS) regulates our responsivity to stress and emotional behavior, including the neuroendocrine and behavioral aspects of stress, seeking to inhibit stress and reduce its negative impacts [21, 24]. The ECS is also involved in the regulation of mood, anxiety, reward, and extinction of fear learning (which becomes dysregulated in post-traumatic stress disorder) [20]. When there is disruption of endocannabinoid signaling, it recapitulates many of the effects of stress such as HPA axis activation [24].

Animal research indicates that endocannabinoid signaling is altered by stress as well as mediating or modulating stress responses [55], with mobilization of 2-AG occurring downstream of glucocorticoid receptor activation [56] and AEA increases occurring in response to corticotropin-releasing hormone receptor activation, secondary to FAAH inhibition [57, 58]. The endocannabinoid/CB1 receptor signaling can inhibit the activation of the HPA axis by stress and also enhance recovery following termination of the stress response [58].

## Several Lines of Evidence that the ECS Is a Regulator of the Stress Response

Several lines of evidence provide support for contention that the ECS is an important regulator of the stress response, including the following:

- Cannabis consumption in humans is associated with reduced anxiety and perceptions of stress and greater relaxation [24].
- Animal studies indicate that disruption of endocannabinoid signaling produces a neurobehavioral phenotype which displays characteristics of the stress response including increased anxiety, activation of the HPA axis, hypervigilance, and impaired cognitive flexibility [24].
- Components of the ECS (AEA, 2-AG, their degradative enzymes, and CB1 receptors) are structures found in the corticolimbic system and HPA axis [24].
- Evidence of presence of the CB1 receptors in sympathetic neuron terminals and cells of the adrenal medulla [6].

Research suggests that both the sympathetic nervous system stress response and the neuroendocrine stress response (mediated by the HPA axis) are regulated by the ECS [6, 58].

## Bidirectional Relationship Between Stress and the ECS

However, the relationship between the ECS and stress is not unidirectional. In addition to mediating and modulating the effects of stress on the brain, the ECS is altered by exposure to stress, and there is much animal research evidencing the roles of the endocannabinoids and CB1 receptor in brain adaptations as a result of exposure to repeated stress. Chronic stress exposure can increase an individual's vulnerability to mental illness, and because of the association of the ECS to our stress systems, it may be an important therapeutic target for prevention and treatment of mental illnesses associated with stress [6].

## ECS and the Autonomic Nervous System Stress Response

There is evidence that the ECS is involved in modulation of the sympathetic nervous system (SNS) stress response, as CB1 receptors have been found on sympathetic neuron terminals and cells of the adrenal medulla and CB1 receptor agonists have been shown to inhibit the release of the norepinephrine and epinephrine from these, as well as inhibit vasoconstriction and inflammation, both mediated by the SNS [6]. As yet though, the source and trigger for endocannabinoids innervating CB1 receptors on SNS terminals are not yet known [6]. Circulating levels of AEA and 2-AG in the peripheral circulation are increased with stress exposure [58]. As occurs in the CNS, the ECS in the periphery is activated by exposure to a stressor and serves to buffer the response through inhibition of release of catecholamines epinephrine and norepinephrine [6].

## ECS, the Corticolimbic System, and the HPA Axis

The ECS is involved in the homeostasis of the corticolimbic system, and signaling in corticolimbic structures is critical for regulating emotional behaviors like anxiety and stress in adults [19]. ECS involvement is evidenced by the fact that CB1 receptors are widely expressed and the two key endocannabinoids, anandamide (AEA) and 2-arachidonylglycerol (2-AG), are synthesized in particular in the BLA (and also in the central nucleus), as well as in the hippocampus, medial PFC, and nucleus accumbens [24, 59, 60].

The basolateral amygdala (BLA) is believed to be an important site for ECS regulation of the HPA axis, acting as a "gatekeeper," though there may be other sites also involved [24]. When experiments injecting CB1 receptor antagonists into the PVN or the mPFC were performed, no effect on basal corticosterone levels was found, but when injected into the BLA, an increase in HPA axis activity was demonstrated, supporting the BLA's important role in HPA axis regulation [24].

The ECS does play an important role within the PFC, maintaining top-down regulatory mechanisms that serve to dampen stress and thereby cultivate resilience to effects associated with exposure to stress [6]. The ECS is also a negative regulator of amygdalar reactivity through CB1 receptors located in the amygdala [6].

We also find that CB1 receptors are expressed and AEA and 2-AG are synthesized in the hypothalamus, including in the PVN portion which, as we saw earlier, plays a central role in the neuroendocrine stress response via the HPA axis [29]. On a related note, research in rats also suggests that CB1 receptors in the ventromedial hypothalamus play a role in modulating the unconditioned fear-related defensive behavioral reactions [61].

## ECS and Regulation of the HPA Axis

The ECS regulates the HPA axis in the maintenance of basal and stress-induced responses [25]. The ECS regulates basal and circadian HPA axis activation: for example, AEA levels in the hypothalamus are highest between 7.00 am and 11.00 am and low between 15.00 and 3.00 am [62].

There is a bidirectional relationship between the ECS and the HPA axis. Endocannabinoid signaling contributes to the regulation of the HPA axis, and conversely, the HPA axis helps regulate endocannabinoid signaling [3]. AEA is believed to represent the "tonic" signal, while 2-AG represents the "phasic" signal of the ECS [24]. Endocannabinoid tone, specifically AEA tone in the BLA in particular, provides a steady-state *inhibition* of the HPA axis, mediated via glutaminergic neurons, contributing to maintenance of low basal glucocorticoid levels during basal conditions and limiting HPA axis activity, and if this is disrupted, the HPA axis is activated [3, 25, 63].

The postulated mechanism by which AEA regulates the HPA axis is that a tonic level of AEA/CB1 receptor signaling in the BLA "gates" glutaminergic inputs to key neurons in the BLA, suppressing activation of the HPA axis [3]. Disruption of this AEA tone by stress activates the HPA axis with the resultant secretion of glucocorticoids [24]. Once the HPA axis is activated, the negative feedback mechanism comes into play to reduce the amounts of circulating glucocorticoids and reduce the HPA axis activity, thereby bringing the body back into balance.

The potential mechanism for glucocorticoid-mediated "fast feedback" inhibition of the HPA axis (this can occur in minutes) involves glucocorticoids inducing endocannabinoid signaling through a rapid process in CRH neurons of the PVN [3]. Glucocorticoids induce G-protein-dependent release of endocannabinoids and nitric oxide which inhibit glutaminergic inputs and enhance GABAergic inputs to CRH neurons in the PVN [2, 64]. In this way, they decrease the excitatory drive to the HPA axis [3].

Interestingly, there may be hormonal cross-talk occurring in PVN cells (in the hypothalamus) between glucocorticoids (which stimulate endocannabinoid synthesis and release) and leptin (which blocks glucocorticoid-induced endocannabinoid synthesis and suppression of excitation in the PVN) which may modulate synaptic excitation via endocannabinoid release in the hypothalamus. This could represent a mechanism for integration of the neuroendocrine regulation of energy homeostasis, fluid balance, and the stress response [29].

Let's now look in more detail at what happens to the components of the ECS under conditions of acute and chronic stress.

## How Is the ECS Involved in Acute and Chronic Stress?

In general, stress reduces levels of AEA and increases levels of 2-AG in most corticolimbic brain regions that have been studied. Current evidence suggests that AEA contributes to a tonic-like mechanism, regulating the basal synaptic transmission, while 2-AG acts as a phasic signal, activating CB1 receptors in a burst-like manner [24]. The purpose of the increase in 2-AG is to buffer and limit the detrimental effects of stress on the brain, and it plays a role in terminating the stress-induced HPA axis activation. It also contributes to habituation to stress [24].

However, as we saw in Chap. 2, the concept of the ECS has been extended to include the extended ECS, termed the "endocannabinoidome" which refers to bioactive derivatives, enzymes, transporters, and a plethora of receptor targets modulated by ECS components [65, 66]. We also find evidence that several components of theendocannabinoidome come into play in stress. We will now look at how the key components of the ECS are involved in acute and chronic stress.

### Acute Stress

Stress regulates both AEA and 2-AG levels. Glucocorticoids rapidly increase synaptic concentrations of 2-AG via membrane glucocorticoid receptors that are coupled to 2-AG synthesis, and in this way, activation of the HPA axis is directly linked to increased 2-AG levels [6].

Acute stress triggers a delayed increase in 2-AG levels: a moderate increase in 2-AG content in the medial PFC and a greater increase in 2-AG content in the hypothalamus [24]. However, some animal experiments using restraint stress have found there is no change in 2-AG levels in the amygdala, at least immediately after a certain time period of such stress [24, 67]. Differences in findings of such studies may reflect differences in stress models used. Elevated levels of corticosterone levels (corticosterone in animals is the correlate of cortisol in humans) are understood to mediate the increase in 2-AG in response to stress, but how it elevates AEA is still not understood [24].

In contrast, stress decreases AEA levels via its catabolic enzyme FAAH [6]. In response to acute stress, CRH is released, and this binds with the G-protein-coupled receptor CRH receptor 1, resulting in a fast increase in fatty acid amide hydrolase (FAAH, the enzyme responsible for AEA degradation) activity following activation of receptors on glutaminergic neurons in the BLA [6, 57]. Since FAAH degrades AEA, levels of AEA drop, leading to disinhibition of BLA neurons and increased output from neurons in the amygdala, which then impacts downstream, activating the HPA axis [3, 25]. Since AEA synthesis is constitutive and probably exerts tonic activation of CB1 receptors (i.e., maintaining low levels of neurotransmitter release at synapses that are regulated in this way), the removal of the AEA-induced tone (i.e., the decrease in AEA signaling) leads to reduced CB1 receptor signaling and *increased* neurotransmitter release (remember that the principal way in which endocannabinoids work is to inhibit the release of neurotransmitters), which then facilitates activation of the HPA axis and increases emotional and anxiety-like behavior, impairment of fear extinction, and suppression of cell proliferation in the neurogenic region of the hippocampus [6, 24, 25].

Animal studies indicate that acute stress reduces AEA content in the BLA and the hippocampus; however, its effect on the medial PFC is more complex and evidence is less consistent in the literature, with some experimentally induced stress experiences reducing AEA content and others not altering it or in the case of a mechanical stress like foot-shock (often used in mice experiments), elevating it [24].

There have been few investigations of the effect of acute stress on CB1 receptors in those regions of the brain associated with stress regulation. One study found that there was no effect of acute stress on density of CB1 receptors in the amygdala [27].

## Chronic Stress

Chronic stress can downregulate the ECS, with resultant excessive stress responses and poor adaptation [6]. The sequela of chronic stress, in particular prolonged exposure to stress hormones (e.g., cortisol), is often illness, including depression, cardiovascular disease, and cancer [8, 68].

Various animal experiments suggest that under conditions of chronic stress, the endocannabinoid signaling in the paraventricular nucleus (PVN, of the hypothalamus) is impaired, resulting in impaired "fast-feedback" inhibition of the HPA axis, something that may help explain the elevated glucocorticoid levels in chronic stress [3, 69].

Under chronic stress, the following changes in the ECS occur:

- **CB1 receptors are downregulated:** Generally, a downregulation of CB1 receptor expression in most parts of the brain involved in the stress response occurs, with the exception of the medial prefrontal cortex (where research indicates homotypic and heterotypic stressors increase CB1 receptor expression at the level of mRNA, protein, and receptor binding).
- **AEA is decreased:** Sustained exposure to glucocorticoids upregulates CRH signaling which consequently maintains increased FAAH and therefore decreased AEA levels. This contributes to the activation of the HPA axis, manifestation of anxiety, impairment of fear extinction, suppression of cell proliferation in the neurogenic region of the hippocampus, and development of anhedonia and hyperalgesia.
- **2-AG is increased:** Increases in 2-AG levels (found in acute stress) are amplified under conditions of chronic (repeated) stress, possibly mediated by reductions in MAGL (which degrades 2-AG) [13], leading to habituation of corticosterone responses (in animals, the equivalent of cortisol in humans). Increased 2-AG levels help terminate the stress-induced activation of the HPA axis as well as contribute to habituation to stress [24].

In animal experiments which are where much of our knowledge of mechanisms of action are gleaned, the effects of chronic stress on AEA, 2-AG, and CB1 receptors depend on the nature of the stress experienced, including whether it is homotypic (repeated exposure to the same stressor, e.g., restraint stress, social defeat stress) or heterotypic stress (exposure to different types of stress) [24]. Table 3.1 sets out the different effects of chronic homotypic stress and heterotypic stress on the endocannabinoids and CB1 receptors.

Mice experiments have demonstrated that stress-induced development of anxiety-like behavior is accompanied by the transient appearance of 2-AG-mediated long-term depression at GABAergic synapses in the basolateral amygdala (BLA, involved in motivation, affective regulation, and emotional learning) which is mediated partly by downregulation of MAGL. It appears that endocannabinoid synaptic plasticity at inhibitory synapses within the amygdala and increases in 2-AG levels prevent the behavioral and synaptic adaptations to chronic stress and suggests the possibility that pharmacological enhancement of 2-AG levels might be a useful approach to treating stress-induced mental health disorders [13].

**Table 3.1** Effect of chronic homotypic and heterotypic stress on the ECS (from [24])

| Type of chronic stress<br>Endocannabinoid | Chronic homotypic stress | Chronic heterotypic stress |
|---|---|---|
| **Level of 2-AG** | Levels increased; may be mediated by reduced levels of MAGL (the enzyme that degrades 2-AG) [24, 25]<br>Progressively enhanced levels in forebrain circuits which may mediate adaptation to stress and habituation of HPA axis [24] | Effects on 2-AG in various corticolimbic structures not consistent [24]<br>2-AG levels reduced in the hippocampus [70] |
| **Level of AEA** | Levels reduced in the amygdala, hippocampus, medial prefrontal cortex, and hypothalamus (Hill et al. [3] in Morena), in response to increased FAAH (at least within the amygdala) [24]<br>Changes in AEA and FAAH probably mediated by chronic exposure to corticosterone, mediated through a CRH mechanism [24] | Effects on AEA and FAAH not consistent across animal studies<br>General sense that AEA signaling, especially in the amygdala and hippocampus, is compromised [24] |
| **CB1 receptors** | Downregulation of CB1 receptor expression in the hippocampus, hypothalamus, striatum, and dorsal root ganglion [24]<br>Increased CB1 expression in medial prefrontal cortex [59, 71]<br>Desensitization of CB1 receptors on GABAergic terminals in BLA [72].<br>Effects mediated by corticosterone [24] | Downregulation of CB1 receptor expression in the hippocampus, hypothalamus, striatum, and dorsal root ganglion<br>Increased CB1 expression in medial prefrontal cortex [59, 71] |

## The Endocannabinoidome (Extended ECS) and Stress

As mentioned previously, the extended ECS has been termed the "endocannabinoidome" (be careful of the spelling; it is not –"diome" as in gut microbiome). The endocannabinoidome refers to bioactive derivatives, enzymes, transporters, and a plethora of receptor targets modulated by ECS components [65, 66]. Members of the extended ECS are also involved in responses to stress. For example, TRPV1 plays an important role in regulating CNS function in response to stress. There is evidence that TRPV1 can modulate glial and neuronal activity, mediating several pathways including glial reactivity, cytokine release, synaptic transmission and plasticity [73]. Another example is that peroxisome proliferator-activated receptor γ (PPARγ) is expressed in brain regions involved in regulation of psychological stress and aging such as the hippocampus, and may play a role in preventing the effects of aging and stress on the brain. It is also known that PPARγ agonists are able to reduce the physiological stress response [74]. These are only two examples to simply indicate that the ECS involvement in stress regulation extends beyond the classic cannabinoid receptors.

## Genes, Stress, and the Endocannabinoid System

Polymorphisms in genes coding for components of the ECS may influence an individual's stress responses. Single nucleotide polymorphisms (SNPs) in CNR1, the gene that codes for CB1 receptors, have been found to be associated with stress-induced activation of the ventromedial PFC (the brain region which plays an important role in regulation of emotions) as measured using magnetic resonance imaging, while under non-stress conditions, this genotype was associated with enhanced cross-talk with the vmPFC and amygdala. Research suggests that there may be a protective effect of this particular genotype of the CB1 receptor polymorphism (CNR1; rs1049353) against stress-related psychopathologies [75].

### Social Isolation

Rat experiments in which rats were socially isolated from weaning to adulthood found that the expression levels of CB1 receptors, DAGL-α, DAGL-β, MAGL, and NAPE-PLD mRNA, were significantly higher in several brain areas particularly the prefrontal area, cortical layers, and several thalamic regions. DAGL-β mRNA levels were significantly higher in the substantia nigra and ventral tegmental area, while FAAH mRNA expression was significantly lower in several prefrontal areas, cortical layers, and the caudate putamen [76].

### Environmental Enrichment

Animal research (in mice) indicates that exposure to environmental enrichment during early life stages was associated with differential regulation of genes encoding for various components of the ECS. An experiment compared expression of CB1, receptors, FAAH, and MAGL in various brain regions in mice reared under conditions of environmental enrichment compared to standard environments, from weaning to adulthood. They found that environmental enrichment increased CB1 receptor mRNA levels in the hypothalamus and BLA but decreased them in the basomedial amygdala. They also found that FAAH mRNA levels were higher in the hypothalamus and BLA in mice reared under environmental enrichment conditions (no change in the basomedial amygdala), but MAGL mRNA levels were not affected in any of the brain regions investigated. The researchers surmised that these regional changes induced by environmental enrichment could indicate that early exposure to environmental enrichment can induce changes in the ECS that may result in reduced responses to stress, something they confirmed in findings that environmentally enriched mice had reduced stress responses (as measured in a novelty-induced suppression of feeding test) [77].

## Early Life Stress and the Endocannabinoid System

The endocannabinoid receptors in the corticolimbic structures are critical to normal development, and if these receptors are altered by early life stress, brain development can be altered resulting in emotional and cognitive dysfunction. Animal and human research indicates that environmental stress during periods of high neural plasticity (e.g., during pregnancy, childhood, and adolescence) can cause emotional disturbances [19, 21, 78–81]. The effects of early life stress may emerge later in life, during adolescence or adulthood [21, 79]. For example, early life stress is associated with post-traumatic stress disorder (PTSD) and major depression in adulthood [78].

### Early Life Stress, Corticolimbic System, and HPA Axis Development

Early life stress influences the development of the corticolimbic system and the HPA axis [21, 79] and increases vulnerability to adult psychopathology [79]. The corticolimbic system plays a key role in mediating the effects of early life stress on brain dysfunction later in life, and early life stress is a long-term risk factor for dysfunctional development of those limbic structures involved in stress and emotion regulation [79].

Severe early stress produces a chain of events involving stress-induced programming of glucocorticoid, noradrenergic, and vasopressin-oxytocin stress systems which augment stress responses. These then produce effects on neurogenesis, synaptic over production and pruning, and nerve myelination during sensitive developmental periods, resulting in reductions in size of areas of the brain (mid-portions of the corpus callosum); attenuated development of areas including the left neocortex, hippocampus, and amygdala; and abnormal frontotemporal electrical activity and decreased functional activity of the cerebellar vermis. These changes may be the mechanism through which early stress increases the risk of developing mental health conditions including depression, PTSD, ADHD, and others [82].

## Stress Responsivity

The ECS plays a crucial role in regulating stress responsivity and emotional behavior during the child's development and is sensitive to early life stress in a sex- and region-dependent way. The effect of early life stress on the ECS is bidirectional, that is, the ECS can reduce stress through its anxiolytic activity and environmental stress can alter the ECS anxiolytic capacity [21].

## Findings from Animal Models

Animal experiments have demonstrated that maternal deprivation and social isolation in early life affect several parts of the ECS in neonate, adolescent, and adult rat brains, including altering CB1 mRNA expression and producing changes of cannabinoid receptors in corticolimbic and striatal brain areas [19, 21, 81]. In a rat experiment, using a maternal deprivation as a model for early life stress, researchers measured the expression of genes coding for CB1 and CB2 receptors, TRPV1 and GPR55 receptors, FAAH, MAGL, and enzymes involved in endocannabinoid synthesis (N-acyl phosphatidyl-ethanolamine phospholipase D and diacylglycerol lipase) in various brain regions: frontal cortex, ventral and dorsal striatum, dorsal hippocampus, and amygdala. They found that maternal deprivation increased the expression of all genes measured in the frontal cortex in adolescent male rats, but in females this increase was in the hippocampus [81].

Since ECS signaling in the amygdala plays an important role in production of anxiety and excitation of the HPA axis, it is possible that impairment of CB1 receptor signaling may sensitize the person to stress [21, 79].

## Early Life Stress and Genetic Patterns in Humans

Early life stress in humans has been associated with specific genetic patterns including CACNA1C which encodes for an essential calcium channel that is part of ECS signaling. This channel relates to neuronal excitability, plasticity, and neurogenesis and was associated with childhood trauma leading to vulnerability to anxiety and depression [83]. Single nucleotide polymorphisms (SNPs) in CNR1 (gene coding for CB1 receptors) and the gene encoding for FAAH (specifically the genetic variant rs324420) are associated with bipolar disorder and major depression [84]. And even variants in CNR2 (codes for CB2 receptors) and the FAAH gene (functional polymorphism C385A) interact with childhood trauma and in anxious and depressive phenotypes [85]. Furthermore, Juhasz et al. [86] found that variants in the CNR1 gene are associated with high neuroticism and low agreeableness and interact with recent negative life events to predict current depressive symptoms. It would therefore appear evident that genes play a significant potential role in defining susceptibility to life stresses, personality types, and behavioral responses. More research is needed to define the exact influence of the various endocannabinoidome permutations on personality and psychopathology.

## Sex Differences in How Early Life Stress Affects the ECS

In a similar way that there are sex differences between the stress response along the HPA axis, evidence suggests that there are sex differences in the ECS. Greater CB1R G-protein has been found in the hippocampus in males than females, but females showed greater CB1R G-protein activation, implying a more sensitive response of CB1Rs. It is possible that sex differences in the ECS could explain different responses to stressors [87].

Research indicates that early life stress decreases CB1 receptors in adulthood in males in the striatum, PFC, and amygdala (findings in females are not as clear) and increases gene expression for enzymes involved in endocannabinoid degradation in various brain regions (frontal cortex, striatum, hippocampus, and amygdala). Males also showed increased dorsal hippocampus prostaglandin products of arachidonic branch of the ECM.

In a rat experiment, early life stress demonstrated regional and sex-specific effects including:

- Impairing peripheral basal corticosterone (adult males only)
- Decreasing 2-AG and AEA in the cerebellar interpositus nucleus (males only)
- Decreasing 2-AG in the cerebellar Crus (females only)
- Increasing dorsal hippocampus prostaglandins (males only)
- Impairing social preference (females only) [87]

## The Gut and Stress

The gut is understood to play a critical role in the functioning of the immune system, influencing inflammation and the nervous system [88]. The gut "microbiome" refers to the microorganisms within the gut which form part of a multidirectional communication network with the brain, the microbiome-gut-brain axis [89]. The ECS is an important translational mediator for this communication.

The gut microbiota play a key role in the regulation of the gut-brain axis [90]. Vagal and spinal afferent pathways provide the means of communication between the gut microbes and the central nervous system [90]. The gut microbiota also modulate immune signaling from the gut to the brain via the induction of various cytokines [90].

### The Gut Microbiome and Stress

The gut microbiome is involved in the stress response. There is increasing evidence that the gut microbiome and brain and immune and endocrine systems are all in constant communication, and the gut microbiome is a key player in the stress response [8]. The microbiome-gut-brain axis is believed to mediate the interaction between stress, the HPA axis, and the immune system [91] and to regulate moods and emotions. Stress can modulate the microbiota, and the microbiota can alter the set point for stress sensitivity [89].

The gut microbiota regulates the production of many neurotransmitters and their precursors including GABA, dopamine, acetylcholine, tryptophan, serotonin, and norepinephrine, and neurotransmitter imbalances or deficiencies are associated with mental health problems including depression and anxiety [89, 90]. Changes in GABA receptor expression are implicated in the pathogenesis of anxiety and depression, both of which are associated with functional bowel problems [92]. The gut microbiota can also secrete and upregulate essential proteins and metabolites involved in neuropeptide and gut hormone release, such as short-chain fatty acids and brain-derived neurotrophic factor [90].

## Microbiota Changes and Stress

Several preclinical studies have demonstrated clear links between stress and gut microbiota changes [8]. For example:

- Germ-free mice have an exaggerated HPA axis response to restraint stress which was reversed by mono-colonization with *Bifidobacterium infantis* [93].
- Lack of normal gut microbiota in mice is associated with decreased expression of BDNF in the hippocampus, a key protein involved in neuronal plasticity and cognition [94].
- Absence of the gut microbiota in rats has been found to exacerbate behavioral responses to acute stress and was associated with an altered neurotransmitter turnover rate in areas of the brain known to regulate reactivity to stress and anxiety-like behavior [95].
- Treatment of mice with *Lactobacillus rhamnosus* (JB-1) induced changes in GABA mRNA expression in areas of the brain and reduced stress-related corticosterone and anxiety and depression-related behavior, with the vagus nerve implicated as the major modulatory pathway between the gut and the brain [92].

Research also indicates that depression is associated with dysregulated gut microbiota composition [89].

## The Gut Regulates the HPA Axis

Evidence indicates that gut microbes may be involved in the development and functioning of the HPA axis [90, 93, 96]. As we have seen, dysregulation of the HPA axis occurs in stress, as well as in anxiety and depression. The gut microbiota can contribute to increased cortisol and inflammation, and inflammation can also feed into microbiota alterations through its negative effects on the gastrointestinal system [90, 97].

## Leaky Gut and Mental Health

The gut has an important role in regulating intestinal permeability and maintaining the intestinal barrier. Deficits in intestinal permeability may be an etiological factor in chronic low-grade inflammation that can occur in some individuals suffering depression [98]. Gastrointestinal disorders, including exacerbations of their symptoms/signs, are often associated with stress.

Normally the intestine maintains tight junctions between the cells lining it. If these are compromised, the intestine lining becomes permeable or "leaky" [88], the so-called "leaky gut." When there are high levels of cortisol and inflammatory mediators, these can increase the intestinal permeability, and Gram-negative bacteria (which have an additional lipopolysaccharide [LPS] exterior membrane) can move into the bloodstream [90]. This can then induce chronic inflammation in the CNS [90, 99]. Inflammatory gastrointestinal conditions such as irritable bowel syndrome, understood to involve compromised intestinal permeability, often co-exist with high rates of mental health conditions such as depression [100], lending further credence to the role of the gut in regulation of moods and emotion via the gut-brain axis [90].

A US study found that the prevalence and median levels of serum IgM and IgA against LPS of enterobacteria were significantly higher in patients with major depression than in controls [52]. Their results suggest that increased gastrointestinal permeability (leaky gut) with increased translocation of Gram-negative bacteria is involved in the pathophysiology of depression [52]. Systemic LPS and administration of proinflammatory cytokines can cause chronic central neuroinflammation, and central neuroinflammation is known to induce a sickness behavior complex that is similar to the symptoms of major depression (e.g., anorexia, malaise, loss of interest, etc.) [52].

## The Endocannabinoidome, the Gut, and Links to Mental Health

There is a growing body of data that suggests that the gut, the brain, and the ECS are all interlinked when it comes to, at least some, mental health conditions. It is clear that the ECS plays a critical role in the functioning of the gut, given its wide distribution in the gut where it regulates most gut functions:

- Gastrointestinal motility
- Gastrointestinal inflammation and gut permeability
- Nausea and vomiting
- Visceral sensation
- Immune homeostasis in the gut
- Energy balance
- Appetite/ hunger signaling [101–103]

ECS dysfunction is associated with pathology in the gut including inflammatory bowel disease (IBD), irritable bowel syndrome, and obesity [102], and of course these conditions are inflammatory in nature. For example, CB1 receptor activation in the intestinal epithelium contributes to development of obesity and metabolic disease [104], and polymorphisms in the CNR1 gene (encodes for CB1 receptors) have been found to be associated with forms of irritable bowel syndrome [105]. Ulcerative colitis, one of the types of IBD, has been found to induce changes in the expression of the ECS in human colonic tissue [106].

Patients with visceral (abdominal) pain often find this is exacerbated by stress, and there is now evidence that the ECS modulates chronic stress-associated visceral hyperalgesia [103, 107]. CB1 receptors in sensory ganglia (that innervate the gut) control visceral sensation, and transcription of CNR1 (the gene encoding for CB1 receptors) is modified through epigenetic processes under conditions of chronic stress. There appears a potential mechanism to explain the link between stress and abdominal pain: chronic stress induces visceral hyperalgesia through region-specific changes in endocannabinoid and endovanilloid (endogenous ligand for TRPV1) pathways in sensory neurons that innervate the pelvic viscera [103].

## Inflammation, the Gut, and the ECS

It appears that the gut, the ECS, and at least some mental health conditions (e.g., depression) may be linked, and this may be through inflammation. We have already seen that the gut microbiome plays a critical role in the functioning of the immune system, thereby influencing inflammation and the nervous system [88], and we also know that the gut is involved in the stress response. We also find that depression is associated with dysregulation of the gut microbiota composition, and in a later chapter, we will see that the ECS is altered in depression. There is also evidence that inflammation is involved in the pathogenesis of several other mental health conditions, including anxiety, autism spectrum disorder, and Alzheimer's disease (discussed in later chapters). If inflammation is indeed involved in the pathophysiology of mental health conditions such as depression [52], then since one of the roles of the ECS is to control inflammation, it stands to reason that the ECS may play a role in those mental health conditions [50], and where "leaky gut" is part of the pathogenesis of a mental health condition such as depression, it would not be unreasonable to posit that the ECS within the gut may be important in the body's attempts to bring the gut back into balance.

Understanding the potential or indeed likely link between the gut microbiome, the ECS, stress, and mental health reminds us that when treating mental health conditions such as depression, we should address any deficiency or dysfunction of the gut microbiota as part of a holistic treatment approach. This generally includes examining a patient's diet and bacterial and possibly parasite exposures carefully. Of course, this is an area where more research is needed.

The role of the ECS in the gut and how it links with regulation of stress, emotions, and mental health conditions are an area of research that will no doubt expand in the future. In Chinese medicine, the link between emotions and dysfunction of organ systems, including (but not confined to) the digestive system, forms an important part of its theoretical model of physiological functioning of the body [108]. Biomedical research is in the process of elucidating the mechanisms of how emotions and the body are interrelated, albeit through the lens of its own (biomedical) model.

## Cannabis Exposure and Stress Responsivity

Research indicates that the use of cannabis (i.e., typically containing high levels of tetrahydrocannabinol, the exogenous cannabinoid that is associated with dose-dependent intoxication) during adolescence, a time of maturation of the stress response system, can cause long-term alterations in stress responsivity, and cannabis use in adolescence has been associated with mental health conditions including depression and substance abuse disorder in adulthood in some preclinical and human studies [109, 110, 111] (discussed more in other chapters). For this reason, the recreational use of cannabis in adolescents should be avoided—this is a time of much neural plasticity and development of the brain and the ECS; therefore, exposure to any environmental toxins that can negatively impact on the synaptic pruning and refining occurring during this sensitive developmental phase should be prevented.

## Conclusion

Stress is an increasing feature of our westernized lifestyles, and there is evidence linking it to many diseases including increased risk of cardiovascular disease, cancer, and mental health problems including anxiety and depression, sleep problems, and substance abuse. Stress impacts on the sympathetic nervous system and the HPA axis, and increasingly evidence implicates inflammation which may provide a common underlying pathway linking stress and stress-related illnesses. The ECS is involved in the regulation of stress and emotions, and when there is chronic stress, we also see changes in the ECS. The gut has gained increased importance within the scientific community, and it is clear that the ECS is critical in its homeostatic regulation. It is therefore not surprising that there is increasing evidence linking the gut microbiome, the ECS, and the stress response. Inflammation appears to be one underlying factor linking some mental health illnesses, stress, the gut microbiome, and the ECS. In treating mental health conditions, it therefore is prudent to remember to address any dysfunction in the gut.

**Summary of Changes Associated with Acute and Chronic Stress**

- Acute and chronic stress: AEA is reduced and 2-AG increased.
- Reduction of AEA occurs relatively quickly in response to stress and is mediated by CRH activating CRHR1 receptors to increase hydrolysis of AEA by increased FAAH.
- Under chronic stress: ongoing exposure to glucocorticoids upregulates CRH signaling, and the FAAH increases and AEA decreases are maintained.
- In acute stress, decreased AEA signaling contributes to anxiety, activation of the HPA axis, impairment of fear extinction, and suppression of cell proliferation in the hippocampus, and additionally, under chronic stress conditions, the more sustained reduction in AEA also contributes to anhedonia and hyperalgesia.
- Increase in 2-AG is delayed and likely to be mediated by increased corticosterone. Amplification of 2-AG responses under conditions of repeated stress, which also results in habituation of corticosterone responses, may be mediated by reduced MAGL [24, 25]

## References

1. Selye H. A syndrome produced by diverse nocuous agents. Nature. 1936;138(3479):32.
2. Herman JP, Nawreen N, Smail MA, Cotella EM. Brain mechanisms of HPA axis regulation: neurocircuitry and feedback in context Richard Kvetnansky lecture. Stress. 2020;23(6):617–32.
3. Hill MN, Patel S, Campolongo P, et al. Functional interactions between stress and the endocannabinoid system: from synaptic signalling to behavioral output. J Neurosci. 2010;30(45):14980–6.
4. Pearlin L. Stress and mental health: a conceptual overview. In: Horwitz AV, Scheid TL, editors. A handbook for the study of mental health: social contexts, theories and systems. Cambridge University Press; 1999. p. 161–75.
5. Chiang JJ, Turiano NA, Mroczek DK, Miller GE. Affective reactivity to daily stress and 20-year mortality risk in adults with chronic illness: findings from the National Study of Daily Experiences. Health Psychol. 2018;37:170–8.
6. deRoon-Cassini T, Stollenwerk RM, Beatka M, Hillard CJ. Meet your stress management professionals: the endocannabinoids. Trends Mol Med. 2020;26(10):953–68.
7. CAMH. Stress. CAMH, 2021. Available at: www.camh.ca. Accessed 5 Jan 2021.
8. O'Brien K, Sali A. A Clinician's guide to integrative oncology: what you should be talking about with Cancer patients and why? US: Springer; 2017.
9. Dinan TG. Stress: the shared common component in major mental illnesses. Eur Psychiatry. 2005;20(S3):S326–8.

10. Weymar M, Schwabe L, Löw A, Hamm AO. Stress sensitizes the brain: increased processing of unpleasant pictures after exposure to acute stress. J Cognitive Neuroscience. 2012;24(7):111–1518.
11. Jovanovic T, Ressler KJ. How the neurocircuitry and genetics of fear inhibition may inform our understanding of PTSD. Am J Psychiatry. 2010;167(6):648–62.
12. McEwen BS. Protection and damage from acute and chronic stress: allostasis and allostatic overload and relevance to the pathophysiology of psychiatric disorders. Ann N Y Acad Sci. 2004;1032:1–7.
13. Sumislawski JJ, Ramikie TS, Patel S. Reversible gating of endocannabinoid plasticity in the amygdala by chronic stress: a potential role for monoacylglycerol lipase inhibition in the prevention of stress-induced behavioral adaptation. Neuropsychopharmacology. 2011;36:2750–61.
14. McEwen BS. Physiology and neurobiology of stress and adaptation: central role of the brain. Physiol Rev. 2007;87(3):873–904.
15. Willis MA, Haines DE. The Limbic System. In: Haines DE, Mihailoff GA, editors. Fundamental neuroscience for basic and clinical applications. 5th ed. Philadelphia: Elsevier; 2018.
16. Prager E. The corticolimbic system in health: implications for learning, memory and disease. Advanced Science News. Jan 27, 2017. Available at: https://www.advancedsciencenews.com/corticolimbic-system-health-disease/. Accessed 18 Jan 2021.
17. Rusbridge C. Neurobehavioral disorders: the corticolimbic system in health and disease. Vet Clin North Am Small Anim Pract. 2020;50(5):1157–81.
18. Thompson JM, Neugbauer V. Cortico-limbic pain mechanisms. Neurosci Lett. 2019;702:15–23.
19. Dow-Edwards D, Silva L. Endocannabinoids in brain plasticity: cortical maturation, HPA axis function and behaviour. Brain Res. 2017;1654:157–64.
20. Korem N, Zer-Aviv TM, Ganon-Elazar E, et al. Targeting the endocannabinoid system to treat anxiety-related disorders. J Basic Clin Physiol Pharmacol. 2016;27(3):193–202.
21. Goldstein Ferber S, Trezza V, Weller A. Early life stress and development of the endocannabinoid system: a bidirectional process in programming future coping. Dev Psychobiol. 2019;00:1–10.
22. Hubner C, Bosch D, Gall A, et al. Ex vivo dissection of optogenetically activated mPFC and hippocampal inputs to neurons in the basolateral amygdala: implications for fear and emotional memory. Front Behav Neurosci. 2014;8:64.
23. Waddell J, Bangasser DA, Shors TJ. The basolateral nucleus of the amygdala is necessary to induce the opposing effects of stressful experience on learning in males and females. J Neurosci 2008;28:5290–4.
24. Morena M, Patel S, Bains JS, Hill MN. Neurobiological interactions between stress and the endocannabinoid system. Neuropsychopharmacology. 2016;41:80–102.
25. Parker LA. Cannabinoids & emotional regulation. In: Cannabinoids and the brain. Massachusetts: MIT Press; 2017.
26. Herman JP, Figueiredo HF, Mueller NK, et al. Central mechanisms of stress integration: hierarchical circuitry controlling hypothalamic-pituitary-adrenocortical responsiveness. Front Neuroendocrinol. 2003;24:151–80.
27. Hill MN, McLaughlin RJ, Morrish AC, et al. Suppression of amygdalar endocannabinoid signalling by stress contributes to activation of the hypothalamic-pituitary-adrenal axis. Neuropsychopharmacology. 2009;34:2733–45.
28. Pecoraro N, Dallman MF, Warne JP, et al. From Malthus to motive: how the HPA axis engineers the phenotype, yoking needs to wants. Prog Neurobiol. 2006;79:247–340.
29. Malcher-Lopez R, Di S, Marcheselli VS, et al. Opposing crosstalk between leptin and glucocorticoids rapidly modulates synaptic excitation via endocannabinoid release. J Neurosci. 2006;26:6643–50.
30. Stevens FL, Robin A, Hurley RA, Taber KH. Anterior cingulate cortex: unique role in cognition and emotion. J Neuropsychiatry Clin Neurosci. 2011;23:2.

31. Larkin KT, Brown LA, Tiani AG. Chapter 5. The autonomic and neuroendocrine response to stress. In: Chantler PD, Larkin KT, editors. Cardiovascular implications of stress and depression. Academic Press; 2020. p. 87–110.
32. Andreassi JL. Psychophysiology: human behavior & physiological response, 5th ed. In: Larkin KT, Brown LA, Tiani AG, editors. Chapter 5. The autonomic and neuroendocrine response to stress. Academic Press; 2007. p. 87–110.
33. Ney LJ, Matthews A, Bruno R, Felmingham KL. Cannabinoid interventions for PTSD: where to next? Prog Neuropsychopharmacol Biol Psychiatry. 2019;93:124–40.
34. Herman JP. Regulation of adrenocorticosteroid receptor mRNA expression in the central nervous system. Cell Mol Neurobiol. 1993;13(4):349–72.
35. Ulrich-Lai YM, Herman JP. Neural regulation of endocrine and autonomic stress responses. Nat Rev Neurosci. 2009;10:397–409.
36. Patel R. HPA axis dysfunction explained: the facts you need to know. WebFMD. Nov 3, 2019. Available at: https://webfmd.com/hpa-axis-dysfunction/. Accessed 11 Jan 2021.
37. Goel N, Workman JL, Lee TT, et al. Sex differences in the HPA axis. Compr Physiol. 2014;4:1121–55.
38. Davis M, Emory E. Sex differences in neonatal stress reactivity. Child Dev. 1995;66:14–27.
39. McEwen BS, Stellar E. Stress and the individual. Mechanisms leading to disease. Arch Intern Med. 1993;153(18):2093–101.
40. Chida Y, Stepto A. Greater cardiovascular responses to laboratory mental stress are associated with poor subsequent cardiovascular risk status: a meta-analysis of prospective evidence. Hypertension. 2010;55(4):1026–32.
41. Panaite V, Salomon K, Jin A, Rottenberg J. Cardiovascular recovery from psychological and physiological challenge and risk for adverse cardiovascular outcomes and all-cause mortality. Psychosom Med. 2015;77(3):215–26.
42. Lovallo WR. Do low levels of stress reactivity signal poor states of health? Biol Psychol. 2011;86(2):121–8.
43. Lumley MA, Chi W, Wiholm C, et al. The relationship of chronic and momentary work stress to cardiac reactivity in female managers: feasibility of a smart phone-assisted assessment system. Psychosom Med. 2014;76:512–8.
44. Uchino BN, Kiecolt-Glaser JK, Cacioppo JT. Age-related changes in cardiovascular response as a function of a chronic stressor and social support. J Pers Soc Psychol. 1992;63(5):839–46.
45. Raison C. Introduction: the inflammation connection. Psychiatric Times. Apr 2018. Available at: https://www.psychiatrictimes.com/special-reports/introduction-inflammation-connection. Accessed 8 Jan 2020.
46. Liu Y-Z, Wang Y-X, Jiang C-L. Inflammation: the common pathway of stress-related diseases. Front Hum Neurosci. 2017;11:316. https://doi.org/10.3389/fnhum.2017.00316.
47. Lutgendorf SK, Sood AK. Biobehavioral factors ad cancer progression: physiological pathways and mechanisms. Psychosom Med. 2011;73:724–30.
48. Maes M, Song C, Lin A, et al. The effects of psychological stress on humans: increased production of pro-inflammatory cytokines and a Th1- like response in stress-induced anxiety. Cytokine. 1998;10(4):313–8.
49. Maes M, Lin AH, Delmeire L, et al. Elevated serum interleukin-6 (IL-6) and IL-6 receptor concentrations in posttraumatic stress disorder following accidental man-made traumatic events. Biol Psychiatry. 1999;45(7):833–9.
50. Reiche EM, Nunes SO, Morimoto HK. Stress, depression, the immune system and cancer. Lancet Oncol. 2004;5(10):617–25.
51. Song C, Kenis G, van Gastel A, et al. Influence of psychological stress on immune-inflammatory variables in normal humans. Part II. Altered serum concentrations of natural anti-inflammatory agents and soluble membrane antigens of monocytes and T lymphocytes. Psychiatry Res. 1999;85(3):293–303.
52. Maes M, Kubera M, Leunis J-C. The gut-brain barrier in major depression: intestinal mucosal dysfunction with an increased translocation of LPS from gram negative enterobacteria (leaky gut) plays a role in the inflammatory pathophysiology of depression. Neuroendocrinol Lett. 2008;29(1):117–24.

53. Miller MH. Five things to know about inflammation and depression. Psychiatric Times. Apr 30, 2018. Available at: https://www.psychiatrictimes.com/special-reports/five-things-know-about-inflammation-and-depression. Accessed 8 Jan 2020.
54. Wirtz PH, von Känel R. Psychological stress, inflammation, and coronary heart disease. Curr Cardiol Rep. 2017;19:111.
55. Hillard CJ. Stress regulates endocannabinoid-CB1 receptor signalling. Semin Immunol. 2014;26:380–8.
56. Di S, Malcher-Lopes R, Marcheselli VL, et al. Rapid glucocorticoid-mediated endocannabinoid release and opposing regulation of glutamate and GABA inputs to hypothalamic magnocellular neurons. Endocrinology. 2005;146:4292–301.
57. Gray JM, Vecchiarelli HA, Morena M, et al. Corticotropin-releasing hormone drives anandamide hydrolysis in the amygdala to promote anxiety. J Neurosci. 2015;35:3879–92.
58. Hillard CJ. Circulating endocannabinoids: from whence do they come and where are they going? Neuropharmacology. 2018;43:155–72.
59. Hill MN, Carrier EJ, McLaughlin RJ, et al. Regional alterations in the endocannabinoid system in an animal model of depression: effects of concurrent antidepressant treatment. J Neurochem. 2008;106(6):2322–36.
60. Ramikie TS, Nyilas R, Bluette RJ, et al. Multiple mechanistically distinct modes of endocannabinoid mobilization at central amygdala glutaminergic synapses. Neuron. 2014;81:1111–25.
61. Khan AU, Falconi-Sobrinho LL, Dos Anjos-Garcia T, et al. Cannabidiol-induced panicolytic-like effects and fear-induced antinociception impairment: the role of the CB 1 receptor in the ventromedial hypothalamus. Psychopharmacology (Berl) 2020;37(4):1063–79.
62. Liedhegner ES, Sasman A, Hillard CJ. Brain region-specific changes in N-acylethanolamine contents with time of day. J Neurochem. 2014;128:491–506.
63. Steiner MA, Marsicano G, Nestler EJ, et al. Antidepressant-like behavioural effects of impaired cannabinoid receptor type 1 signalling coincide with exaggerated corticosterone secretion in mice. Psychoneuroendocrinology. 2008;33:54–67.
64. Di S, Malcher-Lopes R, Halmos KC, Tasker JG. Nongenomic glucocorticoid inhibition via endocannabinoid release in the hypothalamus: a fast feedback mechanism. J Neurosci. 2003;23(12):4850–7.
65. Di Marzo V, Wang J, editors. The endocannabinoidome. The world of endocannabinoids and related mediators. US: Elsevier Inc; 2014.
66. Piscitelli F, Carta G, Bisogno T, et al. Effect of dietary krill oil supplementation on the endocannabinoidome of metabolically relevant tissues from high-fat-fed mice. Nutr Metab (Lond). 2011;8:51.
67. Patel S, Roelke CT, Rademacher DJ, Hillard CJ. Inhibition of restraint stress-induced neural and behavioural activation by endogenous cannabinoid signalling. Eur J Neurosci. 2005;21:1057–69.
68. Chrousos GP. Stress and disorders of the stress system. Nat Rev Endocrinol. 2009;5(7):374–81.
69. Wamsteeker JI, Kuzmiski JB, Bains JS. Repeated stress impairs endocannabinoid signaling in the paraventricular nucleus of the hypothalamus. J Neurosci. 2010;30:11188–96.
70. Hill MN, Patel S, Carrier EJ, Rademacher DJ, et al. Downregulation of endocannabinoid signalling in the hippocampus following chronic unpredictable stress. Neuropsychopharmacology. 2005;30:508–15.
71. Lee TT, Hill MN. Age of stress exposure modulates the immediate and sustained effects of repeated stress on corticolimbic cannabinoid CB(1) receptor binding in male rats. Neuroscience. 2013;249:106–14.
72. Patel S, Kingsley PJ, Mackie K, et al. Repeated homotypic stress elevates 2-arachidonoylglycerol levels and enhances short-term endocannabinoid signalling at inhibitory synapses in basolateral amygdala. Neuropsychopharmacology. 2009;34:2699–709.
73. Ho KW, Ward NJ, Calkins DJ. TRPV1: a stress response protein in the central nervous system. Am J Neurodegener Dis 2012;1(1):1–14.
74. Ulrich-Lai YM, Ryan KK. PPARγ and stress: implications for aging. Exp Gerontol 2013;48(7):671–6.

75. Wirz L, Reuter M, Felten A, Schwabe L. An endocannabinoid receptor polymorphism modulates affective processing under stress. Soc Cogn Affect Neurosci. 2018;13(11):1177–89.
76. Robinson SA, Loiacono R, Christopoulos A et al. The effect of social isolation on rat brain expression of genes associated with endocannabinoid signalling. Brain Research 2010;1343:153–67.
77. El-Rawas R, Thiret N, Nader J, et al. Early exposure to environmental enrichment alters the expression of genes of the endocannabinoid system. Brain Res. 2011;1390:80–9.
78. Davidson RJ, McEwan BS. Social influences on neuroplasticity: stress and interventions to promote well-being. Nat Neurosci. 2012;15(5):689–95.
79. Hill MN, Eiland L, Lee TT, et al. Early life stress alters the developmental trajectory of corticolimbic endocannabinoid signalling in male rats. Neuropharmacology. 2019;146:154–62.
80. Marco EM, Viveros MP. The critical role of the endocannabinoid system in emotional homeostasis: avoiding excess and deficiencies. Mini Rev Med Chem. 2009;9:1407–15.
81. Marco EM, Echeverry-Alzate V, Lopez-Moreno JA, et al. Consequences of early life stress on the expression of endocannabinoid-related genes in the rat brain. Behav Pharmacol. 2014;25:547–56.
82. Teicher MH, Andersen SL, Polcari A, et al. Developmental neurobiology of childhood stress and trauma. Psychiatr Clin North Am. 2002;25(2):397–426.
83. Lazary J, Eszlari N, Kriko E, et al. Genetic analyses of the endocannabinoid pathway in association with affective phenotypic variants. Neurosci Lett. 2021;744:135600.
84. Monteleone P, Bifulco M, Maina G, et al. Investigation of CNR1 and FAAH endocannabinoid gene polymorphisms in bipolar disorder and major depression. Pharmacol Res. 2010;61:400–4.
85. Lazary J, Eszlari N, Juhasz G, Bagdy G. A functional variant of CB2 receptor gene interacts with childhood trauma and FAAH gene on anxious and depressive phenotypes. J Affect Disord. 2019;257:716–22.
86. Juhasz G, Chase D, Pegg E, et al. CNR1 gene is associated with high neuroticism and low agreeableness and interacts with recent negative life events to predict current depressive symptoms. Neuropsychopharmacology. 2009;34:2019–27.
87. Moussa-Tooks, et al. Long-term aberrations to cerebellar endocannabinoids induced by early-life stress. Sci Rep. 2020;10:7236.
88. Perlmutter D. Brain maker. Great Britain: Yellow Kite; 2015.
89. Sherwin E, Rea K, Dinan TG, Cryan JF. A gut (microbiome) feeling about the brain. Curr Opin Gastroentero. 2016;32(2):96–102.
90. Simpson CA, Diaz-Arteche C, Eliby D, et al. The gut microbiota in anxiety and depression – a systematic review. Clin Psychol Rev. 2021;83:101943.
91. De Palma G, Collins SM, Bercik P, Verdu EF. The microbiota-gut-brain axis in gastrointestinal disorders: stressed bugs, stressed brain or both? J Physiol. 2014;592(Part 14):2989–97.
92. Bravo JA, Forsythe P, Chew MV, et al. Ingestion of Lactobacillus strain regulates emotional behaviour and central GABA receptor expression in a mouse via the vagus nerve. Proc Natl Acad Sci U S A. 2011;108(38):10650–5.
93. Sudo N, Chida Y, Aiba Y, et al. Postnatal microbial colonization programs the hypothalamic-pituitary-adrenal system for stress response in mice. J Physiol. 2004;558(Pt1):263–75.
94. Mayer EA, Knight R, Mazmanian SK, et al. Gut microbes and the brain: paradigm shift in neuroscience. J Neurosci. 2014;34(46):15490–6.
95. Crumeyrolle-Arias M, Jaglin M, Bruneau A, et al. Absence of the gut microbiota enhances anxiety-like behavior and neuroendocrine response to acute stress in rats. Psychoneuroendocrinology. 2014;42:207–17.
96. Foster JA, Rinaman L, Cryan JF. Stress & the gut-brain axis: Regulation by the microbiome. Neurobiol Stress 2017;7:124–36.
97. Kamada N, Seo SU, Chen GY, Nunez G. Role of the gut microbiota in immunity and inflammatory disease. Nat Rev Immunol. 2013;13(5):321–35.

98. Kelly JR, Kennedy PJ, Cryan JF, et al. Breaking down the barriers: the gut microbiome, intestinal permeability and stress-related psychiatric disorders. Front Cell Neurosci. 2015;9:932.
99. Huang TT, Lai JB, Du YL, et al. Current understanding of gut microbiota in mood disorders: an update of human studies. Front Genet. 2019;10:98. https://doi.org/10.3389/fgene.2019.00098.
100. Simpson CA, Schwartz OS, Simmons JG. The human gut microbiota and depression: widely reviewed, yet poorly understood. J Affect Dis. 2020;274:73–5.
101. Acharya N, Penukonda S, Shcheglova T, et al. Endocannabinoid system acts as a regulator of immune homeostasis in the gut. Proc Natl Acad Sci U S A. 2017;114(19):5005–10.
102. DiPatrizio NV. Endocannabinoids in the gut. Cannabis Cannabinoid Res. 2016;1:1.
103. Sharkey KA, Wiley JW. The role of the endocannabinoid system in the brain-gut axis. Gastroenterology. 2016;151(2):252–66.
104. Cani PD. Crosstalk between the gut microbiota and the endocannabinoid system: impact on the gut barrier function and the adipose tissue. Clin Microbiol Infect. 2012;18(4):50–3.
105. Camilleri M, Kolar GJ, Vazquez-Roque MI, et al. Cannabinoid receptor 1 gene and irritable bowel syndrome: phenotype and quantitative traits. Am J Phys. 2013;304:G553–60.
106. Marquez L, Suarez J, Iglesias M, et al. Ulcerative colitis induces changes on the expression of the endocannabinoid system in the human colonic tissue. PLoS One. 2009;4:e6893.
107. Storr MA, Sharkey KA. The endocannabinoid system and gut-brain signalling. Curr Opin Pharmacol. 2007;7:575–82.
108. O'Brien KA, Xue CC. The theoretical framework of Chinese medicine. In: Leung P-C, Xue CC, Cheng Y-C, editors. A comprehensive guide to Chinese medicine. 2nd ed. New Jersey: World Scientific Press; 2016.
109. Andersen SL, Teicher MH. Desperately driven and no brakes: development stress exposure and subsequent risk for substance abuse. Neurosci Behav Rev. 2009;33(4):516–24.
110. McCormick CM, Green MR. From the stressed adolescent to the anxious and depressed adult: investigations in rodent models. Neuroscience. 2013;249:242–57.
111. Lee TTY, Gorzalka BB. Timing is everything: evidence for a role of corticolimbic endocannabinoids in modulating hypothalamic–pituitary–adrenal axis activity across developmental periods. Neuroscience. 2012;204:17–30.

# Overview of Medicinal Cannabis

# 4

## Introduction

There is clear evidence from population studies that cannabis is commonly used to alleviate common mental health conditions, including depression, anxiety and stress [1, 2]. For example, in a 1986 survey, 72% of daily cannabis users reported use of cannabis to relax or relieve tension [3]. In another study, 50% medical cannabis patients using cannabis to treat pain reported it also provided relief from anxiety and stress [4]. A Washington State survey found the most frequently reported conditions for cannabis use were as follows: pain (61%), anxiety (58%), depression (50%), headache/migraine (35%), nausea (27%) and muscle spasticity (18%). On average, those surveyed reported an 86% reduction in symptoms and 59.8% of medical users used cannabis as alternative to pharmaceutical prescriptions [5]. In a recent survey by the USA Arthritis Foundation, 79% surveyed are currently using CBD, have used it in the past or are considering using it; 87% of those currently using CBD do so to manage their arthritis, with pain being the primary reason in 94% [6].

Further afield in Australia, in a survey of 1748 Australians using cannabis for medical reasons, prior to legalisation in 2016, the most frequent reasons for medical cannabis use were as follows: anxiety (50.7%), back pain (50.0%), depression (49.3%), sleep problems (43.5%), neck pain (25.6%) and post-traumatic stress disorder (22.9%). More than 80% respondents indicated that medicinal cannabis effectively managed their target symptom [7]. There is also evidence for its use in war veterans to manage symptoms associated with post-traumatic stress disorder [8–10].

Whilst cross-sectional surveys only give a snapshot in a particular population at a specific point in time, nonetheless they are a form of evidence that this plant may be beneficial in a range of mental health conditions. The remaining chapters of this book will delve more deeply into the preclinical and clinical research, exploring mechanisms of action and evidence of efficacy in relation to several common mental health conditions.



K. O'Brien, P. Blair, *Medicinal Cannabis and CBD in Mental Healthcare*,
https://doi.org/10.1007/978-3-030-78559-8_4

**This Chapter**
In Chap. 2 we learned about our own endocannabinoid system and in Chap. 3 we focused on the endocannabinoid system's involvement in stress. These set the stage, to an extent, to understand why this plant called cannabis has beneficial effects as we make our own cannabinoids (endocannabinoids) and have a whole regulatory system, the endocannabinoid system, which has a range of receptors with which many of the constituents of cannabis interact. In this chapter, we will take a look at what medicinal cannabis is. This chapter will describe the taxonomy of the plant, its historical uses, and a little about the regulations, then delve into understanding the key active constituents (cannabidiol, tetrahydrocannabinol, terpenes) and their therapeutic actions and mechanisms of actions, as well as the different forms of medicinal cannabis.

## Definition of Medicinal Cannabis

We define medicinal cannabis as:

***Cannabis or cannabis products used specifically to treat illness and/or to promote wellness, and individualised to the patient.***

Medicinal cannabis includes the raw herb, as well as proprietary forms of medicines which include whole herb products, extracts of active constituents of the *Cannabis sativa* plant, as well as synthetic cannabinoid products (which we consider as pharmaceuticals). Medicinal cannabis can be both an herbal medicine and a pharmaceutical. Both forms have a valid place in health and medical care.

Ideally medicinal cannabis should be prescribed by a knowledgeable healthcare practitioner, in particular if a patient is taking pharmaceuticals that it could potentially interact with.

## Taxonomy: What Is in a Name?

Cannabis is plant and in its natural form, it is clearly an herbal medicine. It grows in the ground. There has been debate within the literature as to the taxonomy or nomenclature of *Cannabis*. The genus is *Cannabis* and the family Cannabaceae [11]. A taxonomy adopted by Small and Cronquist, based on combining morphological and chemical characters (fruit morphology and tetrahydrocannabinol, of which we learn about shortly), recognises four distinct taxa of the species *Cannabis sativa*. There are two main subspecies: *C. sativa* subspecies sativa and *C. sativa* subspecies indica, each of which have two different varietates [11].

According to this biphasic approach to taxonomy the varietates belonging to the subspecies sativa[1] are common in North America, Europe and Asia. They show a limited intoxicant potential and are cultivated for fibre and oil. In contrast, the

[1] *Cannabis sativa* L. subsp. *sativa* var. *sativa;* and *Cannabis sativa* L. subsp. *sativa* var. *spontanea* Vavilov

varietates of the subspecies indica[2] have high intoxicant potential (due to the presence of tetrahydrocannabinol, abbreviation THC, the only constituent in cannabis which is potentially intoxicating) and grow mainly in the Asiatic Continent [11, 12]. A more recent taxonomy recognises six different groups of cultivars- see [11] for discussion. There are hundreds of strains or 'cultivars' or 'chemovars' of the cannabis plant, the term 'chemovar' being preferred by some as it more accurately relates to the chemical constituents. The different cultivars have varying amounts of phytocannabinoids (the most well researched being THC and cannabidiol, abbreviation CBD) plus other active constituents, described shortly. Those strains or cultivars grown for the recreational or 'adult use' market are high in THC, specifically because THC is potentially intoxicating, producing a euphoric state of mind in sufficient doses.

## Hemp

The term 'hemp' is used to describe those strains of cannabis which have very low amounts of THC. In the USA, the upper limit of THC in those plants designated as hemp is 0.3%. Typically, hemp varieties are grown for the clothing, building, ropes, food and cosmeceutical industries; however, hemp can be used to produce CBD medicines in some countries such as the USA. Suffice to say at this point in the book, hemp is still the plant cannabis but when you look at hemp cultivars, you will notice they are often larger and taller plants compared to cannabis cultivars used to produce flowers predominantly for the adult-use and medicinal markets. Quite simply, this is because it is the stems and leaves of the plant that are used for industrial use (the more the better).

## Hemp Oil and Hemp Seed Oil

Another distinction needs to be made: the term 'hemp oil' is often used in the USA to refer to CBD oil derived from hemp, CBD being a phytocannabinoid with medicinal properties which is produced in glandular structures predominantly on the flowers (less so on other parts like leaves) of female plants. The term 'hemp oil' can also be used to denote the food stuff made from the hemp *seeds*, which do not contain phytocannabinoids (including CBD) unless as a contaminant from processing. It is our preference to delineate the two different kinds of products very clearly, using the term *hemp seed oil* to denote oil derived from the seeds, and the term *hemp-derived CBD oil* to denote the oil extracted from the buds/flowers and leaves of the hemp cultivars.

[2] *Cannabis sativa* L. subsp. *indica* Small & Cronquist var. *indica* (Lam) Wehmer; and *Cannabis sativa* L. subsp. *indica* Small & Cronquist var. *kafiristanica* (Vavilov) Small & Cronquist

## Historical Use of Cannabis as Medicine

Cannabis has been used medicinally for thousands of years. Neolithic evidence of cannabis use has been found 12,000 years ago [13], and cannabis has also been discovered in 2500-year-old Chinese tombs in Eastern China [14]. Fruit and seeds macrofossils have been found attached to potsherds in the Okinoshima Mesolithic archaeological site in central Japan dated about 10,000 years ago, during the Jōmon 'cord marked pottery' culture (12500–2300 BCE) [15]. Cannabis was most likely introduced from Central Asia consistent with the origins of various palaeolithic and Bronze Age Siberians/Central Asians who initially populated the Japanese archipelago [16].

## Cannabis in China

Cannabis has a long history of use in Chinese medicine. Given the use of hemp seed as food in ancient China, it was probably natural for the medicinal properties of the plants to be discovered, and it appears the use of cannabis as a form of medicine was a very early development in ancient China [13]. Its medicinal use in treating pain has been traced back to ancient Chinese texts, dating to 2900 B.C. In the ancient herbal medicine text, the Shennong Ben Cao Jing (Divine Husbandman's Classic of Herbal Medicine, written between 200 and 250 CE), indications for the medicinal use of cannabis included constipation, gout, rheumatic pain, female reproductive tract disorders, malaria, beri-beri and absentmindedness [17, 18]. Cannabis was also used with wine in ancient China as an anaesthetic in surgery, when the famous Chinese medicine physician Hua Tuo (117–207 AD) used a decoction called ma-fei-san (hemp-boiling compound) taken with wine as an anaesthetic for abdominal surgery [13]. It is likely to have been much better than nothing!

A little later on in the history of Chinese medicine, we see notations of the difference between hemp seeds and the 'fruits' (ma-fen) in a text written around 500 A.D. where the latter was said to have been used by magicians in combination with ginseng to set forward time to reveal future events [13]. This reference to magicians is explained by the fact that in ancient China, like in many early cultures, medicine had a strong link with magic and medicine men were magicians. The temporal distortions and hallucinations of cannabis were also noted in later dynasties by various authors of Chinese medicine texts such as T'ang Shen-Wei in the tenth century [13].

## Cannabis in Other Ancient Cultures

Records of the medicinal use of cannabis span many different cultures and countries throughout ancient and more modern history including Egypt, Persia, England, Spain and others. Such uses include many different types of clinical conditions including neuralgia, sleep, bipolar disease, anxiety, depression, mood, nervousness, menopause, headache, migraine, tumours, convulsions, pleurisy, gout, post-partum haemorrhage and many more [19].

In ancient India, cannabis has been strongly associated with religious practices, with the Vedas stating that cannabis is *'a source of happiness, donator of joy, and bringer of freedom'* [18] and indeed it is used in a beverage called 'bhang' today in celebrations. It was used in India for a range of conditions including as an analgesic, hypnotic, anti-inflammatory, antibiotic, anti-parasitic, anti-spasmodic, anaesthetic, diuretic, pro-digestive, appetite stimulant, antitussive, expectorant [18] as well as to treat anxiety [14, 19].

In ancient Egypt, use of *C. sativa* as medicine was extensively reported on Assyrian clay tablets and Egyptian Ebers Papyrus (3000 years ago) [20].

Cannabis was considered a sacred plant in several religions. In India and Tibet, it was used to facilitate mediation and communication with spirits, and in the Old Testament, the use of *Cannabis sativa* as incense and a sacred oil was also cited [20].

For a comprehensive chronology of the medicinal use of cannabis throughout history, see Russo [19].

## Medicinal Cannabis in the Western World

The spread of cannabis to western countries was likely to be via African slaves who were brought to the west by the Portuguese, and this is thought to be how cannabis took root in Brazil in the early 1500s. Through contact with African slaves, South American Indians began to smoke cannabis or marijuana and include it in their ceremonies. Cannabis use then spread further throughout Brazil, Mexico, Latin America, the Caribbean, and so too did its medical uses: cannabis tea was used for rheumatism, colic, female problems, toothache and sleep problems. In Europe, originally the focus was on hemp fibre rather than medicine, when in 1533 King Henry VIII ordered English farmers to grow hemp or risk paying fine [21].

As Lee [21] explains, indeed in the era of sea power, hemp fibre was a critical substance and for hundreds of years, the major European maritime powers relied on hemp for their ships (i.e. ropes and sails). It was being grown in the USA, and in 1762 Virginia awarded bounties for hemp culture and manufacture, and imposed penalties on those who did not produce it. Even George Washington in 1765 was said to have grown hemp, and there is some conjecture it may not have just been for the fibre. In 1861, around the time of the American Civil War, hemp fibre was losing commercial value, becoming overtaken by cotton, and the steamship was also overtaking ships powered by sails. However, its value as a medicine was surging and even Sir William Osler, founding father of modern medicine, endorsed the use of cannabis as the best treatment for migraines. Cannabis cigarettes for asthma, the inclusion of hemp in mustard plasters and muscle ointments and the use of cannabis as an analgesic was common [21]. Meanwhile in the UK, the personal physician to Queen Victoria, Sir John Russell Reynolds (1828–1896), prescribed hemp tincture to relieve painful menstrual cramps and also recommended it for insomnia [21].

The introduction of the medical use of cannabis to western medicine in the first half of the nineteenth century is attributed to an Irish physician and a French psychiatrist who spread its medical use from England and France to the rest of Europe then later, to North America [22]. Irish physician William B O'Shaughnessy first encountered cannabis in India and began to study its effects in animals and humans, whilst French psychiatrist Jacques-Joseph Moreau encountered it through Arabs and began his own studies using himself and his students. Moreau stated that hashish was *'a powerful and unique method to investigate the genesis of mental illness'* (Moreau 1845) [22].

For an excellent read about the history of cannabis, see the book *Smoke Signals* by Martin Lee.

## Regulations in the USA

In the USA, cannabis essentially became a prohibited substance for what are probably largely political reasons, with the passing of the *Marijuana Tax Act 1937* that created an exorbitant tax for growing, possession and distribution. The American Medical Association tried to prevent the passing of this Act but to no avail. The plant was demonised by the head of the Federal Bureau of Narcotics and willing political helpers included a significant newspaper magnate, with quite the propaganda campaign levelled against it. It became associated with a type of counter-culture, in particular it was associated with the jazz scene, as well as prominent African Americans including Malcolm X, Satchmo and others. Within 10 years of it being banned, the use of cannabis had almost doubled, such was the usefulness of legislation that criminalised it. See Martin Lee's excellent book *Smoke Signals* [21] for the history.

Much of the misunderstanding or lack of understanding that abounds today is a legacy of the misinformation that has been propagated in the past, and the equating of recreational use ('adult use') of cannabis with medicinal use. As we will see later, cannabis is not one 'thing'. Strains of cannabis bred for the recreational or adult-use market are much higher in one particular active constituent, THC, which produces the characteristic euphoric effects. Safety concerns are largely based on evidence associated with recreational use (which is usually smoking of strains with high THC content). More on this later.

Up until its prohibition in the USA, there were over 100 medical indications listed in the US Pharmacopoeia for cannabis. Yet to this day, under the Federal *United States Controlled Substances Act*, cannabis is considered a Schedule 1 drug. Schedule 1 is the most restrictive of the five schedules, defined as a drug/substance having a high potential for abuse, with no currently accepted medical use in treatment, and a lack of accepted safety for its use under medical supervision. One can see the ridiculousness of the inclusion of cannabis as a Schedule 1 drug. Despite this federal prohibition, to date 33 states and the District of Columbia have legalised its medicinal use, and 10 states plus the District of Columbia have legalised recreational or adult use [23, 24].

## Active Constituents of Cannabis

*Cannabis sativa* has approximately 540 different secondary metabolites, including phytocannabinoids, terpenes and other constituents which are responsible for many of the plant's therapeutic benefits [25].

The main constituents of the plant are as follows:

- Phytocannabinoids: There are more than 120 phytocannabinoids; responsible for defence and interaction with herbivores and pests.
- Terpenes (terpenoids): There are over 200 terpenes. These oils give the particular cultivar its characteristic aroma, for example, limonene gives a lemon smell, alpha-pinene gives a pine aroma
- Other plant nutrients including: Flavonoids, polysaccharides, coumarins, glycosides, phenols, alcohols, steroids [12, 26]

### Where Are the Phytocannabinoids and Terpenes Found?

The secondary metabolites (phytocannabinoids, terpenes) are found in resin produced by glandular structures called trichomes on the flowers (made up of smaller florets), leaves, bracts and stems of the *unfertilised* female plants. The male leaves have few glandular trichomes that can produce small amounts [20]. Female plants produce much higher amounts of phytocannabinoids (reported 20 times higher) than male plants and for this reason they are preferred. Also, it is the seed-free, unfertilised female plants (termed sinsemilla) which produce a higher yield of phytocannabinoids in the flower heads or buds than those that have been pollinated. Thus, in growing them, to avoid pollination the male plants must be removed to ensure the female plants are not exposed to pollination [12].

### Entourage Effect

Whilst the phytocannabinoids have received much of the attention in research and are understood to be responsible for many of the therapeutic actions of the cannabis, the terpenes and the other plant nutrients are understood to provide the '*entourage effect*'. The entourage effect refers to the physiological regulation by which multiple endogenous chemical components of the cannabis plant display a cooperative effect in eliciting a cellular response additional and/or synergistic to the actions of the phytocannabinoids [27]. This is an important point to understand, given the different types of medicinal cannabis products on the market.

According to Russo, practitioner observations indicate that much lower doses of CBD are needed in the treatment of seizures when a small amount of THC, THCA [tetrahydrocannabinolic acid) and linalool (a terpene) are part of the medicinal cannabis product [19, 28]. There is also evidence from animal studies that CBD can enhance the efficacy of THC and mitigate some of its undesirable side effects (discussed later) [29].

It is the authors' opinion that whole plant extracts will be therapeutically more beneficial and have less adverse effects than extracts of isolates of phytocannabinoids or synthetic copies of phytocannabinoids. Nature is not stupid, but humans often are.

## Cannabis Strains/Cultivars and Active Constituent Profiles

Cannabis is a plant. There are literally hundreds of strains or cultivars (cultivated varieties) of *C. sativa*. There is some debate within the literature about the correctness of the term 'strain' compared with 'cultivar' in relation to cannabis varieties. We will simply use the word 'cultivar'. Each cultivar has its own chemical profile, that is to say, each cultivar will vary in the types and amounts of various phytocannabinoids and terpenes. The term 'chemovar' is used to denote a form of classification based on the chemical profile of the plant. These cannabis cultivars have been given rather interesting names including *Afghan #1*, *Jack Herer*, *Gorilla Glue*, *OG Kush* and *Grape Diamonds*. Many are hybrids of different subspecies (e.g. AK-47 variety is a cross between *Cannabis indica ssp. indica* and *Cannabis indica ssp. afghanica*) [30]. Each cultivar has a characteristic phytocannabinoid and terpene profile, taste, aroma, duration of effect and effect on the body. In Michael Backes' book *Cannabis Pharmacy* [30], the characteristics of various cultivars of cannabis are described in terms of aroma, taste, potency, duration of effects, psycho-activity, analgesia, muscle relaxation, dissociation, stimulant and sedation actions.

From the perspective of one of the authors who is trained in Chinese herbal medicine (Kylie O'Brien), there is a wealth of empirical knowledge about the various strains or cultivars that is held by the growers, bud tenders (sellers of cannabis), those for whom cannabis is part of their culture (e.g. in Jamaica, Rasthafarians) and indeed those who have simply sampled a lot of the strains. For example, the aroma of the cultivar of cannabis, due to its terpene composition predominantly, provides an indication of the variety's effects [30]. Those cultivars with a pine aroma (i.e. containing alpha-pinene) are typically varieties that are stimulating, whilst those with a lavender aroma (i.e. from linalool) are associated typically with varieties that are more sedative [30]. This is not unexpected. In Chinese medicine, the taste and temperature characteristics of an herb are at least partly responsible for the therapeutic effects of an herb, and aromatherapy is a whole therapeutic modality based on our sense of smell.

This on-the-ground knowledge is not dissimilar to the way in which empirical knowledge was built up in Chinese herbal medicine, for example. In contrast, what is sold on the proprietary medicinal cannabis market (i.e. oils in bottles, capsules) is focused primarily on CBD and THC content and the relative percentages of each (and sometimes the terpene content). It seems that the variety and subtlety of the varieties of the raw plant have been lost in the production of proprietary medicines, perhaps a product of the reductionistic approach of biomedicine and pharmaceuticals. Yet, understanding the properties and potential therapeutic effects of a wide variety of different whole-plant strains or cultivars scientifically is perhaps something that should be considered. It seems curious that the empirical knowledge of the bud tenders and growers is, largely, not being captured in the proprietary cannabis oil market, at least not yet.

Through chemical and genetic fingerprinting, it is possible to precisely identify each cannabis chemical profile (ie. the chemovar) and genetic profile. Each variety of cannabis contains genes which determine its specific chemical expression, that is, the type and amounts of specific phytocannabinoids and terpenes. Chemical fingerprinting is used to determine the normal range of phytocannabinoids and terpenoids produced by a specific phenotype of a specific cannabis cultivar [30].

### Genes and Environmental Conditions

The two main factors influencing the formation of any cannabis cultivar are its genetics and the environment. The genotype is its blueprint for growth, and the phenotype is the physical expression of the genotype. The environment plays a vital role in inducing these characteristics coded in its genetic blueprint, and the plant's colour, morphology, aroma and resin production are all impacted by the environmental conditions in which it is grown [20].

The phytocannabinoid content of *Cannabis sativa* is influenced by environmental conditions such as humidity, temperature, radiation, photo-period length, soil nutrients, parasites and time of harvest [27, 31]. Phytocannabinoids and several terpenes (in the leaves and flowers) act as a barrier to water loss [20]. Sparse rainfall, low humidity and sunny climate produce a plant rich in psychoactive components (i.e. THC) [20]. Soil nutrients can influence the cannabinoid production, as does humidity: there is increased phytocannabinoid content with decreased humidity [20].

One of the most important growth factors in cultivating cannabis is light: its quality, intensity and photo-period [32]. Exposure to high UV radiation produces significantly greater contents of THC; THC is more stable to UVB radiations compared with the other phytocannabinoids which may be more rapidly degraded on exposure [33].

Phytocannabinoids and terpenes are protective: they block other sources of environmental stress including attacks by bacteria, fungi, insects and competition with surrounding vegetation [20]. Many of the terpenes in the resin such as pinene and limonene repel insects [34], and the resin may also show antibiotic and antifungal properties [35].

## A Word of Caution About Reductionism

The reductionist approach to understanding cannabis seeks to reduce its medicinal benefits to key active constituents, and then try to find out their mechanisms of action and therapeutic benefits, and synthetically copy them. This is the classic drug-discovery model. Such approaches were tried in Chinese herbal medicine last century, with little success. This is primarily because herbs are composed on many active constituents, and the reason that they are therapeutically beneficial is likely to lie in the synergism between these active constituents. We suggest the same caution here with the plant *Cannabis sativa*. It has over 500 active constituents, with hundreds of different cultivars. The 'entourage effect' which describes the synergisms between the active constituents is likely to be the reason it is so beneficial. The terpenes, polyphenols and flavonoids have their own therapeutic actions.

With that said, let us now take a look at some of the key active constituents in the plant.

## Phytocannabinoids: Overview

There are 11 main classes of phytocannabinoids, and over 120 individual cannabinoids [12, 20]. The most well researched of these are tetrahydrocannabinol (THC) and cannabidiol (CBD), described in detail in the next sections. Phytocannabinoids are classified as neutral cannabinoids (without a carboxyl group) and cannabinoid acids (with a carboxyl group) [36].

The main subclasses or types of phytocannabinoids are as follows:

- Trans-Δ-9-tetrahydrocannabinol (Δ9-THC)-type compounds
- Cannabidiol (CBD)-type compounds
- Δ8-THC-type compounds
- Δ-9-tetrahydrocannabivarin (D9-THCV)-type compounds
- Cannabichromene (CBC)-type compounds
- Cannabigerol (CBG)-type compounds
- Cannabinol (CBN)-type compounds
- Cannabicyclol (CBL)-type compounds
- Cannabinodiol (CBDL)-type compounds
- Cannabitriol t(CBTL)-type compounds
- Cannabielsoin (CBE)-type compounds

In the cannabis plant, cannabinoids are biosynthesised and accumulated as cannabinoid acids, and subsequently decarboxylated into their neutral forms [20]. For example, the plant produces cannabidiolic acid (CBDA) and tetrahydrocannabinolic acid (THCA). Heat, light and ageing cause decarboxylation of these compounds producing the decarboxylated species THC & CBD [12]. The acid forms of the main cannabinoids, THCA and CBDA have been found to have potent therapeutic effects also.

Only one of the phytocannabinoids has potentially intoxicating effects, in the sense of producing euphoria and other effects associated with smoking cannabis/marijuana: that phytocannabinoid is THC [37]. Its acid form, THCA, does not have this effect [12]. CBD and indeed the other cannabinoids do not have any intoxicant ability either [38]. However, that is not to say that other constituents of cannabis such as CBD are not psychoactive, as several are such as CBD, which has anxiolytic actions for example. In relation to THC, we use the term 'potentially intoxicating' and we use the word 'potentially' as this euphoric effect is dose-related.

We will now look in depth at two key phytocannabinoids, CBD and THC.

## Cannabidiol

Cannabidiol (CBD) is one of the most well researched of the phytocannabinoids, the other being THC. Cultivars of the plant *Cannabis sativa* that produce CBD include those designated as 'hemp' (as discussed earlier, hemp being defined as a cultivar with a low amount of THC, typically less than 0.3%) as well as cultivars/chemovars that do not fall into the hemp category (typically those containing more than 0.3%

THC, at least in the USA). This is an important point from the perspective of the cannabis industry, in particular in the USA. The passing of the US 2018 Farm Bill appeared to have exempted hemp from the Controlled Substances Act. However, the Drug Enforcement Administration and the Federal Drug Administration have resisted this law and its interpretation and has not officially legalised CBD use or distribution. Other world nations also have diverse and confusing laws and regulations for CBD.

## Therapeutic Actions of CBD

CBD has many therapeutic actions including the following:

- Analgesic
- Anti-nausea, anti-emetic
- Anti-convulsant/ anti-epileptic
- Anti-psychotic
- Anti-inflammatory
- Antioxidant
- Neuroprotective
- Anti-tumoral, anti-cancer
- Anxiolytic
- Antidepressant
- Anti-asthmatic
- Immuno-modulatory
- Anti-bacterial
- Antibiotic [27, 35, 39–43]

### What Conditions Can CBD Potentially Treat?

- There is evidence that CBD could be exploited in the treatment and symptom relief of various disorders including (but not limited to) the following:
- Acne [44, 45]
- Autism [46–48]
- Anxiety [49, 50], depression [51, 52], PTSD [53, 54], psychosis [55]
- Diabetes [56, 57]
- Epilepsy and seizures, including severe forms such as Dravet syndrome and Lennox-Gastaut syndrome [58–63]
- Inflammatory bowel disease (IBD) [64]
- Movement disorders (e.g. Huntington's disease, amyotrophic lateral sclerosis) [65, 66]
- Multiple sclerosis [67]
- Nausea and vomiting [68, 69]
- Neurodegenerative conditions and diseases with proteinopathies, for example, Alzheimer's disease [70]
- Pain and inflammation [71]
- Psoriasis [72, 73]
  and others

## Mechanisms of Action of CBD

Unlike THC, CBD has very low CB1 and CB2 receptor affinity [74, 75], though its effects rely on the integrity of cannabinoid receptors [76, 77]. The actions of CBD are thought to be predominantly via activating the ECS indirectly, and through interacting with other targets [75, 77]. This contention is supported by a meta-analysis of (in vitro and in vivo) studies of mechanisms of action which concluded that CBD does not act *directly* at CB1 receptors [29]. However, whilst many studies indicate that particular effects of CBD occur in the absence of CB1 and CB2 receptors (e.g. in cannabinoid receptor knockout mice which are mice bred to lack these receptors), there are opposing studies that indicate CBD's effects are due to activating CB1 and/or CB2 receptors [78].

Various reports in the scientific literature state that CBD acts as a weak agonist or inverse agonist or even an allosteric modulator of CB1 and CB2 receptors [29, 78–80]. Its action appears to be concentration dependent since in the low nanomolecular range CBD shows antagonism to CB1/2 receptors but has agonist or inverse agonist actions at micromolecular concentrations [81].

CBD does not produce the classic tetrad of actions mediated at CB1 receptors that THC elicits (analgesia, hypo-locomotion, hypothermia and catalepsy) [82]. Instead, it exerts CB1 receptor *agonist-like activity* in some in vitro functional assays in high concentrations likely induced by enhancing endocannabinoid tone [29].

### CBD Modulates Endocannabinoid Tone and Adenosine Tone

CBD can increase AEA levels and the mechanism by which it does so appears to be via inhibition of fatty amide binding protein (FABP) which carries AEA to FAAH [83]. CBD may also enhance endocannabinoid tone by activating phospholipase A2 (PLA2), thereby mobilising arachidonic acid, which is used in the manufacture of AEA and 2-AG [29]. Since AEA does have affinity for CB1 and CB2 receptors (it is a partial agonist) and oxidation products of AEA produce metabolites that also have affinity for CB1 and CB2 receptors, AEA and/or its metabolites might explain reports that CBD is able to act via CB1 and/or CB2 receptors [78]. In this way, we can see that CBD can, via indirect methods, influence or modulate endocannabinoid tone.

In addition to being able to augment endocannabinoid tone, CBD is also able to augment adenosine tone by inhibiting adenosine uptake, acting as an indirect agonist at $A_{2A}$ receptors. This has the opposite action: a consequence of agonism of $A_{2A}$ receptors in post-synaptic cells is *prevention* of glutamate $mGlu_5$ receptor-mediated release of AEA and 2-AG through A2A/$mGlu_5$ heteromers [29]. Thus, there are two opposing actions of CBD: enhancement of endocannabinoid tone (i.e. increased levels of endocannabinoids) and enhancement of adenosine tone (which decreases release of endocannabinoids); however, typically the balance favours enhancement of endocannabinoid tone [29].

### CBD Modulates Multiple Signalling Systems

CBD has been called a 'promiscuous compound' due to the fact that it exerts actions at multiple targets [29]. In addition to its effects on CB1, CB2 receptors, CBD is an allosteric modulator of several other receptors (μ-,δ-opioid, dopamine $D_2$, $GABA_A$, glycine, some positively and some negatively) [29, 54, 79].

According to McPartland et al. [29], the ability of CBD to modulate many different signalling systems as well as augment endocannabinoid levels is likely to produce different effects on the ECS and CB1 receptors, and these effects will depend on the organ or tissue or cell involved, but they are unlikely to be a result of *direct* actions at CB1 receptors [29].

**CBD and TRPV1 Channels**

CBD is an agonist of potential transient vanilloid type 1 (TRPV1) receptors [84]. CBD's ability to bind and desensitise TRPV1 channels which may contribute to its anxiolytic effects [79, 85], and the effects of CBD on immune function may also be mediated by TRPV1 [78, 84].

**CBD and PPAR Receptors**

CBD is a PPAR-ϒ agonist, since in a rat model of Alzheimer's disease, blockade of PPAR-ϒ was found to attenuate the inhibitory effects of CBD on reactive gliosis and consequent neuronal damage [86]. CBD can increase metabolism of palmitoylethanolamide (PEA) and oleoylethanolamide (OEA), both of which are PPAR-α agonists [69, 87] and therefore may indirectly affect PPAR-α.

**CBD and Serotonin Receptors**

CBD's anxiolytic, neuroprotective and antidepressant effects are understood to be mediated by its ability to activate $5\text{-}HT_{1A}$ receptors [83] and possibly also through binding and desensitising TRPV1 [79]. CBD also inhibits synaptosomal uptake of serotonin [88].

**CBD and Orphan G-Protein Receptors**

CBD antagonises the orphan G-Protein Receptor 55 (GPR55), a G-protein coupled receptor which is a member of the class of receptors called metabotropic receptors. When such receptors are activated, a variety of downstream effects in cells are triggered, and the effects depend on the type of cell [89]. GPR55 has been found to be elevated in many different diseases including inflammatory bowel disease, bone remodelling, nervous system excitability, neutrophil migration, mast cell degranulation, systemic vascular resistance and angiogenesis [90–93].

A study in a mouse model of Dravet syndrome (a condition associated with severe epileptic seizures) found that CBD's ability to rescue Dravet syndrome symptoms, reducing seizures, is associated with increased inhibitory neurotransmission and that this is potentially mediated by antagonism (blocking) of GPR55 in the hippocampus (a critical brain region for seizure activity) [94].

Increased levels of GPR55 have also been implicated in inflammatory bowel disease [95] and cancer [90, 93]. Blockade of GPR55 in a mice model of bowel inflammation has been found to reduce inflammation [95], and this could be the mechanism by which CBD may work in inflammatory bowel diseases [89]. Similarly, since studies in cancer cell lines and animal models indicate that elevated

GPR55 is associated with migratory ability in breast cancer cells [93] and has pro-tumour activity [90], agents that are able to block GPR55 may be very important therapeutically.

CBD also acts as a partial agonist and antagonises THC at GPR18 [79]. Heteromer complexes between CB2 receptors and GPR18 in microglia have been implicated in Alzheimer's disease [96].

**CBD and Adenosine Receptors**

The ability of CBD to enhance adenosine signalling by inhibiting uptake of adenosine at $A_{2A}$ receptors, and in this way enhancing the anti-inflammatory effects of adenosine agonists, suggests a potential therapeutic role in pain and inflammation [71].

**CBD and α3 Glycine Receptors**

CBD exerts positive allosteric modulation of α3 glycine receptors which are involved in pain pathways [29]. Results from an animal study suggest α3 glycine receptors mediate CBD-induced suppression of chronic pain, with the CBD-induced analgesic effect absent in α3 glycine receptors knock-out mice (mice bred to lack α3 glycine receptors) [29, 97].

**Other Effects on Receptors and Neurotransmitters**

CBD has antagonist activity on α-1 adrenergic and μ-opioid receptors [88]. CBD inhibits synaptosomal uptake of noradrenaline, dopamine and GABA [88]. It also modulates intracellular calcium levels via mitochondrial $Na^+/Ca^{2+}$ exchange and T-type and L-type voltage-regulated $Ca^{2+}$ channels [29]. It has also been shown to be a Sigma 1 receptor (σ1R) antagonist [98].

CBD's effects on various key receptors are set out in Table 4.1 (see text for references).

## Immunological and Anti-Inflammatory Effects

The evidence clearly supports the notion that CBD is immune suppressive with various mechanisms involved, including direct suppression of activation of different types of immune cells, induction of apoptosis and promotion of regulatory cells which control other immune cell targets [78]. The effects of CBD on the immune system involve both the innate and adaptive immune responses.

Inflammation is typically associated with the innate immune response. Neutrophils, macrophages and other myeloid cells act quickly to destroy invading pathogens and also cause damage to tissues (though many types of calls produce proinflammatory cytokines in response to inflammation) [78]. If the innate response is not sufficient, the adaptive immune system responds, made up of B cells and T cells. T Cells have several actions: they can lyse/induce apoptosis of infected cells, or signal to other cells and recruit or activate them, with communication mediated by cytokines [78].

Current data indicate that immune effects of CBD are mediated through several receptor targets, including CB2 receptors, CB1 receptors, TRPV1, PPAR-ϒ, and adenosine A2A, inhibition of FAAH and blockade of GPR55 receptors [78].

**Table 4.1** CBD's effects on key receptors

| Receptor | CBD effect |
|---|---|
| α-1 adrenergic | Antagonist |
| μ–/δ-opioid | Negative allosteric modulation |
| Noradrenaline | Inhibits synaptosomal uptake |
| Dopamine | Inhibits synaptosomal uptake |
| GABA | Inhibits synaptosomal uptake |
| α3 glycine receptors | Positive allosteric modulation |
| $A_{2A}$ receptors | Inhibits uptake of adenosine at $A_{2A}$ receptors |
| GPR-18 | Partial agonist |
| GPR55 | Antagonises GPR55 |
| $5\text{-HT}_{1A\text{-}2A}$ | Activates $5\text{-HT}_{1A}$ receptors |
| PPAR-ϒ | Agonist |
| TRPV1 | Agonist |
| PPAR-α | Indirect action: increases PEA & OEA (known PPAR-α agonists) |
| Sigma 1 receptor (σ1R) | Antagonist |

For example, when activated, CB2 receptors (located in abundance in cells and organs of the immune system) attenuate pro-inflammatory responses such as cytokine release and immune cell responses. Although CBD has been found to be an inverse agonist of CB2 receptors, CBD use consistently leads to the reduction in pro-inflammatory markers including TNF-α, iNOS and COX-2 [29, 99]. In this case and others, CBD cellular action was blocked by CB2 receptor antagonists suggesting an agonist or allosteric function in different cell types [29, 100]. The contradiction may be explained by the formation of paired receptor-receptor heteromers leading to a unique signalling expression. This was shown in the case of CBD, a known agonist of the serotonin $5\text{-HT}_{1A}$ receptor, which binds to a CB2 receptor-$5HT_{1A}$ heteromer to manage neonatal hypoxic-ischemic brain damage [101].

CBD can reduce nitric oxide (NO) production in acute and chronic inflammation models and various disease models in animals, and several studies have shown that it inhibits many different inflammatory cytokines and transcription factors including IL-1β, IL-2, IL-6, IL-12, IL-17, TNF-α, INF-γ, CCL3, CCL4 and NF-κB and increase anti-inflammatory cytokines such as IL-4 and IL-10 [29, 78, 79]. Studies indicate CBD mobilises AA by stimulating phospholipase A2 (PLA2) activity [79]; however, what happens next is not certain. Some studies have found CBD can inhibit the metabolism of AA to leukotriene B4 (LTB4) by 5-lipoxygenase, and other studies have found that CBD blocks the metabolism of AA to PGE1 or TxB2 (via COX-1) or PGE2 (via COX-2) [29, 79].

For a summary of the many ways CBD regulates immune responses, see Nichols and Kaplan [78].

### Antioxidant Activity

Research indicates that CBD is a strong antioxidant. In general, CBD can reduce reactive oxygen species (ROS) in healthy cells (where ROS has been stimulated by particular agents) and induce ROS in cancer cells, which is an anti-cancer mechanism by which CBD induces cell apoptosis [29]. In glutamate neurotoxicity CBD was a more potent antioxidant than either ascorbate (vitamin C) or tocopherol (vitamin E) [102]. However, there are cases of the converse being reported. For example, CBD at very low, sub-micromolar concentrations can also inhibit ROS formation induced by $H_2O_2$ in some cancer cells [103], and in the liver microsomes the metabolic derivative CBD hydroxyquinone has been found to be able to induce cytotoxicity by generating ROS [29]. And yet, liver toxicity from pharmaceutical CBD doses have been related to cholestatic patterns and not oxidative stress [104].

### Anti-Bacterial Effect

CBD also shows much promise in treatment of bacterial infections [41], including methicillin-resistant bacterial strains (Gram-positive bacteria *Staphylococcus aureus*) [35, 39], other types of Gram-positive bacteria (including *Streptococcus pneumoniae* and *Clostridioides difficile*) and certain types of Gram-negative bacteria including *Neisseria gonorrhoeae* (causes gonorrhoea) [39].

Part of the anti-bacterial mechanism may involve its effects on bacterial membrane vesicles (MVs), of which there are many types. MVs are released from Gram-negative (Gm –ve) and Gram-positive (Gm +ve) bacteria to communicate with other bacteria as well as forming part of the host-pathogen interactions. MVs are important in biofilm formation and dissemination of toxins within the host. MVs may be involved in antibiotic resistance, for example by protecting biofilms from antibiotics via increased vesiculation. They are released in greater abundance from Gm –ve than Gm +ve bacteria and are vital for bacterial survival.

CBD has been found to be a strong inhibitor of MV release from Gram -ve (*E. coli* VCS257) but not from Gm +ve bacteria (*S. aureus* subsp. aureus Rosenbach). Cell line research found that CBD is able to increase the bacterial action of several antibiotics in Gm -ve bacteria when used in combination, and also increased antibiotic effects of kanamycin in Gram +ve bacteria (without affecting MV release). CBD also changed the protein profiles of MVs released from *E. coli* after 1 h of CBD treatment. These findings suggest that CBD could be a useful adjuvant to selected antibiotics, depending on bacterial species, to increase antibiotic activity and help reduce antibiotic resistance [41].

### Cellular Benefits in the Central Nervous System

CBD has a range of benefits in the central nervous system (CNS), set out in Table 4.2. CBD is neuroprotective and its anti-inflammatory and antioxidant properties may underpin this [105].

Animal and human research has demonstrated therapeutic properties of CBD for brain function and neuroprotection, through direct effects on the ECS and influencing the endogenous endocannabinoids [42]. Such beneficial effects include decreasing production of inflammatory cytokines, influencing microglial cells to return to a ramified state, preserving cerebral circulation during ischemic events and decreasing vascular changes and neuroinflammation [106].

**Table 4.2** Effects of CBD on central nervous system

| Effects in neurons | Effects in endothelial cells | Effects in microglia | Effects in oligodendrites |
|---|---|---|---|
| Decreased mTOR<br>Increased AEA, PPARα<br>Increased apoptosis<br>Enhanced antioxidant and neuroprotection<br>Improved plasticity and BDNF | Decreased pro-inflammatory cytokines<br>Decreased vascular cell adhesion molecule 1 (VCAM-1) | Decreased pro-inflammatory cytokines, pro-inflammatory mediators NF-κB and inducible NO synthase release<br>Slows microglial cell migration | Enhanced antioxidant<br>Decreased endoplasmic reticulum stress |

Maroon and Bost [42]

Animal studies indicate CBD can attenuate brain damage associated with neurodegenerative and/or ischaemic conditions outside the endocannabinoid system. CBD appears to be able to stimulate synaptic plasticity and facilitate neurogenesis, which may help explain its effects in attenuating psychotic, anxiety and depressive behaviours [42]. How it does this involves multiple cellular targets to elevate brain-derived neurotropic factor (BDNF) levels, reduce microglia activation and decrease levels of proinflammatory mediators [42].

## Effects on Cardiovascular System

CBD has been found to be able to cause vasorelaxation in human mesenteric arteries in an endothelium-dependent manner which involves CB1 receptor activation as well as TRPV channel activation, release of nitric oxide and potassium hyperpolarisation [81]. CBD has also been found to inhibit lipopolysaccharide-induced arteriolar and venular vasodilation. At concentrations above 100 nM, CBD has also been found to cause time-dependent vasorelaxation in rat aortae which was inhibited by a PPAR γ receptor antagonist and a superoxide dismutase inhibitor. CBD has been found to be a weak/partial agonist at the PPARγ receptor and PPARγ ligands have been shown to induce Cu/Zn-SOD (increased SOD activity reduces reactive oxygen species and thereby promotes vasorelaxation) [81].

GPR55 is closely involved with ox-LDL-induced foam cells. Foam cells form from macrophages overwhelmed by the abnormal uptake of modified (oxidised) low density lipoproteins (LDL) by way of scavenger LDL receptors. Modulating GPR55 could manage atherosclerosis and other related cardiovascular diseases. Furthermore, in acute coronary syndrome, CBD could block the effects l-α-lysophosphatidylinositol (LPI), an endogenous ligand for GPR55, that is elevated in this condition by acting as a GPR55 antagonist [107].

There is a growing body of evidence indicating that CBD can assist in conditions associated with endothelial dysfunction, for example, diabetes. CBD can decrease monocyte adhesion and trans-endothelial migration, which are part of the pathogenesis of atherosclerosis, (though this effect is not mediated through CB1 or CB2 receptors). In animal models, CBD has been found to be neuroprotective against stroke, reducing infarct volume (an effect independent of CB1 or TRPV1 channels but possibly mediated by 5HT1A since this was sensitive to a 5HT1A receptor antagonist). Neuroprotective mechanisms in stroke also include the ability of CBD to increase cerebral blood flow and reduce vascular permeability in the brain [81].

Finally, CBD can influence various blood cells. It can increase phospholipase A2 expression and lipoxygenase products in platelets, and inhibit adenosine or norepinephrine or collagen-induced platelet aggregation. It can also influence the survival and death of white blood cells, and white blood cell migration. Such abilities may be part of the reason as to why CBD can delay or prevent cardiovascular disorders [81].

### Anti-Cancer Activity and Exosomes

CBD has been shown to have anti-cancer activity in many preclinical studies, though it is beyond the scope of this chapter to focus on those. However, we want to discuss one of the potential mechanisms of action of CBD which may involve exosomes and microvesicles (EMV) as it illustrates an important mechanism of action of CBD.

EMVs are lipid bilayer-enclosed structures which are released by cells. EMVs mediate intercellular communication through the transfer of proteins and genetic material and can affect many physiological and pathological processes including cell migration, differentiation and angiogenesis. Increased EMV release has been found in cancer, in particular in association with resistance to chemotherapy and in the active transfer of pro-oncogenic factors. Resistance to chemotherapeutic drugs may be partly due to EMV shedding from cancer cells which aids increased active drug efflux [40].

CBD is effective in several pathologies linked to EMVs including cancer, and appears to modulate mitochondrial function, including ATP, ROS, proton leak, and uptake and release of calcium. CBD has been found to significantly inhibit the release of EMVs in three cancer cell lines: prostate cancer (PC3), hepatocellular carcinoma (HEPG2) and breast adenocarcinoma (MDA-MB-231), in a dose-dependent manner. The mechanism of action may be associated with changes in mitochondrial function (specifically modulation of STAT3 and prohibitin expression). CBD was shown to sensitise cancer cells to cisplatin and significantly increased cisplatin-mediated apoptosis [40], suggesting a potential adjuvant role in those undergoing chemotherapy with this drug.

## CBD Antagonism and Potentiation of THC

CBD has been found to both antagonise and potentiate the actions of THC in many different animal and human studies.

### Potentiation

In both animal and human studies, CBD has been found to interact with THC in an additive or synergistic manner, to potentiate some of the effects of THC and mitigate some of the side effects [29]. As explained by McPartland et al. [29], in animal models of MS, muscle spasticity, epilepsy, chronic pain and inflammation, diabetes, metabolic syndrome, anorexia and nausea, CBD has been shown to enhance the efficacy of THC, as well as mitigate side effects in various models of psychosis, anxiety and depression-anhedonia [29].

CBD's ability to potentiate some THC effects may be additive or synergistic [29]. In human glioblastoma cells, CBD synergistically enhanced the inhibitory effect of THC on cell growth and survival [108]. Treatment of glioblastoma cells with the combination of CBD and THC significantly modulated the cell cycle and induction of reactive oxygen species (ROS) and apoptosis, and also modulated extracellular signal-regulated kinase (ERK) and caspase activities, effects that were not achieved with either THC or CBD alone [108]. McPartland et al. [29] propose several different non-CB1 receptor mechanisms by which CBD may potentiate the behavioural effects of THC. One is via pharmacokinetic mechanisms, as CBD has been found to increase the area under the curve of THC in the brain and in blood [109]. However, there are many other possible mechanisms. For example, CBD reduces inflammation and pro-inflammatory cytokines through TRPV1, $A_{2A}$ and PPAR-ϒ receptor mechanisms whilst THC reduces inflammation via actions mediated by CB1 and CB2 receptors. Another example is that CBD inhibits FAAH (the enzyme that breaks down AEA), thereby increasing the amount of AEA which suppresses pain via peripheral mechanisms, whilst THC's analgesic effects are mediated via central CB1 receptors [29]. Thus, CBD is acting either in an additive or synergistic manner to the actions of THC. See McPartland et al. [29] for further mechanisms by which CBD may potentiate the action of THC.

### Antagonism

Despite the low binding affinity to the CB receptors, CBD acts as a CB1 inverse agonist or even antagonist at low molecular nM level in the presence of THC, attenuating the THC-associated adverse effects (e.g. anxiety, hunger, tachycardia and sedation) [27, 110]. Clinically, this is an important point as the combination of CBD and THC serves to help mitigate the euphoric effect of THC that is not always desirable for patients.

As explained by McPartland et al. [29], in terms of the ability of CBD to antagonise the effects of THC, CBD does not appear to directly block the effects of THC like the drug rimonabant (CB1 receptor antagonist). A systematic review found that the functional antagonism of THC by CBD may be mediated by non-CB1 receptor mechanisms which include the following:

- CBD augmenting AEA levels: Since CBD and AEA are TRPV1 agonists and pre-synaptic TRPV1 channel activation augments release of glutamate in the brain and spinal cord, this might counteract/antagonise the inhibitory action of pre-synaptic CB1 receptors that co-localise on glutaminergic neurons.
- CBD inhibiting adenosine uptake, acting as an indirect agonist at adenosine receptors, inhibits CB1 receptor-mediated effects.
- CBD acting as a direct and indirect agonist at $5\text{-}HT_{1A}$ receptors, facilitating anxiolytic effects (THC has anxiogenic effects in higher doses) [29].

## Cannabidiolic Acid (CBDA)

The cannabinoid acids are precursors of the natural cannabinoids. The acids of CBD and THC cannabidolic acid and tetrahydrocannabinolic acid (CBDA and THCA, respectively) are PPARγ agonists with potent neuroprotective actions, showing promise in the treatment of Huntington's disease and other neurodegenerative/inflammatory diseases [111]. CBDA may also demonstrate anticonvulsant activity which may be due to serotonergic activity [28].

In general, there is much more research evidence in relation to CBD than CBDA in terms of its pharmacological actions. However, there is evidence that like CBD, CBDA can activate the transient receptor potential cation channels, TRPV1 and TRPA1, and can antagonise TRPM8 [112, 113]. CBDA shows a distinct advantage over CBD in that it produces these effects with much less potency (than CBD) [68]. CBDA also shows 100-fold greater affinity for the 5-$HT_{1A}$ receptor compared with CBD [28, 68]. Animal studies indicate that CBDA is 1000 times more potent than CBD in reducing acute and anticipatory nausea [114].

Whilst CBDA's actions may be more potent than CBD [68], in turn the methyl ester of CBDA may be more efficacious than CBDA itself [115]. The greater efficacy of CBDA and its methyl ester suggests that lower doses may be able to be used. This might also translate into a potential reduction in cost to the end user.

The research into the potential benefits of CBDA is largely preclinical: in vitro and animal research. Such research has elucidated the potential mechanisms of action of CBDA and demonstrated its efficacy in a range of health conditions. There are several promising areas of application which include the following:

- Anxiety [116]
- Depression [117]
- Inflammatory diseases [118]
- Diabetes [119]
- Cancer [120]
- Nausea and vomiting [68, 114]
- Seizures [28]

## Tetrahydrocannabinol (THC)

Δ-9 Tetrahydrocannabinol, abbreviated as THC, is the phytocannabinoid in cannabis that is 'potentially intoxicating', in the sense that it is responsible for the euphoria and other effects on the mind that are commonly experienced when smoking cannabis. The term 'potentially intoxicating' is more accurate than 'psychotropic', and as stated previously, the word 'potentially' is included because any intoxicating effect associated with THC is *dose dependent* and depends on the individual. There is much variation in how individuals metabolise cannabis and its active constituents including THC.

It should be remembered that the cannabis plant in its natural form contains the acid form of THC, tetrahydrocannabinolic acid (THCA). THCA has no intoxicating effect on the body. Thus, if you ingest the raw plant by juicing, for example, you will be ingesting THCA. As mentioned previously, it is only with exposure to light, age or on heating that the THCA is converted to THC via a process of decarboxylation (loss of the carboxylic acid group) [12].

## Therapeutic Actions of THC

THC has many therapeutic actions including the following:

- Analgesic
- Anti-inflammatory
- Bronchodilator
- Muscle relaxant, for example, for spasticity, spasms
- Antipruritic in cholestatic jaundice
- Neuroprotective antioxidant
- Anti-nausea and vomiting
- Anti-cancer
- Anxiolytic (dose dependent), depression, PTSD
- Stimulates appetite
- Relieves insomnia
- Anti-bacterial including methicillin-resistant bacterial strains
- Anti-ageing [27, 35, 69, 121–128].

THC has been found to have 20 times the anti-inflammatory power of aspirin and two times that of hydrocortisone [122].

## Mechanism of Action of THC

THC mimics anandamide and 2-AG by acting as a partial agonist at both cannabinoid receptors, CB1 receptors and CB2 receptors which are found in high concentration in many types of tissue in the body [129]. This underlies many of its activities as a psychoactive agent, analgesic, muscle relaxant and anti-spasmodic [27].

As discussed in Chap. 2, CB1 receptors are found in most areas of the brain and the peripheral nervous system, as well as many organs. Pre-synaptic activation of CB1 receptors in neural tissue inhibits the release of neurotransmitters such as gamma-aminobutyric acid (GABA) and glutamate, causing inhibition of voltage-gated calcium channels and vesicle release. Whilst activation of CB1 receptors usually inhibits the release of neurotransmitters, studies in rats have conversely found that activation of CB1 with THC can increase the release of acetylcholine, dopamine and glutamate in various brain regions [130–133]. This may be due to selective antagonism by THC of endocannabinoids, which has been reported when observing the anti-anxiolytic effects of THC in mice [134]. This dual inhibitory-stimulatory modulation of neurotransmitter release mediated by THC is believed to be responsible for the depressant and excitatory effects of cannabis [110].

The brain's endocannabinoid system has extensive interconnections with many neurotransmitter systems including dopamine, GABA, opioid and norepinephrine (NE). Activation of the endocannabinoid system by THC may have widespread indirect effects on the modulatory endocannabinoid-induced regulation of these other neurotransmitters [37].

### Anti-Inflammatory Effects

THC has strong anti-inflammatory effects on macrophages, NK cells and T lymphocytes including suppression of mitogen-stimulated proliferation, IL2 production, T-cell-dependent antibody responses and secretion of TNF-$\alpha$ [135]. THC has 20 times the anti-inflammatory power of aspirin and 2 times that of hydrocortisone [122]. It is able to regulate the Th1/Th2 type cytokine balance in activated human T cells, polarising the immune response towards the Th2 phenotype which is beneficial in inflammatory conditions [135, 136].

### Anti-Ageing Effects

Mice studies demonstrate that THC may have potential therapeutic uses in reversing age-related cognitive decline. Micro-dosing (i.e. use of low doses) with THC reversed age-related declines in cognitive performance of aged mice and was associated with enhanced expression of synaptic marker proteins. Expression of three synaptic marker proteins was lower in mature mice compared to young mice, indicative of age-related loss of synaptic connectivity, but THC treatment increased the levels of two of these markers (synapsin I and synaptophysin) in mature animals to levels observed in young mice (untreated with THC). THC also increased hippocampal spine density and altered the balance of inhibitory compared with excitatory synapses. THC was also found to affect molecular processes involved in cell plasticity and signalling in mature animals. THC treatment was also associated with changes in gene profiles, and these changes and the associated improvements in cognitive function lasted for several weeks after the treatment was stopped [121].

THC was found to restore hippocampal gene transcription patterns such that the expression profiles of 12-month-old mice treated with THC were similar to mice aged 2 months (not treated with THC), and they further found that transcriptional effects of THC were dependent on glutaminergic CB1 receptors and histone acetylation (histone acetylation promotes cognitive functions), since blocking these prevented the beneficial actions of the THC. Transcripts which were upregulated included Klotho (Kl) (which extends lifespan in different species and improves cognition), transthyretin (gene believed to be protective against Alzheimer's disease) and brain-derived neurotrophic factor (enhances synapse formation and cognitive functions). Transcripts which were downregulated after THC treatment were genes associated with ageing: caspase-1 (involved in age-related impairments in cognition), and connective tissue growth factor (Ctgf) (which enhances the pro-apoptotic activity of transforming growth factor β). This experiment, albeit in an animal model, suggests that restoration of CB1 signalling in old age might possibly be effective in treating cognitive changes associated with age [121].

This study is not an isolated one. In another mice study, old female mice (24 months old) were injected with a very low dose (0.002 mg/kg) of THC. They performed significantly better than untreated young mice aged 2 months in tests of memory and learning with the effects lasting for at least 7 weeks. A single injection of THC increased the level of Sirtuin1 in the hippocampus and frontal cortex in old mice for at least 7 weeks also (Sirtuin 1 is an enzyme shown to be involved in neuroplasticity and neuroprotection). Various brain regions were shown to have a larger volume and higher tissue density in old mice treated with THC [137].

Both studies indicate promise for the use of low doses of THC for safe and effective treatment of cognitive decline in humans. An advantage is that very low doses of THC will not produce the characteristic potentially intoxicating effects associated with higher doses.

## THCA-A

The term 'THCA' refers indistinctly to several acid derivatives of THC. More specifically, $\Delta^9$-tetrahydrocannabinolic acid A (THCA-A) is the acidic precursor of $\Delta^9$-THC. Biosynthesised from cannabigerolic acid, it accumulates in the glandular trichomes on flowers and leaves, representing up to 90% of the total THC contained in the cannabis plant. THCA-A slowly decarboxylates to form THC during storage and fermentation and can further degrade to cannabinol (CBN), due to temperature, light and auto-oxidation). Decarboxylation also occurs rapidly during baking of edibles, smoking, or vaporising.

In vitro research indicates that THCA-A interacts with several molecular targets and has anti-inflammatory, immunomodulatory, neuroprotective and anti-neoplastic properties. Some research seems to indicate that THCA-A acts via CB1 and CB2 receptors [138–140] though other research found that THCA has immune-modulating properties that were not mediated through CB1 and CB2 receptor pathways [141].

Cannabinoid acids bind and activate PPARγ (with higher potency than their decarboxylated products) [111]. PPARγ is a nuclear receptor and key regulator of lipid and glucose homeostasis [142] and is also expressed in many other tissues and cell types [111]. It plays an important role in inflammatory processes and neurodegenerative diseases including Huntington's disease [143].

Cell research indicates that THCA-A may exert immunomodulatory, anti-inflammatory, neuroprotective and anti-neoplastic effects [140]. In vitro and/or in vivo research into THCA-A indicates promise in the following areas:

- Anti-obesity [144]
- Neuroprotection [111] including Parkinson's disease [145]

- Nausea and vomiting [139].
- Anti-inflammatory [146]
- Anti-cancer [103, 147]

## Other Phytocannabinoids

### Cannabichromene (CBC)

In addition to CBD and THC, cannabichromene (CBC) is one of the most abundant cannabinoids in cannabis [27]. Indeed in some strains, it is the second most abundant phytocannabinoid [148]. In terms of mechanisms of action, CBC inhibits endocannabinoid cellular reuptake and is a weak inhibitor of monoacylglycerol lipase (MAGL), the key enzyme that hydrolyses 2-AG [112, 148]. CBC can potently activate transient receptor potential (TRP) ankyrin 1-type (TRPA1) channels [112].

Research has shown CBC to have the following effects: antimicrobial, anti-inflammatory, analgesic and antidepressant-like activity in rodents (see Izzo et al. [148]). CBC also seems to have some anti-cancer activity [103].

CBC appears to play a role in anti-nociception by stimulating the descending anti-nociception pathway in the dorsal ventrolateral periaqueductal grey via several different mechanisms [148]. These mechanisms may include activation of TRPA1, blocking the breakdown of endocannabinoids (and thereby increasing local endocannabinoid levels), and possibly also by potentiating adenosine signalling [149].

In a mice model of gut inflammation, CBC reduced inflammation-induced (by croton oil) gut hypermotility (upper gastrointestinal transit); however, the mechanism of action was not found to be dependent on cannabinoid receptors or TRPA1 [148]. CBD did not affect upper gastrointestinal transit, colonic propulsion or whole gut transit in healthy mice [148].

### Tetrahydrocannabivarin (THCV)

Tetrahydrocannabivarin (THCV) is another cannabinoid which shows promise in the control of blood sugar and management of diabetes and obesity [150]. THCV suppresses appetite, increases satiety and can upregulate energy metabolism. It has been shown to reduce fasting plasma glucose compared with placebo and has also been shown to provide neuroprotection. It is an inverse agonist/selective or neutral antagonist of the CB1 receptor (though unlike the drug rimonabant which was also an inverse agonist/selective antagonist of CB1 receptors but was removed from the market due to unacceptable psychological side effects), THCV has not been found to cause the adverse effects of rimonabant [150].

THCV acts as an agonist or antagonist at CB2 receptors, depending on dose. It appears that THCV may prevent the psychological effects associated with THC; however, at this point the mechanism of action by which it does this remains unknown [150]. Mice studies indicate THCV produces hypophagic effects in fasted and non-fasted mice [151] and THCV has been shown to decrease food intake and reduce body weight in mice models, indicating its anti-obesity effect is via food aversion [152]. Thus, THCV may potentially be useful in the management of obesity as well as type 2 diabetes [150].

## Terpenes

The terpenes, the essential oils of *Cannabis sativa*, are a complex mixture of organic (hydrocarbon) chemicals. Key essential oils include terpenes and oxygenated compounds such as alcohols, esters, ethers, aldehydes, ketones, lactones, phenols and phenol ethers [12]. Terpenes are usually the predominant, essential oils in cannabis and give the various cultivars their characteristic aroma [12, 26]. Terpenes are made up of units of isoprene: CH2 = C(–CH3)–CH=CH2. Monoterpenes consist of two isoprene units, whilst sesquiterpenes consist of three. The term 'terpenoids' indicates related compounds, though this term is often used interchangeably with 'terpenes' [12]. Monoterpenoids usually make up most of the essential oils of cannabis [12].

Terpenes are produced in the same secretory glandular trichomes of the cannabis flower in which the cannabinoids are produced. The phytocannabinoids and the terpenes together make up the resinous secretion of the glands [12]. Terpenes serve a protective function for the plant and have various therapeutic actions [153].

There are over 200 terpenoids in the plant *Cannabis sativa* [27]; however, none are unique to cannabis [12]. Many other plants produce terpenes also. For example, when one walks in a pine forest, the α-pinene in the pine needles contributes to the relaxing feeling that typically is experienced. α-pinene is one of the terpenes found in cannabis.

Note that different cannabis strains/cultivars will produce a different 'terpene profile', that is, there will be particular terpenes in particular amounts in different strains or cultivars of cannabis. It is the monoterpenes, limonene and pinene (which often comprise over 75% of the volatile constituents) that are mainly responsible for the characteristic smells of the different strains/cultivars of cannabis. For example, where there is a predominance of the terpene limonene, the plant will have a lemon scent [12]. The two most abundant terpenes in *Cannabis sativa* are the two monoterpenes α-pinene and limonene, followed by myrcene [12]. However, monoterpenes evaporate, faster than other components, and the composition of the essential oils in the harvested plant may differ from that of the fresh plant, as may the odour [12].

### Actions of Terpenes

Terpenes are lipophilic and have many sites of action including neurotransmitter receptors, muscle and neuronal ion channels, G-protein receptors, enzymes, cell membranes and second messenger systems [26]. Several terpenes such as α-humulene, geraniol, linalool and β-pinene have been found to produce cannabinoid tetrad behaviors in mice (antinociception, hypolocomotion, catalepsy, and hypothermia), suggesting they behave like cannabinoids (ie. they have cannabimimetic activity). In vitro experiments also showed that these same terpenes all activated the CB1 receptor, while some activated other targets such as A2a receptors [154]. Terpenes may influence the binding of THC to CB1 receptors. They can also interact with other neurotransmitter receptors that contribute to cannabinoid-mediated analgesia effects [26]. Terpenes, in particular, are thought to contribute to the 'entourage effect' in which there is synergism between active constituents which are likely to be responsible for the therapeutic efficacy of cannabis and mitigation of side effects of dominant active ingredients such as THC [155]. This notion of an entourage effect finds support in recent research that found that the cannabinometic activity demonstrated in mice (cannabinoid tetrad behaviours) treated with α-humulene, geraniol, linalool, and β-pinene were selectively additive with a CB1 receptor agonist (WIN55,212), suggesting terpenes can increase cannabinoid activity [154].

Most of the research evidence in relation to the therapeutic actions of terpenes comes from preclinical research (cell lines, animals). Terpenes have several

**Table 4.3** Key terpenes and their therapeutic actions

| Terpene | Therapeutic actions |
|---|---|
| **α-pinene** | Anti-cancer, anti-inflammatory, antioxidant, analgesic, anxiolytic and hypnotic effects<br>Can increase non-rapid eye movement (NREM) sleep without affecting the REM and delta activity<br>In humans, it has been found to be a bronchodilator at low levels and a broad-spectrum antibiotic against methicillin-resistant *Staphylococcus aureus* [153]. |
| **β-caryophyllene** | Cardio-protective, hepatoprotective, gastroprotective, neuroprotective, nephroprotective, anti-convulsive, anti-inflammatory, anti-cancer, analgesic, anxiolytic, antidepression and immunomodulatory actions [26, 153, 156, 157, 158, 159, 153, 160]. Potent anti-inflammatory via PGE-1; gastric cytoprotective activities [161]<br>Anti-fungal, anti-bacterial (*S. aureus*), anti-malarial, anti-pruritic in contact dermatitis and can inhibit colitis in a mice model [26]<br>Selectively binds to CB2 receptors [161]. It is the only terpene that can act as an agonist of CB2 receptors, though it also acts on other receptors also [153]<br>Can sensitise cancer cells to conventional cancer drugs [159, 162]<br>Shows promise in treatment of Parkinson's disease [153]<br>PPAR alpha agonist [163]<br>PPAR gamma agonist [163] |
| **umulene (α-caryophyllene)** | Anti-cancer, anti-allergic, anti-bacterial, anti-nociceptive, analgesic<br>Strong anti-inflammatory properties [26, 153] |
| **Limonene** | Anxiolytic, antidepressant, stress reducing<br>Anti-convulsant<br>Anti-cancer and anti-tumour actions in several cancer cell lines<br>Can promote wound healing and anabolism<br>Reduces inflammation, oxidative stress<br>Ameliorates viral infections<br>Immuno-stimulating properties [153, 161] |

**Table 4.3** (continued)

| Terpene | Therapeutic actions |
|---|---|
| **Linalool** (also found in lavender) | Research suggests that linalool is the active ingredient in lavender that confers its anti-inflammatory, anti-nociceptive, anti-bacterial, antioxidant, neuroprotective, hepato-protective, analgesic, sedative, anti-tumour, anti-convulsive, anti-microbial, antidepressant, sedative, anti-stress, anxiolytic and mood-stabilising effects [26, 153]<br>Several anti-cancer effects [153] |
| **Myrcene**[a] | Anti-inflammatory, antioxidant, analgesic, sedative, hypnotic, sleep promoting, muscle relaxant, anxiolytic, neuroprotection, anti-ulcer (gastric), anti-mutagenic<br>Protects the skin against photo-ageing<br>Potential anti-osteoarthritic action [26, 153] |
| **Nerolidol** (also present as a low-level component in orange and other citrus peels) [27] | Sedative effect [164]<br>Enhances skin penetration of 5-fluorouracil [165]<br>Inhibits growth of leishmaniasis [166]<br>Anti-parasitic [167], anti-fungal [168], antimicrobial [169]<br>Anti-cancer actions found in two human carcinoma cell lines [170]; cytotoxic to human leukaemia HL60 cells [171] and found to inhibit colon carcinogenesis in a rat model [172] |

[a]A review did not support the notion that the combination of myrcene and THC induces a strong sedative effect ('couch lock') [153].

therapeutic actions including anti-inflammatory, anxiolytic, inducing apoptosis in breast cancer cells, broad-spectrum antibiotic and others [27]. Research indicates that terpenes may –increase blood-brain barrier permeability – this has led to a patent for a transdermal cannabinoid patch using a terpene as permeation agent [26].

There are several terpenes which have an effect on our emotions. For example, D-limonene has been found to be anxiolytic (human studies), reduces stress, depression, whilst B-myrcene has been found to be anxiolytic, sedative, hypnotic and sleep promoting, as well has having many other therapeutic actions [26, 153]. Table 4.3 sets out some of the terpenes and their therapeutic actions.

## Forms of Medicinal Cannabis

Medicinal cannabis comes in many forms. It may be used raw, for example, juiced. It may be dried and smoked, just as it is when used for 'adult use'. The dried buds may also be vaped (placed in a vaporising unit) and inhaled that way. Major proprietary forms of medicinal cannabis include the following:

1. Cannabis-based liquid extracts: nabiximols (a combination of equal parts THC and CBD)
2. Phytocannabinoid botanicals: dense cannabis extracts manufactured as capsules, pills, sublingual sprays, suppositories, transdermal patches and topical ointments
3. Single molecule drugs: synthetic or semi-synthetic prescription drugs (e.g. nabilone, dronabinol which are FDA-approved) [14].

Many proprietary forms of medicinal cannabis products contain a mixture of two of the main active constituents, THC and CBD in varying ratios. Some contain CBD alone (no THC) commonly referred to as an 'isolate' product. Whole plant medicines (phytocannabinoid botanicals) typically contain other cannabinoids, terpenes and other plant constituents. Similarly, 'full spectrum' extracts will contain a whole plant blend while 'broad spectrum' generally means whole plant but with no appreciable THC.

## Oils Are Not Oils

Much has been written about the 'entourage effect' discussed previously. This term essentially means that those other active constituents, such as terpenes and other phytocannabinoids (other than THC, CBD), contribute to the overall therapeutic action of the key active constituent(s). Such a concept is the basis for understanding how herbal medicines work. It is the synergism between active constituents within a plant that are probably the reason for its efficacy. In Chinese herbal medicine, where typically several different herbs are prescribed in a medicinal formula (tailored for the individual in terms of dosage and types of herbs), it is also the synergy between the herbs that is responsible for the therapeutic efficacy of the formula [173].

The problem that we see with the medicinal cannabis industry, at least in some countries where the industry is less mature, is the lack of knowledge by prescribers about the differences, therapeutically speaking, of different varieties or cultivars of cannabis and the lack of differentiation of cannabis oil products by cannabis companies. This is certainly evident in Australia (which only legalized medicinal use of cannabis in 2016) in relation to cannabis oil products where the ratio of CBD to THC is often the main differentiating factor (though some companies are making a feature of their minor phytocannabinoids and terpenes). Yet, one only has to listen to a good budtender or read Michael Backe's book *Cannabis Pharmacy* to realise that various cultivars have quite different effects, and it is likely this is due to more than the THC and CBD ratios. Things are changing fast in Australia, however, with a rise in popularity of vaporizing cannabis flower as a route of delivery over the past two years. This is likely to be patient-driven. In Australia we are now seeing cannabis companies advertising the relative proportions of 'sativa' and 'indica' in their flower strains as well as key terpenes, with descriptions of their various effects. Sativa-dominant varieties/strains are understood to have a more energizing and uplifting effect whilst indica-dominant strains are understood to be more calming, relaxing and sedative, however Backes argues that the descriptors are correct but the nomenclature wrong [30]. His argument is based on taxonomy. Nonetheless, this nomenclature appears to have stuck, for the time being at least.

The future is likely to be genetic testing to identify single nucleotide polymorphisms (SNPs, pronounced 'snips') for particular genes coding for various parts of the endocannabinoid system, as well as those that indicate a propensity to anxiety, depression and other states, and the matching of cultivars or strains in cannabis products to such SNPs.

## A Gap in Our Knowledge: Lack of Studies in Whole Plant Extracts

Much of the data we have on efficacy and safety come from RCTs assessing synthetic forms of medicinal cannabis (e.g. dronabinol) or limited forms of proprietary medicinal cannabis medicines such as nabiximols (combination of CBD and THC in an almost 1:1 ratio) rather than whole plant extracts of specific cultivars. Animal research tends to use pure isolates of CBD and THC in their investigations, reflective of a reductionist approach that typifies the drug-discovery model. The research focus on synthetic forms is understandable since pharmaceutical companies are able to patent these (and they have deep pockets).

There is a dearth of studies which have compared a whole plant extract with a plant isolate or a pharmaceutical drug (e.g. dronabinol, synthetic THC) in terms of efficacy and safety, though one meta-analysis has attempted to do so [174]. Such study designs are needed, albeit these are more complex and therefore more costly. Psychological effects have been found to occur more frequently with THC than whole cannabis [175]. This is likely to be due to the fact that other constituents of cannabis such as CBD and tetrahydrocannabivarin (THCV) work to mitigate the undesirable effects of THC as well as improving its therapeutic capacity [29].

### Superiority of Whole Spectrum CBD Over Pure CBD Isolate Demonstrated

A study in mice compared the effects of pure CBD isolate compared to a standardised CBD-rich plant extract in terms of its ant-inflammatory and analgesic effects. Mice were given these either intraperitoneally or orally. In terms of anti-inflammatory and anti-nociceptive effects, the pure CBD isolate was associated with a bell-shaped dose-response curve, whereas the dose-response curve for the plant extract was linear, with increasing responses on increasing doses (both oral and intraperitoneal administration). The plant extract reduced zymosan-induced paw swelling and pain in the mice and prevented in vivo TNF-α production and was more efficient in alleviating pain than the pure CBD isolate ($p = 0.01$). Significant pain relief was obtained at a dose of around 10 mg/kg CBD for the plant extract, whereas 25 mg/kg of pure CBD isolate was needed to achieve the same effect. The authors concluded that the other components in the plant synergise with CBD to achieve the anti-inflammatory and analgesic actions noted [176].

### Dangers of Meta-Analyses

There is a danger with meta-analyses in relation to summarising evidence about medicinal cannabis. Meta-analysis is a statistical method of pooling data from separate RCTs to answer, from a statistical point of view, a question. Typically, this question is around efficacy, but it can also be applied to safety. In medicine, meta-analyses are considered the 'gold standard' in a hierarchy of evidence; however, both RCTs and meta-analyses are fundamentally limited in terms of applicability and methodological issues, including various forms of bias [177–179]. Synthetic cannabinoids and single isolates are likely to act very differently in the body to whole plant extracts and if meta-analyses aggregate data from different forms, then we can lose very valuable information and reach erroneous conclusions.

We will investigate what the literature says in relation to efficacy (and where available, safety) of whole plants versus isolates and synthetic cannabinoids for different mental health conditions in the individual chapters.

## Routes of Delivery and Pharmacokinetics

The topic 'Routes of Delivery and Pharmacokinetics' is covered extensively in Chap. 11. What follows here is a quick summary of key points.

The various forms of delivery include the following:

1. **Inhaled:** smoking, vaporising (vaping)
2. **Oral:** liquid, edibles, tablets, capsules, sprays, fresh juice
3. **Topical:** creams, balms, patches
4. **Other:** intranasal, suppositories (rectal, vaginal)

Each of these delivery methods has particular advantages, depending on the clinical condition involved and the patient's preference. Essentially, for a rapid action, routes that bypass the first-pass mechanism of the liver and deliver the active ingredients of the medicinal cannabis product into the bloodstream (e.g. inhalation, sublingual wafers or sprays, oromucosal sprays, intranasal sprays) are preferred. For a longer duration of action, oral routes of delivery are preferred and are convenient.

### Inhalation

Smoking heats cannabis to high temperatures, 600–900 °C. Smoking cannabis is associated with toxic by-products including tar, PAH (polycyclic aromatic hydrocarbons), carbon monoxide (CO) and ammonia (NH3). Chronic use has been found to be associated with respiratory symptoms including cough, bronchitis and increased phlegm, but there is no evidence that it causes lung cancer or chronic obstructive airway disease (COPD) [124, 125].

Vaporising or vaping heats cannabis at a lower temperature (160–230 °C). It has some advantages over smoking in that there is no side stream smoke (and thus fewer concerns about passive smoking), it has fewer toxins (CO is reduced, though PAHs are not completely eliminated), it produces much less harmful by-products and fewer pulmonary symptoms are reported [124].

Advantages to smoking and vaporising are that the active constituents pass quickly into the bloodstream via the highly vascularised lung tissue, bypassing the 'first-pass mechanism' of the liver. Thus, onset of action is faster than with the oral route which may be advantageous for treating acute exacerbations of symptoms/signs (e.g. pain and nausea).

## Oral Route

Oral routes of delivery of cannabis include oils, capsules, tinctures, lozenges, edibles, juicing fresh plants and cannabis teas. Nabiximols is an oromucosal spray which delivers a standardised dose of CBD and THC [124]. Sublingual wafers that deliver via the sublingual blood vessels are also on the market. The oral route has the advantage of convenience, and their duration of action is much longer than smoking/vaporising. Thus, these may be more advantageous for treatment of chronic illnesses.

## Topical Route, Other Routes

Topicals are ideal for localised symptoms including skin conditions and arthritis, though there is less research available with respect to efficacy [124]. Suppositories may be indicated for treatment of specific conditions (e.g. rectal cancer). However, there is variable absorption [124]. The intranasal route is another potential delivery form.

## Bioavailability of CBD

Bioavailability of CBD are much higher with inhalation compared with oral administration [110]. CBD bioavailability following inhalation has been found in one study to be 31% [180]. Other studies have suggested it is similar to that of THC [181]. CBD has a low and highly variable oral bioavailability, estimated at 6–10% due to the first-pass mechanism of the liver [110], though some studies have reported figures of 13–19% [182]. In a study of the intranasal delivery of CBD in rats, bioavailability was 34–46% [183].

## Bioavailability and Onset and Duration of Action of THC

The bioavailability for inhalation of THC is variable, somewhere between 10 and 35% [155, 161, 180, 184–186]. The bioavailability of oral consumption of THC is between 4% and 20% and is lower than for inhalation [187], due to the fact that the cannabinoids undergo extensive first-pass metabolism by CYP450 genes in the liver, prior to entering the systemic circulation [110].

Onset of action of inhaled THC (5–10 min) is much quicker than the oral route (between 30 and 80 min) [124]. Duration of effects are longer for oral administration of THC (6–8 h) compared with inhalation (2–4 h) [124, 188], and this can be an advantage in treating more chronic conditions.

See the Chap. 12 at the back of this book for a comprehensive exploration of metabolism and pharmacokinetics of cannabis.

## Safety

The topic of safety is covered extensively in Chap. 11.

## Going Forward: The United Nations and the Single Convention

Statutory forms of regulation should be about safety, and not about political agendas. More broadly on the world level, cannabis and cannabis resin were until recently included in Schedule IV, with extracts and tinctures included in Schedule I of the Single Convention on Narcotic Drugs, as amended by the 1972 Protocol (the 'Single Convention') [189].

The majority of the member countries of the United Nations (UN), including Australia, are parties or signatories to the 'Single Convention'. This convention is an international treaty to control the production, trade and use of specific drugs, that is, narcotics and drugs with similar effects. Parties to the Single Convention are required to establish or adjust national legislation to conform to the requirements of the Single Convention.

The Single Convention's Schedules of drugs range from most to least restrictive, in this order: Schedule IV, Schedule I, Schedule II, Schedule III. Under the Single Convention, Schedule IV drugs [189] are those with strong addiction-producing properties or have a high liability of abuse that cannot be offset by medical benefits or that poses a risk too great to public health to hazard using them commonly in medical practice. Drugs in Schedule IV are subject to the same controls applicable to Schedule I drugs [190].

In June 2018, the World Health Organization (WHO) Expert Committee on Drug Dependence (ECDD) recommended that preparations considered to be pure CBD not be placed under international drug control as the substance was not found to have psychoactive properties and presents no potential for abuse or dependence [191].

At the end of 2020, the Commission on Narcotic Drugs voted to remove cannabis and cannabis resin from Schedule IV of the Single Convention, though it remains on Schedule I. They rejected the WHO recommendation that CBD (with 0.2% or less THC) should not be subject to international controls (https://news.un.org/en/story/2020/12/1079132).

We thus still have some ways to go.

## Conclusion

Cannabis has been used for thousands of years medicinally by humans. It is a valuable herbal medicine. Key active constituents include phytocannabinoids, terpenes and other plant nutrients. It is likely that the synergy between the active constituents is responsible for its therapeutic actions. Medicinal cannabis comes in many different forms. Medicinal cannabis is not one 'thing'. There are cannabis-based products, whole plant extracts and synthetic copies of key molecules such as THC. Proprietary products tend to differ in the amounts of key phytocannabinoids, THC and CBD. There are different methods of delivery including inhalation, oral administration, external application and others. Ideally, the choice of product and delivery route will depend on the condition and individual preference.

Cannabis has been demonised in the USA and other western countries over the past hundred years, unfairly so, and the political fighting continues around the world. Regulatory changes are occurring worldwide, with more countries opening up access, at least to medicinal cannabis.

## References


1. Hyman SM, Sinha R. Stress-related factors in cannabis use and misuse: implications for prevention and treatment. J Subst Abus Treat. 2009;36(4):400–13.
2. Korem N, Zer-Aviv TM, Ganon-Elazar E, et al. Targeting the endocannabinoid system to treat anxiety-related disorders. J Basic Clin Physiol Pharmacol. 2016;27(3):193–202.
3. Johnston LD, O'Malley PM. Why do the nations's students use drugs and alcohol? Self-reported reasons from nine national surveys. J Drug Issues. 1986;16(1):29–66.
4. Webb CW, Webb SM. Therapeutic benefits of cannabis: a patient survey. Hawaii J Med Public Health 2014;73(4):109–11.
5. Sexton M, Cuttler C, Finnell J, Mischley L. A cross-sectional survey of medical cannabis users: patterns of use and perceived efficacy. Cannabis Cannabinoid Res. 2016;1:131–8.
6. Arthritis Foundation. Patients tell us about CBD use. Available at: http://blog.arthritis.org/news/patients-tell-us-cbd-use/. Accessed 3 Dec 2019.
7. Lintzeris N, Davis J, Elias N, et al. Medicinal cannabis in Australia 2016: the Cannabis as Medicine Survey (CAMS-16). Med J Aust. 2018;209(5):211–6.
8. Bonn-Miller MO, Vujanovic AA, Drescher KD. Cannabis use among military veterans after residential treatment for posttraumatic stress disorder. Psychol Addict Behav. 2011;25:485–91.
9. Cougle JR, Bonn-Miller MO, Vujanovic AA, et al. Posttraumatic stress disorder and cannabis use in a nationally representative sample. Psychol Addict Behav. 2011;25(3):554–8.
10. Kervorkian S, Bonn-Miller MO, Belendiuk K, et al. Associations among trauma, posttraumatic stress disorder, cannabis us, and cannabis use disorder in a nationally representative epidemiologic sample. Psychol Addict Behav. 2015;29:633–8.
11. Pollio A. The name of *cannabis*: a short guide for nonbotanists. Cannabis Cannabinoid Res. 2016;1(1):234–8.
12. World Health Organization (WHO). World Health Organization Expert Committee on drug dependence pre-review. Cannabis plant and cannabis resin. Geneva: World Health Organization; 2018a.
13. Li H. An archaeological and historical account of cannabis in China. Econ Bot. 1974;28:437–48.
14. Jarvis S, Rassmussen S, Winters B. Role of the endocannabinoid system and medical cannabis. JNP. 2017;13(8):525–31.
15. Okazaki H, Kobayashi M, Momohara A, et al. Early Holocene coastal environment change inferred from deposits at Okinoshima archeological site, Boso Peninsula, central Japan. Quat Int. 2011;230:87–94.
16. Pisanti S, Bifulco M. Medical Cannabis: a plurimillennial history of an evergreen. J Cell Physiol. 2019;234(6):8342–51.
17. Abel EL. Marijuana, the first twelve thousand years. New York: Plenum Press; 1980.
18. Touwn M. The religious and medicinal uses of cannabis in China, India and Tibet. J Psychoactive Drugs. 1981;13:23–34.

19. Russo EB. The pharmacological history of cannabis. 2014. Available at: https://www.researchgate.net/publication/312414874_The_pharmacological_history_of_cannabis#fullTextFileContent. Accessed 21 Jan 2021.
20. Boninni SA, Premoli M, Tambaro S, et al. Cannabis sativa: a comprehensive ethnopharmacological review of a medicinal plant with a long history. J Ethnopharmacol. 2018;117:300–3015.
21. Lee MA. Smoke signals: a social history of Marijuana - Medical, recreational and scientific. US: Scribner; 2012.
22. Pamploma FA, Takahashi RN. Psychopharmacology of the endocannabinoids: far beyond anandamide. J Psychopharmacol. 2012;26(1):7–22.
23. Lava N. Medical Marijuana FAQ. WebMD Medical Reference Sources. 15 Dec 2018. Available at: https://www.webmd.com/a-to-z-guides/qa/what-us-states-have-legalized-medical-marijuana. Accessed 5 Sept 2019.
24. Marijuana Break. How many states is recreational marijuana legal in? 30 July 2019. Available at: https://www.marijuanabreak.com/how-many-states-have-recreational-weed. Accessed 5 Sept 2019.
25. Amin MR, Ali DW. Pharmacology of medical cannabis. Adv Exp Med Biol. 2019;1162:151–65.
26. Baron EP. Medicinal properties of cannabinoids, terpenes, and flavonoids in cannabis, and benefits in migraine, headache, and pain: an update on current evidence and cannabis science. Headache. 2018;58:1139–86.
27. Russo EB. Taming THC: potential cannabis synergy and phytocannabinoid-terpenoid entourage effects. Brit J Pharmacol. 2011;163:1344–64.
28. Russo EB. Cannabis therapeutics and the future of neurology. Front Integr Neurosci. 2018;12:51.
29. McPartland JM, Duncan M, Di Marzo V, Pertwee R. Are cannabidiol and Δ9-tetrahydrocannabivarin negative modulators of the endocannabinoid system? A systematic review. Br J Pharmacol. 2015;172:737–53.
30. Backes M. Cannabis pharmacy. New York: Black Dog & Leventhal Publishers; 2017.
31. Rahn B. Cannabis genotypes and phenotypes: what makes a cannabis strain unique? 14 April, 2014. Available at: https://www.leafly.com/news/growing/cannabis-genotypes-and-phenotypes-what-makes-a-strain-unique. Accessed 9 Aug 2020.
32. Magagnini G, Grassi G, Kotiranta S. The effect of light spectrum on the morphology and cannabinoid content of Cannabis sativa L. Med Cannabis Cannabinoids. 2018;1:19–27.
33. Pate DW. Chemical ecology of cannabis. J Int Hemp Assoc. 1994;2(29):32–7.
34. McPartland JM. Cannabis as repellent and pesticide. J Int Hemp Assoc. 1997;4:87–92.
35. Appendino G, Gibbons S, Giana A, et al. Antibacterial cannabinoids from Cannabis sativa: a structure activity study. J Nat Prod. 2008;71:1427–30.
36. Hanus LO, Meyer SM, Munoz E, et al. Phytocannabinoids: a unified critical inventory. Nat Prod Rep. 2016;33(12):1357–92.
37. World Health Organization (WHO). World Health Organization Expert Committee on drug dependence pre-review. Delta-9-Tetrahydrocannabinol. Geneva: World Health Organization; 2018b.
38. Lafaye G, Karila LM, Blecha L, Amine B. Cannabis, cannabinoids, and health. Dialgoues Clini Neurosci. 2017;19:309–16.
39. Blaskovich MAT, Kavanagh AM, Elliott AG, et al. The antimicrobial potential of cannabidiol. Commun Biol. 2021;4:7. https://doi.org/10.1038/s42003-020-01530-y.
40. Kosgodage US, Mould R, Henley AB, et al. Cannabidiol (CBD) is a novel inhibitor for exosome and microvesicle (emv) release in cancer. Cancer Front Pharmacol. 2018;9:889.
41. Kosgodage US, Matewele P, Awamaria B, et al. Cannabidiol is a novel modulator of bacterial membrane vesicles. Front Cell Infect Microbiol. 2019;9:324. https://doi.org/10.3389/fcimb.2019.00324
42. Maroon J, Bost J. Review of the neurological benefits of phytocannabinoids. Surg Neurol Int. 2018;9:91.

43. World Health Organization (WHO). World Health Organization Expert Committee on Drug Dependence. Cannabidiol (CBD) Critical Review Report. Expert Committee on Drug Dependence Fortieth Meeting Geneva, 4–7 June 2018. World Health Organization (WHO), 2018c. Available at: https://www.who.int/medicines/access/controlled-substances/CannabidiolCriticalReview.pdf.
44. Olah A, Toth BI, Borbiro I, et al. Cannabidiol exerts sebostatic and anti-inflammatory effects on human sebocytes. J Clin Invest. 2014;124(9):3713–24.
45. Spelman L, Sinclair R, Freeman M, et al. The safety of topical cannabidiol (CBD) for the treatment of acne. J Investig Dermaol. 2018;138(5):S180.
46. Aran A, Cassuto H, Lubotzky A. Cannabidiol based medical cannabis in children with autism- a retrospective feasibility study. Neurology. 2018;90(15 Suppl):P3.318.
47. Barchel D, Stolar O, De-Haan T, et al. Oral cannabidiol use in children with autism spectrum disorder to treat related symptoms and co-morbidities. Front Pharmacol. 2018;9:1521.
48. Bar-Lev Schleiber L, Mechoulam R, Saban N, et al. Real life experience of medical cannabis treatment in autism: analysis of safety and efficacy. Sci Rep. 2019;9(1):1–7.
49. Bergamaschi MM, Queiroz RH, Chagas MH, et al. Cannabidiol reduces the anxiety induced by simulated public speaking in treatment-naïve social phobia patients. Neuropsychopharmacology. 2011;36(6):1219–26.
50. Shannon S, Lewis N, Lee H, Hughes S. Cannabidiol in anxiety and sleep: a large case series. Perm J. 2019;23:18–041.
51. Carroon J, Philips JA. A cross-sectional study of cannabidiol users. Cannabis Cannabinoid Res. 2018;3(1):152–61.
52. Sales AJ, Carlos CC, Guimares FS, Joca RL. Antidepressant-like effect induced by Cannabidiol is dependent on brain serotonin levels. Prog Neuropsychopharmacol Biol Psychiatry. 2018;86:255–61.
53. Das RK, Kamboj SK, Ramadas M, et al. Cannabidiol enhances consolidation of explicit fear extinction in humans. Psychopharmacology. 2013;226(4):781–92.
54. Zlebnik N, Cheer JF. Beyond the CB1 receptor: is cannabidiol the answer for disorders of motivation? Annu Rev Neurosci. 2016;39:1–17.
55. Leweke FM, Mueller JK, Lange B, Rohleder C. Therapeutic potential of cannabinoids in psychosis. Biol Psychiatry. 2016;79(7):604–12.
56. Kusminski CM, Mcternan PG, Kumar S. Role of resistin in obesity, insulin resistance and Type II diabetes. Clin Sci. 2005;109(3):243–56.
57. Stanley CP, Wheal AJ, Randall MD, Sullican SE. Cannabinoids alter endothelial function in the Zucker rat model of type 2 diabetes. Eur J Pharmacol. 2013;720:376–82.
58. Devinsky O, Cilio MR, Cross H, et al. Cannabidiol: pharmacology and potential therapeutic role in epilepsy and other neuropsychiatric disorders. Epilepsia. 2014;55:791–802.
59. Devinsky O, Marsh E, Friedman D, et al. Cannabidiol in patients with treatment-resistant epilepsy: an open-label interventional trial. Lancet Neurol. 2016;15(3):270–8.
60. Devinsky O, Cross JH, Laux L, et al. Trial of cannabidiol for drug-resistant seizures in the Dravet syndrome. N Engl J Med. 2017;376:2011–20.
61. Devinsky O, Nabbout R, Miller I, et al. Long-term cannabidiol treatment in patients with Dravet syndrome: an open-label extension trial. Epilepsia. 2019;60(2):294–302.
62. Hofmann ME, Frazier CJ. Marijuana, endocannabinoids and epilepsy: potential and challenges for improved therapeutic intervention. Exp Neurol. 2013;244:43–50.
63. Jones NA, Hill AJ, Smith SA, et al. Cannabidiol displays antiepileptiform and antiseizure properties in vitor and in vivo. J Pharmacol Exp Ther. 2010;332(2):569–77.
64. Irving PM, Iqbal T, Nwokolo C, et al. A randomised double-blind, placebo-controlled, parallel group, pilot study of cannabidiol-rich botanical extract in the symptomatic treatment of ulcerative colitis. Inflamm Bowel Dis. 2018;24:714–24.
65. de Lago E, Fernandez-Ruiz J. Cannabinoids and neuroprotection in motor-related disorders. CNS Neurol Disord Drug Targets. 2007;6(6):377–87.
66. Iuvone T, Esposito G, De Filippis D, et al. Cannabidiol: a promising drug for neurodegenerative disorders? CNS Neurosci Ther. 2009;15(1):65–75.

67. Lakhan SE, Rowland M. Whole plant cannabis extracts in the treatment of spasticity in multiple sclerosis: a systematic review. BMC Neurol. 2009;9:59.
68. Bolognini D, Rock EM, Cluny NL, et al. Cannabidiolic acid prevents vomiting in *Suncus murinus* and nausea-induced behaviour in rats by enhancing 5-$HT_{1A}$ receptor activation. Br J Pharmacol. 2013;168(6):1456–70.
69. Parker LA. Cannabinoids & emotional regulation. In: Cannabinoids and the brain. MIT Press; 2017.
70. Dash R, Ali C, Jahan I, et al. Emerging potential of cannabidiol in reversing proteinopathies. Ageing Res Rev. 2021;65:101209.
71. Carrier EJ, Auchampach JA, Hillard CJ. Inhibition of an equilibrative nucleoside transporter by cannabidiol: a mechanism of cannabinoid immunosuppression. Proc Natl Acad Sci. 2006;103:7895–900.
72. Pucci M, Rapino C, Di Francesco A, et al. Epigenetic control of skin differentiation genes by phytocannabinoids. Br J Pharmacol. 2013;170:581–91.
73. Wilkinson JD, Williamson EM. Cannabinlids inhibit human keratinocyte proliferation through a non-CB1/CB2 mechanism and have a potential therapeutic value in the treatment of psoriasis. J Dermatol Sci. 2007;45(2):87–92.
74. Bih CI, Chen T, Nunn AVW, et al. Molecular targets of cannabidiol in neurological disorders. Neurotherapeutics. 2015;12(4):699–730.
75. Pisanti S, Malfitano AM, Ciaglia E, et al. Cannabidiol: state of the art and new challenges for therapeutic applications. Pharmacol Ther. 2017;175:133–50.
76. Campos AC, Moreira FA, Gomes FV, et al. Multiple mechanisms involved in the large-spectrum therapeutic potential of cannabidiol in psychiatric disorders. Philos Trans R Soc Lond Ser B Biol Sci. 2012;367(1607):3364–78.
77. Ney LJ, Matthews A, Bruno R, Felmingham KL. Cannabinoid interventions for PTSD: where to next? Prog Neuropsychopharmacol Biol Psychiatry. 2019;93:124–40.
78. Nichols JM, Kaplan BLF. Immune responses regulated by cannabidiol. Cannabis Cannabinoid Res. 2019;5(1):12–31. https://doi.org/10.1089/can.2018.0073.
79. Ligresti A, De Petrocellis L, Di Marzo V. From phytocannabinoids to cannabinoid receptors and endocannabinoids: pleiotropic physiological and pathological roles through complex pharmacology. Physiol Rev. 2016;96(4):1593–659.
80. Mechoulam R, Peters M, Murillo-Rodriguez E, Hanus L. Cannabidiol-recent advances. Chem Biodivers. 2007;4(8):1678–92.
81. Stanley CP, Hind WH, O'Sullivan SE. Is the cardiovascular system a therapeutic target for cannabidiol? Br J Clin Pharmacol. 2012;75(2):313–22.
82. Long LE, Chesworth R, Huang X-F, et al. A behavioural comparison of acute and chronic $\Delta^9$-tetrahydrocannabinol and cannabidiol in C57BL/6JArc mice. Int J Neuropscychopharmacol. 2010;13(7):861–76.
83. Elmes MW, Kaczocha M, Berger WT, et al. Fatty acid-binding proteins (FABPS) are intracellular carriers for $\Delta^9$-Tetrahydrocannabinol (THC) and Cannabidiol (CBD). J Biol Chem. 2015;290(14):8711–21.
84. Bisogno T, Hanus L, de Petrocellis L, et al. Molecular targets for cannabidiol and its synthetic analogues: effects in vanilloid VR1 receptors and on the cellular uptake and enzymatic hydrolysis of anadamide. Br J Pharmacol. 2001;134:845–52.
85. Iannotti FA, Hill CL, Leo A, et al. Nonpsychotropc plant cannabinoids, cannabidivarin (CBDV) and cannabdiol (CBD) activate and desensitize transient receptor potential vanilloid 1 (TRPV1) channels in vitro: potential for the treatment of neuronal hyperexcitability. ACS Chem Neurosci. 2014;5(11):1131–41.
86. Esposito G, Scuderi C, Valenza M, et al. Cannabidiol reduces Aβ-induced neuroinflammation and promotes hippocampal neurogenesis through PPARγ involvement. PLoS One. 2011;6(12):e28668.
87. Tutunchi H, Ostadrahimi A, Saghafi-Asl M, Maleki V. The effects of oleoylethanolamide, an endogenous PPAR-α agonist, on risk factors for NAFLD: A systematic review. Obes Rev. 2019;20(7):1057–69.

88. Brown JD, Winterstein AG. Potential adverse drug events and drug-drug interactions with medical and Consumer Cannabidiol (CBD) use. J Clin Med. 2019;8(7):989.
89. Kaplan J. What is the GPR55 receptor and why is it important in CBD's benefits? April 4, 2018. Leafly. Available at: https://www.leafly.com/news/science-tech/health-benefits-cbd-on-g-protein-coupled-receptor-55. Accessed 3 Dec 2019.
90. Hasenoehrl C, Feuersinger D, Sturm EM, et al. G protein-coupled receptor GPR55 promotes colorectal cancer and has opposing effects to cannabinoid receptor 1. Int J Cancer. 2018;142(1):121–32.
91. Lanuti M, Talamonti E, Baccarrone M, Chiurchiu V. Activation of GPR55 receptors exacerbates oxldl-induced lipid accumulation and inflammatory responses, while reducing cholesterol efflux from human macrophages. PLoS One. 2015;10(5):e0126839.
92. Wlodarczyk M, Sobolewska-Wlodarczyk A, Cygankiewicz AI, et al. G protein-coupled receptor 55 (GPR55) expresses differently in patients with Crohn's disease and ulcerative colitis. Scand J Gastroenterol. 2017;52(6–7):711–5.
93. Zhou XL, Guo X, Song YP, et al. The LPI/GPR55 axis enhances human breast cancer cell migration via HBXIP and p-MLC signaling. Acta Pharmacol Sin. 2018;39(3):459–71.
94. Kaplan JS, Stella N, Catterall WA, Westenbroek RE. Cannabidiol attenuates seizures and social deficits in a mouse model of Dravet syndrome. PNAS. 2017;114(42):11229–34.
95. Stancic A, Jandl K, Hasenohrl E, et al. The GPR55 antagonist CID16020046 protects against intestinal inflammation. Neurogastroenterol Motil. 2015;27(10):1432–45.
96. Reyes-Resina I, Navarro G, Aguinaga D et al. Molecular and functional interaction between GPR18 and cannabinoid CB 2 G-protein-coupled receptors. Relevance in neurodegenerative diseases. Biochem Pharmacol. 2018;157:169–79.
97. Xiong W, Cheng K, Cui T, et al. Cannabinoid potentiation of glycine receptors contributes to cannabis-induced analgesia. Nat Chem Biol. 2011;7:296–303.
98. Rodríguez-Muñoz M, Onetti Y, Cortés-Montero E, Garzón J, Sánchez-Blázquez P. Cannabidiol enhances morphine antinociception, diminishes NMDA-mediated seizures and reduces stroke damage via the sigma 1 receptor. Mol Brain. 2018;11(1):51.
99. Castillo A, Tolón MR, Fernández-Ruiz J, Romero J, Martinez-Orgado J. The neuroprotective effect of cannabidiol in an in vitro model of newborn hypoxicischemic brain damage in mice is mediated by CB2 and adenosine receptors. Neurobiol Dis. 2010;37:434–40.
100. McKallip RJ, Jia W, Schlomer J, Warren JW, Nagarkatti PS, Nagarkatti M. Cannabidiol-induced apoptosis in human leukemia cells: a novel role of cannabidiol in the regulation of p22phox and Nox4 expression. Mol Pharmacol. 2006;70(3):897–908.
101. Franco R, Villa M, Morales P, et al. Increased expression of cannabinoid CB2 and serotonin 5-HT1A heteroreceptor complexes in a model of newborn hypoxic-ischemic brain damage. Neuropharmacology. 2019;152:58–66.
102. Hampson AJ, Grimaldi M, Axelrod J, Wink D. Cannabidiol and (−)Delta9-tetrahydrocannabinol are neuroprotective antioxidants. Proc Natl Acad Sci U S A. 1998;95(14):8268–73.
103. Ligresti A, Moriello AS, Starowicz K, et al. Antitumour activity of plant cannabinoids with emphasis on the effect of cannabidiol on human breast carcinoma. J Pharmacol Exp Ther. 2006;318:1375–87.
104. Huestis M, Solimini R, Pichini S, et al. Cannabidiol adverse effects and toxicity. Curr Neuropharmacol. 2019;17(10):974–89.
105. Scuderi C, Filippis DD, Iuvone T, et al. Cannabidiol in medicine: a review of its therapeutic potential in CNS disorders. Phytother Res. 2009;23(5):597–602.
106. Camposa AC, Fogac MV, Sonegoa AB, Guimarãesa FS. Cannabidiol, neuroprotection and neuropsychiatric disorders. Pharmacol Res. 2016;112:119–27.
107. Robertson-Gray O, Walsh SK, Ryberg E, et al. l-α-Lysophosphatidylinositol (LPI) aggravates myocardial ischemia/reperfusion injury via a GPR55/ROCK-dependent pathway. Pharmacol Res Perspect. 2019;7(3):e00487.
108. Marcu JP, Christian RT, Lau D et al. Cannabidiol enhances the inhibitory effects of delta9-tetrahydrocannabinol on human glioblastoma cell proliferation and survival. Mol Cancer Ther. 2010;9(1):180–9.

109. Klein C, Karanges E, Spiro A, et al. Cannabidiol potentiates Δ9-tetrahydrocannabinol (THC) behavioural effects and alters THC pharmacokinetics during acute and chronic treatment in adolescent rats. Psychopharmacology. 2011;218:443–57.
110. Nahtigal I, Blake A, Hand A, et al. The pharmacological properties of Cannabis. J Pain Manag. 2016;9(4):481–91.
111. Nadal X, Del-Rio C, Casano S, et al. Tetrahydrocannabinolic acid is a potent PPARγ agonist with neuroprotective activity. Br J Pharmacol. 2017;174(23):4263–76.
112. De Petrocellis L, Ligresti A, Moriello AS, et al. Effects of cannabinoids and cannabinoid-enriched Cannabis extracts on TRP channels and endocannabinoid metabolic enzymes. Br J Pharmacol. 2011;163(7):1479–94.
113. De Petrocellis L, Vellani V, Aniello Schiano-Moriello A, et al. Plant-derived cannabinoids modulate the activity of transient receptor potential channels of ankyrin type-1 and melastatin type-8. J Pharmacol Exp Ther. 2008;325(3):1007–15.
114. Rock EM, Limebeer CL, Navaratnam R, et al. A comparison of cannabidiolic acid with other treatments for anticipatory nausea using a rat model of contextually elicited conditioned gaping. Psychopharmacology. 2014;231:3207–15.
115. Pertwee RG, Rock EM, Guenther K, et al. Cannabidiolic acid methyl ester, a stable synthetic analogue of cannabidiolic acid, can produce $5\text{-HT}_{1A}$ receptor-mediated suppression of nausea and anxiety in rats. Br J Pharmacol. 2018;175(1):100–12.
116. Rock EM, Limebeer CL, Petrie GN, et al. Effect of prior foot shock stress and $\Delta^9$-tetrahydrocannabinol, cannabidiolic acid, and cannabidiol on anxiety-like responding in the light-dark emergence test in rats. Psychopharmacology. 2017;234(14):2207–17.
117. Hen-Shoval D, Amra S, Shbiro L et al. Acute oral Cannabidiolic Acid Methyl Ester reduces depression-like behaviour in two genetic animal models of depression. Behav Brain Res 2018;351;1–3.
118. Rock EM, Limebeer CL, Parker LA. Effect of cannabidiolic acid and $\Delta^9$-tetrahydrocannabinol on carrageenan-induced hyperalgesia and edema in a rodent model of inflammatory pain. Psychopharmacology. 2018;235(11):3259–71.
119. Smeriglio A, Giofre SV, Galati EM, et al. Inhibition of aldose reductase activity by Cannabis sativa chemotypes extracts with high content of cannabidiol or cannabigerol. Fitoterapia. 2018;127:101–8.
120. Takeda S, Okajima S, Miyoshi H, et al. Cannabidiolic acid, a major cannabinoid in fiber-type cannabis, is an inhibitor of MDA-MB-231 breast cancer cell migration. Toxicol Lett. 2012;214(3):314–9.
121. Bilkei-Gorzo A, Albayran O, Draffehn A, et al. A chronic low dose of $\Delta^9$-tetrahydrocannabinol (THC) restores cognitive function in old mice. Nat Med. 2017;23(6):782–7.
122. Evans FJ. Cannabinoids: the separation of central from peripheral effects on a structural basis. Planta Med. 1991;57:S60–7.
123. Lutz B, Marscicano G, Maldonado R, Hillard CJ. The endocannabinoid system in guarding against fear, anxiety and stress. Nat Rev Neurosci. 2015;16:705–18.
124. MacCallum CA, Russo EB. Practical considerations in medical cannabis administration and dosing. Eur J Internal Med. 2018;49:12–9.
125. National Academies of Sciences, Engineering and Medicine. Report. The health effects of cannabis and cannabinoids. Washington DC: The National Academies Press; 2017.
126. Rock EM, et al. Cannabinoid regulation of acute and anticipatory nausea. Cannabis Cannabinoid Res. 2016;1(1):113–21.
127. Russo EB. Cannabinoids in the management of difficult to treat pain. Ther Clin Risk Manag. 2008;4(1):245–59.
128. Torres S, Lorente M, Rodriguez-Formes F, et al. A combined preclinical therapy of cannabinoids and Temozolamide against glioma. Mol Cancer Ther. 2011;10(1):90–103.
129. Mechoulam R, Fride E, Di Marzo V. Endocannabinoids. Eur J Pharmacol. 1998;359:1–18.
130. Gardner EL. Endocannabinoid signaling system and brain reward: Emphasis on dopamine. Pharmacol Biochem Behav. 2005;81:263–84.

131. Pertwee RG, Ross RA. Cannabinoid receptors and their ligands. Prostaglandins Leukot Essent Fatty Acids. 2002;66:101–21.
132. Pisanu A, Acquas E, Feno S, et al. Modulation of A9-THC-induced increase of cortical and hippocampal acetylcholine release by ir opioid and D1 dopamine receptors. Neuropharmacology. 2006;50:661–70.
133. Pistis M, Ferraro L, Pira L, et al. A9-Tetrahydrocannabinol decreases extracellular GABA and increases extracellular glutamate and dopamine levels in the rat prefrontal cortex: an in vivo microdialysis study. Brain Res. 2002;6:155–8.
134. Patel S, Hillard CJ. Pharmacological evaluation of cannabinoid receptor ligands in a mouse model of anxiety: further evidence for an anxiolytic role for endogenous cannabinoid signaling. J Pharmacol Exp Ther. 2006;318:304–11.
135. Jenny M, et al. The potential role of cannabinoids in modulating serotonergic signaling by their influence on tryptophan metabolism. Pharmaceuticals. 2010;3:2647–60.
136. Yuan M, Kiertscher SM, Cheng Q, et al. Delta 9-Tetrahydrocannabinol regulates Th1/Th2 cytokine balance in activated human T cells. J Neuroimmunol. 2002;133:124–31.
137. Sarne Y, Toledano R, Rachmany L, et al. Reversal of age-related cognitive impairments in mice by an extremely low dose of tetrahydrocannabinol. Neurobiol Aging. 2018;61:177–86.
138. Rosenthaler S, Pöhn B, Caroline Kolmanz C et al. Differences in receptor binding affinity of several phytocannabinoids do not explain their effects on neural cell cultures. Neurotoxicol Teratol 2014;46:49–56.
139. Rock EM, Kopstick RL, Limebeer CL, Parker LA. Tetrahydrocannabinolic acid reduces nausea-induced conditioned gaping in rats and vomiting in Suncus murinus. Br J Pharmacol. 2013;170(3):641–8.
140. Moreno-Sanz G. Can You Pass the Acid Test? Critical Review and Novel Therapeutic Perspectives of Δ 9-Tetrahydrocannabinolic Acid. Cannabis Cannabinoid Res. 2016;1(1):124–30.
141. Verhoeckx KC, Korthout HA, van Meeteren-Kreikamp AP et al. Unheated Cannabis sativa extracts and its major compound THC-acid have potential immuno-modulating properties not mediated by CB1 and CB2 receptor coupled pathways. Int Immunopharmacol. International Immunopharmacology 2006; 6(4): 656–65.
142. Tontonoz P, Spiegelman BM. Fat and beyond: the diverse biology of PPAR gamma. Annu Rev Biochem. 2008;77:289–312.
143. Quintanilla RA, Utreras E, Cabezas-Opazo FA. Role of PPAR gamma in the differentiation and function of neurons. PPAR Res. 2014;2014:768594.
144. Palomares B, Ruiz-Pino F, Garrido-Rodriguez M, et al. Tetrahydrocannabinolic acid A (THCA-A) reduces adiposity and prevents metabolic disease caused by diet-induced obesity. Biochem Pharmacol. 2020;171:113693.
145. Moldzio R, Pacher T, Krewenka C, et al. Effects of cannabinolids Delta(9)-tetrahydrocannabinol, Delta(9)-tetrahydrocannabinolic acid and cannabidiol in MMP+ affected murine mesencephalic cultures. Phytomedicine. 2012;19:819–24.
146. Ruhaak LR, Feith J, Karlsson PC, et al. Evaluation of the cyclooxygenase inhibiting effects of six major cannabinoids isolated from Cannabis sativa. Biol Pharm Bull. 2011;34: 774–8.
147. De Petrocellis L, Ligresti A, Schiano Moriello A, et al. Non-THC cannabinoids inhibit prostate carcinoma growth in vitro and in vivo: pro-apoptotic effects and underlying mechanisms. Br J Pharmacol. 2013;168:79–102.
148. Izzo AA, Capasso R, Aviello G, et al. Inhibitory effect of cannabichromene, a major non-psychotropic cannabinoid extracted from Cannabis sativa, on inflammation-induced hypermotility in mice. Br J Pharmacol. 2012;166:1444–60.
149. Maione S, Piscitelli F, Gatta L, et al. Non-psychoactive cannabinoids modulate the descending pathway of antinociception in anaesthetized rats through several mechanisms of action. Br J Pharmacol. 2011;162(3):584–96.

150. Abioye A, Ayodele O, Marinkovic A, et al. Δ9-Tetrahydrocannabivarin (THCV): a commentary on potential therapeutic benefit for the management of obesity and diabetes. J Cannabis Res. 2020;2:6.
151. Riedel G, Fadda P, McKillop-Smith S, et al. Synthetic plant-derived cannabinoid receptor antagonists show hypophagic properties in fasted and non-fasted mice. Br J Pharmacol. 2009;156:1154–566.
152. Wargent ET, Zaibi MS, Silvestri C, et al. The cannabinoid D(9) tetrahydrocannabivarin (THCV) ameliorates insulin sensitivity in two mouse models of obesity. Nutr Diabetes. 2013;3(5):e68.
153. Nuutinen T. Medicinal properties of terpenes found in *Cannabis sativa* and *Humulus lupulus*. Eur J Med Chem. 2018;157:198–228.
154. LaVigne JE, Hecksel R, Keresztes A, Streicher JM. Cannabis sativa terpenes are cannabimimetic and selectively enhance cannabinoid activity. Nature Scientific Reports. 2021;11:8232.
155. McPartland JM, Russo EB. Cannabis and cannabis extracts: greater than the sum of their parts? J Cannabis Ther. 2001;14:103–32.
156. Bahi A, Al Mansouri S, Al Memari E, et al. β-Caryophyllene, a CB2 receptor agonist produces multiple behavioral changes relevant to anxiety and depression in mice. Physiol Behav. 2014;135:119–24.
157. Baldissera MD, Souza CF, Grando TH, et al. B-caryophyllene reduces atherogenic index and coronary risk index in hypercholesterolemic rats: the involvement of cardiac oxidative damage. Chem Biol Interact. 2017;270:9–14.
158. de Oliveira CC, de Oliveira CV, Grigoletto J, et al. Anticonvulsant activity of beta-caryophyllene against pentylenetetrazol-induced seizures. Epilepsy Behav. 2016;56:26–31.
159. Fidyt K, Fiedorowicz A, Strzadala L, Szumny A. B-carophyllene and β-carophyllene oxide-natural compounds of anticancer and analgesic properties. Cancer Med. 2016;5:3007–17.
160. Sharma C, Al Kaabi JM, Nurulain SM, et al. Polypharmacological properties and therapeutic potential of β-caryophyllene: a dietary phytocannabinoid of pharmaceutical promise. Curr Pharm Des. 2016;22:3237–64.
161. Cyr C, Arboleda MF, Aggarwal SK, et al. Cannabis in palliative care: current challenges and practical recommendations. Ann Palliat Med. 2018;7(4):463–77. https://doi.org/10.21037/apm.2018.06.04.
162. Di Giacomo S, Di Sotto A, Mazzanti G, Wink M. Chemosensitizing properties of beta-caryophyllene and beta-caryophyllene oxide in combination with doxorubicin in human cancer cells. Anticancer Rec. 2017;37:1191–6.
163. Youssef DA, El-Fayoumi M, Mahmoud MF. Beta-caryophyllene protects against diet-induced dyslipidemia and vascular inflammation in rats: Involvement of CB2 and PPAR-γ receptors. Chemico-Biological Interactions 2019;297:16–24.
164. Binet L, Binet P, Miocque M, Roux M, Bernier A. Recherches sur les proprietes pharmcodynamiques (action sedative et action spasmolytique) de quelques alcools terpeniques aliphatiques. Ann Pharm Fr. 1972;30:611–6.
165. Cornwell PA, Barry BW. Sesquiterpene components of volatile oils as skin penetration enhancers for the hydrophilic permeant 5-fluorouracil. J Pharm Pharmacol. 1994;46: 261–9.
166. Arruda DC, D'Alexandri FL, Katzin AM, Uliana SRB. Antileishmanial activity of the terpene nerolidol. Antimicrob Agents Chemother. 2005;49(5):1679–87.
167. Abou Laila M, Sivakumar T, Yokoyama N, Igarashi I. Inhibitory effect of terpene nerolidol on the growth of *Babesia* parasites. Parasitol Int. 2010;59(2):278–82.
168. Lee SJ, Han JI, Lee GS, et al. Antifungal effect of eugenol and nerolidol against Microsporum gypseum in a guinea pig model. Biol Pharm Bull. 2007;30(1):184–8.
169. Brehm-Stecher BF, Johnson EA. Sensitization of *Staphylococcus aureus* and *Escherichia coli* to Antibiotics by the Sesquiterpenoids Nerolidol, Farnesol, Bisabolol, and Apritone. Antimicrob Agents Chemother. 2003;47(10):3357–60.
170. Kubo I, Morimitsu Y. Cytotoxicity of green tea flavor compounds against two solid tumor cells. J Agric Food Chem. 1995;43:1626–8.

171. Nibret E, Wink M. Trypanocidal and antileukaemic effects of the essential oils of *Hagenia abyssinica*, *Leonotis ocymifolia*, *Moringa stenopetala*, and their main individual constituents. Phytomedicine. 2010;17:911–20.
172. Wattenberg LW. Inhibition of azoxymethane-induced neoplasia of the large bowel by 3-hydroxy-3,7,11-trimethyl-1,6,10-dodecatriene (nerolidol). Carcinogenesis. 1991;12:151–2.
173. O'Brien KA, Xue CC. The theoretical framework of Chinese medicine. In: Leung P-C, Xue CC, Cheng Y-C, editors. A comprehensive guide to Chinese medicine. 2nd ed. New Jersey: World Scientific Press; 2016.
174. Black N, Stockings E, Campbell G, et al. Cannabinoids for the treatment of mental disorders and symptoms of mental disorders: a systematic review and meta-analysis. Lancet Psychiatry. 2019; https://doi.org/10.1016/S2215-0366(19)30401-8.
175. Grinspoon L, Bakalar JB. Marihuana, the forbidden medicine. New Haven: Yale University Press; 1997.
176. Gallily R, Yekhtin Z, Hanuš LO. Overcoming the bell-shaped dose-response of can- nabidiol by using cannabis extract enriched in cannabidiol. Pharmacol Pharmacy. 2015;6:75–85.
177. Coulter I. Evidence based complementary and alternative medicine. What role for sociology? Annual Conference Australian Sociological Association, University of New England, Armidale, NSW, Australia, 6 Dec 2003.
178. Lewin DI. Meta-analysis: a new standard or clinical fool's gold? J NIH Res. 1996;8: 310–31.
179. Sterne JAC, Gavagha D, Egger. Publication and related bias in meta-analysis: power of statistical tests and prevalence in the literature. Ann Intern Med. 2000;133:420–9.
180. Grotenhermen F. Pharmacokinetics and pharmacodynamics of cannabinoids. Anesthesiology. 1997;86:24–33.
181. Nadulski T, Pragst F, Weinberg G, et al. Randomized, double-blind, placebo controlled study about the effects of cannabidiol (CBD) on the pharmacokinetics of delta9-tetrahydrocannabinol (THC) after oral application of THC verses standardized cannabis extract. Ther Drug Monit. 2005;27:799–810.
182. Mechoulam R, Gallily R. Cannabidiol: an overview of some pharmacological aspects. J Clin Pharmacol. 2002;42:11–9.
183. Paudel KS, Hammell DC, Agu R et al. Cannabidiol bioavailability after nasal and transdermal application: effect of permeation enhancers. Drug Dev Ind Pharm. 2010;36(9):1088–97.
184. Goulle JP, Saussereau E, Lacroix C. Delta-9- tetrahydrocannabinol pharmacokinetics. Ann Pharm Fr. 2008;66:232–44.
185. McGilveray IJ. Pharmacokinetics of cannabinoids. Pain Res Manag. 2005;10(Suppl A):15A–22A.
186. Ohlsson A, Lindgren JE, Wahlen A, et al. Plasma delta-9 tetrahydrocannabinol concentrations and clinical effects after oral and intravenous administration and smoking. Clin Pharmacol Ther. 1980;28(3):409–16.
187. Huestis MA. Human cannabinoid pharmacokinetics. Chem Biodivers. 2007;4:1770–804.
188. Abramovici H. Information for health care professionals: cannabis (marihuana, marijuana) and the cannabinoids. Health Canada 2013. Available at: http://www.hc-sc.gc.ca/dhp-mps/alt_formats/pdf/marihuana/med/infoprof-eng.pdf.
189. United Nations. The International Drug Control Conventions Schedules of the Single Convention on Narcotic Drugs of 1961 as amended by the 1972 Protocol, as at 24 May 2019. United Nations, New York, 2019. Available at: https://undocs.org/ST/CND/1/Add.1/Rev.5. Accessed 12 Sept 2019.
190. Encyclopedia.com. Single convention on narcotic drugs. Encyclopedia of drugs, alcohol, and addictive behavior. Available at: Encyclopedia.com: https://www.encyclopedia.com/education/encyclopedias-almanacs-transcripts-and-maps/single-convention-narcotic-drugs. Accessed 14 Sept 2019.
191. World Health Organization (WHO). Cannabis Review Questions and Answers. World Health Organization (WHO), 2018d. Available at: http://www.who.int/medicines/access/controlled-substances/Cannabis_Review_QA_26July2018.pdf. Accessed 9 Oct 2018.

# 5 Anxiety

## Introduction

Anxiety and depression are the two most prevalent forms of mental illness, with a heavy burden in terms of personal suffering, as well as socially and economically [1]. Chronic pain, anxiety and depression are often comorbid. Compared with the general population, people suffering from chronic pain are up to four times more likely to meet the diagnostic criteria for mood and anxiety disorders [2].

Surveys indicate that cannabis is commonly used to alleviate anxiety, stress, depression and sleep disorders [3–7]. An early survey published in 1986 found that 72% of daily cannabis users reported the use of cannabis to relax or relieve tension [8]. A US survey found that 50% of medical cannabis patients using cannabis to treat pain reported that it provided relief from anxiety and stress [9]. Another survey of 1429 medicinal cannabis users found that the most frequently endorsed reason for medical cannabis use was managing pain, anxiety and depression (>58% use to manage anxiety and >50% use to manage depression) [10]. Other cross-sectional studies have found that posttraumatic stress disorder (PTSD) patients reported using cannabis to cope with hyperarousal and sleep [11–13]. A systematic review and meta-analysis of empirical studies of patient-reported use of medicinal cannabis for pain, anxiety and depression (13 studies) found that 51.7% of those surveyed use medicinal cannabis for anxiety (34.7% for relief from depression symptoms and 67.2% for pain) [14].

In the USA, where medicinal cannabis is available, prescriptions for anti-anxiety medications have also decreased significantly [15]. Women, it appears, are also more likely to use cannabis to cope with anxiety than men [16]. This study finds support in another study of 1513 patients at a New England medical cannabis dispensary, which found that 71.8% had decreased their use of anti-anxiety medications since they started medicinal cannabis use [17].

Further afield in Australia, the *Cannabis As Medicine Study (CAMS-16)* conducted in 2016 surveyed 1748 Australians who were using cannabis for medical reasons, prior to legalisation of its medical use (recreational use is still illegal in



K. O'Brien, P. Blair, *Medicinal Cannabis and CBD in Mental Healthcare*,
https://doi.org/10.1007/978-3-030-78559-8_5

most states and territories, with the exception of the Australian Capital Territory, which legalised its use early in 2020). The most common reasons for medical cannabis use were anxiety (50.7%), back pain (50.0%), depression (49.3%), sleep problems (43.5%), neck pain (25.6%) and PTSD (22.9%). More than 80% of respondents indicated medicinal cannabis effectively managed their target symptom [18]. The consistency of reported purpose of use for medicinal cannabis in these countries alone suggests that cannabis is not being used for mere recreation or psychotropic effects. Surveys also demonstrate that medicinal cannabis has also been found to improve the quality of life and relieve anxiety [19].

**This Chapter**

Whilst much of the current pharmacological treatment of affective disorders is focused primarily on augmenting monoaminergic (serotonin, dopamine primarily) transmission, there is a growing attention in the literature of the role of neuropeptides, cytokines and bioactive lipids in the pathogenesis of anxiety and mood disorders [20]. The endocannabinoid system (ECS) is a complex and sophisticated signalling system. This chapter will explore how the ECS is involved in anxiety and the preclinical and clinical evidence for the use of medicinal cannabis in its treatment. Whilst we focus on evidence in relation to CBD and THC, we also look at a few of the other plant nutrients including terpenes. We conclude with two case studies from Dr. Blair's practice including dosing tips for clinicians.

A note of caution: much of the preclinical research (animal studies) is conducted using purified isolates of CBD and THC. However, we need to remember that cannabis is a plant with at least 540 secondary metabolites, and other phytocannabinoids and terpenes have a clear role to play in its therapeutic effects, including treatment of anxiety. We therefore should try to keep this in mind when we interpret the research findings that are often largely related to pure isolates and not whole plant medicines. We suggest caution in extrapolating the findings of studies of synthetic copies of single molecules to whole-spectrum plant medicines. Instead, seek to understand if there are differences in efficacy and safety profiles which may then guide your choice in clinical practice. After that brief lecture, let us get on with understanding more about anxiety.

## Anxiety: Overview

Anxiety is a natural and usually short-lived reaction to a stressful situation. Who has not felt a bit anxious before a job interview, an exam, a date or even a visit to the doctor? The American Psychological Association [21] defines anxiety as 'an emotion characterised by feelings of tension, worried thoughts and physical changes like increased blood pressure'. However, anxiety is pathogenic when the emotional response is disproportionate to the cause (i.e. in duration, intensity or frequency) and where it stops a person leading a normal life [22].

Anxiety disorder is characterised by severe, frequent, recurring and persistent anxiety symptoms. Anxiety disorders are very common. They affect around 14% of

Australians each year and are the most common type of mental health disorder in Australia [23]. In the USA, an estimated 19.1% of adults had any anxiety disorder in the past year, and an estimated 31.1% of adults experience any anxiety disorders at some point in their lives [24]. Past year prevalence for any anxiety disorder was higher for females (23.4%) than males (14.3%) [24]. Anxiety disorders share features of excessive fear and anxiety which can cause psychological and physical symptoms that can, in turn, cause significant distress and interfere with functioning in social, occupational or other areas of life [22].

## Types of Anxiety Disorder

Anxiety disorders can manifest in different forms and for varying durations. For example, anxiety may be continuous and daily (generalised anxiety disorder) or can manifest as acute and debilitating episodes of extreme anxiety (panic attack disorder) [25].

There are six main types of anxiety disorder:

- **Generalised anxiety disorder:** characterised by persistent, excessive worry, often about daily life situations, e.g. work, family, health
- **Social anxiety disorder (SAD):** characterised by severe anxiety about being viewed negatively by others or criticised by others, leading the person to avoid social situations
- **Obsessive compulsive disorder (OCD):** characterised by obsessions (recurring, persistent and distressing thoughts, images or impulses) or compulsions (to carry out repetitive behaviours or rituals or mental acts, e.g. repetitive handwashing) or both
- **Panic disorder**: characterised by repeated and unexpected panic attacks which have no apparent trigger
- **Specific phobia**: characterised by extreme fear and anxiety of particular objects or situations, e.g. arachnophobia
- **Agoraphobia:** characterised by intense anxiety in places or situations where the person feels it would be difficult for them to get out of quickly or get help if needed (e.g. being in a crowd) [23]

## Associated Comorbidities

Anxiety is often comorbid with other conditions, including depression, sleep disorders and chronic pain, to name only a few. In a given 12-month period, an estimated 10–20% of adults will visit their primary care physician during an anxiety or depressive disorder episode, with more than half of these suffering from a comorbid second anxiety or depressive disorder [26]. Comorbidity of anxiety and depression is associated with greater chronicity, slower recovery, increased recurrence rates and greater psychosocial disability, plus increased use of medical services [26] and therefore economic and societal cost. An estimated 58% of patients with a major depressive disorder have a lifetime anxiety disorder [27].

Sleep disorders such as insomnia are also comorbid with anxiety disorders. Some studies indicate that where sleep disorders are associated with anxiety disorders, there is increased morbidity. For example, in PTSD patients, insomnia is associated with increased likelihood of suicidal behaviour, depression and substance abuse [28]. Not surprisingly, the relationship between insomnia and anxiety disorders is also affected by the presence of comorbid major depressive disorder [29].

Anxiety is one of several comorbidities of chronic pain. Anxiety can be a response to other symptoms of other diseases, for example, asthma [30], and can manifest in relation to fear of dying, for example, in cancer patients [31].

In western medicine, these conditions are often treated separately, using different medications with often resultant polypharmacy and all the potential for side effects and drug interactions that go along with that, symptomatic of a reductionist approach. The beauty with forms of herbal medicine is that often one herb (in the case of cannabis) or a combination of herbs (as is used in Chinese medicine) can often treat several comorbidities at once. Certainly, *Cannabis sativa* may be able to address several comorbidities at once.

### Treatment of Anxiety

The two main treatment approaches are psychotherapy and pharmaceuticals. Others include lifestyle interventions including exercise, avoiding alcohol, stress management and relaxation techniques, eating healthy foods and ensuring good sleep.

Cognitive behavioural therapy is an effective form of psychotherapy, teaching the patient specific skills to improve symptoms. It involves exposure therapy in which the patient gradually encounters the trigger for their anxiety, building confidence that they can effectively manage the trigger (situation, object) and anxiety symptoms [32].

Commonly used anxiolytic pharmaceuticals include antidepressants (including selective serotonin reuptake inhibitors, tricyclic antidepressants, tetracyclic antidepressants and monoamine oxidase inhibitors), anticonvulsants (e.g. pregabalin) and sedatives (e.g. benzodiazepines and beta-blockers (for short term relief)), all of which act on various physiological pathways [33]. Pharmaceuticals are not always effective and can cause a range of different side effects [34].

## Pathomechanisms Involved in Anxiety

Anxiety is characterised by non-specific and chronic apprehension and arousal associated with the potential occurrence of a future threat [35]. Anxiety disorders may be viewed as maladaptive fear responses resulting from dysregulation of brain circuitry involved in fearfulness generation. Healthy individuals can assess whether a situation is similar to or different from a previously encountered situation and elicit appropriate responses. Those with anxiety disorders often exhibit an overgeneralisation of fear responses in response to emotional stimuli. In anxiety disorders such as PTSD, there is increased reactivity to neutral stimuli that resembles the previous aversive event even in the presence of cues indicating safety [36]. PTSD will be covered in Chap. 6.

Many lines of evidence indicate that anxiety disorders are due to a dysfunction in the regulation of brain circuits that regulate our emotional responses to threatening stimuli [37]. There are several pathomechanisms underpinning anxiety. The neurobiological approach suggests that anxiety is associated with a dysregulation of the normal top-down control exerted by the medial prefrontal cortex (mPFC) over the activity of the amygdala [35]. There is also evidence that inflammation is involved [38], and in some types of anxiety disorder, the noradrenergic system also comes into play. Serotonin and GABA are neurotransmitters also involved.

## Role of the Amygdala and Prefrontal Cortex in Anxiety

The amygdala plays the central role in anxiety regulation. Other brain areas involved are the prefrontal cortex (PFC) and anterior cingulate gyrus, areas of the cortex that receive and send glutaminergic (excitatory) projections to and from the basolateral amygdala (BLA) and are activated at the same time as the amygdala when an emotional stimulus appears [37].

Instinctive reactions to a threat (mediated via the amygdala) and the regulatory processes that occur consequently (mediated by the PFC, which signals the emotional salience of the stimuli) are referred to as 'bottom-up' and 'top-down' responses, respectively. The medial PFC (mPFC) regulates the experience or anxiety by modulating the neuronal activity of the BLA. More dorsal cortical regions are responsible for conscious control of anxiety and more ventral areas for subconscious control. The top-down control by the mPFC normally inhibits the output of the amygdala [37] and is associated with reduced anxiety, which is demonstrated by functional neuroimaging studies that indicate increased PFC and decreased amygdala activity during successful emotional regulation [35].

However, in anxiety the dynamic interactions between the amygdala and the mPFC that allow us to react to stimuli and regulate our emotional responses are compromised or dysregulated [35]. Functional neuroimaging studies demonstrate changes in the prefrontal-cingulate-amygdala circuit, which is involved in emotion regulation [39]. Functional neuroimaging of high trait anxious individuals shows increased amygdala reactivity coupled with reduced activity within the PFC in response to threat, with similar demonstration of alterations in circuit connectivity in anxiety disorders, including hyper-activity of the amygdala and both hyper-activity and hypoactivity of the PFC and cingulate cortex (different studies have found hyper- and hypo-activity of the PFC, depending on the region within the PFC, type of anxiety disorder and study design) [39, 40]. For example, in highly anxious but otherwise healthy people, functional neuroimaging studies have demonstrated increased amygdala activity, and other studies have found decreased activity of the vmPRF and dmPFC (though some have found decreased vmPFC and increased dmPFC activity, suggesting these subregions might play different roles in anxiety) [35]. In some studies of generalised anxiety disorder and PTSD, the mPFC has been found to be hypo-active [37], though other studies indicate that in GAD, the mPFC is hyper-active [40].

In SAD, functional MRI studies showed increased amygdala reactivity when viewing harsh facial expressions as well as neutral faces compared with healthy controls [41–43]. Amygdala reactivity was correlated with symptom severity and trait anxiety in those suffering from SAD [35, 41, 42, 44]. Other studies have found a significantly reduced functional connectivity between the medial orbitofrontal cortex and left amygdala [45], failure to recruit the mPFC [46] and structural changes such as compromised structural integrity of the uncinate fasciculus (white matter fibre tract connecting the amygdala and orbitofrontal cortex) [47], all evidence of a disruption of connectivity between the amygdala and mPFC [35].

The locus coeruleus (LC) is also involved in anxiety, and it is understood that GABA projections carry anxiety-related information from the amygdala to various brainstem centres, including the LC, and the LC provides noradrenergic projections to the hippocampus and amygdala. The interconnections between these brain regions may be important in the regulation of oxidative stress-mediated anxiety, which will be discussed shortly [48].

## Serotonin in Anxiety

Serotonin is known to be a key modulator of emotional regulation and the activity of the PFC-cingulate-amygdala complex as well as the serotonin system (receptors, serotonin transporter) implicated in threat-driven emotion and trait anxiety. The serotonin transporter is the target of selective serotonin reuptake inhibitors (SSRIs), which are used to treat anxiety. Polymorphisms in the serotonin transporter gene have been linked to trait anxiety levels and altered PFC-cingulate-amygdala circuitry [39].

High trait anxiety (predisposition to elevated anxiety and fear) is associated with a higher risk of anxiety disorders (as well as depression). An experiment on primates found an association between anxiety-like behaviour and increased expression of the serotonin transporter in the right ventrolateral PFC and, most strongly, in the amygdala. Anxiety-like behaviour was decreased by blockade of serotonin reuptake in the amygdala (via injection of an SSRI into the amydgala). The authors concluded that their findings suggest that high amygdala serotonin transporter expression contributes to the high trait anxiety phenotype [39].

## Noradrenergic System Involvement in Anxiety

Many studies have investigated the role of the noradrenergic system in anxiety disorders, with many of these focused on panic disorder. A review of clinical studies investigating the role of central noradrenergic dysfunction in anxiety disorders concluded that there is evidence in panic disorder that there is noradrenergic dysfunction, with a higher baseline secretion of noradrenaline, along with increased reactivity shown in response to challenges to the noradrenergic system. However, for other types of anxiety like PTSD, the results are conflicting, and in studies of generalised anxiety disorder, most show no difference between normal subjects and GAD sufferers. Likewise, in obsessive-compulsive disorders, there are no differences, and there is little available evidence in relation to social and other phobias [49].

## GABA Involvement in Anxiety

GABA is another key neurotransmitter involved in emotional regulation, including anxiety. Brain circuits in the amygdala comprise GABAergic interneurons, and GABA plays a key part in modulating anxiety responses under normal and pathological conditions [37]. There are allosteric sites on the $GABA_A$ receptor allowing inhibition of neurons in the amygdala to be precisely regulated. Neuronal inhibition is downregulated in anxiety states, and this may be via changes in the levels of endogenous modulators of these allosteric sites and changes in the composition of the $GABA_A$ receptor [37]. Benzodiazepines, used to treat anxiety, bind to $GABA_A$ receptors, enhancing GABA neurotransmission resulting in anxiolysis, sedation, striated muscle relaxation and anticonvulsant effects [33].

## Immune Dysfunction and Inflammation in Anxiety

There is a growing evidence base supporting a link between inflammation and anxiety as well as depression and whilst the exact causal mechanism is still to be elucidated [50], pieces of the jigsaw puzzle are coming together.

Persistent stress and chronic illness represent conditions of chronic challenge to the immune system, and the inflammatory response may contribute to the pathophysiology of various mental health conditions [38]. The immune system generates the cytokine signalling, which, in turn, plays a role in the brain regulation of moods, synaptic plasticity, neuroendocrine responses and neurotransmitter metabolism. Dysregulation of the immune system in the central nervous system (CNS) may lead to a variety of disorders, including anxiety, depression, sleep disorders and cognitive dysfunction [38]. Research conducted on humans also shows that increased anxiety levels are associated with impaired cellular immunity (cellular and humoral immune responses) (e.g. Zhou et al. [51], Arranz et al. [52], [53]) and increased risk of infections [54]. For example, a study on women found that there was decreased chemotaxis and phagocytosis (as well as decreased NK cell activity, IL-2 release and total antioxidant activity and increased superoxide anion and TNF-α levels and increased plasma cortisol) in anxious women [52].

### Inflammation and Anxiety

Systemic inflammation is accompanied by disturbances in the regulation of emotions that have been related to the pathophysiology of both anxiety and depression [50, 55]. Anxiety increases the risk of inflammatory diseases, and increased inflammatory activity in anxious people may contribute to the increased risk [56]. For example, anxiety increases the risk of cardiovascular disease independent of depression [57].

Inflammation has consistently been found to affect anxiety-related regions of the brain, including the amygdala, insula and anterior cingulate cortex [55]. The source of inflammation may vary for different individuals, but it is thought to be the result of a combination of lifestyle factors (e.g. diet, exercise, weight, sleep), genetic predisposition to inflammation, illness and exposure to stress and/or trauma, with inflammatory signals impacting the brain, leading to anxiety and mood-related symptoms. These inflammatory signals may be local (cytokines activating local inflammatory signalling pathways and microglia) or involve peripheral inflammatory cytokines traveling to the brain, crossing the blood-brain barrier to activate the local immune system [55].

#### Animal Studies Linking Systemic Inflammation, Neuroinflammation and Anxiety

Several animal studies have demonstrated increased anxiety-like behaviour in response to systemic inflammation induced under experimental conditions [58–60], and this appears to be mediated through those parts of the brain involved in emotional regulation (amygdala, insula, PFC) [50]. Animal studies show clear evidence of an association between raised levels of several cytokines and anxiety-like behaviour, including increased IL-6 and TNF-α [61, 62], and genetic deletion of the INF-ϒ gene was found to be associated with increased emotionality in mice [63].

Mice studies demonstrate that activated monocytes and macrophages migrate to the brain in response to chemokines produced by activated microglia (which is produced in response to cytokine signalling from the periphery). These immune cells travel to perivascular and meningeal spaces and may underpin or contribute to anxiety and depression, as evidenced in animal models of stress-induced anxiety and depression [55, 64, 65]. Monocyte trafficking from the spleen to the brain contributes to re-establishment of anxiety in stress-sensitised mice, demonstrating that neuroinflammation promotes mood disturbances following stress sensitisation and suggesting that neuroimmune interactions may underlie recurrent anxiety disorders (e.g. PTSD) [65].

In other mice experiments, repeated social defeat in mice enhanced the inflammatory capacity of $CD11b^+$ cells in the brain, promoting anxiety-like behaviour in a manner that is dependent on interleukin (IL)-1 and β-adrenergic receptors [64]. When socially defeated mice were injected with lipopolysaccharide, it resulted in increased inflammatory CNS macrophages, exaggerated microglia activation and prolonged social withdrawal [64].

**Human Studies Linking Inflammation and Anxiety**

Evidence from human studies confirms that inflammation is linked to anxiety. High levels of inflammation have been observed in patients with generalised anxiety disorder [66], panic disorder [67] and PTSD [55, 67, 68]. Positive correlations have been demonstrated between anxiety and several inflammatory cytokines, including TNF-α, IL-6 and C-reactive protein [52, 69]. For example, a study on cardiovascular disease-free subjects found that anxiety score was significantly positively correlated with C-reactive protein, TNF-α, homocysteine and fibrinogen levels in men, whereas in women, it was positively correlated with CRP, white blood cell count, IL-6, homocysteine and fibrinogen levels, showing that anxiety is associated with inflammation and coagulation markers [69]. Increased state anxiety has been found to occur in response to experimental immune challenge, as reflected in the increased levels of pro-inflammatory cytokines [70, 71].

An RCT sought to investigate the neural mechanisms underpinning inflammation-induced anxiety by inducing transient systemic inflammation in 43 healthy men (low-dose lipopolysaccharide injection compared with saline in the control group) and performing resting-state functional resonance imaging before and 3.5 h after injection. Their study demonstrated that acute systemic inflammation alters temporal variance and functional connectivity in the brain regions/networks involved in emotional regulation [50].

**What Are the Mechanisms by which Inflammation May Cause Anxiety?**

The potential mechanisms of action linking inflammation to anxiety and other mood disorders are described well by Felger [55]. She explains that in patients with anxiety and mood disorders, inflammation is increased in response to stress, diet, lifestyle factors and illness.

The innate immune system becomes activated, a process involving intracellular signal transduction pathways and pro-cytokine oligomers (inflammasomes), releasing inflammatory cytokines. These cytokines are associated with increased oxidative stress and production of reactive oxygen species (ROS) and reactive nitrogen species (RNS), which in turn contribute to oxidation of tetrahydrobiopterin (BH4). BH4 is needed for the synthesis of monoamines via particular enzymes (phenylalanine hydroxylase, tryptophan hydroxylase and tyrosine hydroxylase). Reduced BH4 then leads to reduced synthesis of the monoamines, serotonin (5-HT), dopamine and norepinephrine [55].

Inflammatory cytokines can also increase the enzyme indoleamine-2,3-dioxygenase (IDO), leading to increased kynurenine and its neurotoxic metabolites, which then impacts glutamate signalling. As a result of inflammation in the brain or neuroinflammation, glutamate is released from microglia, whilst uptake is reduced by astrocytes leading to excesses in glutamate stimulation. Neurocircuits within the brain are altered, including those in the basal ganglia, PFC and motor circuits and those brain regions associated with anxiety and fear (amygdala, prefrontal and insular circuitry), which may then contribute to symptoms of anxiety as well as depression [55].

### Oxidative Stress

Oxidative stress occurs when the levels of oxidants generated within the body (e.g. hydrogen peroxide, superoxide, nitric oxide) exceed the cellular capacity to scavenge oxidants and repair damage [38, 72]. This can be due to increased generation of ROS or RNS or impaired defence against them (e.g. depletion of enzymatic antioxidants, including superoxide dismutase, catalase and glutathione peroxidase or depletion of non-enzymatic antioxidants such as glutathione, vitamin C, vitamin A, vitamin E and selenium [72]). Consequences of oxidative stress in the brain include impaired neuronal signalling, mitochondrial dysfunction and inhibition of neurogenesis, each of which can contribute further to increased oxidative stress, a vicious cycle [72].

Both human and animal research indicates that oxidative stress is involved in anxiety. A study on mice demonstrated evidence of oxidative stress in the central and peripheral systems of anxious mice, finding an imbalance in oxidative status in neuronal and glial cells in the cerebellum and hippocampus, neurons in the cerebral cortex and peripheral leukocytes in mice displaying anxiety-like behaviour [73]. Another study in a rat model of foetal alcohol spectrum disorders found that anxiety- and depression-like behaviours were accompanied by increased oxidative stress and that physical exercise provided a protective effect [74].

Human research also supports the involvement of altered oxidative stress-related mechanisms in anxiety, with several studies demonstrating increases in oxidative stress markers, increased activity of antioxidant enzymes (such as superoxide dismutase) and reductions in the blood levels of antioxidants (including glutathione, vitamin E and selenium) in association with anxiety (see Hovatta et al. [72]).

This reminds us of the importance of diet and lifestyle providing essential nutrients whilst avoiding oxidised foods and detrimental substances and exposures for ensuring optimal functioning of our bodies, including the ability to combat oxidative stress.

For a deeper dive into the role of inflammation and oxidative stress in anxiety, see Hovatta et al. [72] and Salim et al. [38].

## Neurogenesis and the Hippocampus

Neurogenesis is the process by which new neurons are formed, whilst neuroplasticity is the process by which the brain reorganises itself, forming new connections [75]. In mammals, significant levels of adult neurogenesis occur in two brain regions: the olfactory bulb (newborn neurons migrate from the subventricular zone of the lateral ventricles to the olfactory bulb) and the dentate granule cell layer of the hippocampus (newborn neurons are generated locally within the subgranular zone and migrate into the granular cell [GC] layer of the dentate gyrus and become glutamatergic dentate GCs in the hippocampus) [76, 77].

The dentate gyrus of the hippocampus plays a role in emotions, mood, anxiety, stress response and memory and learning. The striatum is involved in not only motor coordination but also regulation of reward, pleasure, motivation and aversion [78]. Adult neurogenesis takes place in a 'neurogenic niche', which refers to the complex local environment that supports neural precursor cells. Self-renewing neural stem cells within the subgranular zone of the hippocampus give rise to new neurons and astrocytes [77].

As they mature, these newborn neurons develop neurites (which are extensions from the cell body) in a process called 'neuritogenesis', and these eventually develop into axons and dendrites [79]. Synaptogenesis is the process of forming new synapses.

### Adult Hippocampal Neurons and the Stress Response

Research has demonstrated that adult-born hippocampal neurons are necessary for the normal expression of the stress response, both endocrine and behavioural aspects [80]. Neurogenesis is thought to buffer the stress response by activating the hippocampus-induced feedback on the hypothalamus-pituitary-adrenal axis (HPA) and influencing memory and learning [80, 81].

Stress is known to cause changes in hippocampal function, though the specific mechanisms are not completely understood. It is thought to involve maladaptive plasticity changes associated with neuronal atrophy or loss, changes in dendrites (decreased length, complexity) and decreased 'spine' density found in animal models of chronic stress (a 'spine' is a small protrusion from a neuron's dendrite that receives input from an axon at a synapse) [81].

Various studies have shown that chronic stress can disrupt neuroplasticity mechanisms in the limbic system, and this has been associated with the onset of anxiety and mood disorders [81, 82]. Stress can impair neurogenesis [81]; studies in depression indicate reduced dendritic complexity and the expression of proteins involved in synaptogenesis and survival in the hippocampus [83]. Findings from studies such as these (in depression) may also be relevant to anxiety. CBD may have a role to play in addressing this particular pathomechanism underpinning anxiety, as we will see later.

The 'neurogenic theory of depression' which posits that impaired adult hippocampal neurogenesis (AHN) triggers depression (and that restoration of function leads to recovery from depression) has been extended to include anxiety [84].

This has some support from findings that adult hippocampus neurogenesis has been found to be impaired in many animal models of depression (and anxiety) and social stress models in primates and that patients with anxiety and depression have smaller dentate gyri (found on MRI and on post-mortem), suggestive of impaired AHN [84, 85].

### Neuritogenesis and Anxiety

As explained earlier, neuritogenesis is the formation of new axons and dendrites on neuron cell bodies [79]. Neurogenesis, synaptogenesis and neuronal survival are partly mediated by glycogen synthase kinase 3β signalling, and GSK3β and synaptic proteins such as synapsin a/b and post-synaptic density protein 95 are also involved in dendritic remodelling [81].

This process of neuritogenesis, vital to reprogramming our brain to learning and new experiences, may play a significant role in anxiety and depression. This finds support in preclinical research. For example, in a detailed study of primary neuron neuritogenesis and spine morphology, behavioural tests in mice with decreased spine density in the mPFC caused anxiety-like behaviours and sensorimotor deficits [79]. In a study using an autism model, genetic deletion of the Auts2 gene in mice resulted in defects in neuronal migration and neuritogenesis in the developing cerebral cortex, which were found to correlate with behavioural abnormalities in anxiety-related emotions and memory functions [86].

## The Endocannabinoid System in Anxiety

Animal and human research indicates that the ECS is involved in our stress response and in anxiety. The corticolimbic region of the brain includes the PFC, amygdala (especially the BLA) and hippocampus. These areas are all involved in our stress response, emotions, emotional memory, reward and anxiety-related behaviours, and the ECS is widely distributed in these regions, including CB1 receptors, anandamide (AEA), 2-arachidonoyl glycerol (2-AG) and fatty acid amide hydrolase (FAAH) [4, 87–89]. Interestingly, the 'runner's high', which is a feeling of euphoria and anxiolysis, was generally attributed to the production of endogenous endorphins. However, it is now known that the blood levels of both endorphins and AEA are elevated after running and that the resulting associated anxiolysis relies on intact CB1 receptors in GABAergic neurons in the forebrain [90].

The role of the serotonergic system in anxiety regulation is well known. The association between the ECS and the serotonergic system is demonstrated by findings that there is cross-talk between the CB1 receptors and 5-HT receptors in rat cerebellar and bovine synaptic membranes, as well as co-expression of CB1 receptors and different 5-HT receptor subtypes in neuronal subpopulations in the cerebellum and forebrain [91].

To understand the effects of cannabinoids on anxiety, much research has been conducted using drugs that selectively target the ECS as well as genetic knockout mice models (bred to be deficient in, for example, CB1 receptors). Such research provides evidence that the ECS, via CB1 receptor activation, is involved in the regulation of emotional behaviour. Treatment of rats with CB1 receptor antagonist rimonabant (taken off the market due to unacceptable psychological side effects) produced anxiogenic responses [92]. CB1 receptor agonists have been found to have bimodal effect. Lower doses have been found to be anxiolytic and higher doses anxiogenic, with similar bimodal effects found using CB1 receptor antagonists [93].

Some studies using CB1 receptor knockout mice have found anxiogenic responses in anxiety models [93], for example, demonstrating an increase in the basal level of anxiety [94]. However not all experiments have found this. The apparent contradictions could relate to the fact that there are CB1 receptors on glutaminergic (excitatory) and GABAergic (inhibitory) neurons and whether the experimental conditions predominantly modulate one or the other. In addition, the anxiolytic and anxiogenic effects of pharmacological enhancement of the ECS in animal models have been found to differ depending on the different brain regions involved. An example is that when THC is injected into the PFC, it promotes anxiolytic effects but when injected into the BLA, it causes an anxiogenic response [93].

Thus, the body of knowledge about the role of the ECS in the modulation of moods including anxiety is not complete and is seemingly contradictory. We are still learning about various pathways and nuances of how this cell signalling system helps us regulate our emotions. The best approach for grasping the fundamentals of ECS is to embrace the concept of modulation or regulation by phyto- and endocannabinoids as opposed to a single monolithic action (agonism, antagonism) in all tissues in all physiologic states.

Let us look at some of the research on how the ECS is involved in anxiety, knowing that the picture is not perfect, and with the awareness that the body of evidence is growing as we speak.

## HPA Axis in Anxiety

The HPA plays an important role in stress, anxiety and depression, and the ECS is involved. The activation of the HPA is common to all kinds of threats. The system is designed to mitigate short-duration threats, but exposure to prolonged stress can induce a loss of the regulatory negative feedback mechanism, inducing sustained increases in the glucocorticoid levels that alter brain neuroplasticity and neurogenesis [95, 96]. The implications are that stress could lead to altered or reduced neuroplasticity, which has been linked to anxiety and major depressive disorders [95, 97].

According to Balsevich et al. [98], glucocorticoids immediately affect the global shift of the membrane lipid metabolism towards metabolic pathways for the synthesis of the anti-inflammatory AEA and 2-AG and away from inflammatory arachidonic acid production. Inhibition of the cyclooxygenase-2 (COX2) synthesis by glucocorticoids helps this mechanism by suppressing the synthesis of pro-inflammatory prostaglandins as well as endocannabinoid-derived prostanoids [99]. However, chronic stress and chronic glucocorticoid exposure appears to adversely affect neuronal architecture, causing atrophy of dendritic branches and reduction of dendritic spine density and changes in spine morphology [100].

Qin and colleagues [101] found that chronic stress-induced glucocorticoids downregulated endocannabinoid signalling and that the emergence of anxiety was associated with genomic shift in productions at the nuclear level (epigenetic).

## Endocannabinoids, Cannabinoid Receptors and Anxiety

Exposure to stress decreases AEA levels in several limbic areas of the brain [102, 103]. This suggests that deficits in AEA signalling contribute to anxiety-like behaviour induced by stress [20]. Stress-induced AEA deficiency has been found to correlate with anxiety-like behaviour [20]. In healthy human volunteers, the levels of circulating AEA and related fatty acid ethanolamides were found to increase with acute psychosocial stress [104].

### Enzymes of the ECS

Various studies have sought to manipulate the enzymes involved in the synthesis and degradation of the endocannabinoids and have shown significant therapeutic responses. In mice, the anxiety levels were increased, and the whole brain AEA levels were suppressed 24 h after foot shock. Pre-treatment with a FAAH inhibitor (remember that FAAH is the enzyme that degrades AEA) prevented the drop in AEA produced by acute stress and prevented enhanced anxiety-like behaviour, mediated by the action of AEA at the CB1 receptors [20].

Inhibition of the enzyme that degrades 2-AG, MAGL, also reduces anxiety [105–107]. But, a deficiency in DAGL (diacylglycerol lipase α, the enzyme which is involved in the synthesis of 2-AG) leads to increased anxiety associated with a marked decrease in brain 2-AG. MAGL inhibitors prevented this decrease in 2-AG and increased anxiety. However, MAGL inhibitors that elevate 2-AG (which is a full agonist at CB1 receptors compared with AEA which is a partial agonist) can also cause receptor desensitisation [108].

### TRPV1

The regulation of anxiety is not simply through CB1 receptor-dependent processes, however [93]. AEA has been found to have biphasic or bimodal properties: it acts as an anxiolytic on CB1 receptors at lower doses and as an anxiogenic agent on the transient receptor potential vanilloid type 1 (TRPV1) channel at higher doses [109, 110]. TRPV1 is expressed in many parts of the brain, including the hippocampus, basal ganglia and cortex [111]. CB1 receptors and TRPV1 channels have opposite effects on anxiety regulation, with CB1 receptors being activated and TRPV1 channels being antagonised to produce anxiolytic responses in mice [112]. Maintaining the balance between CB1 receptor activation and TRPV1 channel activation is thus critical in regulating anxiety [113].

## Scientific Evidence: CBD in the Treatment of Anxiety

Preclinical evidence supports acute administration of CBD for several types of anxiety including generalised anxiety, panic disorder, SAD, obsessive-compulsive disorder and PTSD; however few studies have studied chronic dosing of CBD [114]. There is a growing body of clinical research evidence that also supports the contention that CBD may have a place in the treatment of anxiety in humans, though again much of the research has been limited to acute dosing. More studies are needed in longer-term use of CBD for the treatment of anxiety and within the different subpopulations of anxiety.

In this section, we will explore the potential mechanisms of action by which CBD may work as an anxiolytic and then look at animal and human studies of efficacy.

## Mechanisms of Action of CBD in Anxiety

The mechanisms of action of CBD as an anxiolytic have not been fully elucidated. The regulation of anxiety and learned fear processing is understood to involve 5-HT1A receptors, TRPV1 channels and endocannabinoid signalling [113]. CBD is agonistic at the 5-HT1A receptor and shares similar mechanisms with lithium, supporting a potential role for CBD in the treatment of mood disorders [115].

However, CBD interacts with several other receptors that regulate fear and anxiety-related behaviours, including CB1 receptors, CB2 receptors and GPR55 [114, 116]. Further research is needed to investigate the involvement of other potential mechanisms by which CBD might affect behaviour, including inhibition of adenosine uptake, inverse agonism at CB2 receptors, CB1 receptor antagonism, GPR55 antagonism, PPAR $\gamma$ receptor agonism, intracellular calcium increase [117], FAAH inhibition [81] and TRPV1 activation [118].

Overall, the research evidence suggests that the CBD acute anxiolytic effects are likely due to the facilitation of 5-HT1A-mediated neurotransmission in the key brain regions related to defensive properties, such as the dorsal periaqueductal grey (DPAG), bed nucleus of the stria terminalis and medial PFC. In contrast, other actions of CBD, including anti-compulsive, increased fear extinction, and impaired reconsolidation of aversive memories, blockade of anxiogenic consequences of chronic unpredictable stress and facilitation of AHN may be due to the potentiation of AEA-mediated neurotransmission, whilst TRPV1 activation may be involved in its anti-psychotic action [117].

This is a complex picture that is not yet complete. Here are some of the research findings.

### CBD and the Serotonergic System

Although CBD is able to interact with several receptors, evidence points to its anxiolytic effect being due to its action on the serotonergic system, probably via a direct action on 5-HT1A receptors in the midbrain DPAG area which controls the autonomic and behavioural responses to threat [119, 120]. Research indicates that the anxiolytic effect induced by injections of CBD, either systemic or into the inter-DPAG region in rats was blocked by a 5-HT1A receptor antagonist [119, 121]. Other areas of the brain related to the control of anxiety are also involved in the attenuation of anxiety responses [122, 123].

The acute effects of CBD on anxiety are dose-dependent, with low and intermediate doses but not high doses found to be effective. The effects of low and intermediate doses were blocked by 5-HT1A receptor antagonists. When researchers blocked TRPV1 receptors, this allowed high doses of CBD to be also effective. This suggests that the anxiolytic effects of low and intermediate doses of pure CBD involve the 5-HT1A receptors, whilst higher doses activate the TRPV1 channels [113]. The activation of TRPV1 channels promotes anxiety, so this might cancel out any anxiolytic effect via 5-HT1A receptors, thereby explaining why higher doses are not effective [124].

But things are not so simple. Whilst research on cells indicates that CBD acts as a 5HT1A agonist [125], other studies suggest that this is not the case under in vivo conditions [126]. Other studies found that the ability of CBD to facilitate 5HT1A-mediated neurotransmission does not appear to involve blockade of its 5HT reuptake nor do changes in 5HT1A mRNA expression in the DPAG region following chronic administration appear to be responsible [127]. Thus, it appears that CBD's modulation of 5HT1A is quite complex and may involve allosteric interactions [126, 128].

CBD may also regulate anxiety, directly or indirectly, PPAR-γ, equilibrative nucleoside transporters, additional TRP channels and glycine receptors [114]. The anxiolytic effect of CBD may also be by activating adenosine receptors that play a significant role in cardiovascular function as well as exerting broad anti-inflammatory effects on the body [129, 130].

A biphasic effect of CBD (and THC) was also demonstrated in the mitogen-induced degradation of tryptophan, catalysed by the enzyme IDO. At nanomolar levels, CBD and THC both enhanced the enzyme activity of IDO in PBMC (i.e. CBD and THC enhanced the degradation of tryptophan), and this was via CB1 and CB2 activation, but at higher (micromolar) levels, THC and CBD both downregulated the mitogen-stimulated tryptophan degradation (suppressed IDO activity), and this was independent of CB1 and CB2 receptor involvement. CBD was found to be 2–4 times stronger than THC in suppressing IDO activity. Research suggests a link by which CBD (and THC) might affect the serotonergic system, and disturbances of serotonergic activity have been shown to play a role in neuropsychiatric disorders, including mood disorders and depression. Tryptophan plays a role in cell mediated immune responses, but it is of course also the precursor for the biosynthesis of serotonin (5HT). CBD and THC has been found to suppress the degradation of tryptophan mediated by the enzyme IDO. This suppression of IDO-mediated degradation of tryptophan by CBD and THC may be an additional mechanism by which the anti-depressive effects of CBD and THC are linked to the serotonergic system [131]. It may be an important mechanism of action by which THC and CBD improve mood disturbances and quality of life, in particular in those who have diseases underpinned by inflammation [131].

### CBD and the HPA

In stress studies of animals, CBD has been found to be able to modulate the HPA factors coordinating the brain's management of stress. In *unstressed* animals administered CBD, there was no effect on the HPA. However acute restraint stress induced opposite effects on the *5-HTR1A* gene expression, depending on the brain region:

there was an increase in the *5-HTR1A* relative gene expression in the hippocampus that was absent (i.e. was blocked) in mice pre-treated with CBD (5, 15 and 30 mg/kg doses), but there was a decrease in the *5-HTR1A* gene expression in the amygdala that was only blocked by a pre-treatment dosage of 5 mg/kg CBD. Pure CBD also blocked the effects of acute stress on corticotropin-releasing factor, proopiomelanocortin (sleep related) and glucocorticoid receptor gene expression. Interestingly, most of the effects were seen in a limited dosage range of CBD between 5 and 15 mg/kg, consistent with other studies of pure CBD [132].

### CBD, Neurogenesis and Neuritogenesis

Another effect of CBD that may involve the ECS is its ability to increase AHN, an impairment of which has been associated with the pathogenesis of anxiety disorders [133, 134]. This is one of the pathomechanisms discussed in an earlier section.

The anxiolytic effect of CBD in chronically stressed mice was demonstrated to depend on hippocampal neurogenesis [81, 133]. Studies on antidepressant treatments in mice have shown that intact AHN plays a role in their anxiolytic effects [135]. In a Parkinson's disease model, CBD also appears to promote neuritogenesis by modulating several key substances involved. CBD increased cell viability, differentiation and the expression of axonal (GAP-43) and synaptic (synaptophysin and synapsin I) proteins [136]. The mechanism involved the activation of tyrosine kinase receptors (trkA) and occurred even in the absence of the endogenous agonist, nerve growth factor [136].

Interestingly, research has also demonstrated that a key terpene of cannabis, beta caryophyllene, can also activate trkA receptors and induce neuritogenesis, and it appears to do so via a mechanism that is independent of cannabinoid receptors or nerve growth factor [137].

A mice study using a chronic unpredictable stress model of anxiety showed that after 14 days, CBD injections were anxiolytic in stressed rats. This effect was blocked by CB1 and CB2 receptor antagonists but not by a 5HT-1A receptor antagonist (indicating that the effects were mediated by cannabinoid receptors). Importantly, they found that these effects were associated with increased hippocampal neurogenesis and spine density in the dentate gyrus of the hippocampus, and this effect was reduced more by the CB2 receptor antagonist. In the stressed rats, CBD decreased FAAH (the enzyme responsible for the breakdown of AEA) and increased the expression of glycogen synthase kinase 3β (p-GSK3β), a protein that partly mediates neurogenesis, synaptogenesis and neuronal survival. This effect was reduced by the CB2 antagonist. The study authors concluded that CBD is able to reduce the effects of chronic unpredictable stress in this animal model through the facilitation of endocannabinoid signalling (endocannabinoid activation and CB1/CB2 receptor activation) and recruitment of intracellular/synaptic proteins that play roles in neurogenesis and dendritic remodelling [81].

### CBD and Endocannabinoid Degradation

CBD interferes with the uptake and degradation of endocannabinoids, though the relevance in relation to anxiolytic effects is not clear [126]. CBD has been found to have an indirect effect on CB1 receptors by preventing the enzymatic breakdown of AEA, thereby allowing it to stay in the system longer [130]. Elevated AEA in the cerebrospinal fluid has been found to be inversely correlated with psychotic symptoms [130]. In a randomised controlled trial (RCT), CBD treatment was accompanied by a significant increase in serum AEA levels, which was significantly associated with clinical improvement in patients with acute schizophrenia, suggesting that the inhibition of AEA breakdown might contribute to CBD's anti-psychotic effects [130].

### CBD, Inflammation and Immune Function

As mentioned previously, inflammation may underpin both anxiety and depression [55]. Therefore, CBD's anti-inflammatory effects may be relevant and could contribute to its anxiolytic action.

CBD and THC show a biphasic effect, that is, they have both inhibitory and stimulatory effects on the cells of the immune system. Both THC and CBD can decrease TNFα production in human NK cells in peripheral blood mononuclear cells (PBMCs), but THC can increase TNFα production in human monocytes. In many cases, the effects of CBD and THC seem to depend on their concentration: the stimulatory actions have been reported at lower (nanomolar) doses, whilst inhibitory actions have been reported at higher (micromolar) doses. For example, low doses of THC and CBD (similar to doses of smoking cannabis) stimulated INFγ production, but higher doses suppressed INFγ production [43]. Similarly, there appears to be a concentration-dependent effect of both CBD and THC on Th1- and Th2-type cytokines [131].

Both CBD and THC have been found to regulate mitogen-induced Th-1-type immune responses in PBMCs. Treatment of PBMC with either CBD or THC can dose-dependently suppress the mitogen-induced production of neopterin (marker of cellular immunity). Pre-treatment of PBMCs with low (nanomolar) doses of THC or CBD increased the production of the pro-inflammatory cytokine INF-γ, whilst it suppressed its production when high doses were used, demonstrating the biphasic response mentioned previously [131]. For more information on CBD's anti-inflammatory effects, see Chap. 4.

### CBD, Sleep and Anxiety

The anxiolytic effect of CBD appears to be involved in the alleviation of sleep disorders associated with anxiety. Animal studies suggest that CBD may block anxiety-induced REM sleep deprivation through its anxiolytic effect on the brain [138].

## Animal Research: Efficacy of CBD in Anxiety

Several rodent studies have established the anxiolytic effects of CBD, similar to anxiolytic drugs, in various experiments [139–144].

## Animal Models of Anxiety: Elevated Plus Maze

Models of anxiety in mice and rats often use an elevated plus maze (EPM) as a method of measuring anxiety. The EPM is typically constructed with two opposite arms surrounded by walls (closed arms) and two arms devoid of enclosing walls (open arms), which are elevated. The EPM test is able to detect both anxiolytic and anxiogenic drug effects in rats [145]. It is based on the animal's aversion to open spaces and preference for closed spaces. The height and lack of enclosing walls are anxiety-producing for the animals. In this EPM model, anxiety is expressed by the rodent spending more time in the enclosed arms of the maze and less time in the open arms of the maze. Thus, an anxiolytic effect would be indicated by an increase in the proportion time spent in the open arms (i.e. time in open arms/total time in open plus closed arms) and an increase in the proportion of entries in the open arms (no. of entries into open arms/total entries into open plus closed arms).

## Anxiety Studies in Rodents

In one study that used an EPM model of anxiety in rats, doses of 2.5, 5.0 and 10.0 mg/kg of pure CBD significantly increased the entry ratio (open/total number of entries), indicating an anxiolytic effect. Diazepam (2.0 mg/kg) also produced an anxiolytic effect. This study also found that CBD at a higher dose of 20.0 mg/kg was no longer effective. None of the CBD doses altered the total number of entries (measure of total exploratory activity). The conclusion of the study was that CBD causes a selective anxiolytic effect, within a limited range of doses, in the EPM [139]. A limited range of effects is common in studies of pure CBD without its naturally associated plant compounds.

In another rat study, CBD was found to induce an anti-anxiogenic effect in a fear-potentiated plus maze test, a model of contextual conditioned fear [145]. It has also been shown to reduce behavioural and autonomic stress-induced responses in rats [143]. Male rats were given i.p. injections of vehicle (placebo) or pure CBD (1, 10 or 20 mg/kg) and 30 min later subjected to 60 min of restraint during which cardiovascular responses were measured. In the second experiment, the rats received i.p. injections of a $5\text{-HT}_{1A}$ receptor antagonist before the CBD treatment and exposure to restraint. Twenty-four hours later, the rats were tested in the EPM. Exposure to the restraint stress predictably increased the blood pressure and heart rate of the rats and induced an anxiogenic response in the EPM 24 h later. CBD was found to attenuate these effects, and the $5\text{-HT}_{1A}$ receptor antagonist blocked the effects of CBD. This led to the conclusion that CBD can attenuate the acute autonomic responses to stress and the emotional consequences of anxiety by facilitating $5\text{-HT}_{1A}$ receptor-mediated neurotransmission [143].

## Animal Studies of Chronic CBD Administration

Only a few studies have assessed the effects of chronic CBD administration. In one study, treatment with pure CBD for 21 days attenuated inhibitory avoidance acquisition in rats [146]. In another study, chronic but not acute administration of pure

CBD was found to have a moderate anxiolytic effect on mice at low (1 mg/kg) and high doses (50 mg/kg) [147].

A few studies have found no effect of CBD on anxiety-like responses in rats. For example, a study of acute and chronic dosing (14 days) of rats with rimonabant, CBD, CBG and THC (dose of 2.5 mg/kg) found that rimonabant (CB1 receptor antagonist/inverse agonist) and THC (CB1 receptor agonist) both induced anxiogenic-like responses, whilst neither acute nor chronic dosing of CBD and CBG altered anxiety-like responses (i.e. showed neither anxiolytic nor anxiogenic responses) [148]. In another study, rats were acutely or chronically treated for 14 days with CBD (15, 30 and 60 mg/kg) or saline (control) or imipramine (30 mg/kg), and their behaviour was assessed using the forced swimming test (used to assess depression-like behaviour) and open-field tests (used to assess anxiety-like behaviour). Afterwards, the levels of BNDF in the hippocampus, PFC and amygdala were assessed. This study found that CBD at the dose of 30 mg/kg reduced depression-like behaviour and increased the BDNF levels in the rat amygdala, relevant to depression, but had no impact on the open-field test [149].

Another experiment found something totally contrary to what other studies have found, i.e. that chronic dosing of CBD (10 mg/kg) for 14 days actually increased anxiogenic responses and reduced BDNF expression in the hippocampus and frontal cortex (no change in the striatum) and significantly reduced TfkB expression in the hippocampus and significantly reduced phosho-ERK1/2 expression [150]. What does all that mean? It seems in this experiment that CBD *decreased* the expression of proteins that antidepressants and anxiolytic drugs would normally enhance. However, this study has been criticised on two main counts [151]. Firstly, it only used a single dose of CBD (10 mg/kg) instead of a range of doses in order to obtain a clearer dose-response profile. Secondly, the reporting of only part of the test of anxiety used (reporting total distance travelled but not time spent in the inner and outer zones of activity boxes) was queried, with a suggestion that more relevant tests of anxiety (e.g. EPM) should have been used as well [151].

Thus, one can see that the nuances of animal experiments need to be understood if we are to make sense of the outcomes of such experiments.

The contrast in the dose-response relationships for acute versus chronic CBD exposure suggests that some anxiolytic effects of CBD are indirect and related to shifts in the balance of endocannabinoid ligands or receptors. It is important to keep in mind that animal experiments are, at best, an approximation of what might occur in humans. Again, we should also remember that animal studies tend to use pure CBD isolate, and it is very likely that whole plant CBD medicines (containing other phytocannabinoids, terpenes and other plant nutrients) will have quite a different effect on the body. We shall now look at effects of pure CBD in anxiety.

## Pure CBD Isolate and the Bell-Shaped Dose-Response Curve in Animal Studies

Various animal studies assessing the anxiolytic effect of *pure* CBD have shown that the dose-response relationship appears to follow a bell-shaped curve, where the anxiolytic effects are found using moderate doses of CBD, but not at lower or higher doses [139, 152–154]. Injection of CBD into the DPAG, one of the areas involved in the control of anxiety, in rats was also associated with a bell-shaped curve [119]. Other studies of acute systemic application of CBD without prior stress found anxiolytic effects or no effect [140, 145].

Up to this point in time, no anxiogenic effects have been found to be associated with acute systemic administration of CBD in animal models of general anxiety [124]. In other words, CBD may reduce anxiety, but it does not cause it. This is in contrast with tetrahydrocannabinol (THC), which appears to be anxiogenic in higher doses (discussed later).

**Why Might Higher Doses of CBD Be Ineffective?**

Why higher doses of (pure) CBD are ineffective as an anxiolytic may be due to the activation of TRPV1 receptors at higher doses. CBD is able to activate TRPV1 receptors [155], and these receptors appear in several brain regions related to the control of defensive and stress responses, including the mPFC, hippocampus, hypothalamus, dorsolateral PAG and LC [156]. CBD acts as a TRPV1 agonist at high concentrations, potentially interfering with AEA inactivation [155]. Another study found evidence to support the idea that high doses of CBD activate TRPV1 receptors in the PAG and that activation of these receptors may be involved in the bell-shaped dose-response curves observed in CBD [119]. Since the activation of TPPV1 receptors has anxiogenic effects, this would prevent the anxiolytic effect [124], thereby effectively cancelling it out.

Incidentally, this bell-shaped curve has also been demonstrated in a clinical study of 60 healthy participants: subjective anxiety measures were reduced with 300 mg CBD, but not with 100 mg or 900 mg CBD in the post-speech phase of a simulated public-speaking test [126]. This study also used pure CBD (not whole-spectrum CBD).

## Animal Study of Pure CBD Versus Whole Plant CBD

A 2015 animal study compared the shape of the dose-response curves for anti-inflammatory and anti-nociception effects using whole plant CBD and pure CBD isolate in rats. The study found that purified CBD was associated with an inverted U-shaped (bell-shaped) dose-response curve, whereas whole plant CBD showed a linear dose-response curve for anti-nociception [157]. When the study looked at the anti-inflammatory effects of pure CBD versus whole plant CBD, again, the paw thickness dose-response curve showed a U-shaped curve for the pure CBD and a linear dose-response curve for the whole plant. The results for the pure CBD isolate suggest a narrow therapeutic window, outside of which pure CBD may not be as effective (at least in terms of reducing inflammation or reducing pain). But the whole plant CBD extract pharmaceutically acts very differently, in a dose-dependent manner (that intuitively might be expccted).

Until such experiments are replicated in anxiety, in both animals and in humans, comparing pure isolate with whole plant CBD, we can perhaps only speculate – could there be a similar effect for anxiety? We do know that many of the terpenes have anxiolytic actions, so this may be possible.

## Animal Research of CBDA in Anxiety

Research in rats indicates that cannabidiolic acid (CBDA), the acid precursor of CBD, has anxiolytic actions that can be reversed by a 5-hydroxytryptamine 1A (5-$HT_{1A}$) receptor antagonist [158]. In a rat study investigating the neuromotor tolerability profile of CBDA as a potential anti-nausea agent, the researchers found that CBDA had no adverse effects on performance in any neuromotor tolerability test and found evidence of anxiolytic effects of CBDA in a habituated open field test. CBDA was found to be well tolerated and devoid of the sedative side effect profile of benzodiazepine anxiolytics, which are often used to treat anticipatory nausea (they have limited efficacy and significant side effects and induce dependency) [159].

In an anxiety model in rats, HU-580 (the methyl ester of CBDA), but not CBDA, reversed the effect of foot shock on the anxiety-like response. Anxiety in the rodents is generally reflected in decreased time spent in the light box. They found that HU-580 increased the time foot-shocked rats spent in the light compartment of a light-dark box. The effect was blocked by the 5-HT1A antagonist WAY100635, suggesting mediation by 5-HT1A receptors [160]. Further research into the acid form of CBD may be something to watch for in the future.

## Human Research: Efficacy of CBD in Anxiety

The anxiolytic effects of CBD on humans were first demonstrated in the reversal of anxiogenic effects of THC when administered simultaneously [161, 162]. Human studies generally support an anxiolytic role of CBD, but such evidence tends to be limited to acute dosing [114]. However one study of psychiatric patients, which will be discussed later, reported anxiogenic effects in some patients [163].

### Surveys

As discussed at the start of the chapter, there are many surveys suggesting that individuals are using medicinal cannabis including CBD for a range of diagnosed health conditions, and anxiety is one of the most common [3–7, 18]. One longitudinal, cross-sectional web-based survey conducted on patients and caregivers of patients with a diagnosed health condition registered with the Realm of Caring Foundation (not-for-profit organisation) compared 808 cannabis users with 468 non-cannabis users. The study found that compared with non-users, cannabis users self-reported significantly lower anxiety and depression, better sleep, better quality of life, greater health satisfaction and lower average of pain severity ($p < 0.05$) and used 14% less prescription medications. Medicinal cannabis use was associated with positive ratings of health and quality of life across several domains. CBD-dominant products were found to be used at a higher rate than THC-dominant products, with mean doses of CBD of 79 mg/day (adjusted for body weight: 1.4 mg/kg; median 0.6 mg/kg; range 0.01–15.7 mg/kg) and mean doses of THC 3 mg/day (adjusted for body weight: 0.05 mg/kg; median 0.02 mg/kg; range <0.01–0.6 mg/kg) [19].

### Regional Cerebral Brain Flow Studies: Anxiety and CBD

A study conducted in 2004 on 10 healthy males investigated the effects of CBD on regional cerebral blood flow (rCBF) using single-photon emission computed tomography (SPECT). The study randomised participants to receive either 400 mg of CBD or placebo and used a crossed, double-blind study design. This was 99.9% pure CBD dissolved in corn oil. There were two experimental sessions, with an interval of 1 week. A Visual Analogue Mood Scale (VAMS) was used to assess anxiety[1]. The participants were given either the placebo or CBD and then exposed to a potential stressful or anxiety-provoking exercise, a public-speaking test. The effects on rCBF using SPECT were assessed. It was found that 400 mg of CBD significantly reduced subjective anxiety and that the brain activity increased in the left para-hippocampal gyrus and decreased in the left amygdala-hippocampus complex, extending into the hypothalamus and also into the left posterior cingulate gyrus. The anxiolytic effects were detected before the anxiety-evoking situation, indicating that CBD can reduce anticipatory anxiety [164].

This study design was repeated in 2011, and 10 participants who suffered from SAD were enrolled. The participants were again randomised to receive CBD (400 mg, 99.9% pure, dissolved in corn oil) or placebo in a crossed, double-blind design, which had two experimental sessions separated by an interval. The VAMS was used to assess subjective anxiety. The results indicated that compared with placebo, a single dose of CBD (400 mg) significantly reduced subjective anxiety measures before and after SPECT (anticipatory anxiety, $p < 0.001$) [165]. SPECT showed reduced uptake of the brain activity marker (ethyl-cisteinate dimer labelled with technetium-99 m [ECD]) in the left para-hippocampal gyrus (indicating decreased activity) in contrast to the earlier study of healthy males [164], which found increased activity, reflecting a difference between healthy patients and patients with SAD. SPECT also found reduced ECD uptake in the inferior temporal gyrus and increased ECD uptake in the right posterior cingulate gyrus ($p < 0.001$, uncorrected) [165].

A third study (double-blind, randomised, placebo-controlled trial) also looked at regional brain flow using functional MRI in 15 healthy males viewing faces that elicited anxiety. Each scanning session was preceded by intake of either 10 mg THC, 600 mg CBD (both approximately 99.6% and 99.9% pure, respectively) or placebo as gelatin capsules. The main outcome measures included regional brain activation (which was dependent on blood oxygenation), electrodermal activity (skin conductance response (SCR)) and objective and subjective anxiety ratings. Pre-treatment with 600 mg of CBD was associated with reduced anxiety, reduced number of fluctuations in SCR and suppression of blood oxygenation level-dependent signals in the amygdala and anterior and posterior cingulate cortex whilst viewing intensely fearful faces (with the suppression of amygdalar and

[1] Double-blinded studies are those in which the participants and the researcher doing the measuring do not know which study medication the participant is taking: in this case, the CBD or the placebo. In this way, bias is minimised. A cross-over design simply means that each participant got to experience both the CBD and the placebo (though they would not know in which order).

anterior cingulate responses being correlated with the concurrent reduction in SCR fluctuations). This led the researchers to conclude that CBD's effects on activation in the limbic and paralimbic regions of the brain may contribute to its anxiolytic effect. THC increased anxiety and the level of intoxication, sedation and psychotic symptoms and appeared to mainly modulate activation in other brain regions, specifically in the frontal and parietal areas of the brain. The study concluded that the effects of CBD on limbic and paralimbic regions may contribute to its ability to reduce autonomic arousal as well as subjective anxiety, whilst the anxiogenic effects associated with THC could be related to its effects on other brain areas [166].

As you can see, all these three studies used almost pure CBD, whereas the last study used pure THC. It would be interesting if these studies were repeated with whole-spectrum CBD and THC medicinal cannabis products.

### Observational Study: CBD and Anxiety

An observational study of 670 people used an application (Releaf App™) that recorded the effects of cannabis flower consumption; it was conducted from 2016 to 2019. It found a decrease in symptom intensity levels in 95.1% of cannabis use sessions (with an increase in 2.32% of the sessions and no change in 2.16% of the sessions). On average, users experienced a symptom intensity reduction of 3.47 points for anxiety, 3.98 for stress and 4.33 points for agitation/irritability (on a −5 to + 5 visual analogue scale). Medium and high THC levels were the primary independent predictor of increased symptom relief, and this was statistically significant in relation to anxiety only. Interestingly, the CBD levels were in general not associated with changes in symptom intensity levels. Cannabis users reported anxiogenic effects (e.g. feeling anxious, irritable, paranoid or restless or having a rapid pulse) in less than 13% of cannabis use sessions, but in majority (around 66%) of the sessions, they reported anxiolytic effects, including feeling relaxed, happy, peaceful and optimistic [167].

### Case Studies and Case Series

There are currently only a few published case studies in the literature. Examples of these studies are as follows.

#### Paediatric Case Study: CBD and Anxiety in a PTSD Sufferer

A case study was published of a 10 year-old girl suffering from PTSD, who displayed anxiety, aggressiveness, disobedience, impulsivity, sexually inappropriate behaviours, low self-esteem and poor sleep. She was initially treated with the following supplements to assist with anxiety and sleep: melatonin (5 mg/night), magnesium (300 mg/d) and diphenhydramine (25 mg/night). These medications helped slightly, but she was still having outbursts at school and at home, and her anxiety continued. She was trialled on CBD supplements (25 mg) at bedtime plus 6–12 mg of sublingual spray during the day as needed for anxiety. Sleep and anxiety were measured using the Sleep Disturbance Scale for Children and the Screen for Child Anxiety-Related Disorders (SCARED).

The child experienced a gradual increase in sleep quality and quantity as well as decrease in anxiety, with no side effects. The scores of both the scales used to measure sleep disorders and anxiety were reduced after the first month and continued to decrease over the 6-month period of monitoring. The 'SCARED score' was 34 at baseline, 24 at 2 months, 19 at 4 months, 16 at 5 months and 18 at 6 months. The Sleep Disturbance Scale for Children scores were 59 at baseline, 42 at 2 months, 41 at 4 months, 37 at 5 months and 38 at 6 months. This data indicates that within two months, she was benefiting in terms of reduced anxiety and better sleep. Anxiety scores continued to decrease over 6 months of monitoring, whereas sleep scores tended to plateau after 2 months.

After 5 months she was able to sleep in her own room and was handling school well. The therapeutic strategy was to eventually taper off the CBD and transition her into lifelong coping strategies, including meditation and yoga [168].

**Retrospective Case Series: CBD for Psychiatric Patients**

A large retrospective case series was conducted over 3 months at an outpatient psychiatric clinic investigating the effect of CBD for anxiety and sleep problems, as an adjunct to regular treatment [163]. This study was conducted on a final sample of 72 patients, 47 whose main complaint was anxiety and 25 whose main complaint was sleep problem. Anxiety was measured using the Hamilton Anxiety Rating (HAM-A) Scale, which has 14 questions, and sleep was assessed using the Pittsburgh Sleep Quality Index. The side effects and tolerability were also assessed. The average age of patients with anxiety was 34 years (18–70 years), and for those with sleep disorders, 36.5 years (18–72 years). The study doses used ranged from 25 mg/day to 175 mg/day.

Overall, the anxiety scores showed a larger decrease (improvement) over the study period compared with the sleep scores which showed a mild decrease (improvement). The anxiety scores decreased within the first month and then remained decreased for the remainder of the study.

- At the first monthly assessment, 79.2% (57/72) of patients experienced an improvement in anxiety, whilst 11/72 (15.3%) experienced worsening of anxiety.
- At the 2-month assessment, 56.5% (23/41) of patients reported improvement in anxiety compared with the previous monthly visit, whilst 19.5% (8/41) reported worsening compared with the previous month.
- In those with anxiety ($n = 47$), the mean HAM-A score at baseline was 23.87 +/ 9.87, 1 month (18.02 +/ 7.56), 2 months (16.35 +/ 8.80) and 3 months (16.36 +/ 9.80).
- In those whom sleep disorder was the predominant complaint ($n = 25$), the mean HAM-A score at baseline was 22.18 +/ 7.55, 1 month (17.82 +/ 9.72), 2 months (17.36 +/ 10.91) and 3 months (13.78 +/ 7.86).

The sleep scores improved within the first month in 48 patients (66.7%); however they fluctuated over time. CBD was found to be well tolerated in all but three patients (two of which discontinued CBD treatment within the first week due to fatigue and the third due to increased sexually inappropriate behaviour, which were thought to be related to disinhibition as the patient's anxiety had responded dramatically) [163].

### What Do We Learn Here?

What might we learn from this study? First, the results indicate that CBD was helpful in reducing subjective anxiety in a reasonable percentage of patients for whom anxiety was identified as a predominant issue as well as in patients who identified sleep as the predominant issue. In both groups, subjective anxiety scores reduced (improvement) over the 3 months. There was also a trend within both groups indicating improvements in sleep as measured by the PSQI. The study did not assess if the reductions were statistically significant.

There were some patients in which anxiety increased rather than decreased. There is no analysis in the study of why that might have been the case. There was no information on the types of CBD medicines that patients were given. Most patients were also taking psychiatric medication. This was an unblinded study – an 'open-label study' which means that the patients knew they were taking CBD. Therefore, the placebo effect could have contributed to the results.

We also know from clinical experience that medicinal cannabis needs to be individualised to the patient. Most patients were given 25 mg/day of CBD in capsule form. A small number were given 50 mg/day or 75 mg/day, with one patient given a CBD dosage that was gradually increased to 175 mg/day (this patient has history of trauma and schizoaffective disorder). Thus, the results largely pertain to a dosage of 25 mg/day of CBD. The study authors stated that the doses used in the study (25–175 mg/day) were much lower than those reported in other studies (300–500 mg/day) because in their experience, lower doses seem to produce an adequate response, and higher doses, e.g. 600 mg/day, would make the cost too expensive [163]. It is unknown if increasing this dosage could have been associated with greater reductions in anxiety. We also do not know if, for the patients who dropped out, reducing the dose to 25 mg/day would have allowed them to continue in the study and show anxiety and sleep improvements. Nonetheless, the results indicate a positive effect of CBD, at relatively low doses, on anxiety (and sleep) and that it was well tolerated by the study sample.

## Randomised Controlled Trials: CBD for Treatment of Anxiety

CBD may be efficacious in alleviating certain types of anxiety. Social anxiety disorder (SAD) has been the type of anxiety most studied to date. In particular, clinical studies indicate that CBD can reduce the anxiety associated with simulation of public speaking, an anxiety- inducing activity [169]. In such studies using a task of a simulated public speech as a stressor, CBD has been found to reduce anticipatory anxiety, post-stress anxiety and performance anxiety. However, a real-world public-speaking task increases heart rate, systolic blood pressure and diastolic blood pressure significantly more than the simulated public-speaking test [170] and might be a better method for research in future studies, since it would be interesting to see if CBD also affected these other physiological variables.

Table 5.1 sets out several studies on humans that have assessed the efficacy of CBD in anxiety, many of which have been on participants with SAD. Some of these are regional brain flow studies, one is a case series and there are several randomised controlled trials (RCTs).

### Systematic Reviews: CBD and Anxiety Treatment

A systematic review [172] based on one RCT on 24 patients with generalised SAD [169] reported that a single 600 mg dose of CBD was associated with a significantly greater improvement in anxiety compared with placebo in a simulated public-speaking test (see Table 5.1). This systematic review included four RCTs (232 patients) of chronic pain, which also reported on anxiety symptoms. The cannabinoid medicines studied were dronabinol, nabilone and nabiximols, with length of studies varying. The review concluded that the RCTs suggested greater short-term benefit with cannabinoids than placebo for self-reported anxiety symptoms [172].

A 2019 meta-analysis stated that: 'Most of the included studies were done among individuals in whom depression or anxiety was secondary to another medical condition, and in these studies we found no impact of pharmaceutical THC (with or without CBD) on depression symptoms, and a small reduction in anxiety symptoms'. This systematic review concluded that 'Of the few studies in which participants had an anxiety disorder, we did not see a significant benefit of CBD on symptoms of anxiety' [173]. This is curious, as they cite Bergamaschi et al. [169] and Crippa et al.'s [165] studies in relation to this statement; however both these studies actually did find significant benefits of CBD over placebo, and Bergamaschi et al.'s [169] study is the one reported in Whiting et al.'s [172] systematic review, which confirms the efficacy of CBD. We will come back to this study later in the section on THC.

It is always advisable to look at the individual studies. Systematic reviews and meta-analyses might be deemed the 'gold standard' of evidence in medicine, but those who understand research and statistics are aware of their limitations. They often do not include study designs that nonetheless have value, and when you combine numbers from different studies, you often lose information. It is also good to check any affiliations that authors might have with companies that might have vested interests in particular outcomes. Medicine is a political world.

## Scientific Evidence: THC in the Treatment of Anxiety

According to the World Health Organization (WHO) reports on THC [174] and cannabis and its resins [175], anxiety, panic and psychosis are known to be adverse side effects of cannabis and THC in some individuals. Yet one of the main effects of THC and cannabis is a euphoric mood. Does this mean that THC should be avoided in people with anxiety disorders or depression? Not necessarily. The dosage of THC is a key consideration. One of the difficulties is that much of the data on cannabis use relates to recreational use, usually smoking or vaping, and strains grown for the

**Table 5.1** Human studies of CBD in anxiety

| Reference | Participants (No.) | Details of study | Results |
|---|---|---|---|
| Zuardi et al. [162] | Healthy volunteers, $N = 40$ participants (mean age 22.8 years) | Double-blind RCT. Investigation of the effects of ipsapirone and CBD on healthy volunteers submitted to a simulated public-speaking (SPS) test compared with benzodiazepine diazepam and placebo<br>4 groups of 10: CBD (300 mg), diazepam (10 mg), ipsapirone (5 mg) or placebo as gelatin capsules (CBD was dissolved in corn oil, whist the other drugs were mixed with starch)<br>Subjective anxiety measured using the Visual Analogue Mood Scale (VAMS) and State-Trait Anxiety Inventory (STAI) | CBD significantly decreased anxiety after the SPS test (i.e. post-stress anxiety); ipsapirone attenuated SPS-induced performance anxiety (measured in the middle of the speech). Diazepam was anxiolytic before and after the SPS test but had no effect on the increase in anxiety induced by the speech test. Only ipsapirone attenuated the increase in systolic blood pressure induced by the test. Significant sedative effects were found only in the diazepam group |
| Crippa et al. [164] | $N = 10$ healthy males | Effects of CBD on regional cerebral blood flow (rCBF) in healthy volunteers using single-photon emission computed tomography (SPECT)<br>CBD (400 mg, 99.9% pure, dissolved in corn oil) or placebo, crossed, double-blind design, 2 experimental sessions with an interval of 1 week<br>Visual Analogue Mood State (VAMS) used to assess anxiety | CBD significantly reduced subjective anxiety<br>Brain activity increased in the left-para-hippocampal gyrus and decreased in the left amygdala-hippocampus complex, extending into the hypothalamus and also into the left posterior cingulate gyrus<br>Anxiolytic effects were detected before the anxiety-evoking situation, indicating that CBD can reduce **anticipatory anxiety** |

**Table 5.1** (continued)

| Reference | Participants (No.) | Details of study | Results |
|---|---|---|---|
| Crippa et al. [165] | *N* = 10 patients with Social Anxiety Disorder (SAD) | Effects of CBD on regional cerebral blood flow (rCBF) in patients with SAD investigated using single-photon emission computed tomography (SPECT)<br>CBD (400 mg, 99.9% pure dissolved in corn oil) or placebo, crossed, double-blind design, 2 experimental sessions<br>Visual Analogue Mood State (VAMS) used to assess anxiety | Compared with placebo, a single dose of CBD (400 mg) significantly reduced subjective anxiety measures before and after SPECT (**anticipatory anxiety**, $p < 0.001$)<br>SPECT showed reduced ECD uptake in the left para-hippocampal gyrus (indicating decreased activity) in contrast to Crippa et al.'s [164] study on healthy adults that found increased activity, which may reflect the difference between healthy patients and patients with SAD. SPECT also found reduced ECD uptake in the inferior temporal gyrus and increased ECD uptake in the right posterior cingulate gyrus ($p < 0.001$, uncorrected)<br>The results suggest that CBD reduces anxiety in SAD, and this is related to the effects on activity in the limbic and paralimbic brain areas. |

(continued)

**Table 5.1** (continued)

| Reference | Participants (No.) | Details of study | Results |
|---|---|---|---|
| Fusar-Poli et al. [166] | $N = 15$ healthy males | Randomised, double-blind, placebo-controlled study to investigate the effects of THC and CBD on regional brain function during emotional processing. Participants were assessed on 3 separate occasions using event-related functional MRI whist viewing faces that elicited different anxiety levels. Each session was preceded by intake of either 10 mg THC, 600 mg CBD (both approximately 99.6% and 99.9% pure, respectively) or placebo. The main outcome measures: regional brain activation (blood oxygenation level-dependent response), electrodermal activity (skin conductance response [SCR]) and objective and subjective ratings of anxiety | THC associated with increased anxiety, levels of intoxication, sedation and psychotic symptoms. Trend towards reduced anxiety associated with CBD. The number of SCR fluctuations during processing of intensely fearful faces increased following THC administration but decreased after CBD administration. CBD attenuated blood oxygenation level-dependent signal in amygdala and the anterior and posterior cingulate cortex whilst men were processing intensely fearful faces; suppression of the amygdalar and anterior cingulate responses was correlated with concurrent reduction in SCR fluctuations. THC mainly modulated activation in the frontal and parietal areas. |
| Bergamaschi et al. [169] | Patients with social anxiety disorder (SAD) ($n = 24$), 12 healthy controls | Double-blind study, $n = 24$ Px with SAD compared with $n = 12$ healthy controls<br>SAD patients randomised into 2 groups, 600 mg CBD or placebo<br>Outcome variable: performance of simulated public-speaking test | Pre-treatment with CBD in SAD patients significantly reduced anxiety, cognitive impairment and discomfort in speech performance and significantly decreased alert levels in anticipatory speech compared with healthy controls<br>SAD+ Placebo group: higher anxiety, cognitive impairment, discomfort and alert levels compared with healthy controls during the simulated public-speaking test |

**Table 5.1** (continued)

| Reference | Participants (No.) | Details of study | Results |
|---|---|---|---|
| Zuardi et al. [126] | $N = 60$ healthy subjects, both sexes (18–35 years) | Double-blind, placebo-controlled RCT. Subjects randomised into 5 groups: placebo, clonazepam (1 mg) and CBD (100, 300 and 900 mg). Subjects then were required to speak in front of a group formed by the remaining participants. Participants completed the anxiety and sedation factors of the visual analogue mood scale, and heart rate and blood pressure were measured. Each session had four steps following the administration of the treatment or placebo: -5 (baseline), 80 (pre-test), 153 (speech) and 216 (post-speech). | Pure CBD used (99.6% purity). 300 mg of CBD was found to attenuate anxiety in the post-speech phase; however neither 100 mg nor 900 mg was able to do so. Results of animal studies confirmed that CBD induced anxiolytic effects with a dose-dependent inverted U-shaped curve in healthy subjects in the post-speech phase.<br>300 mg of CBD did not reduce SBP or DBP |
| Masataka [171] | 37 Japanese teenagers aged 18–19 years with social anxiety disorder (SAD) and avoidant personality disorder | Double-blind, placebo-controlled RCT. Participants randomised to receive cannabis oil containing 300 mg of CBD or placebo. SAD symptoms were measured at the beginning and end of the treatment period of 4 weeks, using the Fear of Negative Evaluation Scale and the Liebowitz Social Anxiety Scale | CBD significantly decreased anxiety as measured by both scales; reduction in symptoms comparable to paroxetine (drug used commonly to treat this condition) |
| Shannon et al. [163] | Retrospective case series at psychiatric clinic (3 month study)<br>$N = 72$ patients:<br>$n = 47$ main concern anxiety;<br>$n = 25$ main concern poor sleep | CBD adjunct to normal treatment for anxiety and sleep disorders (most 25 mg/day in capsule: if anxiety predominantly, dosing was after breakfast; if sleep problems predominant, dosing in evening after dinner) | Anxiety scores decreased within the 1st month in 57 patients (79%) and remained decreased.<br>Sleep scores improved within the 1st month in 48 patients (67%), but scores fluctuated over time.<br>CBD was well tolerated, and few reported side effects (2 discontinued in the 1st week – fatigue; 1 discontinued – sexually inappropriate behaviour) |

recreational market are typically those high in THC. Let us look at what the preclinical and clinical research says.

## Preclinical Research: Effects of THC on Anxiety

Preclinical studies suggest that there is a biphasic or bimodal response associated with THC: in low doses, THC is anxiolytic, but chronic administration of high doses produces anxiogenic effects [176–178]. Animal research has found that acute administration of higher doses of THC under conditions of high stress increases anxiety by increasing neuronal activity in the limbic system and especially in the amygdala [124, 179]. Further potential mechanisms of action have been elucidated using genetic knockdown mice models (selectively knocking out CB1 receptors in either GABA or glutamate neurons). Such studies have found an anxiolytic effect of cannabinoids at low doses, mediated by the CB1R activation of cortical glutamatergic neurons (thereby decreasing the release of this excitatory neurotransmitter) and an anxiogenic effect at high doses, mediated by the CB1R activation of forebrain GABAergic neurons (thereby decreasing the release of this inhibitory neuron) [108, 177]. CB1 receptor stimulation by low-dose THC in anxiety-related brain regions (e.g. PFC, amygdala and hippocampus) of rats was found to activate different signalling pathways, including those involving CREB function/activity (thought to regulate anxiety-like behaviour in rats), and this may underlie also THC's anxiolytic effect [180]. Several other preclinical studies have found that THC may have an anxiolytic action [20, 91, 181–183]. Some of these are set out in Table 5.2.

However, it is not so simple to say that low doses are anxiolytic and high doses are anxiogenic. The effects of THC may depend on whether the animals were stressed or not. In one experiment, both low and high doses of THC exerted anxiolytic effects on non-stressed rats, whereas in rats subjected to chronic unpredictable stress, the low dose induced anxiogenic effects, whilst the high dose of THC induced an anxiolytic effect [182]. These experiments invariably used pure THC.

### Anti-inflammatory Effects

THC shows strong anti-inflammatory and immunosuppressive effects on several types of immune cells, including macrophages, natural killer (NK) cells and T lymphocytes. This includes suppression of mitogen-stimulated proliferation, IL2 production, T-cell-dependent antibody responses and secretion of (pro-inflammatory) TNF-α [131]. THC can also regulate the Th1/Th2-type cytokine balance in activated human T cells, which can skew the immune response towards a Th2 phenotype (beneficial in diseases characterised by inflammation) [184]. As with CBD, THC may also play a role in reducing or alleviating anxiety through its anti-inflammatory effects.

**Table 5.2** Preclinical research into THC and anxiety

| Reference | Aim of study | Details and results of study |
|---|---|---|
| Fokos and Pagini [182] | To examine how exposure to chronic unpredictable stress will affect reward function and anxiety after acute administration of THC in rats | Male rats were exposed to no stress or 10 days of chronic, unpredictable stress. Alterations in brain reward function were assessed with the intracranial self-stimulation paradigm. Anxiety responses were measured with the EPM.<br>Chronic unpredictable stress did not affect the baseline brain stimulation reward thresholds, and THC was not associated with reinforcing actions in the ICSS paradigm in non-stressed or stressed rats. In non-stressed animals, the low and high doses of THC both exerted anxiolytic-like effects. In stressed rats only the high dose of THC induced an anxiolytic-like response, whilst the low dose induced anxiogenic effects |
| Rubino et al. [180] | To investigate the effects of low-dose THC on anxiety and elucidate neuroanatomical substrates and cellular mechanisms underlying the anxiolytic effect of THC | Anxiolytic effect obtained in doses of 0.075–1.5 mg/kg (dose of 0.75 mg/kg was the most effective).<br>Pre-treatment with CB1R antagonist fully reversed THC's effect, suggesting CB1R involvement. The CFos expression in rats exposed to EPM: THC significantly lowered the amount of cFos in PFC and amygdala (but not other cerebral areas). As CREB function regulates anxiety-like behaviour in rats, phosphorylated CREB was measured in the same brain areas (PFC, amygdala, hippocampus, nucleus accumbens). Rats treated with THC showed a significant increase in CREB activation in PFC (linked to increased ERK activation) and hippocampus (linked to decreased CAMKII activity- kinase that inhibits CREB activation), effects that were reversed by pre-treatment with the CB1R antagonist (suggests that CB1Rs are critically involved) |
| Berrendero and Maldonado [181] | To investigate the possible involvement of different opioid receptors in the anxiolytic-like responses induced by THC | Mice study using light-dark box as means of measuring anxiety.<br>Administration of low-dose THC (0.3 mg/kg) produced anxiolytic responses in the light-dark box. Pre-treatment with the CB1 receptor antagonist completely blocked the anxiolytic response, suggesting that the effect is mediated by the CB1 receptors. Pre-treatment with μ-opioid receptor antagonist and δ-opioid receptor antagonist but not the κ-opioid antagonist blocked the THC anxiolytic effects<br>The results suggest that the endogenous opioid system is involved in the regulation of anxiety by cannabinoids |

(continued)

**Table 5.2** (continued)

| Reference | Aim of study | Details and results of study |
|---|---|---|
| Braida et al. [91] | To assess the in vivo involvement of 5-$HT_{1A}$ subtype receptors on the anxiety-like behaviour induced by acute injection of AM 404 and THC in Sprague–Dawley rats | Rats given THC (0.075–0.75 mg/kg i.p.) 30 min before and AM 404 (0.75–1.25 mg/kg i. p.) 60 min before the EPM test exhibited a dose–response anxiolytic effect (as evidenced by an increase in the percentage of total entries and time spent in the open and decrease in total entries and time spent in the closed arms) The anxiolytic effect obtained with the maximal active dose of both THC (0.75 mg/kg) and AM 404 (1.25 mg/kg) was blocked by a 5-$HT_{1A}$ receptor antagonist. The combination of an ineffective dose of THC (0.015 mg/kg) or AM 404 (0.015 mg/kg) on anxiety-related responses with an ineffective dose of the 5$HT_{1A}$ receptor agonist led to a synergistic effect<br>The results suggest that the anxiolytic effect produced by endo- and phytocannabinoids is modulated by the 5-$HT_{1A}$ receptors |
| Liu and Burnham [183] | To test the effects of THC, CBD and a combination of CBD and THC (15:1 ratio) in mice models of anxiety (the EPM) and depression (forced swimming test, FST) | **Anxiety Expt.** Male CD1 mice (30–35 g) were injected i.p. with CBD (0, 3, 6, 12, 24, 48 and 96 mg/kg), THC (0, 0.2, 0.4, 0.8, 1.6, 3.2 and 6.4 mg/kg), CBD + THC (0, 3 + 0.2, 6 + 0.4, 12 + 0.8, 24 + 1.6, 48 + 3.2, 96 + 6.4 mg/kg) or diazepam (positive control, 0 and 2.5 mg/kg). They were then tested in the EPM for 5 min<br>Results: CBD did not have significant anxiolytic effects at any dose. THC caused a significant increase in time spent in open arms of EPM at 3.2 and 6.4 mg/kg (more time spent in the open arms of the EPM where height and openness of the elevated arm are typically anxiety-producing indicates less anxiety)<br>Combination of CBD + THC was no different from THC alone<br>**Depression Expt.**<br>Adult, male CD1 mice (30–35 g) were injected i.p. with CBD (0, 7.5, 15, 30, 60 and 120 mg/kg), THC (0, 0.5, 1, 2, 4 and 8 mg/kg), CBD + THC (0, 7.5 + 0.5, 15 + 1, 30 + 2, 60 + 4, 120 + 8 mg/kg) or imipramine (positive control, 0 and 30 mg/kg). Mice tested in FST (6 min) or open field arena (60 min). CBD was injected 60 min before testing; THC was tested 30 min before testing. Mice were tested only once ($n$ = 10–15 for each dose)<br>Results: CBD did not have significant anti-depressive effects at any dose.<br>THC significantly decreased immobility time in FST at 2 mg/kg without affecting the open-field activity (suggests an antidepressant effect)<br>Combination of CBD + THC was no different from THC alone<br>Conclusion: THC had both anxiolytic and antidepressant effects at some doses |

## Human Research: Effects of Cannabis and THC on Anxiety

There is a small number of human studies that have assessed the effects of cannabis and THC in relation to anxiety. These include brain imaging studies, observational studies and a small number of RCTs. Some of these published studies are as follows.

### Brain Imaging Studies

Several studies have used functional imaging to assess the effects of THC on various brain regions, as well as on the levels of anxiety. These lend support to the notion that the ECS is involved in the regulation of anxiety; these also provide information on the effects of THC on anxiety and which brain regions appear to be involved.

In a study of 15 healthy male volunteers, regional brain activity was measured, and anxiety was rated subjectively on three separate occasions. Volunteers randomly received either 10 mg THC, 600 mg CBD or placebo. The study found that the 10 mg oral THC increased anxiety and other negative emotions compared with placebo, in contrast to oral CBD (600 mg), which led to a small decrease in anxiety, which did not quite reach statistical significance ($p = 0.06$). THC administration was associated with an increase in activity in the precuneus and primary motor cortex and reduced activity in the bilateral middle frontal gyrus and posterior cingulate cortex [166].

Another imaging study that focused on changes in the amygdala in non-daily users found that 7.5 mg THC reduced amygdala responses to threatening faces and anterior cingulate responses to negative emotional images [185].

In another study of healthy volunteers, the effects of acute dosing of THC (two doses, 7.5 mg and 15 mg) compared with placebo were examined in separate testing sessions. The volunteers received the THC or placebo before assessing facial emotion recognition and emotional responses to pictures of emotional scenes. THC was found to impair recognition of facial fear and anger significantly but only slightly impaired recognition of sadness or happiness. The effect on emotional evaluation was not clearly associated with THC's mood-altering effects [186].

In a later imaging study of healthy males, performance and brain activity in several regions were assessed during a task of matching of stimuli with negative images (fearful faces) and positive images (happy faces) after placebo or THC (9 mg) administration. In this study, the task activated many brain regions, including the amygdala, orbital frontal gyrus, hippocampus, PFC, parietal gyrus and occipital cortex. They found an interaction between THC and the emotional content of the images – brain activity associated with processing of happy images was reduced, and that associated with processing of the fearful faces was increased after THC administration [187]. This study did not find any significant alteration in amygdala activity in association with the viewing of different faces; however an interaction between THC and activity was observed in several other brain regions, including the right PFC, left hippocampus, left and right occipital cortex, vermis, right superior parietal gyrus and right supplementary motor area, which were all statistically significant [187]. This study was interesting as it was the first to show opposite effects of THC for processing stimuli with positive and negative emotional contents across several brain regions and suggests that THC shifts the brain's apparent bias for negative emotional stimuli towards positive emotional stimuli, thereby adding further evidence of the ECS involvement in the regulation of emotions [187].

It should be noted that in all of these studies, the participants were healthy adults. These were not conducted on people diagnosed with anxiety.

### Survey of Whole Plant Cannabis: Are Some Strains Better in Alleviating Anxiety?

Few clinical studies have been conducted to ascertain whether particular cannabis strains might be more effective than others in alleviating various medical conditions. This is also true for anxiety. In addition, most of the preclinical research focuses on purified cannabinoids, such as purified CBD or THC. One study sought to investigate which cannabis strains might be more effective in treating anxiety by surveying 442 medical cannabis patients receiving organically grown cannabis from a single source. The study found that more than 50% of the respondents (266/442) reported anxiety as a symptom for which they use medicinal cannabis, and 15% reported being diagnosed with a specific anxiety disorder. Around 14% of participants reported anxiety as an adverse reaction to medicinal cannabis [25].

A total of 260 participants rated the effectiveness of cannabis in alleviating anxiety on a Likert scale of 0–10 (0 = not effective, 10 = extremely effective). The mean score was 8.03 (95% CI 7.83–8.22 CI, $p = 0.05$; median 8). Patients were asked to identify which strains were most effective in relieving anxiety. A total of 219 and 189 participants gave responses for the most effective strain and the least effective strain, respectively.

- The top four strains/cultivars voted to be the most effective were Bubba Kush ($n = 44$, 20.1%), Skywalker OG Kush ($n = 39$, 17.8%), Blueberry Lambsbread ($n = 36$, 16.4%) and Kosher Kush ($n = 33$, 15.1%).
- The top four chemovars voted to be the least effective were Chocolope ($n = 22$, 11.6%), Blueberry Lambsbread ($n = 16$, 8.5%), CBD Shark ($n = 16$, 8.5%) and Tangerine Dream ($n = 15$, 7.9%).

Interestingly, Blueberry Lambsbread (a myrcene-dominant strain) was included the top four of chemovars voted to be the least *and* most effective. The study authors suggest that this might arise from the differences in the biochemistry between patients or different symptom aetiologies, which may require different pharmacological approaches. In the most effective strains, the following terpenes were found to be most abundant: trans-nerolidol, followed by myrcene and β-caryophyllene.

The active constituents of these eight cultivars (four voted to be the most effective and four voted to be the least effective) were then analysed using high-performance liquid chromatography (HPLC-MS/MS) and GC-MS to investigate whether there were any correlations between phytocannabinoids and terpenes and anxiolytic action. They found that THC and the terpene trans-nerolidol were (statistically) significantly correlated with increased anxiolytic activity, whilst the following (all terpenes) were significantly correlated with decreased anxiolytic activity: guaiol, eucalyptol, γ-terpinene, α-phellandrene, 3-carene and sabinene hydrate [25].

The interesting fact about this study is that it recognises that there are differences in efficacy, in this case for anxiety, between the different strains of cannabis. Different strains have different chemical profiles (phytocannabinoids, terpenes), which are responsible for the therapeutic action on the body. Moreover, in this study, not only the phytocannabinoids but also the terpenes are investigated.

## Observational Studies

In a study of chronic dosing, investigating only inhaled methods of consuming cannabis (smoking, vaping, concentrates, dab bubbler, dab portable), a total of 561 medical cannabis users (299 women and 262 men, mean age 33, std dev. 10 years) used an application to track changes in anxiety ($n = 770$), depression ($n = 561$) and stress ($n = 726$) [188]. The mean number of sessions tracked was 13.15 per person (std dev. 38.48; range 1–972 sessions). A total of 11,953 tracked inhalation sessions were included in the final data analysis (it included only those who re-rated their symptoms within 4 h of inhalation).

The results were as follows:

- Cannabis significantly reduced ratings of anxiety (58% reduction), depression (50% reduction) and stress (58% reduction).
- Anxiety symptom ratings were reduced in 93.5% of tracked sessions, exacerbated in 2.1% of sessions and no change in 4.4% sessions; women perceived a significantly greater reduction in anxiety ratings than men.
- Stress was reduced in 93.3% of tracked sessions, increased in 2.7% and no change in 4% of sessions (no difference between genders).
- Depression symptom ratings were reduced in 89.3% of tracked sessions, exacerbated in 3.2% and no change in 7.5% of sessions (no difference between genders).
- High THC (e.g. >26.5%)/high CBD (e.g. >11%) cannabis best for reducing perceived symptoms of stress.
- Low THC (e.g. <5.5%)/high CBD (e.g. >9.5%) cannabis best for reducing perceived symptoms of depression

There was no apparent dose effect found for anxiety or depression; they found that two puffs were just as effective at reducing anxiety ratings as 10 or more puffs (but two puffs were better than one). For depression, one puff was just as effective as 10 or more puffs. For stress, there was a positive linear relationship between the number of puffs and reduction of stress ratings, with 10 or more puffs producing the largest perceived decreases in stress. One must remember that this study included five different inhalation methods, which could have influenced results. The baseline ratings of anxiety and stress were relatively stable across tracked sessions; however the baseline ratings of depression significantly increased over sessions or time [188].

This study is important in that it focused on a very common method of consuming medicinal cannabis, at least in the USA: inhalation [189]. A US survey indicated that over 92% of medical and non-medical use was through this method, whilst a much lower percentage (8%) was via oral administration [10]. In contrast, many other studies on humans have investigated the oral route of administration. Ideally research is needed in all routes of administration.

**Retrospective Study: Medicinal Cannabis Reduced Benzodiazepine Use**
Benzodiazepines are commonly used in the treatment of anxiety and insomnia, as well as neurological conditions. A retrospective study was conducted on 146 medicinal cannabis patients (average age 47 years, 61% female and 54% reporting prior cannabis use) who reported the use of benzodiazepines at the initiation of cannabis therapy. The patients were using benzodiazepines for pain (47.9%), neurological (7.5%), psychiatric (31.9%) and other (12.7%) conditions. After 2 months of medicinal cannabis use, 30.1% had discontinued use of benzodiazepines, and by 4 and 6 months, 44.5% and 45.2% of patients had discontinued benzodiazepine use, respectively. There was no significant difference in the proportions of CBD and THC in the cannabis used by those who discontinued or did not discontinue benzodiazepines. The study did not assess strain of cannabis used or the method of administration [190].

### Randomised Controlled Trials

In one double-blind RCT of 24 healthy cannabis users, the effects of smoking low and high doses of THC (1.8% and 3.6%, respectively) were compared with placebo on subjective ratings of anxiety. In four blinded sessions, the participants smoked cannabis cigarettes containing placebo, THC with low or high levels of cannabichromene (0.1% vs 0.5%) and low or high levels of CBD (0.2% vs 1.0%). The participant ratings of anxiety increased after smoking cannabis compared with placebo ($p < 0.05$), and the ratings did not differ between the high and low THC strains. In addition, during tests of working memory and episodic memory, compared with placebo, active THC cigarettes were associated with a decrease in performance, reduction in EEG power and reduction in ERP components, which reflected attention-related processes [191].

In a double-blind, placebo-controlled study of healthy adults, low doses (7.5 mg) of oral THC attenuated self-reported negative emotional effects of a psychosocial stressor, but high doses (12.5 mg) increased subjective distress, anxiety and depression [192].

### Systematic Reviews

Finally, a systematic review (7 studies, $n = 252$) found that pharmaceutical THC with or without CBD improved anxiety symptoms among people with other medical conditions (mainly chronic non-cancer pain and MS), though the quality of the evidence was judged to be low [173]. The authors stated the following:

> 'Most of the included studies were done among individuals in whom depression or anxiety was secondary to another medical condition, and in these studies, we found no impact of

pharmaceutical THC (with or without CBD) on depression symptoms, and a small reduction in anxiety symptoms'.

This is an important point – studies are generally statistically powered to have enough participants to identify a change in the primary outcome variable but may not be sufficiently powered to identify changes in secondary outcome variables. This means that there may not have been sufficient participant numbers in a study to determine whether the medicine had an effect on anxiety or depression as secondary outcome variables. We also note here that this review was about 'pharmaceutical THC'. Thus, one cannot extrapolate this to whole-spectrum products containing THC.

## Does Adding CBD to THC Lower Its Anxiogenic Effect?

There is some support in both preclinical and clinical studies that CBD may be able to attenuate the less desirable effects of THC, including its anxiogenic effects. Data is mixed in animal studies.

### Preclinical Research

In animal studies, data is mixed as to whether adding CBD to THC can lower the anxiogenic effect of THC [193]. The question is complicated by findings that different models of stress and anxiety used in animal experiments have been shown to produce different results in relation to the effects of CBD on anxiety [81, 193].

For example, in one rat study, acute administration of CBD attenuated the THC-induced reduction in social interaction (which is a putative anxiety-like behaviour) [194]. Yet, another rat study found that CBD could augment some of the undesirable effects associated with chronic THC use. In this study, a comparison was made between rats given THC only and rats given CBD and THC. Rats were given ascending doses of THC daily over 21 days (1 mg/kg, then 3 mg/kg, then 10 mg/kg). Some rats were given the equivalent CBD dose 20 min before each THC injection. The addition of CBD was found to inhibit body weight gain associated with chronic THC dosing, but it also mildly augmented the anxiogenic effects and locomotor suppressant effects and decreased social interaction associated with THC. The mechanism of action by which CBD potentiates the psychoactive and physiological effects of THC is likely to involve CYP450 enzymes. CYP450 enzymes metabolise both CBD and THC, so the addition of CBD may have resulted in delayed metabolism and elimination of THC [195].

### Clinical Research

There have been a few clinical studies that have examined whether CBD is able to attenuate some of the undesirable effects of THC, such as anxiety. In an early study using double-blind controlled trial methodology, 40 healthy males were assigned to one of 8 experimental groups receiving (per oral) placebo, 30 mg THC, 15 mg CBD,

30 mg CBD, 60 mg CBD and mixtures of 30 mg THC and either 15, 30 or 60 mg CBD. Pulse rate, time production tasks and psychological reactions were measured at time intervals following ingestion. The study found that only 30 mg THC alone increased pulse rate, disturbed time tasks and induced strong psychological reactions. The psychological reactions usually started within 30–50 min after ingestion, reaching a peak 30–60 min later, and gradually subsided within the next 2–3 h. In general, these symptoms appeared in waves during which the participants reported strong feelings of anxiety (sometimes near a state of panic), between which they were less anxious. Doses of 15–60 mg of CBD alone provoked no such effects; however it was found to be efficient in blocking or attenuating most of the adverse effects of THC when these were used together. All doses of CBD were able to partially block the anxiety component of THC: even 15 mg of CBD was able to considerably reduce psychological reactions induced by 30 mg THC. Adding CBD to THC was associated with not just less anxiety and panic but also more pleasurable effects (associated with the THC) [161].

In a double-blind study in 1982, eight (8) healthy volunteers received 0.5 mg/kg THC, 1 mg/kg CBD, a mixture containing 0.5 mg THC plus 1 mg/kg CBD, placebo (control) and diazepam (control) in different sequences. CBD was found to block the anxiety produced by THC, as well as other effects induced by THC (i.e. the 'marijuana-like' effects). No change was detected in pulse rate measurements [196].

In contrast, a study of nabiximols (combination of THC and CBD) compared with THC alone did not find evidence of a beneficial effect on anxiety by having CBD in the mix. In this study they compared 5 mg THC, 15 mg THC, low-dose nabiximols (5.4 mg THC/5.0 mg CBD) and high-dose nabiximols (16.2 mg THC, 15.0 mg CBD) with placebo. All produced anxiety compared with placebo; however there were no differences between THC alone and the combinations of THC and CBD in the measures of anxiety [197].

In a study of nabilone (synthetic THC), patients taking nabilone for neurogenic pain preferred the cannabis herb (which of course has a broader spectrum of cannabinoids, terpenes and other biologic compounds) and reported that the cannabis herb also relieved the associated anxiety and depression [198]. It is likely that the combination of several cannabinoids and other plant nutrients (e.g. terpenes) improves the therapeutic value [199].

### Systematic Review: The Jury Is Still Out

More recently, in 2019 a systematic review was conducted on whether CBD was able to influence the acute effects of THC. This review contained 16 studies with 466 participants in total, 10 of which had a low risk of bias. The results were mixed. CBD was found to reduce the effects of THC in several, but not all, studies. In some studies (but not all), CBD was found to reduce intense experiences of anxiety or psychosis-like effects of THC and to attenuate some of the impairments on emotion and reward-processing. There was considerable variability across the studies in terms of dose, route of administration and ratio of THC to CBD, which is not surprising in a systematic review. No clear dose-response profile was found. The authors of the review concluded that although the findings were conflicting, the results suggest that CBD may interact with some acute effects of THC [200].

### What Do We Conclude?

The above studies have focused on the potential effects on anxiety of adding CBD to THC. Acute exposure to THC has been shown to cause acute, transient and dose-related impairments in cognitive functioning, including executive functioning, abstract ability, decision making, verbal learning, short-term memory, working memory and attention. Although the results of clinical data are mixed, some studies suggest that CBD may attenuate some of these other undesirable effects on cognition induced by THC, as well as psychosis [193].

We still have a lot more to learn with respect to the potential effects of adding CBD to THC on the less desirable effects induced by THC. A major limitation of the current research is that the majority of animal studies have assessed the potential interactions between CBD and THC using acute dosing rather than chronic dosing. Another issue is that only a limited number of preclinical studies have investigated the effects of injected THC; yet inhalation is the most common method of cannabis use in humans [193].

See Boggs et al. [193] for a good summary of current preclinical and clinical evidence in relation to the potential effects of CBD in attenuating the effects of THC.

## Whole Plant Medicines and Entourage Effects in Anxiety

Much of the research discussed previously relates to CBD and THC, two of the main cannabinoids and certainly the most well researched of the phytocannabinoids. However, cannabis has over 700 secondary metabolites. There is increasing evidence of anxiolytic effects of some of the other phytocannabinoids, as well as the terpenes. Here, we will look at some of these.

### Other Phytocannabinoids with Potential Anxiolytic and Antidepressant Effects

Many of the lesser known and researched phytocannabinoids appear to have anxiolytic and antidepressant effects. Thus, understanding the chemical profile of the cannabis strain used in a cannabis medicine, including minor cannabinoids, is important as these, along with the terpenes, are likely to add synergistically to the therapeutic effect. Here are some examples:

- CBDA (cannabidiolic acid) methyl ester: more potent than CBD in reducing acute stress-induced anxiety-like behaviour in rats;
- CBC (cannabichromene): AEA uptake inhibitor; antidepressant in rodent model;
- CBG (cannabigerol): antidepressant in rodent model [160, 201]

### Terpenes with Anxiolytic Effects

Several terpenes may be anxiolytic, including:

- α-Pinene
- β-Caryophyllene
- Linalool
- Limonene
- Humulene
- Myrcene
- Trans-nerolidol and many others [201]

A distinction needs to be made between something that acts as a sedative and something that acts as an anxiolytic agent. Many of the terpenes have sedative actions, and many sedatives have also anxiolytic actions. This section will look very briefly at just *some* of the research that indicates that many of the terpenes present in *Cannabis sativa* (also present in other plants) may have anxiolytic effects. This is important in the context of whole plant medicines – the terpene profile of the various strains or cultivars of cannabis varies, and therefore, when choosing a strain of cannabis, read the label (or certificate of analysis).

Note that most of the following studies are on terpenes derived from plants other than *Cannabis sativa*.

**α-Pinene** imparts a pine aroma and, not surprisingly, is found in pine trees. It has been shown to have anxiolytic and hypnotic effects via the GABAergic system on inhalation; it can also increase non-rapid eye movement (NREM) sleep without affecting the REM and delta activity [202]. In a mice experiment in which the mice inhaled a therapeutic concentration of α-pinene (either 8μL/L or 32μL/L air essential oil from *Chamaecyparis obtusa* [EOCO]), there were significant increases in the number of visits to open arms and times spent in open arms of the EPM, indicating an anxiolytic response. For the lower concentration of inhaled α-pinene, there was no increase in locomotor activity, which the investigators posit may be due to a low, constant concentration of α-pinene in certain parts of the brain. However, for the higher level of inhaled α-pinene (32μL/L air EOCO), they found an increase in locomotor activity and an increase in the concentration of α-pinene in most parts of the brain [203]. Other mice studies have also found inhaled α-pinene to have anxiolytic actions [203–205].

**β-Caryophyllene** (BCP) is an under-recognised phytocannabinoid. It is a common terpene in cannabis and many other plants and herbs, including black pepper and hops. Mice experiments have demonstrated anxiolytic effects of β-caryophyllene [206] as well as **trans-nerolidol** [207]. BCP is a full agonist at CB2 receptors [206, 208], and CB2 receptors are involved in the regulation of mood disorders and anxiety [209, 210]. This terpene has also been shown to activate nuclear peroxisome proliferator-activated receptors-α (PPAR-α) [211]. Which receptors are involved in mediating the anxiolytic effects associated with BCP is still being elucidated, but research implicates CB2, PPAR-ϒ and 5-HT1A receptors. In one study, the anxiolytic and anti-depressant effects of BCP were found to be fully reversed by treatment with AM630 (CB2 antagonist), suggesting that CB2 receptors were involved

[206]. In another study the anxiolytic, anti-oxidant and anti-inflammatory effects of BCP were found to be mediated by both the PPAR-γ and CB2 receptors, whilst antidepressant and memory improvement was found to be mediated only by the CB2 receptors, mainly by the upregulation of PGC-1α and BDNF [212]. However, in yet another study, the anxiolytic effect of BCP was found to be mediated by the 5-HT1A receptors without involvement of the GABA (A) receptors [213].

**Limonene** is a terpene that imparts a citrus-like taste and aroma and is found in several plants, including citrus fruits like lemons. It activates the adenosine receptor, which is involved in the transmission of dopamine. In a rat study set up to assess the effect of component of lemon essential oil on the monoamine levels in the brain and serum under conditions of physical and psychological stress, R-limonene, citral and γ-terpinene were found to inhibit the elevation of serum corticosterone levels (stress hormone) and cerebral monoamine levels. The stereo-isomer of R-limonene, *S* -limonene, has a stronger effect and inhibited the elevation of brain monoamines on psychological stress, leading the authors to conclude that limonenes, particularly *S* -limonene, have a potent stress-alleviating effect [214].

**Linalool** is a terpene that contributes to lavender's relaxing fragrance and is also found in cannabis. Linalool has anxiolytic, sedative and anti-neoplastic properties, and these may relate to its modulatory activity on glutamate and GABA neurotransmitter systems. Research on mice models of anxiety has found that linalool, specifically the leaf essential oil and its major compound *S*-(+)-linalool, significantly increased the time that mice remained in the centre of the open field test, open arms of the EPM test and the illuminated section of the light-dark test, indicating anxiolytic responses that were without side effects, which affect the motor activity. When the level of monoamines in the brains of the mice was measured, decreased levels of serotonin, dopamine and norepinephrine, were observed, which the authors stated were consistent with the anxiolytic effects [215].

**Myrcene** has been found to protect the brain, heart and skin from inflammation and oxidative damage and also has anti-nociceptive actions [202]. There is weak evidence currently for a sedative effect [202], a study in mice where high doses (200 mg/kg) increased barbiturate-induced sleeping time and motor relaxation [216].

## N-Palmitoylethanolamine (PEA) and Anxiety

N-Palmitoylethanolamine (PEA) may play a role in maintaining cellular homeostasis in the face of external stressors causing inflammation and oxidative stress [217]. Research suggests that it may also play a role in the regulation of emotions.

The activation of PPAR-α by PEA induces biosynthesis in the periphery of allopregnanolone, which is a GABAergic neurosteroid that may be involved in mood disorders. A mouse model of PTSD was used to study the effects of PPARα activation on emotional behaviour. Two groups of mice were investigated – one was a socially isolated group and the other was group-housed mice. In this experiment, the neurosteroid levels were measured before and after PEA treatment using chromatography-mass spectroscopy in various brain regions after exposure to a contextual fear conditioning test (used as a means of measuring PTSD-like behaviour), the EPM test (used as a means of measuring anxiety-like behaviour), forced swimming test (used as a measurement of depressive-like behaviour) and tail suspension test (also used as a measurement of depressive-like behaviour). They also measured the neurosteroidogenic enzyme levels in the hippocampus of mice [218].

They found that PEA facilitated fear extinction and fear extinction retention in the PTSD-simulating test. They also found that PEA induced marked anxiolytic and anti-depressive effects in socially isolated mice, along with decreased allopregnanolone levels. These effects were blocked by PPAR-α deletion, PPAR-α antagonists and neurosteroid enzyme inhibitors, and they were mimicked by PPAR-α agonists. The improvements in behaviour were correlated with PEA-induced upregulation of PPAR-α, neurosteroidogenic enzyme expression and normalisation of allopregnanolone levels in the corticolimbic areas of the brain, leading to the conclusion that PPAR-α is involved in emotional behaviour regulation. Thus, PPAR-α might be a useful therapeutic target for mental health disorders characterised by deficient neurosteroidogenesis, such as PTSD and major depressive disorder [218].

## Diet, ECS and Anxiety

Omega 3 (ω3 or n3) polyunsaturated fatty acids play an important role in nutritional therapy and in the modulation of the ECS as we learned earlier. The relevance of lipids in brain function is illustrated by the fact that the CNS has the highest concentration of lipids in the organism after the adipose tissue (50–60% of the dry weight of the brain) [219]. It is generally considered that humans evolved on a diet with a ratio of Omega 6 (ω6) to Omega 3 (ω3) polyunsaturated fatty acids (PUFAs) equal to approximately 1:1. In mammals, linoleic acid (LA, ω6 PUFA) and alpha linoleic acid (ALA, ω3 PUFA) cannot be synthesised de novo and need to be provided through the diet. These essential PUFAs are metabolised into long-chain bioactive lipids using the same enzymatic pathway, meaning that LA and ALA are in competition for conversion to AA and DHA but also for their entry into the brain [220].

The reduced dietary supply of ω3 PUFAs to the brain is associated with many brain diseases, including depression and anxiety disorders [221]. Supporting clinical observations, preclinical studies conducted on rodents showed that ω3 PUFA-deficient diet consumption induces anxiety-like and depressive-like symptoms as well as abnormal social behaviour in adult offspring [222]. Rats that were fed with a ω3 PUFA-deficient diet displayed HPA hyper-reactivity after stress exposure reflected by increased levels of plasma corticosterone compared with the control diet group [223].

# Is Cannabis Use Associated with Anxiety?

## What Is the Evidence?

The question of whether recreational cannabis use is associated with mood disorders such as anxiety (and depression) has been investigated in many studies. Some of the adverse effects of acute cannabis intoxication include feelings of anxiety and/or paranoia [174, 175]. A number of large cross-sectional surveys have found that cannabis users report a higher incidence of anxiety disorders and symptoms compared with non-cannabis users; however the nature of the association is not definitive [224], and evidence of an association does not imply causality. Let's look at some of these studies.

### Associations Between Cannabis Use, Cannabis Dependence and Anxiety

A systematic review of 31 studies (with prospective cohort or cross-sectional designs using non-institutionalised cases) found positive and statistically significant associations between anxiety and cannabis use (OR 1.24, 95% CI: 1.06–1.45, $p = 0.006$; 15 studies) and between anxiety and cannabis use disorder (OR = 1.68, 95% CI: 1.23–2.31, $p = 0.001$; 13 studies) [225]. Analysis of data from the National Comorbidity Survey in the US indicated that cannabis dependence was associated with an approximate two-fold risk of having mood or anxiety disorder [226]. Another study found that among those with anxiety disorders, the mental health summary scores (on a quality-of-life scale, SF-12) were lower among regular (but not occasional) cannabis users compared with non-users [227]. In an Australian study that analysed data from the 2007 National Survey of Mental Health and Wellbeing, those who had not used cannabis were significantly less likely to have an anxiety disorder than cannabis users without cannabis use disorder (CUD) (OR 0.7, 95% CI 0.50.9), and whilst cannabis users with a CUD were significantly more likely to have an affective disorder than cannabis users without a CUD, they were no more likely to meet the criteria for an anxiety disorder (than cannabis users without a CUD) [228].

One study sought to investigate whether the prevalence of mental disorders differed between frequent cannabis users with and without dependence and the general population. The study included 521 young adults (aged 18–30 years) who were frequent cannabis users. Of these, 252 were diagnosed with DSM-IV cannabis dependence (D+), and 269 were without DSMIV cannabis dependence (D−). These were compared with 1072 young adults from the general population [229]. The study found that both dependent and non-dependent frequent cannabis users were at a higher risk than the general population for having 'any mental disorder' though the risk was much greater for cannabis-dependent than non-dependent frequent users (OR 14.97 and 5.35, respectively, both highly statistically significant). The study found that 'externalising disorders' (an example of an externalising disorder is ADHD) were more prevalent in D− (OR 8.91, $P < 0.001$) and D+ adults (OR 17.75, $p < 0.001$) compared with the general population. 'Internalising disorders' were more prevalent only in the D+ group (mood OR 4.15, $p < 0.001$; anxiety OR 2.20, $p$  0.002) compared with the general population, but not in the D- group. However, when they factored in childhood adversity and substance use other than cannabis, these associations were reduced and often became *non-significant.* For example, there was still a significantly higher risk of having any 12-month disorder and conduct disorders in both frequent cannabis use groups compared with the general population, but there was no difference in 'any mood disorder', major depressive disorder, 'any anxiety disorder' and 'general anxiety disorder' once these confounding factors were taken into account. In other words, childhood adversity and substance use other than cannabis are likely to have explained the differences between the two frequent cannabis use groups and the general population rather than the cannabis use. The prevalence of mental health disorders remained higher in the D+ compared with the D- groups (OR 2.40, $p < 0.001$) [229].

**Cannabis Use in Adolescence and Anxiety**

A systematic review and meta-analysis was conducted of longitudinal and prospective studies that assessed cannabis use in adolescents under 18 years of age and potential association with development of depression, anxiety and suicidality. A total of 11 studies ($n = 23317$ individuals) were included. This study concluded that there was a significantly increased odds of developing depression in young adulthood in cannabis users compared with non-users (OR 1.37, 95% CI 1.16–1.62), increased odds for suicide ideation (OR 1.50) and suicide attempt (OR 3.46) but no significant increased odds for anxiety [230].

In a longitudinal cohort study that spanned 30 years, cannabis use during adolescence was associated with depression and suicidality in adult life, but not anxiety disorders [231].

A longitudinal study on adolescents in New Zealand assessed the outcomes of cannabis use at ages of 15–16 years. The study found that cannabis use between ages 15 and 16 years was significantly associated with anxiety disorders, major depression and suicide attempt (between ages 16 and 18 years) compared with non-use, but when other confounding factors including other individual, family and social factors were factored into the statistical analysis, these associations between cannabis use and anxiety/depression/suicide attempt became statistically insignificant. This indicates that other factors rather than cannabis use were responsible for the increased later risk of these mental health conditions [232]. This again brings home a very important point in research: that potentially confounding factors must be recognised and included in statistical modelling.

In an Australian study which was a state-wide survey of 1601 secondary school students aged 14–15 who were followed up for 7 years, they found that around 60% of participants had used cannabis by the time they were 20, and 7% were daily users. Daily use in young women was associated with a greater than five-fold increase in odds of reporting depression and anxiety (OR 5.6, 95% CI 2.6–12.0). Weekly or greater cannabis use in teenagers was associated with almost doubling of risk for later depression and anxiety (OR 1.9, 95% CI 1.1–3.3). However, depression and anxiety in teenagers did not predict later weekly or daily cannabis use [233].

### Theories to Explain Association Between Cannabis Use and Anxiety

A number of large cross-sectional surveys have found that cannabis users report a higher incidence of anxiety disorders and symptoms compared with non-cannabis users; however the nature of the association is not definitive [224]. There are five main theories that attempt to explain the association between cannabis use and anxiety. These are:

- *Common factor theory*: suggests there are associations because they both have common antecedents, which could include biological, social and environmental factors (e.g. childhood trauma)
- *Self-medication theory*: there is an association because individuals who are anxious are motivated to use cannabis to alleviate their symptoms
- *Direct causal theory*: use of cannabis increases the risk of development of an anxiety disorder
- *Reciprocal feedback loop theory*: simultaneous causation between anxiety and cannabis use arise from common factors; each condition leads to an exacerbation of the other due to direct causality and/or self-medication
- *Stress misattribution theory*: a proportion of the associations found between anxiety and cannabis are due to users misattributing their stress symptomatology to anxiety symptoms [224]

A study of 316 participants who were surveyed about their history of cannabis use and stress and anxiety symptoms did not fully support any of the first four hypotheses; however cannabis users reporting self-medication for anxiety were found to be self-medicating their stress symptoms, lending some support for the stress-misattribution theory [224].

## Guidelines for Treating Anxiety with CBD

### When to Use Medicinal Cannabis

Medicinal cannabis treatment should be considered after a thorough clinical assessment and implementation of a comprehensive treatment plan, including lifestyle modification, diet and behavioural approaches. Anxiety or depression can be primary manifestations of several disease conditions that need to be addressed promptly. Medicinal cannabis treatment might also be considered after failure of usual drug therapy or in conjunction with diseases known to be associated with depression like diabetes, rheumatoid arthritis and malignancy.

## Type of Product (Blends)

Ideal blends are high in CBD and low in THC but need to match the patient's age, level of sensitivity to cannabinoids or THC, urine drug testing requirements, body mass and other associated symptoms. Several terpenes like caryophyllene may be a significant part of the product blend and combine well with hemp phytocannabinoids to complement the effects on both anxiety and depression as well as inflammatory conditions. These blends may represent variations of the 'entourage' that enhance effectiveness and reduce adverse effects. This is in stark contrast with single-component CBD or isolates that have shown a bell-shaped dose-response with a narrow window of effectiveness compared with the linear dose-response of biologically derived source (BDS) CBD.

Not only do BDS cannabinoids allow for lower amounts to achieve benefits; they also cause reduced adverse effects [157]. For example, in human anxiety studies, 300 mg to 600 mg of isolate [234] was used to improve symptoms, whereas in a case study of 47 patients in a mental health facility, dosages of only 25–175 mg were needed to achieve significant improvements of anxiety symptoms in 79% of patients within 4 weeks with side benefits of sleep enhancement in 66% [163]. In another series of clinical cases with PTSD for which anxiety is a significant symptom, symptom control was achieved with average doses of 33–48 mg of BDS CBD within 3 weeks [235].

The notion that CBD in the presence of other plant constituents improves the dose-response, is supported by some recent reports showing that CBD in a standardised cannabis extract is more potent or efficacious than pure CBD, including with respect to its anti-proliferative effect on tumour cells and inhibitory effect on bladder contractility. The higher efficiency of plant extract might be explained by additive or synergistic interactions between CBD and minor phytocannabinoids or non-cannabinoids presented in the extracts. Most research has characterised isolated single constituents of traditional herbal medicine. However, our data provides legitimation of whole plant extracts in contrast with synthetic drugs. The therapeutic synergy observed with plant extracts results in lower amount, with reduced adverse effects [157].

THC has anxiolytic properties, and it also can be anxiogenic in some individuals at different doses. THC is a valuable component of the full spectrum cannabis, but a high concentration does not appear necessary; lower doses avoid possible adverse psychotropic experiences. A good example may be in studies on the drug Sativex®, a cannabinoid mouth spray containing THC and CBD (in a ratio of 1.08:1), which is marketed for the treatment of neuropathic pain, spasticity and overactive bladder. Preliminary clinical studies have not shown this formulation to significantly reduce anxiety (in fact, it was reported to induce a mild yet insignificant increase of this symptom) [236]. Higher THC content may be appropriate in some situations to improve sleep, address pain and reduce the need for larger amounts of CBD since higher THC blends tend to allow for decreased amounts of CBD.

## What Form of Product Should You Use?

The best formulation matches the patients preferred lifestyle and tastes. Capsules have a longer duration of action but sublingual tinctures often provide immediate relief of acute stressful situations. The treatment plan might include both approaches in some patients.

## Dosing Guidelines

Age and body mass are only rough guides for dosing of cannabinoid medicines. Generally, 15–30 mg starting doses are appropriate for people weighing 45 kg or greater and can be adjusted after the first doses for the effects. Patients aged seven years or below should start with ½ usual servings, the same for patients 70 years or older. For individuals known to be sensitive to common medications like paracetamol or aspirin, treatment should start with single drops of liquid into the mouth or on the skin of, for instance, the back of the hand.

The typical response is rapid depending on the route of administration using doses in the lower range of 25–50 mg of a CBD-dominant formulation in a twice-daily schedule. The sublingual route delivers a response typically within 5 min, whereas oral doses may require 60–90 min before calming effects are noted. Frequently, if asked, patients will report a general relaxation across the shoulders.

## Titration and Follow-Up

Symptoms of anxiety (and depression) respond very quickly to cannabinoids even on the first dose. If possible, have a staff member follow up the day of or day after the first doses to guide or review the initial response and begin titration to optimise mood and performance or minimise rare adverse symptoms.

Adjust the daily dose or frequency to best fit the patient's situation. Maintain that dose indefinitely or for 1 month and then consider reducing the dose by as much as half based on continuing need.

Often, as in the case of PTSD, patients can achieve remission. Others may decide that the life-enhancing and transformative benefits of cannabinoids are too valuable to suspend and will make cannabinoid a part of their medical nutritional lifestyle.

## Other Tips to Enhance Therapeutic Action

Cannabinoids are best absorbed with food or fatty snack. Studies show that long-chain triglycerides enhance absorption into the intestinal lymphatics bypassing hepatic first-pass effects providing increased concentrations of 250 times plasma levels [237]. This has important implications in those with inflammation needing immune modulation. In fact, cannabinoids ingested with triglycerides achieved higher concentrations (micromolar) in the intestinal lymphatics, which could not be obtained in general circulation, effectively suppressing inflammatory cytokine-expressing T cells [237].

Sleep disorders are common in anxiety and depression. Most patients report improved depth and quality of sleep, but a few can feel activated mentally with an evening dose. Until the patient has experience using cannabinoid medicines, it is advisable that they avoid medium chain trigylcerides (MCT, often used as a carrier oil in medicinal cannabis products) within 2 h or more of bed time. Have the patient use a smart phone sleep application if they feel they are not getting adequate sleep. Often these software programs actually induce deep sleep, of which the patient is unaware. Characteristically patients may say they slept very little or not at all, but they do not report significant fatigue.

## Drug-Cannabis Interactions

Cannabinoids can interfere with drug metabolism based on the modulation of the cytochrome 450 system, specifically the CYP2C and CYP3A classes of isozymes, in vitro and in animal models. However, the modulation is relative and dose-related, seen only with very large doses of CBD isolate far exceeding customary medicinal cannabis treatment. For example, in a study of 13 subjects (aged 4–19 yrs) with epilepsy, concurrent use of clobazam and CBD (Epidiolex, GW Pharmaceuticals) in doses of 20 mg/kg to 25 mg/kg of CBD was associated with significant elevations in the blood levels of clobazam (incidentally 70% had > 50% reduction in seizures and side effects were found in 77% of subjects which were alleviated with clobazam dose reduction) [238]. Other anti-epileptic drugs (17 tested) may increase or decrease in conjunction with CBD [239]. However, another report regarding warfarin and AEDs showed significant increases in INR only at and above isolate CBD doses of 10 mg/kg/day (i.e. 700 mg CBD for an average person) [240]. Thus, interactions can occur at high-dose schedules typical in resistant epilepsy using isolate products but seldom in BDS CBD.

## Case Studies from Dr. Blair's Practice

### Case 1 Chronic Anxiety

Mary is a 61-year-old woman with chronic anxiety who has had panic attacks for over 10 years, which was controlled with increasing doses of Klonopin. She desires to discontinue this drug at the insistance of her healthcare provider. She also has mild arthritis and uses NSAIDs for control. She has minimal outside activities and very little exercise because of her fear of crowded areas. She is married with two grown children who live in other distant states. She smokes one pack of cigarette per day. Her diet includes some prepared packaged meals and processed food, and she consumes occasional gin and tonic cocktails three times per week.

Past history excludes trauma or abuse. She has no military experience. She has not had any serious infection.

Medications include clonazepam 0.5 mg twice daily, ibuprofen 400 mg three times daily, and lisinopril 10 mg per day. She has tried to discontinue clonazepam on several occasions but experiences severe anxiety and panic symptoms, with sweating, paralysing fear and loose stools.

Regarding cannabis exposure, she reports some experimentation in her early 20s that were associated with some anxiety, but otherwise, no other usage. She was intrigued about the possible use of non-psychoactive CBD to help her stop or reduce her anxiety and allow her to discontinue clonazepam.

Other observations: Physically, her blood pressure is 140/90 mmHg (indicating mild hypertension); pulse, 80 bpm; weight, 80 kg; and height, 177 cm. Her knees are slightly tender, and she walks with a mild limp to the right side. No swelling or leg oedema is present. Cognitively she is clear without indications of depression.

Diagnoses: Panic/anxiety and probable benzodiazepine dependence. Other diagnoses of relevance are osteoarthritis and mild hypertension.

## Treatment Recommendation

Cannabis extract, full spectrum, low THC/CBD ratio (1:20) 25 mg twice daily with option for additional dose with panic episodes.

After controlling residual anxiety and panic symptoms, consider initiating a slow tapering (reduction) in clonazepam whilst increasing CBD as needed to control any symptoms.

Also recommended: A high-quality multivitamin with trace minerals, omega 3 fatty acids DHA/EPA (4 gms/day) and slow-release magnesium supplement (400 mg per day).

## Clinical Course

The initial 25-mg CBD was highly effective for reducing residual anxiety and improving general mood, activity and interest in socialisation. The patient also had decreased knee pain and improved sleep.

After 2 weeks, she felt ready to begin a taper of clonazepam (i.e. systematic reduction in clonazepam). She was asked to decrease her dosage by approximate 1/8 per week and use additional cannabis to control any symptoms.

During the first week, she experienced some insomnia and increased anxiety that were improved with an additional 25-mg CBD per day. After the second week and a decreased dose of clonazepam, her symptoms were too difficult to manage in spite of additional CBD, and she returned to the previous drug dose. After 1 week of respite, she was able to continue the taper on schedule due to the fact that she had confidence in using CBD to control her symptoms as well as greater determination.

After total elimination of the clonazepam, she was able to decrease her CBD dose to 25 mg twice daily and maintain her well-being. Her blood pressure normalised to 120/80 mmHg, and her pulse remained at 80 bpm. She took up daily walking without significant pain in her knees, and she was preparing more meals for herself and her husband from fresh food.

Many older patients are often prescribed benzodiazepines for anxiety symptoms with the assurance that they are not addictive. However, some patients do experience dependency with difficult and challenging withdrawal symptoms. Tapering programs of over 12 months have been suggested and published (see Ho et al. [241] and The Ashton Protocol, https://www.benzowarrior.com/tapering-methods). For many people with anxiety disorders, low THC cannabis is a better option.

## Case 2 Posttraumatic Stress Disorder with Prominent Anxiety

Dan is a 34-year-old trucking business owner and social worker from California with a history of drug abuse as a teenager. He had a sudden episode of panic whilst driving his family home from a distant event. This was associated with tingling in his hands, arms and body along with palpitations and a feeling that he might faint. He recovered after 4 h but continued to have repeated episodes over the next 3 months. A full clinical evaluation found moderate hypertension, and he was placed on losartan (ACEII inhibitor) and diagnosed with panic attacks.

Prior to and during these episodes, his only medication was Zyrtec for seasonal allergies, which was discontinued. He denied any illicit drug use, trauma, injuries, infections or chemical exposures.

His current symptoms included fear of driving, being overly cautious, anxiety and distress related to driving. He had continuous feelings of distress and negative thoughts about himself. His blood pressure was marginally controlled on medications. His sleep was restless. Diet was unremarkable except for being forced to stop drinking his favourite drink (coffee).

Past History: His past history included methamphetamine and cocaine abuse and addiction as a teenager from the age of 17 to 21 years during which time he was homeless and living rough in San Francisco. After seven inpatient rehabilitation attempts, he was successful and transitioned to an online college degree and full employment, eventually owning his own trucking firm, which he sold 4 years prior to these events.

### Cannabis History

His first experience with cannabis was at age 10, but he was not a regular user. A friend suggested the use of hemp CBD, but because of his past history of addiction, he was reluctant to pursue this until now.

### Medical Assessment

The patient self-referred for evaluation and guidance for cannabis therapy, seeking the assistance of a medical professional other than his general practitioner. On evaluation he appeared to have a form of anxiety/panic related to a physiologic event 3 months prior with continued symptoms. Because of his addiction history and knowledge of many current psychotropic therapies as a social worker, he wanted to avoid benzodiazepines and any potentially addictive medications.

Physical Examination: His blood pressure was 140/90 mmHg and pulse, 75 bpm. He had a BMI of 22 and body weight of 77 kg. He was cognitively clear-minded and emotionally sound. He spoke well without indications of depression. His business and personal affairs were in perfect order, including a successful marriage with two children.

### Treatment Recommendations

High CBD, low THC cannabis liquid product was recommended for twice daily use and as needed for disturbing symptoms. His initial dose of 25 mg provided significant relief and calming effect. He was asked to continue this therapy and log several clinical parameters on a daily basis. After 1 week his blood pressure normalised, and he discontinue his blood pressure medications.

After 1 month he returned to his usual activities, including driving and seeing patients as a social worker. He adjusted his cannabis dosing to a single 75 mg at night. Two months later whilst vigorously hiking and hunting in Utah, he recognised that his daily cannabis use prevented soreness of extreme unaccustomed physical exertion. At 4 months he decided to pursue a PhD in psychology and dedicate himself to helping others with addiction using non-psychotropic cannabinoids.

### Comments

Although the diagnosis was not clear, a history of a disturbing event powered by major physiologic symptoms and a background of adverse childhood (adolescent) experiences suggest a form of PTSD with prominent anxiety. This was associated with physiologic blood pressure changes and marginal symptoms of depression. Motivated by addiction avoidance, early therapy allowed for rapid resolution and remission. Continued therapy is now based on life enhancement qualities rather than continued anxiety therapy. Changes in life course towards occupations with a compassionate orientation are common in many individuals with resolving anxiety/stress conditions.

## Conclusion

Epidemiological data indicates that anxiety, stress and depression are common conditions for which people self-medicate with cannabis. The ECS is widely distributed in those regions of the brain involved in our stress response, emotions, emotional memory, reward and anxiety-related behaviours. Research indicates that dysfunction of the ECS is involved as part of the pathomechanism of anxiety. Preclinical research has elucidated how CBD and THC may address some of the underlying mechanisms associated with anxiety. Preclinical and clinical research provides support for the notion that CBD is efficacious in treating anxiety, though much of the research is related to acute dosing. More research into chronic dosing, using whole plant medicinal cannabis medicines, is needed. Pure CBD appears to have a bell-shaped dose-response curve, whilst purified THC appears to have a bimodal action. However, whole plant medicines with other phytocannabinoids, terpenes and other plant nutrients are likely to act very differently from purified isolates. Nature was not stupid, but humans often are. An integrative, multi-disciplinary approach that addresses why anxiety is occurring in the first place is likely to be the best approach to helping people deal with anxiety.

## References


1. Micale V, Di Marzo V, Sulcova A, et al. Endocannabinoid system and mood disorders: Priming a target for new therapies. Pharmacol Ther. 2013;138:18–37.
2. Arrow BA, Hunkeler EM, Blasey CM, et al. Comorbid depression, chronic pain and disability in primary care. Psychosom Med. 2006;68:262–8.
3. Hyman SM, Sinha R. Stress-related factors in cannabis use and misuse: implications for prevention and treatment. J Subst Abus Treat. 2009;36(4):400–13.
4. Korem N, Zer-Aviv TM, Ganon-Elazar E, et al. Targeting the endocannabinoid system to treat anxiety-related disorders. J Basic Clin Physiol Pharmacol. 2016;27(3):193–202.
5. Belenduik KA, Babson KA. Vandrey R, Bonn-Miller MO. Cannabis species and cannabinoid concentration preference among sleep-disturbed medicinal cannabis users. Addict Behav 2015;50:178.
6. Tringale R, Jensen C. Cannabis and insomnia. Depression 2011;4(12):0–68.
7. Turna J, Patterson B. Is cannabis treatment for anxiety, mood, and related disorders ready for prime time? Depress Anxiety 2017;1–12.
8. Johnston LD, O'Malley PM. Why do the nation's students use drugs and alcohol? Self-reported reasons from nine national surveys. J Drug Issues. 1986;16(1):29–66.
9. Webb CW, Webb SM. Therapeutic benefits of cannabis: a patient survey. Hawaii J Med Public Health. 2014;73(4):109–11.
10. Sexton M, Cuttler C, Finnell J, Mischley L. A cross-sectional survey of medical cannabis users: patterns of use and perceived efficacy. Cannabis Cannabinoid Res. 2016;1:131–8.
11. Bonn-Miller MO, Vujanovic AA, Drescher KD. Cannabis use among military veterans after residential treatment for posttraumatic stress disorder. Psychol Addict Behav. 2011;25:485–91.
12. Bremner JD, Southwick SM, Darnell A, Charney DS. Chronic PTSD in Vietnam combat veterans: course of illness and substance abuse. Am J Psychiatry. 1996;153:369–75.
13. Schierenbeck T, Riemann D, Berger M, Hornyak M. Effect of illicit recreational drugs upon sleep: cocaine, ecstasy and marijuana. Sleep Med Rev. 2008;12(5):381–9.
14. Kosiba JD, Maisto SA, Ditre JW. Patient-reported use of medical cannabis for pain, anxiety, and depression symptoms : systematic review and meta-analysis. Soc Sci Med. 2019;233:181–92.
15. Bradford AC, Bradford WD. Medical marijuana laws reduce prescription medication use in Medicare Part D. Health Aff. 2016;35(7):1230–6.
16. Cuttler C, Mischley L, Sexton M. Sex differences in cannabis use and effects: a cross-sectional survey of cannabis users. Cannabis Cannabinoid Res. 2016;1:166–75.
17. Piper BJ, DeKeuster RM, Beals ML, et al. Substitution of medical cannabis for pharmaceutical agents for pain, anxiety and sleep. J Psychopharmacol. 2017;31:569–75.
18. Lintzeris N, Driels J, Elias N, et al. Medicinal cannabis in Australia 2016: the Cannabis as Medicine Survey (CAMS-16). Med J Aust. 2018;209(5):211–6.
19. Schlienz NJ, Scalsky R, Martin EL, et al. A cross-sectional and prospective comparison of medicinal cannabis users and controls on self-reported health. Cannabis Cannabinoid Res. 2020; https://doi.org/10.1089/can.2019.0096.
20. Bluett R, et al. Central anandamide deficiency predicts stress-induced anxiety: behavioral reversal through endocannabinoid augmentation. Transl Psychiatry. 2014;4:e408.
21. American Psychological Association. Anxiety. Available at: https://www.apa.org/topics/anxiety/. Accessed 15 Feb 2020.
22. American Psychiatric Association. Diagnostic and Statistical Manual of Mental Disorders (5th edition). Arlington: American Psychiatric Publishing; 2013.
23. Australian Psychological Society. Anxiety Disorders. Available at: https://www.psychology.org.au/for-the-public/Psychology-topics/Anxiety. Accessed 29 Nov 2018.
24. National Institute of Mental Health. Any Anxiety Disorder. 2017. Available at: https://www.nimh.nih.gov/health/statistics/any-anxiety-disorder.shtml. Accessed 15 Feb 2020.
25. Kamal BS, Kamal F, Lantela DE. Cannabis and the anxiety of fragmentation—a systems approach for finding an anxiolytic cannabis chemotype. Front Neurosci 2018;12:730.

26. Hirschfeld RM. The comorbidity of major depression and anxiety disorders: recognition and management in primary care. Prim Care Companion J Clin Psychiatry. 2001;3(6):244–54.
27. Kessler RC, Berglund P, Demler O, et al. The epidemiology of major depressive disorder: results from the National Comorbidity Survey Replication (NCS-R). JAMA. 2003;289:3095–105.
28. Asnis GM, Caneva E, Henderson MA. Treatment of insomnia in anxiety disorders. Psychiatr Times. 2012; 29(1).
29. van Mill JG, Hoogendijk WJ, Vogelzangs N, et al. Insomnia and sleep duration in a large cohort of patients with major depressive disorder and anxiety disorders. J Clin Psychiatry. 2010;71:239–46.
30. Katon WJ, Richardson L, Lozano P, McCauley E. The relationship of asthma and anxiety disorders. Psychosom Med. 2004;66(3):349–55.
31. Mosher CE, Winger JG, Given BA et al. Mental health outcomes during colorectal cancer survivorship: a review of the literature. Psychooncology 2016;11:1261–1270..
32. Mayo Clinic. Anxiety disorders. 2018-2021. Available at: https://www.mayoclinic.org/diseases-conditions/anxiety/diagnosis-treatment/drc-20350967. Accessed 21 Jan 2021.
33. Fuentes D, Ray SD, Holstege CP. Anxiolytics. In: Wexler, editor. Encyclopedia of Toxicology. Third ed. Elsevier; 2014. p. 280–6.
34. Davis CP. Anti-Anxiety Drugs (Anxiolytics) Side Effects, List of Names, MedicineNet, n.d. Available at: https://www.medicinenet.com/anxiolytics_for_anxiety_drug_class/article.htm#what_are_anti-anxiety_anxiolytic_drugs. Accessed 21 Jan 2021.
35. Kim MJ, Loucks RA, Palmer AL, et al. The structural and functional connectivity of the amygdala: From normal emotion to pathological anxiety. Behav Brain Res. 2011;23:403–10.
36. Kheirbek MA, Klemenhagen KC, Sahay A, Rene H. Neurogenesis and generalization: a new approach to stratify and treat anxiety disorders. Nat Neurosci. 2012;15(12):1613–20.
37. Nuss P. Anxiety disorders and GABA neurotransmission: a disturbance of modulation. Neuropsychiatr Dis Treat. 2015;11:165–75.
38. Salim S, Chugh G, Asghar M. Chapter One - Inflammation in anxiety. Adv Protein Chem Struct Biol. 2012;88:1–25.
39. Quah S, McIver L, Roberts A, Santangelo AM. Trait anxiety mediated by amygdala serotonin transporter in the common marmoset. J Neurosci. 2020;40(24):4739–49.
40. Shin LM, Liberzon I. The neurocircuitry of fear, stress, and anxiety disorders. Neuropsychopharmacology. 2010;35(1):169–91.
41. Cooney RE, Atlas LY, Joormann J, et al. Amygdala activation in the processing of neutral faces in social anxiety disorder: is neutral really neutral? Psychiatry Res. 2006;148:55–9.
42. Stein MB, Goldin PR, Sareen J, Zorrilla LT, Brown GG. Increased amygdala activation to angry and contemptuous faces in generalized social phobia. Arch Gen Psychiatry. 2002;59:1027–34.
43. Yoon KL, Fitzgerald DA, Angstadt M, et al. Amygdala reactivity to emotional faces at high and low intensity in generalized social phobia: a 4-Tesla functional MRI study. Psychiatry Res. 2007;154:93–8.
44. Shah SG, Klumpp H, Angstadt M, Nathan PJ, Phan KL. Amygdala and insula response to emotional images in patients with generalized social anxiety disorder. J Psychiatry Neurosci. 2009;34:296–302.
45. Hahn A, Stein P, Windischberger C, et al. Reduced resting-state functional connectivity between amygdala and orbitofrontal cortex in social anxiety disorder. NeuroImage. 2011;56:881–9.
46. Goldin PR, Manber T, Hakimi S, et al. Neural bases of social anxiety disorder: emotional reactivity and cognitive regulation during social and physical threat. Arch Gen Psychiatry. 2009;66:170–80.
47. Phan KL, Orlichenko A, Boyd E, et al. Preliminary evidence of white matter abnormality in the uncinate fasciculus in generalized social anxiety disorder. Biol Psychiatry. 2009;66:691–4.
48. Salim S, Ashghar M, Taneja M, et al. Potential contribution of oxidative stress and inflammation to anxiety and hypertension. Brain Res. 2011;1404:63–71.
49. Kalk NJ, Nuss DJ, Lingford-Hughes AR. The role of central noradrenergic dysregulation in anxiety disorders: evidence from clinical studies. J Psychopharmacol. 2011;25(1):3–16.

50. Labrenz F, Ferri F, Wrede K, et al. Altered temporal variance and functional connectivity of BOLD signal is associated with state anxiety during acute systemic inflammation. NeuroImage. 2019;184:916–24.
51. Zhou FL, Zhang WG, Wei YC, et al. Impact of comorbid anxiety and depression on quality of life and cellular immunity changes in patients with digestive tract cancers. World J Gastroenterol. 2005;11:2313–8.
52. Arranz L, Guayerbas N, De la Fuente M. Impairment of several immune functions in anxious women. J Psychosom Res. 2007;62:1–8.
53. Godbout J, Glaser R. Stress-Induced Immune Dysregulation: Implications for Wound Healing, Infectious Disease and Cancer. J Neuroimmune Pharmacology. 2006;1(4):421–7.
54. Aviles H, Johnson MT, Monroy FP. Effects of cold stress on spleen cell proliferation and cytokine production during chronic Toxoplasma gondii infection. Neuromodulation. 2004;11:93–102.
55. Felger JC. Imaging the role of inflammation in mood and anxiety-related disorders. Curr Neuropharmacol. 2018;16(5):533–58.
56. O'Donovan A, Hughes BM, Slavich GM, et al. Clinical anxiety, cortisol and interleukin-6: evidence for specificity in emotion-biology relationships. Brain Behav Immun. 2010;24:1074–7.
57. Kubzansky LD, Kawachi I. Going to the heart of the matter: do negative emotions cause coronary heart disease? J Psychosom Res. 2000;48:323–37.
58. Bassi GS, Kanashiro A, Santin FM, etl. Lipopolysaccharide-induced sickness behaviour evaluated in different models of anxiety and innate fear in rats. Basic Clin Pharmacol Toxicol. 2012;110:359–69.
59. Goehler LE, Lyte M, Gaykema RPA. Infection-induced viscerosensory signals from the gut enhance anxiety: implications for psychoneuroimmunology. Brain Behav Immun. 2007;21:721–6.
60. Prager G, Hadamitzky M, Engler A, et al. Amygdaloid signature of peripheral immune activation by bacterial lipopolysaccharide or staphylococcal enterotoxin B. J NeuroImmune Pharmacol. 2013;8:42–50.
61. Fiore M, Alleva E, Probert L, et al. Exploratory and displacement behavior in transgenic mice expressing high levels of brain TNF-alpha. Physiol Behav. 1998;63:571–6.
62. Schrott LM, Crnic LS. Increased anxiety behaviors in autoimmune mice. Behav Neurosci. 1996;110:492–502.
63. Kustova Y, Sei Y, Morse HC, Basile AS. The influence of a targeted deletion of the IFN gamma gene on emotional behaviors. Brain Behav Immun. 1998;12:308–24.
64. Wohleb ES, Fenn AM, Pacenta AM, et al. Peripheral innate immune challenge exaggerated microglia activation, increased the number of inflammatory CNS macrophages, and prolonged social withdrawal in socially defeated mice. Psychoneuroendocrinology. 2012;37(9):1491–505.
65. Wohleb ES, McKim DB, Shea DT, et al. Re-establishment of anxiety in stress-sensitized mice is caused by monocyte trafficking from the spleen to the brain. Biol Psychiatry. 2014;75(12):970–81.
66. Bankier V, Barajas J, Martinez-Rumayor A, Januzzi JL. Association between C-reactive protetin and generalized anxiety disorder in stable coronary heart disease patients. Eur Heart J. 2008;29:2212–7.
67. Hoge EA, Brandstetter K, Moshier S, et al. Broad spectrum of cytokine abnormalities in panic disorder and posttraumatic stress disorder. Depress Anxiety. 2009;26:447–55.
68. Spitzer C, Barnow S, Volzke H, et al. Association of posttraumatic stress disorder with low-grade elevation of C-reactive protein: evidence from the general population. J Psychiatr Res. 2010;44:15–21.
69. Pitsavos C, Panagiotakos DB, Papageorgiou C, et al. Anxiety in relation to inflammation and coagulation markers, among healthy adults: the ATTICA study. Atherosclerosis. 2006;185:320–6.
70. Lasselin J, Elsebbruch S, Lekander M, et al. Mood disturbance during experimental endotoxemia: predictors of state anxiety as a psychological component of sickness behaviour. Brain Behav Immun. 2016;57:30–7.

71. Reichenberg A, Yirmiya R, Schuld A, et al. Cytokine-associated emotional and cognitive disturbances in humans. Arch Gen Psychiatry. 2001;58:445.
72. Hovatta I, Juhila J, Donner J. Oxidative stress in anxiety and comorbid disorders. Neurosci Res. 2010;68(4):261–75.
73. Rammal H, Bouayed J, Younos C, Soulimani R. Evidence that oxidative stress is linked to anxiety-related behaviour in mice. Brain Behav Immun. 2008;22:1156–9.
74. Brocardo PS, Boehme F, Patten A, et al. Anxiety and depression-like behaviours are accompanied by an increase in oxidative stress in a rat model of fetal alcohol spectrum disorders: protective effects of voluntary physical exercise. Neuropharmacology. 2012;62:1607–18.
75. Queensland Brain Institute. What is Neurogenensis? https://qbi.uq.edu.au/brain-basics/brain-physiology/what-neurogenesis [accessed 20 July 2021].
76. Ernst A, Alkass K, Bernard S, et al. Neurogenesis in the striatum of the adult human brain. Cell. 2014;156(5):1072–83.
77. Song J, Olsen RHJ, Sun J, et al. Neuronal circuitry mechanisms regulating adult mammalian neurogenesis. Cold Spring Harb Perspect Biol. 2016;8(8):a018937. https://doi.org/10.1101/cshperspect.a018937.
78. Neurohacker Collective. What is neurogenesis. Definition, mechanisms and its role in bain plasticity. Aug 24, 2018. Available at: https://neurohacker.com/what-is-neurogenesis. Accessed 24 Feb 2021.
79. Li Q, Wang L, Ma Y, et al. P-Rex1 Overexpression results in aberrant neuronal polarity and psychosis-related behaviors. Neurosci Bull. 2019;35(6):1011–23.
80. Snyder JS, Soumier A, Brewer M, et al. Adult hippocampal neurogenesis buffers stress responses and depressive behaviour. Nature. 2011;476:458–61.
81. Fogaca MV, Campos AC, Coelho LD, et al. The anxiolytic effects of cannabidiol in chronically stressed mice are mediated by the endocannabinoid system: Role of neurogenesis and dendritic remodeling. Neuropharmacology. 2018;135:22–33.
82. Post RM. Transduction of psychosocial stress into the neurobiology of recurrent affective disorder. Am J Psychiatry. 1992;149:999–1010.
83. Samuels BA, Hen R. Neurogenesis and affective disorders. Eur J Neurosci. 2011;33:1152–9.
84. Miller BR, Hen R. The current state of the neurogenic theory of depression and anxiety. Curr Opin Neurobiol. 2015;0:51–8.
85. Boorman E, Zajkowska Z, Ahmed R, et al. Crosstalk between endocannabinoid and immune systems: a potential dysregulation in depression? Psychopharmacology. 2016;233:1591–604.
86. Hori K, Nagai T, Shan W, et al. Heterozygous Disruption of Autism susceptibility candidate 2 Causes Impaired Emotional Control and Cognitive Memory. PLoS One. 2015;10(12):e0145979.
87. Dow-Edwards D, Silva L. Endocannabinoids in brain plasticity: cortical maturation, HPA axis function and behavior. Brain Res. 2017;1654:157–64.
88. Hill MN, Patel S, Campolongo P, et al. Functional interactions between stress and the endocannabinoid system: from synaptic signalling to behavioural output. J Neurosci. 2010;30(45):14980–6.
89. Atkinson DL, Abbot JK. Cannabinoids and the brain: the effects of endogenous and exogenous cannabinoids on brain systems and function. In: Compton MT and Manseau MW (Eds). The Complex Connection Between Cannabis and Schizophrenia. Elsevier Science and Technology, 2017.
90. Fuss J, Steinle J, Bindila L, et al. A runner's high depends on cannabinoid receptors in mice. Proc Natl Acad Sci U S A. 2015;112(42):13105–8.
91. Braida D, Limonta V, Malabarba L, et al. 5-HT1A receptors are involved in the anxiolytic effect of Delta9-tetrahydrocannabinol and AM 404, the anandamide transport inhibitor, in Sprague-Dawley rats. Eur J Pharmacol. 2007;555:156–63.
92. Navarro M, Hernández E, Muñoz RM et al. Acute administration of the CB1 cannabinoid receptor antagonist SR 141716A induces anxiety-like responses in the rat. NeuroReport 1997;8(2):491–6.
93. Ruehle S, Rey AA, Remmers F et al. The endocannabinoid system in anxiety, fear memory and habituation. J Psychopharmacology (Oxford) 2012–01;26(1):p.23–39.

94. Haller J, Bakos N, Szirmay M, Ledent C, Freund TF. The effects of genetic and pharmacological blockade of the CB1 cannabinoid receptor on anxiety. Eur. J. Neurosci. 2002;16:1395–98.
95. Briones BA, Gould E. Chapter 7 - Adult Neurogenesis and Stress. Fink F (Ed). Stress: Physiology, Biochemistry, and Pathology. Academic Press, 2019:79–92.
96. Hall BS, Moda RN,Liston C. Glucocorticoid mechanisms of functional connectivity changes in stress-related neuropsychiatric disorders. Neurobiol. Stress 2015;1:174–83.
97. Merkulov VM, Merkulova TI, Bondar NP. Mechanisms of brain glucocorticoid resistance in stress-induced psychopathologies. Biochem Mosc. 2017;82:351–65.
98. Balsevich GN, Petrie GN, Hill MN. Endocannabinoids: effectors of glucocorticoid signaling. Front Neuroendocrinol. 2017;47:86–108.
99. Malcher-Lopes R, Franco A, Tasker JG. Glucocorticoids shift arachidonic acid metabolism toward endocannabinoid synthesis: a non-genomic anti-inflammatory switch. Eur J Pharmacol 2008;583:322–39.
100. Tanokashira D, Morita T, Hayash K et al. Glucocorticoid Suppresses Dendritic Spine Development Mediated by Down-Regulation of Caldesmon Expression. J Neurosci 2012; 32(42):14583–91.
101. Qin Z, Zhou X, Pandey NR et al. Chronic Stress Induces Anxiety via an Amygdalar Intracellular Cascade that Impairs Endocannabinoid Signaling. Neuron 2015; 85(6): 1319–31.
102. Gunduz-Cinar O, Hill MN, McEwan B, Holmes A. Amygdala FAAH and anandamide: mediating protection and recovery from stress. Trends Pharmacol Sci. 2013;34:637–44.
103. Rademacher DJ, Meier SE, Shi L, et al. Effects of acute and repeated restraint stress on endocannabinoid content in the amygdala, ventral striatum, and medial prefrontal cortex in mice. Neuropharmacology. 2008;54:108–16.
104. Dlugos A, Childs E, Stuhr KL, et al. Acute stress increases circulating anandamide and other N-acylethanolamines in healthy humans. Neuropsychopharmacology. 2012;37:2416–27.
105. Kinsey SG, O'Neal ST, Long JZ, et al. Inhibition of endocannabinoid catabolic enzymes elicits anxiolytic-like effects in the marble burying assay. Pharmacol Biochem Behav. 2011;98:21–7.
106. Sciolino NR, Zhou W,Hohmann AG. Enhancement of endo-cannabinoid signaling with JZL184, an inhibitor of the 2-arachidonoylglycerolhydrolyzing enzyme monoacylglycerol lipase, produces anxiolytic effects under conditions of high environmental aversiveness in rats. Pharmacol.Res. 2011;64:226–34.
107. Sumislawski JJ, Ramikie PS, Patel S. Reversible Gating of Endocannabinoid Plasticity in the Amygdala by Chronic Stress: A Potential Role for Monoacylglycerol Lipase Inhibition in the Prevention of Stress-Induced Behavioral Adaptation. Neuropsychopharmacology 2011;36:2750–61.
108. Lutz B, Marscicano G, Maldonado R, Hillard CJ. The endocannabinoid system in guarding against fear, anxiety and stress. Nat Rev Neurosci. 2015;16:705–18.
109. Batista PA, Fogaca MV, Guimaraes FS. The endocannabinoid, endovanilloid and nitrergic systems could interact in the rat dorsolateral periaqueductal gray matter to control anxiety-like behaviours. Behav Brain Res. 2015;293:182–8.
110. Rubino T, Realini N, Castiglioni C, et al. Role in anxiety behavior of the endocannabinoid system in the prefrontal cortex. Cereb Cortex. 2008;18:1292–301.
111. Cristino L, de Petrocellis L, Pryce G et al. Immunohistochemical localization of cannabinoid type 1 and vanilloid transient receptor potential vanilloid type 1 receptors in the mouse brain. Neuroscience. 2006;139:1405–15.
112. Micale V, Cristino L, Tamburella A, et al. Anxiolytic effects in mice of a dual blocker of fatty acid amide hydrolase and transient receptor vanilloid type-1 channels. Neuropsychopharmacology. 2009;34:593–606.
113. Papagianni EP, Stevenson CW. Cannabinoid regulation of fear and anxiety: an update. Curr Psychiatry Rep. 2019;21:38.
114. Blessing EM, Steenkamp MM, Manzanares J, Marmar CR. Cannabidiol as a potential treatment for anxiety disorders. Neurotherapeutics. 2015;12:825–36.
115. Rong C, Lee Y, Carmona DS, et al. Cannabidiol in medical marijuana: research vistas and potential opportunities. Pharmacol Res. 2017;121:213–8.

116. Mechoulam R, Peters M, Murillo-Rodriguez E, Hanus LO. Cannabidiol- recent advances. Chem Biodivers. 2007;4(8):1678–92.
117. Campos AC, Moreira FA, Gomes FV, et al. Multiple mechanisms involved in the large-spectrum therapeutic potential of cannabidiol in psychiatric disorders. Philos Trans R Soc Lond Ser B Biol Sci. 2012;367(1607):3364–78.
118. Iannotti FA, et al. Nonpsychotropic plant cannabinoids, cannabidivarin (CBDV) and cannabidiol (CBD), activate and desensitize transient receptor potential vanilloid 1 (TRPV1) channels in vitro: potential for the treatment of neuronal hyperexcitability. ACS Chem Neurosci. 2014;5(11):1131–41.
119. Campos AC, Guimarães FS. Involvement of 5HT1A receptors in the anxiolytic-like effects of cannabidiol injected into the dorsolateral periaqueductal gray of rats. Psychopharmacology. 2008;199:223–30.
120. De Mello Schier AR, de Oliveira Ribeiro NP. Cardoso de Oliveira Silva A et al. Cannabidiol, a Cannabis sativa constituent, as an anxiolytic drug. Braz J Psychiatry. 2012;34(suppl 1):104–10.
121. Soares V, Campos AC, deBortoli VC et al. Intra-dorsal periaqueductal gray administration of cannabidiol blocks panic-like response by activating 5-HT1A receptors. Brain Behav Res 2010;213(2):225–9.
122. Fogaça MV, Reis FM, Campos AC, Guimaraes FS. Effects of intra-prelimbic prefrontal cortex injection of cannabidiol on anxiety-like behavior: involvement of 5HT1A receptors and previous stressful experience. Eur Neuropsychopharmacol. 2014;24:410–9.
123. Gomes FV, Reis DG, Alves FH, et al. Cannabidiol injected into the bed nucleus of the stria terminalis reduces the expression of contextual fear conditioning via 5-HT1A receptors. J Psychopharmacol. 2012;26:104–13.
124. Parker LA. Cannabinoids and the Brain. Massachusetts: MIT Press; 2018.
125. Russo EB, Burnett A, Hall B, Parker KK. Agonistic properties of cannabidiol at 5-HT1a receptors. Neurochem Res. 2005;30:1037–43.
126. Zuardi AW, Rodrigues NP, Silva AL, et al. Inverted U-shaped dose-response curve of the anxiolytic effect of cannabidiol during public speaking in real life. Front Pharmacol. 2017;8:259.
127. Campos AC, de Paula SV, Carvalho MC, et al. Involvement of serotonin-mediated neurotransmission in the dorsal periaqueductal gray matter on cannabidiol chronic effects in panic-like responses in rats. Psychopharmacology. 2013b;226:13–24.
128. Rock EM, Bolognini D, Limebeer CL, et al. Cannabidiol, a non-psychotropic component of cannabis, attenuates vomiting and nausea-like behaviour via indirect agonism of 5-HT(1A) somatodendritic: autoreceptors in the dorsal raphe nucleus. Br J Pharmacol. 2012;165:2620–34.
129. Lee MA. CBD: how it works. O'Shaughnessy's. 2011. Autumn.
130. Leweke RM, Piomelli D, Pahlisch F, et al. Cannabidiol enhances anandamide signaling and alleviates psychotic symptoms of schizophrenia. Transl Psychiatry. 2012;2:e94.
131. Jenny M, Schrocksnadel S, Uberall F, Fuchs D. The potential role of cannabinoids in modulating serotonergic signaling by their influence on tryptophan metabolism. Pharmaceuticals. 2010;3:2647–60.
132. Viudez-Martínez A, García-Gutiérrez MS, Manzanares J. Cannabidiol regulates the expression of hypothalamus-pituitary-adrenal axis-related genes in response to acute restraint stress. J Psychopharmacol. 2018;32(12):1379–84.
133. Campos AC, Ortega Z, Palazuelos J, et al. The anxiolytic effect of cannabidiol on chronically stressed mice depends on hippocampal neurogenesis: involvement of the endocannabinoid system. Int J Neuropsychopharmacol. 2013a;16(6):1407–19.
134. David DJ, Wang J, Samuels BA, et al. Implications of the functional integration of adult-born hippocampal neurons in anxiety-depression disorders. Neuroscientist. 2010;16(5):578–91.
135. David DJ, Samuels BA, Rainer Q, et al. Neurogenesis- dependent and -independent effects of fluoxetine in an animal model of anxiety/depression. Neuron. 2009;62(4):479–93.
136. Santos NAG, Martins NM, Sisti FM, et al. The neuroprotection of cannabidiol against MPP(+)-induced toxicity in PC12 cells involves trkA receptors, upregulation of axonal and

synaptic proteins, neuritogenesis, and might be relevant to Parkinson's disease. Toxicol in Vitro. 2015;30(1 Pt B):231–40.
137. Santos NAG, Martins NM, Sisti FM, et al. The cannabinoid beta-caryophyllene (BCP) induces neuritogenesis in PC12 cells by a cannabinoid-receptor-independent mechanism. Chem Biol Interact. 2017;261:86–95.
138. Hsiao YT, Yi PL, Li CL, Chang FC. Effect of cannabidiol on sleep disruption induced by the repeated combination tests consisting of open field and elevated plus-maze in rats. Neuropharmacology. 2012;62(1):373–84.
139. Guimarães FS, Chiaretti TM, Graeff FG, Zuardi A. Antianxiety effect of cannabidiol in the elevated plus-maze. Psychopharmacology. 1990;100:558–9.
140. Moreira FA, Aguiar DC, Guimaraes FS. Anxiolytic-like effect of cannabidiol in the rat Vogel conflict test. Prog Neuro-Psychopharmacol Biol Psychiatry. 2006;30(8):1466–71.
141. Onaivi ES, Green MR, Martin BR. Pharmacological characterization of cannabinoids in the elevated plus maze. J Pharmacol Exp Ther. 1990;253:1002–9.
142. Resstel LB, Joca SR, Moreira FA, et al. Effects of cannabidiol and diazepam on behavioural and cardiovascular responses induced by contextual conditioned fear in rats. Behav Brain Res. 2006;172:294–8.
143. Resstel LB, Tavares RF, Lisboa SF, et al. 5-HT1A receptors are involved in the cannabidiol-induced attenuation of behavioural and cardiovascular responses to acute restraint stress in rats. Br J Pharmacol. 2009;156(1):181–8.
144. Lemos JI, resstel LB, Guimaraes FS. Involvement of the prelimbic prefrontal cortex on cannabidiol-induced attenuation of contextual conditioned fear in rats. Behavioural Brain Research 2010;207(1):105–11.
145. Bitencourt RM, Pamplona FA, Takahashi RN. Facilitation of contextual fear memory extinction and anti-anxiogenic effects of AM404 and cannabidiol in conditioned rats. Eur Neuropsychopharmacol. 2008;18(12):849–59.
146. Campos AC, Guimarães FS. Evidence for a potential role for TRPV1 receptors in the dorsolateral periaqueductal gray in the attenuation of the anxiolytic effects of cannabinoids. Prog Neuro-Psychopharmacol Biol Psychiatry. 2009;33:1517–21.
147. Long LE, Chesworth R, Huang XF. A behavioural comparison of acute and chronic Delta9-tetrahydrocannabinol and cannabidiol in C57BL/6JArc mice. Int J Neuropsychopharmacol. 2010;13:861–76.
148. O'Brien LD, Wills KL, Segsworth B, et al. Effect of chronic exposure to rimonabant and phytocannabinoids on anxiety-like behavior and saccharin palatability. Pharmacol Biochem Behav. 2013;103(3):597–602.
149. Réus GZ, Stringari RB, Ribeiro KF, et al. Administration of cannabidiol and imipramine induces antidepressant-like effects in the forced swimming test and increases brain-derived neurotrophic factor levels in the rat amygdala. Acta Neuropsychiatrica. 2011;23:241–8.
150. Elbatsh MM, Assareh N, Marsden CA, Kendall DA. Anxiogenic-like effects of chronic cannabidiol administration in rats. Psychopharmacology. 2012;221(2):239–47.
151. Gururajan A. Comment on: "Anxiogenic-like effects of chronic cannabidiol administration in rats" (Elbatsh MM, Assareh N, Marsden CA, Kendall DA, Psychopharmacology 2012). Psychopharmacology. 2012;222:725–6.
152. Levin R, Peres FF, Almeida V, et al. Effects of cannabinoid drugs on the deficit of prepulse inhibition of startle in an animal model of schizophrenia: the SHR strain. Front Pharmacol. 2014;5:10.
153. Nazario LR, Antonioli R, Capiotti KM, et al. Caffeine protects against memory loss induced by high and non-anxiolytic dose of cannabidiol in adult zebrafish (Danio rerio). Pharmacol Biochem Behav. 2015;135:210–6.
154. Peres FF, Levin R, Suiama MA, et al. Cannabidiol prevents motor and cognitive impairments induced by reserpine in rats. Front Pharmacol. 2016; https://doi.org/10.3389/fphar.2016.00343.

155. Bisogno T, Hanus L, De Petrocellis L, et al. Molecular targets for cannabidiol and its synthetic analogues: effect on vanilloid VR1 receptors and on the cellular uptake and enzymatic hydrolysis of anandamide. Br J Pharmacol. 2001;134:845–52.
156. Mezey E, Toth AE, Cortright DN, et al. Distribution of mRNA for vanilloid receptor subtype 1 (VR1), and VR1-like immunoreactivity, in the central nervous system of the rat and human. Proc Natl Acad Sci U S A. 2000;97:3655–60.
157. Gallily R, Yekhtin Z, Hanuš LO. Overcoming the bell-shaped dose-response of cannabidiol by using cannabis extract enriched in cannabidiol. Pharmacol Pharm. 2015;6:75–85.
158. Rock EM, Limebeer CL, Petrie GN, et al. Effect of prior foot shock stress and $\Delta^9$-tetrahydrocannabinol, cannabidiolic acid, and cannabidiol on anxiety-like responding in the light-dark emergence test in rats. Psychopharmacology. 2017;234(14):2207–17.
159. Brierley DI, Samuels J, Duncan M, et al. Neuromotor tolerability and behavioural characterisation of cannabidiolic acid, a phytocannabinoid with therapeutic potential for anticipatory nausea. Psychopharmacology. 2016;233:243–54.
160. Pertwee RG, Rock EM, Guenther K, et al. Cannabidiolic acid methyl ester, a stable synthetic analogue of cannabidiolic acid, can produce 5-$HT_{1A}$ receptor-mediated suppression of nausea and anxiety in rats. Br J Pharmacol. 2018;175(1):100–12.
161. Karniol IG, Shirakawa I, Kasinski N, et al. Cannabidiol interferes with the effects of delta 9 - tetrahydrocannabinol in man. Eur J Pharmacol. 1974;28:172–7.
162. Zuardi AW, Cosme RA, Graeff FG, Guimaraes FS. Effects of ipsapirone and cannabidiol on human experimental anxiety. J Psychopharmacol. 1993;7(1 suppl):82–8.
163. Shannon S, Lewis N, Lee H, Hughes S. Cannabidiol in anxiety and sleep: a large case series. Perm J. 2019;23:18–41.
164. Crippa JA, Zuardi AW, Garrido GE, et al. Effects of cannabidiol (CBD) on regional cerebral blood flow. Neuropsychopharmacology. 2004;29(2):417–26.
165. Crippa JAS, Derenusson GN, Ferrari TB, et al. Neural basis of anxiolytic effects of cannabidiol (CBD) in generalized social anxiety disorder: a preliminary report. J Psychopharmacol. 2011;25(1):121–30.
166. Fusar-Poli P, Crippa JA, Bhattacharyya S, et al. Distinct effects of {delta}9-tetrahydrocannabinol and cannabidiol on neural activation during emotional processing. Arch Gen Psychiatry. 2009;66(1):95–105.
167. Stith SS, Li X, Diviant JP, et al. The effectiveness of inhaled *Cannabis* flower for the treatment of agitation/irritability, anxiety, and common stress. J Cannabis Res. 2020;2:47. https://doi.org/10.1186/s42238-020-00051-z.
168. Shannon S, Opila-Lehman J. Effectiveness of cannabidiol oil for pediatric anxiety and insomnia as part of posttraumatic stress disorder: a case report. Perm J. 2016;20(4):16.
169. Bergamaschi MM, Queiroz RH, Chagas MH, et al. Cannabidiol reduces the anxiety induced by simulated public speaking in treatment-naïve social phobia patients. Neuropsychopharmacology. 2011;36(6):1219–26.
170. Zuardi AW, Crippa JA, Hallak JE, Gorayeb R. Human experimental anxiety: actual public speaking induces more intense physiological responses than simulated public speaking. Rev Bras Psiquiatr. 2013;35:248–53.
171. Masataka N. Anxiolytic effects of repeated cannabidiol treatment in teenagers with social anxiety disorders. Front Psychol. 2019;10:Article 2466. Available at: https://doi.org/10.3389/fpsyg.2019.02466.
172. Whiting PF, Wolff R, Deshpande S, et al. Cannabinoids for medical use: a systematic review and meta-analysis. JAMA. 2015;313(24):2456–73.
173. Black N, Stockings E, Campbell G, et al. Cannabinoids for the treatment of mental disorders and symptoms of mental disorders: a systematic review and meta-analysis. Lancet Psychiatry. 2019; https://doi.org/10.1016/S2215-0366(19)30401-8.
174. World Health Organization. WHO Expert Committee on Drug Dependence Review. Delta-9-tetrahydrocannabinol. Geneva: WHO; 2018a.
175. World Health Organization. WHO Expert Committee on Drug Dependence Review. Cannabis and Cannabis Resins. Geneva: WHO; 2018b.

176. Moreira FA, Kaiser N, Monory K, Lutz B. Reduced anxiety-like behaviour induced by genetic and pharmacological inhibition of the endocannabinoid-degrading enzyme fatty acid amide hydrolase (FAAH) is mediated by CB1 receptors. Neuropharmacology. 2008;54(1):141–50.
177. Rey AA, Purrio M, Viveros MP, Lutz B. Biphasic effects of cannabinoids in anxiety responses: CB1 and GABA(B) receptors in the balance of GABAergic and glutamatergic neurotransmission. Neuropsychopharmacology. 2012;37(12):2624–34.
178. Viveros MP, Marco EM, File SE. Endocannabinoid system and stress and anxiety responses. Pharmacol Biochem Behav 2005;81:331–42.
179. Patel S, Hill MN, Hillard CJ. Effects of phytocannabinoids on anxiety, mood, and the endocrine system. In: Pertwee RG (ed) Handbook of cannabis. Oxford University Press, Oxford, 2014;89–207.
180. Rubino T, Sala M, Viganò D, et al. Cellular mechanisms underlying the anxiolytic effect of low doses of peripheral Delta9-tetrahydrocannabinol in rats. Neuropsychopharmacology. 2007;32(9):2036–45.
181. Berrendero F, Maldonado R. Involvement of the opioid system in the anxiolytic-like effects induced by Δ9-tetrahydrocannabinol. Psychopharmacology. 2002;163:111–7.
182. Fokos S, Panigis G. Effects of delta9-tetrahydrocannabinol on reward and anxiety in rats exposed to chronic unpredictable stress. J Psychopharmacol. 2009;24(5):767–77.
183. Liu J, Burnham M. The effects of CBD and THC in animal models of depression and anxiety. Clin Neurophysiol. 2019;130(8):e118–9.
184. Yuan M, Kiertscher SM, Cheng Q et al. Delta 9-Tetrahydrocannabinol regulates Th1/Th2 cytokine balance in activated human T cells. J Neuroimmunol 2002;133(1–2):124–31.
185. Phan KL, Angstadt M, Golden J, et al. Cannabinoid modulation of amygdala reactivity to social signals of threat in humans. J Neurosci. 2008;28(10):2313–9.
186. Ballard ME, Bedi G, de Witt H. Effects of delta-9-tetrahydrocannabinol on evaluation of emotional images. J Psychopharmacol. 2012;26(10):1289–98.
187. Bossong MG, van Hell HH, Jager G, et al. The endocannabinoid system and emotional processing: a pharmacological fMRI study with Δ9-tetrahydrocannabinol. Eur Neuropsychopharmacol. 2013;23(12):1687–97.
188. Cuttler C, Spradlin A, McLaughlin RJ. A naturalistic examination of the perceived effects of cannabis on negative affect. J Affect Disord. 2018;235:198–205.
189. Schauer GL, King BA, Bunnell RE, et al. Toking, vaping and eating for health or fun: marijuana use patterns in adults. Am J Prev Med. 2016;50:1–8.
190. Purcell C, Davis A, Moolman N, Taylor SM. Reduction of benzodiazepine use in patients prescribed medical cannabis. Cannabis Cannabinoid Res. 2019;4(3):214–8.
191. Ilan AB, Gevins A, Coleman M, et al. Neurophysiological and subjective profile of marijuana with varying concentrations of cannabinoids. Behav Pharmacol. 2005;16:487–96.
192. Childs E, Lutz J, de Wit H. Dose-related effects of delta-9-THC on emotional responses to acute psychosocial stress. Drug Alcohol Depend. 2017;177:136–44.
193. Boggs DL, Nguyen JD, Morgenson D, et al. Clinical and preclinical evidence for functional interactions of cannabidiol and Δ9-tetrahydrocannabinol. Neuropsychopharmacology. 2018;43(1):142–54.
194. Malone DT, Jongejan D, Taylor DA. Cannabidiol reverses the reduction in social interaction produced by low dose Delta(9)-tetrahydrocannabinol in rats. Pharmacol Biochem Behav. 2009;93(2):91–6.
195. Klein C, Karanges E, Spiro A, et al. Cannabidiol potentiates Delta(9)-tetrahydrocannabinol (THC) behavioural effects and alters THC pharmacokinetics during acute and chronic treatment in adolescent rats. Psychopharmacology. 2011;218:443–57.
196. Zuardi AW, Shirakawa I, Finkelfarb E, Karniol IG. Action of cannabidiol on the anxiety and other effects produced by delta 9-THC in normal subjects. Psychopharmacology. 1982;76:245–50.
197. Karschner EL, Darwin WD, Goodwin RS, et al. Plasma cannabinoid pharmacokinetics following controlled oral delta9-tetrahydrocannabinol and oromucosal cannabis extract administration. Clin Chem. 2011;57(1):66–75.
198. Williamson EM, Evans FJ. Cannabinoids in clinical practice. Drugs 2000;60(6):1303–14.

199. Marco EM, Laviola G. The endocannabinoid system in the regulation of emotions throughout lifespan: a discussion on therapeutic perspectives. J Psychopharmacol. 2011;26(1):150–63.
200. Freeman AM, Petrilli K, Lees R, et al. How does cannabidiol (CBD) influence the acute effects of delta-9-tetrahydrocannabinol (THC) in humans? A systematic review. Neuroscience. 2019;107:696–712.
201. Russo EB. Taming THC: potential cannabis synergy and phytocannabinoid-terpenoid entourage effects. Br J Pharmacol. 2011;163:1344–64.
202. Nuutinen T. Medicinal properties of terpenes found in *Cannabis sativa* and *Humulus lupulus*. Eur J Med Chem. 2018;157:198–228.
203. Kasuya H, Okada N, Kubohara M, et al. Expression of BDNF and TH mRNA in the brain following inhaled administration of α-pinene. Phytother Res. 2015;29:43–7.
204. Kasuya H, Hata E, Satou T, Yoshikawa M, et al. Effect on emotional behavior and stress by inhalation of the essential oil from Chamaecyparis obtusa. Nat Prod Commun. 2013;8:515–8.
205. Satou T, Kasuya H, Maeda K, Koike K. Daily inhalation of α-pinene in mice: Effects on behavior and organ accumulation. Phytother Res. 2014;28:1284–7.
206. Bahi A, Al Mansouri S, Al Memari E, et al. β-Caryophyllene, a CB2 receptor agonist produces multiple behavioral changes relevant to anxiety and depression in mice. Physiol Behav. 2014;135:119–24.
207. Goel R, Kaur D, Pahwa P. Assessment of anxiolytic effect of nerolidol in mice. Indian J Pharm. 2016;48:450–2.
208. Gertsch J. Anti inflammatory cannabinoids in diet: towards a better understanding of CB2 receptor action? Commun Integr Biol. 2008;1:26–8.
209. Ashton JC. Knockout controls and the specificity of cannabinoid CB 2 receptor antibodies. Br J Pharmacol. 2011;163:1113.
210. Hill MN, Gorzalka BB. The endocannabinoid system and the treatment of mood and anxiety disorders. CNS Neurol Disord Drug Targets. 2009;8:451–8.
211. Youssef DA, El-Fayoumi HM, Mahmoud. Beta-caryophyllene alleviates diet-induced neurobehavioral changes in rats. Biomed Pharmacother. 2019a;110:145–54.
212. Youssef DA, El-Fayoumi HM, Mahmoud MF. Beta-caryophyllene alleviates diet-induced neurobehavioral changes in rats: the role of CB2 and PPAR-γ receptors. Chem Biol Interact. 2019b;297:16–24.
213. Galdino PM, Nascimento MVM, Florentino IF, et al. The anxiolytic-like effect of an essential oil derived from Spiranthera odoratissima A. St. Hil. Leaves and its major component, β-caryophyllene, in male mice. Prog Neuro-Psychopharmacol Biol Psychiatry. 2012;38:276–84.
214. Fukumoto S, Morishita A, Furutachi K, et al. Effect of flavour components in lemon essential oil on physical or psychological stress. Stress Health. 2008;24(1):3–12.
215. Cheng B-H, Sheen L-Y, Chang S-T. Evaluation of anxiolytic potency of essential oil and *S*-(+)-linalool from *Cinnamomum osmophloeum* ct. linalool leaves in mice. J Tradit Complement Med. 2015;5(1):27–34.
216. Do Vale TG, Furtado EC, Santos J, Viana G. Central effects of citral, myrcene and limonene, constituents of essential oil chemotypes from Lippia alba (Mill.) NE Brown. Phytomedicine. 2002;9:709–14.
217. Skaper S, Facci L, Bartiertato M, Zusso M. N-Palmitoylethanolamine and neuroinflammation: a novel therapeutic strategy of resolution. Mol Neurobiol. 2015;52(2):1034–42.
218. Locci A, Pinna G. Stimulation of Peroxisome Proliferator-Activated Receptor-α by N-Palmitoylethanolamine Engages Allopregnanolone Biosynthesis to Modulate Emotional Behavior. Biol Psychiatry. 2019;85(12):1036–45.
219. Larrieu T, Layé S. Food for mood: relevance of nutritional omega-3 fatty acids for depression and anxiety. Front Physiol. 2018;9:1047.
220. Bazinet RP, Layé S. Polyunsaturated fatty acids and their metabolites in brain function and disease. Nat Rev Neurosci. 2014;15:771–85.
221. Müller CP, Reichel M, Mühle C, et al. Brain membrane lipids in major depression and anxiety disorders. Biochim Biophys Acta Mol Cell Biol Lipids. 2015;1851:1052–65.

222. Bondi CO, Taha AY, Tock JL, et al. Adolescent behavior and dopamine availability are uniquely sensitive to dietary omega-3 fatty acid deficiency. Biol Psychiatry. 2014;75:38–46.
223. Levant B, Ozias MK, Davis PF, et al. Decreased brain docosahexaenoic acid content produces neurobiological effects associated with depression: interactions with reproductive status in female rats. Psychoneuroendocrinology. 2008;33:1279–92.
224. Temple EC, Driver M, Brown RF. Cannabis use and anxiety: is stress the missing piece of the puzzle? Front Psychiatry. 2014;5:168. https://doi.org/10.3389/fpsyt.2014.00168.
225. Kedzior KK, Laeber LT. A positive association between anxiety disorders and cannabis use or cannabis use disorders in the general population- a meta-analysis of 31 studies. BMC Psychiatry. 2014;14:136.
226. Agosti V, Nunes E, Levin F. Rates of psychiatric comorbidity among U.S. residents with lifetime cannabis dependence. Am J Drug Alcohol Abuse. 2002;28:643–52.
227. Lev-Ran S, Le Foll B, McKenzie K, Rehm J. Cannabis use and mental health related quality of life among individuals with anxiety disorders. J Anxiety Disord. 2012;26:799–810.
228. Teesson M, Slade T, Swift W, et al. Prevalence, correlates and comorbidity of DSM-IV cannabis use and cannabis use disorders in Australia. Aust N Z J Psychiatry. 2012;46(12):1182–92.
229. van de Pol P, Liebregts N, de Graaf R, et al. Mental health differences between frequent cannabis users with and without dependence and the general population. Addiction. 2013;108(8):1459–69.
230. Gobbi G, Atkin T, Zytynski T et al. Association of Cannabis Use in Adolescence and Risk of Depression, Anxiety, and Suicidality in Young Adulthood: A Systematic Review and Meta-analysis. JAMA Psychiatry 2019;76(4):426–34.
231. Hengartner MP, Angst J, Ajdacic-Gross V et al. Cannabis use during adolescence and the occurrence of depression, suicidality and anxiety disorder across adulthood: findings from a longitudinal cohort study over 30 years. J Affect Disorders 2020;272:98–103.
232. Ferguson DM, Horwood LJ. Early onset cannabis use and psychosocial adjustment in young adults. Addiction. 1997;92(3):279–96.
233. Patton GC, et al. Cannabis use and mental health in young people: cohort study. BMJ. 2002;325(7374):1195–8.
234. Laczkovics C, Kothgassner OD, Felnhofer A, Klier CM. Cannabidiol treatment in an adolescent with multiple substance abuse, social anxiety and depression. Neuropsychiatrie. 2019; https://doi.org/10.1007/s40211-020-00334-0.
235. Elms L, Shannon S, Hughes S, Lewis N. Cannabidiol in the treatment of post-traumatic stress disorder: a case series. J Altern Complement Med. 2019;25(4):392–7.
236. Tambaro S, Bortolato M. Cannabinoid-related agents in the treatment of anxiety disorders: current knowledge and future perspectives. Recent Pat CNS Drug Discov. 2012;7(1):25–40.
237. Zgair A. Oral administration of cannabis with lipids leads to high levels of cannabinoids in the intestinal lymphatic system and prominent immunomodulation. Nature. 2017;7(1):14542. https://doi.org/10.1038/s41598-017-15026-z.
238. Geffrey AL, Pollack SF, Bruno PL, Thiele EA. Drug–drug interaction between clobazam and cannabidiol in children with refractory epilepsy. Epilepsia. 2015;56(8):1246–51.
239. Friedman D, et al. The effect of epidiolex (cannabidiol) on serum levels of concomitant anti-epileptic drugs. Am Epilepsy Soc. 2014:Abst 2.309.
240. Grayson L, Vines B, Nichol K, Szaflarski JP. An interaction between warfarin and cannabidiol, a case report. Epilepsy Behav Case Report 2018;9:10–11.
241. Ho TT, Gupta SV, Sanchez-Valle A. Prolonged clonazepam-induced withdrawal symptoms in an NAT2 ultraslow acetylator. Pharmacogenomics. 2019;20(02):69–73. https://doi.org/10.2217/pgs-2018-0145.

# Depression

# 6

## Introduction

As discussed previously, mental health issues including depression and anxiety are some of the top reasons for self-medication with cannabis. A systematic review and meta-analysis of empirical studies of patient-reported use of medicinal cannabis for pain, anxiety, and depression (13 studies) found that 34.7% cannabis users surveyed use medicinal cannabis for relief from depression symptoms whilst 51.7% use it for anxiety (and 67.2% for pain) [1]. It is known that depression, anxiety, and pain are highly comorbid [2, 3]. Importantly, the history of cannabis use for depression goes back five centuries. The use of cannabis to treat depression within the western world is found as far back as 1621 in the text *Anatomy of Melancholy*, authored by Oxford scholar Robert Burton, which includes mention of the use of cannabis to treat depression [4]. But the clinical evidence in the literature for the use of medicinal cannabis for treatment of depression is less robust than for anxiety, for example, and inconsistent.

**This Chapter**

This chapter will examine depression, some of the theories of its pathophysiology, and how the endocannabinoid system is involved. It will also examine scientific evidence (epidemiological, preclinical, clinical) of whether medicinal cannabis and in particular cannabidiol (CBD) and tetrahydrocannabinol (THC) may be efficacious or not in treating depression. It will also investigate whether use of cannabis, in particular recreational use, might be associated with depression in a causative manner. We conclude with two case studies from Dr. Blair's practice including dosing tips for clinicians.

We will focus mostly on major depressive disorder (MDD) though we will present some information in relation to bipolar disorder which, in general, has less scientific evidence associated with medicinal cannabis use than MDD.



K. O'Brien, P. Blair, *Medicinal Cannabis and CBD in Mental Healthcare*,
https://doi.org/10.1007/978-3-030-78559-8_6

## What Is Depression?

According to the Mayo Clinic, depression (also called major depressive disorder or clinical depression) is a mood disorder that causes a persistent feeling of sadness and loss of interest, which affects how one feels, thinks, and behaves and can lead to many emotional and physical problems. Depression can negatively impact on daily activities including work, school, and relationships [5].

Major depressive disorder (MDD) is characterized by depressed mood episodes that last for more than 2 weeks, which may often be associated with feelings of low self-esteem, guilt, and worthlessness and high anxiety. There may also be impaired sleep, memory, appetite, and suicidal thoughts [6]. Some other signs and symptoms include: feelings of sadness, emptiness, or hopelessness; irritability, frustration, or outbursts of anger; loss of interest or pleasure in normal activities; lack of energy; self-blame or fixating on failures; frequent or recurrent thoughts of death or suicide, suicide attempts, or suicide; restlessness; lack of appetite and weight loss or increased food cravings and weight gain; difficulty thinking and concentrating; and unexplained physical problems like headaches or back pain [5, 6].

The global prevalence of depression is estimated at 4.4%, with prevalence varying across regions [7]. For example, prevalence in males in the Western Pacific Region is 2.6%, whilst prevalence in females in the African Region is 5.9% [7]. It is the leading cause of global disability, affecting more than 322 million people worldwide and responsible for 7.5% of all years lived with disability [7]. It affects more women than men and can lead to suicide [7].

Bipolar disorder (BD), previously called "manic depression," is associated with extreme mood swings that include emotional highs or euphoria where the person may feel full of energy or unusually irritable (mania, hypermania) and lows (depression). These mood swings which can occur on rare occasion or several times a year can affect the ability to think clearly and can affect sleep, energy, activity, behavior, and judgment [5]. There may be shared genetic risk between schizophrenia and bipolar disorder [8].

## Comorbidities of Depression

Evidence from epidemiological, cross-sectional, and prospective studies indicate that depression, insomnia, and chronic pain are mutually interacting, and each of these increases the risk for emergence and/or exacerbation of the other [9]. For example, depression is reported in up to 54% of patients seeking treatment for pain [2, 10].

Anxiety and depression are also comorbid [3]. Comorbidity is high: an estimated 58% of patients with a MDD have a lifetime anxiety disorder [11], and this comorbidity is associated with greater chronicity, slower recovery, increased recurrence rates, and greater psychosocial disability, as well as increased use of medical services [12]. An estimated 62% of those with generalized anxiety disorder, the most common form of anxiety disorder, were found to have had MDD in their lifetime, and 59% have had an episode of depression in the past 12 months [3, 13, 14].

### Pharmacological Treatment of Depression

Monoamine oxidase inhibitors (MAOIs) and tricyclic antidepressants were two classes of antidepressants introduced around the 1950s; however, they were not well tolerated and there were toxicity issues. These were largely replaced with selective serotonin reuptake inhibitors (SSRIs), norepinephrine reuptake inhibitors (NRIs), and serotonin norepinephrine reuptake inhibitors (SNRIs) and atypical antidepressants such as mirtazapine [15]. Circadian rhythm dysregulation contributes to or is a sequela of mood disturbance; the melatonergic agonist and 5-HT2C antagonist agomelatine has antidepressant activity with a relatively mild side effect profile and is another type of pharmaceutical used to treat depression [15, 16].

Problems associated with SSRIs and other antidepressant medications are that they can require weeks or months to achieve a therapeutic response, many patients are treatment resistant (up to 33%), and compliance is often poor due to side effects [17, 18]. Furthermore, SSRIs have been shown to actually cause depression, mania, and psychosis and, paradoxically, increase suicide ideation and suicide [19].

## Pathophysiology of Depression

The pathogenesis of depression is complex. The monoamine model of depression has been the basis for pharmacological approaches since the 1950s, but this is clearly not the whole story as research indicates that the pathogenesis also includes immune dysregulation and low-grade inflammation (central, systemic) and that there are neurophysiological and neuromorphometric (quantitative neuroanatomical changes of the volume, shape, or location) abnormalities [20, 21]. Impaired adult hippocampal neurogenesis has also been posited to trigger depression, with restoration of neuron development from neuro stem cells leading to recovery [22]. Other factors include HPA axis dysfunction, blunted stress reactivity, NMDA receptor involvement, and changes in BDNF levels. We will explore some of the key factors involved in pathogenesis and then investigate how the ECS is involved.

### Neuromorphometric Changes in Depression

Depression has been found to be associated with changes in brain morphology. Imaging studies have found that the mean gray matter volume is abnormally decreased in several brain regions. Here are some of the research findings:

- Reductions in volume in the hippocampus have been found in association with depression [23–26] though the direction of causation is not definitively known with some studies suggesting episodes of MDD lead to reductions in hippocampal volume and other studies supporting the role of small hippocampal volumes in the etiology of depression [25].

- In patients with MDD and bipolar disorder, reductions in gray matter were found in prefrontal cortex (PFC) ventral to the genu of the corpus callosum (subgenual anterior cingulate cortex) due to a reduction in number of glial cells [27, 28], and decreased brain activity was also found in this region too in both types of depression [27].
- A meta-analysis found significantly smaller volumes in the prefrontal (especially orbitofrontal) and anterior cingulate cortices, as well as in the caudate nucleus and putamen in patients with MDD, with the subgenual anterior cingulate and orbitofrontal cortices being significantly smaller in antidepressant-free individuals compared with those on medication [29]. Another meta-analysis found that in comparison to healthy brains, MDD was associated with lateral ventricle enlargement, larger cerebrospinal fluid volume, and smaller volumes of several brain regions including the basal ganglia, thalamus, hippocampus, frontal lobe, orbitofrontal cortex, and gyrus rectus. In addition, significantly smaller hippocampal volumes were found in patients during MDD episodes compared with patients during remission [30].
- In patients with bipolar disorder, a meta-analysis of 21 studies (660 bipolar disorder patients compared with 770 healthy controls) found that gray matter reductions occurred in several anterior limbic regions compared with healthy normal controls [31].

## Monoamine Theory of Depression

According to the monoamine theory of depression, the basis of depression is a depletion in levels of norepinephrine (NE), serotonin, and/or dopamine in the CNS [32]. According to this model, these neurotransmitters interact with signaling proteins inside the cell membrane in a manner that allows receiving cells to process signals from glutamate and GABA; however, a disruption/depletion of levels of NE, serotonin, or dopamine alters the neuronal signaling in particular brain regions associated with mood [33]. This theory was supported by findings that antidepressant drugs (monoamine oxidase inhibitors, tricyclic antidepressants) which increase levels of these brain neurotransmitters were shown to help alleviate depressive symptoms [32]. The rationale was that if chemicals can reverse symptoms of depression, then depression must be due to chemical abnormalities in the brain [15].

Unfortunately, research has not found strong evidence of a primary dysfunction of a specific monoamine system in people with MDD [34] and the exact role that a deficiency in monoamine systems might play in depression is still unknown. Depletion of monoamines in depressed patients who don't take their medication does not cause any worsening of symptoms, and in healthy volunteers without depressive illness, monoamine depletion doesn't cause depression [32]. Also, use of monoamine-based antidepressants can take weeks to reduce depressive symptoms, something that may indicate neural adaptation occurring downstream is occurring [33]. Although the monoamine model of depression is still the predominant model (and primary target for pharmacological interventions) [15], other more current factors appear to be involved.

## Immune System Function, Inflammation, and Depression

Research indicates that the immune function of people with depression is abnormal, with chronic activation of the innate immune system occurring [35]. Inflammatory cytokines and acute-phase proteins have been found to be elevated in a significant proportion of patients with MDD, bipolar disorder, anxiety, and PTSD [36]. The endocannabinoid system (ECS) and immune system have separately been associated with the pathophysiology of depression, and these systems closely regulate each other. Dysregulated cross-talk between the ECS and the immune system could be implicated in the onset and continuance of depression, though there is a lack of studies examining both the ECS and immune system (at the same time) in depression [20].

### Evidence for Involvement of Immune System and Inflammation in Depression

Boorman et al. [20] and Savitz et al. [21] summarize current evidence for the involvement of the immune system and inflammation in depression, summarized below. Key evidence includes the following:

- Associations have been found between diseases of autoimmune or inflammatory basis such as multiple sclerosis, diabetes, psoriasis, and cardiovascular disease and mood disorders [37–41].
  - In one study of 86 patients with MS, at least 80% showed at least one psychiatric symptom, and the most frequent were depression (59%), sleep disturbance (48%), emotional lability or irritability (42%), and apathy (31%) [39].
  - In a study of psoriasis, those psoriasis patients with depression were 37% more likely to develop psoriatic arthritis than those without [42].
  - A study found that patients diagnosed with MDD had a 32% higher risk of psoriasis than those without [37].
  - A systematic review found that depression was an independent risk factor for onset of a variety of CVDs and that MDD was the most important risk factor for developing CVD [41].
- Studies including meta-analyses have found increased levels of inflammatory markers (including IL-6, IL-1, TNF-α, C-reactive protein) in peripheral blood, serum, plasma, and cerebrospinal fluid of people with depression, compared with healthy individuals, with severity of symptoms in clinically depressed people were directly associated with levels of proinflammatory cytokines [43].
- Depressed people demonstrate increased production of neurotoxic kynurenine metabolites such as quinolinic acid, an agonist of N-methyl-D-aspartate

receptors which is believed to mediate the transition from sickness to depression [44].

- Interferon (IFN-α), used to treat hepatitis C, has been found to cause depression [45] with figures suggesting that 30% of chronic hepatitis C patients treated with IFN-α develop depression [46].
- Healthy individuals given endotoxin were found to develop depression [47]; typhoid injections were found to increase IL-6 and significantly reduce mood in healthy volunteers compare with placebo. Inflammation-associated mood deterioration was found to correlate with enhanced activity in the subgenual anterior cingulate gyrus (sACC, area of brain implicated in depression etiology) during an emotional face processing task, as well as correlated with reduced connectivity of the sACC to the amygdala, medial prefrontal cortex, nucleus accumbens, and superior temporal sulcus, modulated by peripheral IL-6 [48].
- Several anti-inflammatory drugs have been found to be effective in reducing symptoms of depression (e.g., aspirin, celecoxib) [49], and many antidepressants have anti-inflammatory effects and modulate cytokine production (e.g., tricyclic antidepressants, SSRIs); serotonin-noradrenalin antidepressants have also been found to inhibit production and/or release of proinflammatory cytokines and stimulate the production of anti-inflammatory cytokines [50].

Although there is evidence of an association between depression and systemic inflammation, including raised blood levels of inflammatory cytokines in some individuals with depression, it is not known if this is the cause or effect of depression [51].

### Possible Link Between Immune System Activity and Depression Pathogenesis

Activation of indoleamine-2,3-dioxygenase (IDO) enzyme activity may be a link between the immune system activity and pathogenesis of depression, described by Jenny et al. [52]. They explain that IDO-mediated degradation of tryptophan is part of the antimicrobial and antiproliferative immune response and it is also part of the process by which serotonin is produced (tryptophan is the precursor for the biosynthesis of serotonin, 5HT). Disturbance of serotonergic activity plays a role in neuropsychiatric disorders such as depression. In human macrophages, T-cell-derived IFN-γ also involves stimulation of IDO, converting tryptophan to an intermediate which is finally converted to kynurenine, thereby limiting the availability of tryptophan in the circulation. This limitation of tryptophan in the circulation inhibits protein synthesis and thereby the growth of bacteria, viruses, parasites, and highly proliferating tumor cells, and it suppresses T-cell responsiveness. There have been associations found between accelerated tryptophan degradation and blood levels of IFN-γ and neopterin in some diseases associated with an activated cell-mediated response (e.g., cancer, autoimmune conditions), and lower levels of tryptophan have been found to be associated with increased risk of depression in patients with cancer (known to be underpinned by inflammation) or being treated with proinflammatory cytokines [52].

### CNS Inflammation

Studies suggest central nervous system (CNS) inflammation and oxidative stress are also involved in the pathogenesis of depression [20, 53]. Inflammation and oxidative stress are key contributors to the "neuroprogression" seen in MDD, evidenced by increased inflammatory and oxidative stress biomarkers [53]. CNS neuroinflammation may lead to alterations in neurotransmitter metabolism and neuroendocrine function that typically occur in depression [53]. Microglia play roles in initiation and maintenance of neuroinflammation as well as have repair and neuroprotective functions, with activation of microglia being on a continuum between proinflammatory (M1) and anti-inflammatory (M2) [51]. In the CNS, microglial activation is thought to play a role in depression, supported by findings that animal models of depression have demonstrated altered expression of microglial activation markers and time-dependent fluctuations in concentration of microglia in brain areas associated with regulation of mood [20]. Further support comes from findings of significant microgliosis in brains of suicide victims at post-mortem [20, 54], with various studies finding such changes associated with particular brain regions [54].

In addition, in studies of suicide ideation, there appears to be an association between the tryptophan-kynurenine pathway and suicide, with higher reports of plasma tryptophan and kynurenine in MDD patients with suicide attempts compared with MDD patients without suicide attempts [54].

However, it is worth noting that not all studies have confirmed that neuroinflammation is associated with depression, as demonstrated by one study which used PET imaging and found that individuals with mild-moderate depression do not show evidence of neuroinflammation as measured by level of neuroinflammation marker translocator protein compared with those without depression [51].

## Malfunction of Lymphatic Vessels in the CNS Could Be Involved in Depression

Functional lymphatic vessels have been found lining the dural sinuses, which can carry fluid and immune cells from the cerebrospinal fluid and are connected to the deep cervical lymph nodes [55]. Malfunction of these lymphatic vessels may be involved in several neurological disorders in which altered immunity is a key factor, like Alzheimer's disease [55]. It has been speculated that the CNS lymphatic system could also be involved in the pathogenesis of depression via neuroinflammation [20], though this is yet to be substantiated. Research would be needed to ascertain one way or another.

## HPA Axis Dysfunction and Depression

Another popular line of thought, along with the monoamine theory, has been the idea that dysfunction of the HPA axis, specifically an overactivity, plays a key role in depression [56].

There is much in the literature to support this theory, including some of the following:

- Evidence of hypersecretion of corticotrophin-releasing hormone (CRH): CRH immunoreactivity is upregulated in CSF of patients with depression, as well as in the locus coeruleus and peripherally (plasma).
- Elevated basal cortisol levels (CSF, blood) have been found in association with depression; imaging studies indicate that depression is associated with adrenal hypertrophy and more cortisol is produced per molecule of ACTH in depressed patients compared with normal controls. Also, diseases like Cushing's disease which are associated with hypercortisolemia display symptoms similar to major depressive disorder.
- CRHR-1 receptors are downregulated in the prefrontal cortex of depressed persons (in response to hypersecretion of CRH), and glucocorticoid receptors are downregulated in the periphery in depressed people.
- Depressed patients show an attenuation of the normal suppression of CRH activity shown in those without depression (that is part of the negative feedback loop), demonstrated on the dexamethasone suppression test (in non-depressed people, the synthetic glucocorticoid dexamethasone activates a negative feedback loop in the pituitary gland, hypothalamus, and hippocampus, leading to suppression of CRH activity and decrease in HPA axis activity, evidenced by a decrease in cortisol). Depressed patients show a blunting of the CRH-elicited ACTH response in the dexamethasone-CRH test (see Hill and Gozalka [57] for individual studies).

## Exaggerated and Blunted Autonomic and Neuroendocrine Stress Responses

The *reactivity hypothesis* of Krantz and Manuck [58] suggested that stress causes a cascade of events that include an exaggerated autonomic nervous system (ANS) and neuroendocrine response which can promote atherosclerosis, and findings of exaggerated reactions in patients with depression may help explain how depression is associated with increased cardiovascular disease (CVD) risk [59]. Studies have found that excess cortisol may induce MDD and basal cortisol levels may be higher and the post-awakening surge in cortisol may be elevated in individuals at risk of MDD [60]. In a study in caregivers of patients with Alzheimer's disease, those with depressive symptoms had higher levels of plasma norepinephrine in response to a psychological stressor than those with lower depression levels [61].

However, there is both evidence of an exaggerated and a blunted stress response associated with MDD [59, 61, 62]. Blunted reactivity to stress has been demonstrated in people with MDD demonstrated by lower heart rate, systolic blood pressure, and cardiac output reactivity [63], and impaired recovery is also demonstrated, with a meta-analysis finding that the blunted recovery pattern was more pronounced in more severely depressed patients and in older people [64]. Other studies have demonstrated blunted cortisol reactivity in association with depression [65], and blunted heart rate response profiles have been found to be associated with worsening of depressive symptoms [66], this last study suggesting this blunted response pattern is not just a result of depression [59]. A study in Vietnam War veterans found that individuals with MDD and those with comorbid MDD and generalized anxiety disorder (GAD) had lower basal cortisol levels than those with GAD alone or no diagnosis [62]. Depressed individuals were found to have blunted reactivity compared to depressed individuals in remission [67]. Reactivity is often associated with an upregulation of immunity, but blunted reactivity may be associated with a downregulation and compromised ability to fight infection [68].

It would appear difficult to reconcile how depression might be associated with both an exaggerated and a blunted stress response; however, the blunted reactions might occur at a later time, as a result of adaptation to environmental stress [59]. We find other diseases such as diabetes which show an analogous pattern, i.e., there are high insulin levels initially in diabetes, but as the disease progresses over many years, insulin levels decline as beta cell de-differentiation occurs [69].There are other moderating factors in how an individual responds though, and it may be possible that the ECS signaling is involved in directing whether an exaggerated or blunted response occurs. We can only hypothesize at this point.

## Genetic Abnormalities in Depression and a Link with Inflammation

There appears to be a genetic predisposition to development of depression and mood disorders. For example, a study analyzed peripheral blood mononuclear cells and found that 12 protein coding genes were differentially expressed between 29 unmedicated people with depression (8 with bipolar, 21 with major depressive disorder) and 24 healthy controls, with many of them implicated in neurological disorders and/or apoptosis. They found two major gene networks, one of which centered around TNF with NFKβ, TGFβ, and ERK connections, whilst the other featured cell cycle and/or kinase signaling abnormalities. Functional MRI scanning was conducted while participants viewed images of faces displaying different emotions: those with depression demonstrated a greater hemodynamic response in the right amygdala, left hippocampus, and ventromedial prefrontal cortex to sad faces compared with happy faces than healthy controls. mRNA levels of particular genes were significantly correlated with the hemodynamic responses in the amygdala, hippocampus, and ventromedial PFC to sad compared with happy faces, and these differentially expressed gene transcripts correlated significantly with volume of the hippocampus and caudate and the thickness of the left subgenual ACC. This suggests a potential mechanism by which inflammation can lead to depression [21].

Other studies have linked various genetic variations with bipolar disorder [70, 71].

## Neuroplasticity in Depression

The neuroplasticity hypothesis of MDD posits that dysfunction of neural plasticity is the key mechanism underpinning depression. Stress, pain, and cognitive impairment can lead to both depression and neural plasticity changes [24, 72]. Most studies suggest that depression and dysregulated neural plasticity influence each other; however, there is no consensus as to which comes first [73].

The effects of depression on neural plasticity are complex and involve many parts of the brain including the hippocampus, PFC, and amygdala and many signaling pathways including NMDA, glutamate, and glucocorticoids [24].

Studies suggest that impairment of synaptic plasticity (neurogenesis, axon branching, dendritogenesis, and synaptogenesis) in key areas of the CNS, especially the hippocampus, is involved in the pathophysiology of depression and that altered neural plasticity may be associated with alterations in neurotrophic factors such as brain-derived neurotrophic factor (BDNF) [72]. Environmental stressors trigger the HPA axis, exposing the brain to corticosteroids, and this can strongly downregulate hippocampal neurogenesis [72]. Let's look at some key areas that may be involved.

### Altered Synaptic Plasticity in the Hippocampus

There is substantial evidence to support the idea that depression involves alterations to plasticity, in particular, in the hippocampus, and this region has been well studied. We have already discussed some of the studies earlier in this chapter which indicated volumetric changes in the hippocampus in association with MDD. Part of the limbic system, it has a high degree of connectivity to the emotion-related brain regions of PFC and amygdala, it contains high levels of glucocorticoid receptors and glutamate, and it regulates the HPA axis [24], making it particularly susceptible to stress and depression [24].

Animal research supports the link between depression and altered hippocampal synaptic plasticity. For example, in animal models of depression, chronic and severe stress were found to impair hippocampus-dependent memory, an effect explained by changes in hippocampal synaptic plasticity [24]. In other studies, stress has been found to impair activity-dependent persistent increases in synaptic efficacy and increase persistent decreases in synaptic efficacy in the hippocampus of rats [74]. Stress can also decrease dendritic branching and plasticity in the hippocampus, as well as trigger activation of the HPA axis, increased corticosteroids, and downregulation of hippocampal neurogenesis [24].

Changes in synaptic plasticity caused by depression have been found to be associated with hippocampus structural and functional changes [24]. As discussed previously, there is evidence that depression is associated with reduced volume in the hippocampus, as well as the PFC [23–26, 30], and this may also be due to atrophy of neurons and glia in depression [24]. Animal and human studies demonstrate a reduction in total volume of neurons and loss of neurons in stress and depression in adult hippocampi which can be reversed with chronic antidepressant treatment [75]. A bidirectional relationship between depression and hippocampal apoptosis has also been demonstrated (in rodent, other mammal, and human studies), i.e., depression can induce hippocampal apoptosis, and hippocampal apoptosis can lead to depression [24].

### Changes in Synaptic Plasticity in the Prefrontal Cortex and Amygdala

Changes in synaptic plasticity in depression have also been found in the other areas of the limbic system, the PFC, and the amygdala. Depression and stress appear to increase synaptic plasticity in the amygdala, in contrast to what occurs in the hippocampus and PFC. In depression, fMRI studies have found hyperactivity in the ventromedial PFC and hypoactivity in the dorsolateral PFC, and the opposite was found in the recovery from depression in response to medications or psychotherapy [24]. Other brain regions involved in depression include the ventral striatum (reward center). Hypothalamus-hypothalamic synaptic plasticity in depression may be due to increased mRNA expression of synapsin 1 which can contribute to HPA axis hyperactivity and depression-like behaviors in rat models (see Liu et al. [24] for studies).

### Bidirectional Relationship Between Depression and Altered Neural Plasticity

Despite the large number of studies implicating a correlation between depression and altered neural plasticity and some of the mechanisms involved, the neurobiological mechanisms are still not well understood [24]. There is evidence of a bidirectional relationship between depression and neuroplasticity, i.e., that depression might lead to changes in neural plasticity and conversely that changes in neural plasticity, e.g., due to stress, contribute to the initiation and development of depression [24]. The fact that many treatments for depression, including antidepressant medications, appear to exert their effects in ways associated with neural plasticity also lends support to the neuroplasticity model [24]. For a good discussion on this theory, see Liu et al. [24].

### Reduced Brain-Derived Neurotrophic Factor Levels and Depression

As discussed above, it has been proposed that MDD is associated with disruption of neuronal plasticity [24]. Neuronal plasticity involves various neurotrophic factors, including one called brain-derived neurotrophic factor (BDNF), and this may play an important part in neuronal plasticity, including recovery from depressed mood [72, 75]. BDNF is found in the brain and, peripherally, in human serum and plasma and is involved in modulation of neuronal networks [75]. BDNF binds and activates tropomyosin-related kinase B (TrkB) receptors, leading to several intracellular signaling cascades, including those regulated by mammalian target of rapamycin complex 1 (mTORC1), which causes fast protein synthesis and synaptogenesis [18].

Stress and depression have been shown to reduce BDNF levels and expression of its receptor TrkB in the hippocampus and PFC [18], including in animal models of depression and in humans with MDD [75]. In animal studies, reductions in BDNF expression or activity in the hippocampus induced by stress were shown to be prevented by antidepressants [75]. Similarly, clinical studies also demonstrated reduced serum or plasma BDNF levels in untreated MDD patients and restoration of BDNF function as a result of antidepressant treatment [75]. Antidepressants have been found to promote BDNF activity and neuronal plasticity including neurogenesis, synaptogenesis, and maturation of neurons [75].

## Neurogenic Theory of Depression

In humans, approximately 700 newborn granule cells are added each day within the adult hippocampal dentate gyrus. Another model of depression is the *neurogenic theory of depression*, first formally posed in 2000 [22]. It posits that impaired adult hippocampal neurogenesis (AHN) triggers depression, and the restoration of function leads to recovery from depression [22]. This neurogenic theory has been extended to include anxiety [22].

Although still speculative, this theory finds support in several findings including the following:

- Adult hippocampus neurogenesis has been found to be impaired in many animal models of depression (and anxiety) and social stress models in primates.
- Antidepressants can boost adult hippocampus neurogenesis in animal models when the animals are stressed.
- Patients with depression (and anxiety) have smaller dentate gyrus (found on MRI and on post-mortem), suggestive of impaired AHN.
- Depressed patients on medication have a greater number of total dentate granule cells and dentate gyrus size compared to non-medicated patients on post-mortem, though studies of postmortem human brains measure AHN indirectly and find inconsistent effects of antidepressants.
- Increased glucocorticoids can trigger depression and impair AHD [20, 22].

However, impairment of adult hippocampus neurogenesis is only one of several structural changes in the hippocampus found to correlate with depression as well as anxiety, and it is not clear if the relationship is causal or simply an indicator of general gyrus dysfunction [22]. This theory requires greater research.

## The Glutaminergic System, N-Methyl D-Aspartate (NDMA), and Depression

Glutamate is a major excitatory neurotransmitter, and evidence evidence has linked the glutaminergic system and MDD and bipolar disorder. NMDA receptors are a subtype of glutamate receptors, and alterations in NMDA receptor signaling are also thought to play an important role in the pathogenesis of depression and other mood disorders [33, 76]. For example, both these illnesses have been found to be associated with changes in levels of glutamate and abnormal N-methyl-D-aspartate (NDMA) receptor gene expression/concentration/function [33]. Pharmaceuticals that modulate NMDA receptors, for example, ketamine (non-competitive NMDA receptor antagonist), have shown positive effects in patients suffering both these disorders [76]. Also, conventional antidepressants have been shown to be able to modulate NMDA function [33].

Several studies have found raised glutamate levels in peripheral serum, plasma or blood (e.g., [77, 78]) and cerebrospinal fluid [79] associated with MDD, and others (using MRI or other scanning technology) have found reduced glutamate/glutamine levels in several of the brain regions associated with processing of moods and emotions including the hippocampus, amygdala, PFC, anterior cingulate cortex (and others) [33, 78, 80]. Research has also demonstrated reduced levels of major brain inhibitory neurotransmitter γ-aminobutyric acid (GABA) in the prefrontal brain region [80]. It has been thought that the significant reduction in perineuronal oligodendrocytes in the PFC of those suffering MDD and bipolar disorder might explain the relationship between the glutaminergic system and disorders of mood [33, 81]. The argument is that oligodendrocytes in the PFC express glutamine synthetase required to metabolize glutamate and if the numbers of these cells are reduced, this could result in excitotoxicity [33].

Several lines of evidence suggest NMDA involvement in MDD and bipolar disorder including changes found in NMDA receptor functioning, expression and protein levels in various brain regions in patients suffering these illnesses and single nucleotide polymorphisms (SNPs) in the NMDA receptor subunit genes [33].

## Disturbances of Serotonin in Depression

Disturbance of serotonergic activity has been shown to play a role in neuropsychiatric disorders including mood disorders and depression. The essential amino acid tryptophan is a precursor for serotonin production [52]. As Jenny et al. [52] explain, accelerated tryptophan degradation is found in many patients with chronic inflammatory conditions, and patients with chronic inflammation have an increased susceptibility to depression, which suggests that cytokine-induced indoleamine 2,3-dioxygenase (IDO) may play a role in psychiatric illness [52].

An association between increased tryptophan degradation and susceptibility to depression is found in people with chronic diseases underpinned by inflammation such as cancer [82] and those undergoing INF-α therapy (which is proinflammatory) [83]. Therefore, Jenny et al. [52] argue, it is possible that in inflammatory conditions, activation of IDO (which breaks down tryptophan and thereby limits serotonin biosynthesis) could be the link between the immune system and pathogenesis of depression.

### Serotonin-Kynurenine Hypothesis of Depression and the Link to Inflammation

The serotonin-kynurenine hypothesis of depression links the serotonin theory of depression to common inflammatory disorders, integrating stress, inflammation, the kynurenine pathway, serotonergic neurotransmission and glutaminergic transmission.

There are two metabolic pathways of tryptophan:

1. **Methoxyindole pathway** (5% of tryptophan metabolism): tryptophan is metabolized by enzyme tryptophan hydroxylase to produce serotonin, which is a substrate for production of N-acetylserotonin (NAS) which then forms melatonin.
2. Kynurenine pathway (95% of tryptophan metabolism): tryptophan is broken down by enzymes indoleamine 2,3-dioxygenase (IDO) and tryptophan 2,3-dioxygenase (TDO) to kynurenines and their metabolites [84].

IDO inhibits metabolism in several systems within mammals including reproduction, viruses, stem cells, and the nervous system, and there are actually two IDO enzymes, IDO1 (about which much more is known) and IDO2 (the physiological role of which remains unclear) [52].

First proposed last century by Prof. IP Lapin, the serotonin-kynurenine theory of depression suggested that in depression, the cortisol-inducible activation of the enzyme TDO (located in the liver) diverts tryptophan away from producing serotonin and toward kynurenine production, thereby causing a serotonin deficiency. He discovered that kynurenine and its metabolites affect brain function and proposed that neurokynurenines were involved in the pathogenesis of depression [85]. It is now known that there is another rate-limiting enzyme involved in the kynurenine pathway of tryptophan metabolism, IDO.

As explained by Oxenkrug and colleagues [85], upregulation of the tryptophan-kynurenine pathway increases serotonin deficiency, and this then impacts on formation of NAS and melatonin (via the methoxyindole pathway of tryptophan metabolism). Kynurenine is further broken down via two pathways: the kynurenine (KYR)-kynurenic acid (KYNA) pathway and KYR-nicotinamide adenine dinucleotide (NAD) pathway. The KYR-NAD pathway metabolites include NMDA agonists (quinolinic acid, picolinic acid) and free radical generators, and increased NMDA agonist formation has been associated with hyperglutamatergic status which may be associated with depression [86]. KYNA may be involved in cross-talk between melatonin and kynurenine pathways and may contribute to cognitive impairment in depression, dementia, and other illnesses [85].

According to Oxenkrug and colleagues [85], upregulation of the kynurenine pathway is believed to underpin several mental health conditions including depression-associated anxiety, psychosis, and cognitive decline. Stress hormones can induce TDO, and proinflammatory cytokines can induce IDO activation. This upregulation of the kynurenine pathway, then, links depression with conditions associated with chronic inflammation including CVD, obesity, diabetes, psychiatric disorders (e.g., vascular cognitive impairment), HCV, and psoriasis and conditions associated with aging. Genetic and hormonal factors regulate the kynurenine pathway, suggesting that this pathway mediates genetic and environmental mechanisms of depression [85].

The intricacies of this theory have been expanded somewhat by Ramirez et al. [87]. They state that the "serotonergic and immunological hypothesis of depression" proposes that certain types of stress, e.g., infection or psychological stress, activate toll-like receptors (e.g., TLF-4), NF-kB, the inflammasome NLRP3, and secretion of IL-1β, IL-6, and other factors of the innate immune response, which then cause general symptoms of inflammation which are also characteristic of depressive illness (e.g., dysphoria, anhedonia). If the stimulus continues or recurs within 24 h, IDO is activated which then triggers the kynurenine metabolic pathway, leading to decreased serotonin synthesis and increased synthesis of quinolinic acid. Quinolinic acid then activates NDMA receptors in the CNS, stimulating release of proinflammatory mediators including IL-6 and IL-1β and causing hyperactivity of the HPA axis including cortisol, thereby reinforcing the kynurenine metabolic pathway (and therefore production of quinolinic acid and reducing serotonin synthesis) and thereby reinforcing depression [87].

Biosynthesis of IDO1 and the kynurenine pathway of tryptophan metabolism may be a new target for prevention and treatment of depression as well as neurodegenerative diseases (e.g., Alzheimer's disease, Huntington's disease) since tryptophan degradation has been linked to the onset of these [85, 88].

As we will see later, some of the active constituents of cannabis may impact on one of the enzymes involved in the kynurenine pathway of tryptophan metabolism.

### Multi-receptor Involvement

Perhaps not surprisingly, there are a number of receptors or ligands that appear to be involved in the pathophysiology of depression. In addition to 5HT1A receptors and cannabinoid receptors (discussed in the next section), other receptors include PPARγ, GABAA, TRPV1 and mu-opioid receptors. Research into these has demonstrated involvement in antidepressant effects [89]. A full discussion of this is beyond the scope of this book, and readers are thus referred to other sources, such as [89], for more detail.

## The Endocannabinoid System in Depression

The endocannabinoid system (ECS) is well-known to be involved in regulation of mood and depression, as well as modulation of the CNS serotonergic system [52]. The notion of its involvement in mood and emotional behavior, including depression, finds its basis in observations of the effects that cannabis has on mood [34, 90]. As we know, cannabis has been used by humans throughout history for its mood-elevating or euphoric effects, the euphoria associated with tetrahydrocannabinol (THC) in particular [90, 91]. The argument is that given the euphoric effects of cannabis are mediated via CB1 receptor activation, this suggests that (endogenous) promotion of CB1 receptor signaling can facilitate positive effects on mood and may exert antidepressant effects [90]. The extension of this is that disruption of cannabinoid receptor signaling in some way may be involved in the pathogenesis of mood disorders, like depression.

There is much evidence to implicate the involvement of the ECS in the pathophysiology of depression: (1) there is an anatomical basis; (2) studies in which cannabinoid receptors are manipulated indicate involvement; (3) there is evidence of imbalance of the ECS in depression; (4) polymorphisms in genes for CB1 receptors and FAAH may be associated with depression and mood disorders; (5) many antidepressants appear to be able to alter the ECS; (6) there appears to be cross-talk between the immune system and the ECS occurring in depression; (7) the ECS may play a part in the neurogenesis model of depression; and (8) research links ECS activity and underlying pathomechanisms in depression (many of which are described in Gorzalka and Hill [34]). We will look at each one of these briefly.

## Anatomical Basis

Endocannabinoid receptors, both CB1 and CB2 receptors, are distributed in those brain areas involved in the stress response and regulation of mood, emotional reward, and cognition, and these regions are often reported to be altered in those with MDD [34, 92]. These include the corticolimbic area (PFC, hippocampus, amygdala), the hypothalamus, and the cerebellum [15].

In the brain, CB1 receptors highly concentrated in the basal ganglia, frontal cortex, hippocampus, and cerebellum. They are also present in other areas such as the periaqueductal gray (PAG), amygdala, nucleus accumbens, thalamus, and medulla (moderate-low concentration). CB1 receptors are also found in non-neural cells such as microglia, astrocytes, and oligodendrites [15]. We also find CB1 receptors in the dorsal raphe nucleus (brainstem nucleus located in the midbrain and pons, major source of serotonin) and the locus coeruleus (nucleus composed of noradrenergic neurons located in the dorsal pontine tegmentum provides the major source of noradrenalin/norepinephrine to the cerebrum, brainstem, cerebellum, and spinal cord) [15, 93].

Within the cortex, two neuronal subpopulations with opposing actions are the (inhibitory) GABAergic interneurons (high CB1 receptor levels) and the (excitatory) glutaminergic neurons (relatively low CB1 receptor levels). As argued by Micale et al. [15], it is thought that the direct or indirect modulation of the monoamine activity or of GABAergic and glutaminergic neurons, respectively, could underlie the psychotropic and non-psychotropic effects associated with CB1 receptor activation.

### Interconnection of the ECS and Brain Regions in Mood Regulation

How the various brain regions and the ECS are interconnected in the regulation of mood and emotions is quite complex. The following explanation, from Hill et al. [90], goes that glutaminergic pyramidal neurons in the PFC (which express CB1 receptors) send axons to serotonergic (5-HT) neurons and GABAergic interneurons in the dorsal raphe nucleus. Activation of both of these increases 5-HT firing and release of 5-HT (serotonin). The 5-HT neurons innervate the corticolimbic region of the brain involved in depressive symptoms (i.e., amygdala, PFC, hippocampus). The hippocampus sends afferents to the pituitary gland which regulates the HPA axis, known to be dysregulated in depression. In addition, CB1 receptors are expressed on noradrenergic neurons in the locus coeruleus and nucleus prepositus hypoglossi (whose axons terminate on locus coeruleus noradrenergic neurons). The locus coeruleus innervates the dorsal raphe and the corticolimbic regions. Finally, dopaminergic neurons in the ventral tegmental area send their axons to the dorsal raphe nucleus too [90].

AEA, 2-AG, CB1 receptors, FAAH, and MAGL have been found to be present in serotonergic (5-HT) neurons in the dorsal raphe, and in addition to their localization in monoaminergic neurons, they are also expressed in glutaminergic (excitatory) and GABAergic (inhibitory) neurons throughout the cerebral cortex [90].

CB1 receptor signaling has been found to modulate dorsal raphe 5-HT neuronal activity. A rat study demonstrated that the CB1 receptor agonist THC exerted antidepressant effects and modulated 5-HT activity through a CB1 receptor-dependent mechanism [94].

## Evidence from Animal Studies Manipulating Cannabinoid Receptors

Animal research in which cannabinoid receptors and their activity are manipulated in some way provide another line of evidence of involvement of the ECS in the pathophysiology of depression. We will look at just some of the findings.

### Evidence of CB1 Receptor Involvement in Regulation of Emotions and Depression

Involvement of endocannabinoid signaling operating via CB1 receptors in the regulation of moods and emotional behavior finds support in studies investigating what happens when the function of CB1 receptors is blocked. Several studies have found the genetic and pharmacological blockade of CB1 receptors causes a depression-like phenotypic state in animal models, including reduced responsiveness of reward stimuli, deficits in extinction of aversive memories, higher anxiety, and greater stress sensitivity [95–97].

In studies of genetic CB1 receptor knockout mice, the mice have shown depressive-like behavior in several studies utilizing different ways to measure depressive behavior, e.g., sensitivity to rewarding stimuli, forced swim test, and tail suspension test [97–100]. In one study, for example, CB1 knockout mice demonstrated depressive-like behaviors under conditions of chronic unpredictable stress [101]. The depressive phenotype seems to involve several potential mechanisms of action, and this is probably consistent with how we understand the ECS to operate. That is, it is a neuroregulatory system with effects on many different pathways in the body. Thus, if there are deficiencies in one of its key components like the CB1 receptor, this might be expected to impact in several different ways. For example, in one study in CB1 receptor knockout mice, increased despair was associated with BDNF impairment in the hippocampus [98], and in another, CB1 receptor knockout mice displayed hyperactivity of the HPA axis, as indicated by increased corticosterone levels after exposure to stress (in comparison with control mice) [97, 102].

CB1 receptor blockade with the drug rimonabant in rats induced a depressive phenotype, and chronic treatment was associated with decreased serotonin levels in the frontal cortex; marked reductions in hippocampal cell proliferation, survival, and BDNF levels; and elevated proinflammatory cytokines [96]. In humans, rimonabant was removed from the market as it caused serious psychiatric side effects including increased depression, anxiety, and suicide [52, 103, 104].

### Evidence of Role of Adipocyte CB1 Receptors in Depression

Obesity is underpinned by inflammation, and it is associated with depression [105]. In a study in obese rats compared with normal rats, genetic knockout of the adipocyte CB1 receptor was found to alleviate depressive-like behavior, memory deficits, neuroinflammation, and impairment of adult neurogenesis, all of which were associated with obesity. It also reduced obesity-induced inflammation, gliosis, and apoptosis in specific brain regions. Improvements in metabolism (including normalization in insulin resistance and glucose intolerance) were accompanied by normalization of depressive-like behavior, increased adult neurogenesis, and reduced inflammation in the hippocampus and hypothalamus [106]. This study supports the role of adipocyte-brain cross-talk in which adipocyte-specific CB1 receptors are found to be involved in obesity-induced depressive-like behavior, neuroinflammation, and impaired adult neurogenesis in the hippocampus and hypothalamus [106]. The results of this study might seem diametrically opposite to what has been found when CB1 receptors are blocked in the CNS.

Earlier we noted that CNS CB1 receptor knockout mice actually showed depressive-like behavior in several studies [97–100]. And CB1 receptor blockade with the drug rimonabant in rats induced numerous depressive changes specific to the hippocampus [96]. Yet in the study mentioned in the previous paragraph in obese rats [106], peripheral CB1 receptor knockout on adipocytes had the opposite effects—it was associated with alleviation of depression and reduced gliosis and therefore neuroinflammation. The linking mechanism by which this occurs is not understood—was this via metabolic effects (e.g., blocking peripheral adipocytes helped normalize glucose intolerance and insulin resistance) and if so, how? More research in the future will no doubt elucidate more about the crucial role of endocannabinoid system in facilitating the cross-talk that mediates such profound physiological and behavioral changes.

### CB2 Receptors in Emotion Processing and Depression

CB2 receptors may also play a role in emotion processing and have been implicated in anxiety and depression [107]. CB2 receptors are mainly found in the cells, tissues, and organs of the immune system, as well as in inflammatory cells, in glial cells, and in some regions of the brain, e.g., the cerebral cortex, hippocampus, amygdala, hypothalamus, and cerebellum (though in much lower concentrations than CB1 receptors) [15] which we can see are some of the brain regions involved in regulation of emotions.

Again, studies in mice where CB2 receptors are manipulated in multiple ways provide evidence of CB2 receptor involvement. Several studies reviewed in Marco and colleagues provide support for the contention that CB2 receptors are involved in regulation of moods and play a role in normalization of reduced BDNF expression in mice exposed to chronic unpredictable stress [97]. In one study, mice bred to overexpress CB2 receptors showed greater resistance to depression and decreased depressive-like behaviors following stressful situations (as demonstrated in the tail suspension test and novelty-suppressed feeding test) compared with normal mice [108]. This depression-resistant endophenotype was associated with changes in BDNF levels [108]. You will recall that low levels of BDNF in the hippocampus have been associated with depression [109] and are seen as a biochemical marker for depression [97].

Studies in CB2 knockout mice (i.e., lacking CB2 receptors) show increased vulnerability to stress and increased depressive-like behavior demonstrated in a range of experimental tests [97, 110]. In humans, the Q63R polymorphism in the CB2 receptor gene has been found to be associated with depression in a Japanese study [111], lending further support to the involvement of CB2 receptors in depression [97].

Other support for CB2 receptor involvement in depression comes from a study in rats, where β-caryophyllene, a strong CB2 receptor agonist, was found to reduce anxiety and depressive-like behavior, an effect blocked by a CB2 receptor antagonist [107]. You will remember that β-caryophyllene is one of the terpenes found in the cannabis plant, with antioxidant and other beneficial actions.

CB2 receptors are involved in regulation of pain and inflammation [15], and we should remember that part of the pathophysiology of depression involves inflammation and that depression and pain are very often comorbid.

## Evidence of ECS Imbalance in Depression

There is evidence of imbalance of the ECS in depression with many preclinical (animal) and human studies indicating a hypo-function [20, 34]. Gorzalka and Hill [34] have argued that loss of endocannabinoid signaling produces physiological and behavioral effects characteristic of depression and that if this is blocked in humans, this can lead to symptoms of depression and changes in reward sensitivity as well as cognitive-emotional processing, findings that are supported by both animal models of depression and human studies in those with depression. They hypothesized that a deficiency in endocannabinoid signaling can contribute to susceptibility to depression or development of a depressive episode [34].

A significant body of preclinical evidence has shown that loss of endocannabinoid signaling (e.g., by CB1 receptor blockade) can result in phenotypic changes that are similar to symptoms of depression in humans (discussed previously). Other lines of evidence supporting the notion that an endocannabinoid deficiency may underpin depression include findings that stress can downregulate endocannabinoid activity and that some antidepressants can increase endocannabinoid activity [57].

## Preclinical (Animal) Studies Implicating ECS Dysregulation in Depression

There is preclinical evidence to support the notion that there is hypo-functioning of ECS signaling involved in depression, at the level of receptors and endocannabinoids [93]. Some of the research findings are set out in Table 6.1. However, to complicate matters, not all animal models of depression have found decreased levels of endocannabinoids or cannabinoid receptors. Some have found increased levels of both, depending on the brain region.

### Cannabinoid Receptor Changes

In animal models of depression, the effects of experimental stress on CB1 receptor density can depend on the brain region studied [93]. Some animal models of depression have demonstrated a significant increase in CB1 receptor density and binding in the PFC and a significant decrease in the ventral striatum, hypothalamus, midbrain, and hippocampus [15, 93]. In a rat model of depression involving bilateral

**Table 6.1** Examples of preclinical studies supporting hypo-functioning of ECS in depression

| Type of hypoactivity | Study findings |
|---|---|
| CB1R hypoactivity | Genetic CB1 receptor knockout mice (i.e., bred without CB1 receptors) had significantly greater depressive-like behaviors than normal mice and can serve as an animal model for investigating depression [112]<br>Mice treated with CB1 receptor antagonist rimonabant exhibited increased depressive-like behavior, and chronic treatment produced decreases in frontal cortex serotonin levels; marked decreases in hippocampal cell proliferation, survival, and BDNF levels; and increases in proinflammatory cytokines [113]<br>Chronic unpredictable stress in mice caused decreased CB1 receptor functioning and consequent impairment of endocannabinoid-mediated signaling in the nucleus accumbens [114] |
| CB2R hypoactivity or decreased receptor expression | Mice bred to overexpress CB2 receptors showed greater resistance to depression and decreased depressive-like behaviors following stressful situations compared with normal mice [108]. This would then suggest that underexpression of CB2 receptors could be associated with depression<br>A CB2 receptor agonist (β-caryophyllene) administered to mice intraperitoneally lowered depression and anxiety, and this was reversed when a CB2 antagonist was used [107]<br>Reduction in CB2 receptors in the striatum, midbrain, and hippocampus is reported in animal models of depression [111] |
| Deficits in endocannabinoids | Significantly reduced AEA levels were found in brain areas associated with depression-like behavior, such as the hippocampus, hypothalamus, amygdala, and ventral striatum [115]<br>Reduced levels of 2-AG were found in the hippocampus of rats under chronic unpredictable stress conditions though no effect was found in the limbic region [116]<br>FAAH inhibition in mice leads to a reduction in depressive behavior [117–119] including depressive behavior induced by neuropathic pain [120] |

olfactory bulbectomy, there were upregulation and hyper-functionality of CB1 receptors in the PFC which are normalized by chronic treatment with an SSRI [94]. Chronic unpredictable stress increases CB1 receptor protein and mRNA expression in the PFC, though this may be a compensatory effect of reduced endocannabinoid signaling in response to decreased AEA in the PFC [115].

A few studies suggest that changes in availability of CB2 receptors may be involved in depression too [107, 108, 111]. A study reported that there was a reduction of CB2 receptors in the striatum, midbrain, and hippocampus in animal models of depression [111].

**Endocannabinoid Level Changes**

Whilst several studies have found significant decreases in AEA levels under different stress conditions (e.g., chronic unpredictable stress, restraint stress) [115, 121], other studies found no change in AEA levels in various brain regions of rats [117, 122].

Several studies of 2-AG levels in animal depression models have found increased levels, whilst others have found no change or decreases in levels depending on brain region involved (see Micale et al. [15, 93] for individual studies). The differing effects of depression on AEA and 2-AG levels may relate to different functional actions of the two main endocannabinoids. See Boorman et al. [20] and Micale et al. [15, 93] for good summaries of preclinical research.

Administration of drugs which inhibit endocannabinoid uptake or metabolism and CB1 receptor agonists and FAAH inhibitors has been found to induce antidepressant effects in animal models [57, 118, 123, 124]. For example, a rat study found that an FAAH inhibitor (URB557) and a CB1 receptor agonist reduced depressive-like behavior at levels comparable to the tricyclic antidepressant imipramine, effects blocked by the CB1 antagonist rimonabant, which suggests that these effects are mediated by CB1 receptors [124]. Acute or repeated administration of the same FAAH inhibitor was associated with increased firing of serotonergic neurons in the dorsal raphe nucleus and of noradrenergic neurons in the nucleus locus coeruleus, both effects mediated via CB1 receptors (which were also blocked by rimonabant) [118].

Further evidence that hypo-functioning of the ECS may be involved in depression is that upregulation/enhancement of endocannabinoid signaling results in antidepressant and anxiolytic outcomes, potentially acting in similar ways to conventional antidepressants, e.g., by enhancing serotonergic and noradrenergic transmission, dampening the stress response via actions on the HPA axis, enhancing hippocampal 5-HT1A receptor tonic activity, reducing signaling through the 5-HT2A receptor, promoting neurogenesis, and increasing cellular plasticity and neurotropin expression in the hippocampus [90].

Overall, it seems that hypo-functioning of the ECS is involved in animal models of depression [15], or at the very least we can say there is ECS involvement.

## Human Studies: Changes in the ECS in Depression

Several human studies support involvement of the ECS in depression, though results are somewhat variable, with some suggesting hypo-functioning and others suggesting hyper-functioning of the ECS. What is not necessarily clear is whether hyper- or hypo-functioning is a contributing part of the etiology of depression or a reaction to the many changes occurring (the underlying pathomechanisms) in an attempt to bring the system back into balance.

**Cannabinoid Receptor Changes in Depression in Humans**

Some studies suggest an upregulation of CB1 receptors, and others have found a decrease in receptor density [93]. For example, CB1 receptors have been found to be upregulated in postmortem examinations of brains of depressed individuals [125], and in depressed suicide victims, a study found a 24% greater CB1 binding site density and greater CB1 receptor protein in the dorsolateral PFC compared with controls [126]. Yet, in another study, there was no difference in neuronal CB1 receptor density in patients with bipolar disease or schizophrenia compared with controls, but the density of CB1 receptors was significantly less in gray matter glial cells in those with MDD [127].

Rimonabant, the CB1 receptor antagonist drug, was removed from the market due to an increase in depressive symptoms and more serious psychiatric events including suicides [128], underlining the importance of endocannabinoid signaling at CB1 receptors in mood regulation.

Despite a few animal studies suggesting CB2 receptor involvement in regulation of depression [107, 108], human research has not yet demonstrated any changes in CB2 receptors in people with depression, despite their presence in brain regions associated with the stress response [93].

**Human Studies of Endocannabinoid Compound Changes in Depression**

Similarly, there have been some studies which suggest lower levels and others suggesting higher levels of endocannabinoids are associated with depression. For example, a study in women with depression found that basal serum levels of AEA and 2-AG were significantly reduced compared with matched controls, suggesting a deficiency in peripheral endocannabinoid activity associated with depression [129]. Another study found that plasma levels of AEA, palmitoylethanolamide (PEA), and oleoylethanolamine (OEA) correlated with depressive symptomatology in patients with burning mouth syndrome [130]. However, in alcoholics with depression, tissue content of AEA and 2-AG in the dorsolateral prefrontal cortex was higher compared to alcoholics without depression [131].

**Blood Pressure, Endocannabinoids, and Depression**

A study found a positive correlation between serum levels of AEA and 2-AG and diastolic blood pressure and mean arterial pressure in ambulatory, medication-free females suffering depression (compared with age- and ethnicity-matched controls) [132]. Interestingly, they found that diastolic blood pressure was positively correlated with 2-AG (but not AEA) in minor depression and with AEA (but not 2-AG) in major depression, which suggests there may be a differential role of AEA and 2-AG in depression [132].

**Study in Women with Minor and Major Depression: Different Findings**
In a clinical study of women with minor and major depression compared with controls, serum levels of 2-AG were significantly decreased in those with major depression, and this reduction in 2-AG was correlated negatively with duration of the depressive episode (i.e., the longer the depressive episode, the lower the level of 2-AG). In contrast, in women with major depression, levels of AEA were not associated with major depressive symptoms; however, AEA levels were strongly negatively correlated with anxiety (i.e., patients with high anxiety had low serum AEA levels) [133]. The opposite was found in women with minor depression: 2-AG levels were nonsignificantly increased and AEA levels were significantly increased compared to controls. The study authors posit that this could suggest a neuroprotective or compensatory mechanism in patients with less severe depressive symptoms, that is, the endocannabinoids are acting as a buffer against progression to a more severe manifestation of the illness [133].

**Brain-Derived Neurotrophic Factor and Endocannabinoid Activity**
Exercise has been shown to help reduce depression [134], and increasing BDNF may be a potential mechanism by which AEA exerts antidepressant effects [93]. Intense exercise increases both circulating AEA and BDNF levels, and these increases were found to be correlated at the end of an exercise period and after 15 min recovery [135]. This suggests that the increase in AEA during exercise may be one of the factors involved in the increase in peripheral BDNF levels found to be induced by exercise and that increased AEA levels may delay the return of BDNF after exercise to their basal levels [135]. We know that BDNF may play an important part in neuronal plasticity, including recovery from depressed mood [75].

## Genetic Variations and Depression

Genetic variants of the genes coding for cannabinoid receptors (CNR1-CB1 receptors, CNR2-CB2 receptors) can change the gene transcription and protein expression, thereby altering the function of the cannabinoid receptors [136]. Human studies of genetic polymorphisms suggest genetic differences in the ECS may predispose individuals to depression, or conversely, bestow resistance [137].

Barrero et al. [138] found a significant association between polymorphisms in CNR1 (gene coding for the CB1 receptor) and depression in patients with Parkinson's disease. Other studies suggest that genetic variations in CB1 receptor function and FAAH may influence the development of depression and the response to antidepressant medications [139–141]. For example, a study in 256 Caucasian patients with major depression found that a CNR1 gene variation (specifically the CNR1 rs1049353 G allele) conferred an increased risk of antidepressant treatment resistance, in particular in females with high comorbid anxiety. In a subset of 33 patients, they also conducted fMRI scans whilst presenting various emotional faces to them to measure activity in various parts of the brain. They found that CNR1 rs1049353

G allele carriers had weaker bilateral amygdala, putamen, and pallidum activity and left lateralized caudate and thalamus activity in response to masked happy faces. This study suggests that a variation in the CNR1 gene may play a role in both depression and anxiety, and this may be mediated by subcortical hypo-responsiveness to social reward stimuli [139].

Another study assessed single nucleotide polymorphisms (SNPs) in CNR1 and in the gene coding for FAAH in Caucasian patients with recurrent major depression (83 patients) and bipolar disorder (134 patients), compared with 117 healthy individuals. Patients with major depression had a significantly higher frequency of CNR1 1359 G/A gene variants compared with controls. Bipolar and major depressive patients had a nonsignificant and slightly higher frequency of the FAAH gene variant (AC phenotype). Overall, it suggests that variations in genes coding for CB1 receptors and FAAH may contribute to susceptibility to mood disorders [141].

However, the results of associations between genetic variations of CNRs and predispositions to depressive disorders have been somewhat contradictory [136]. In a recent meta-analysis designed to clarify whether particular genetic variants, specifically whether CNR1rs1049353, CNR1 AAT triplet repeat, and CNR2rs2501432 polymorphisms are associated with a greater risk for depressive disorder, it was found that the first two had no association with depression susceptibility whilst there was a significant association between CNR2rs2501432 and depression [136].

## Antidepressant Drugs Affect the ECS

Preclinical research evidence indicates that many antidepressants can modify CB1 receptor expression and endocannabinoid levels and signaling in those areas of the brain associated with mood and emotion, lending support to the contention that the ECS is involved in depression. Various types of antidepressants appear to be able to modify the endocannabinoid tone in different ways, depending on the type of drug and brain region. CB1 receptor upregulation, at least in some parts of the brain, seems to be involved in antidepressant effects of drugs [142]. Agonist trafficking may explain the variable responses found in different animal experiments [142].

Here are some results from rat studies:

- Tricyclic antidepressant imipramine decreased CB1 receptor binding in the midbrain, hypothalamus, and ventral striatum, but increased CB1 in the amygdala, whilst desipramine increased CB1 receptor binding in the hippocampus and hypothalamus [115, 143].
- MAO inhibitor tranylcypromine reduced AEA levels (in the prefrontal cortex, hippocampus, hypothalamus) whilst increasing CB1 receptor binding and 2-AG levels (in prefrontal cortex, hippocampus) [144].
- SSRI fluoxetine increased CB1 binding density in the PFC but had no effect on AEA or 2-AG levels in the brain [144]. SSRIs have been found to either increase or decrease CB1 receptor binding, depending on the drug and brain region involved [93].

## Cross-Talk Between the Immune System and ECS in Depression

Endocannabinoids are immunomodulators, involved in many signaling pathways, and the ECS and the immune system tightly regulate each other's activities. Immunocompetent and endocannabinoid-related cells can influence each other—they can suppress and enhance each other's activities in the CNS and peripheral nervous system. The ECS and immune systems have individually been implicated in the pathogenesis of depression. Now there are studies suggesting these two are related and that dysregulation in the cross-talk or communication between the immune system and the ECS may be involved in the pathophysiology of depression [20]. More studies are needed to further investigate this possibility.

## Endocannabinoid System and the Neurogenesis Model of Depression

The adult mammalian brain produces new neurons through the process of adult neurogenesis, occurring mainly in the hippocampal dentate gyrus (DG) and subventricular zone (SVZ). There is evidence that both BDNF signaling and CB1/CB2 receptors independently modulate neurogenesis, but how they interact is not understood [145].

As we saw earlier, according to the neurogenic model of depression, impaired adult hippocampal neurogenesis occurs in depression [22]. Evidence that the ECS influences hippocampal neurogenesis includes findings that blockade of CB1 receptors resulted in suppression of dentate gyrus progenitor proliferation and reduced BDNF in the hippocampus, whilst increased endocannabinoid signaling increased BDNF, leading to increased neurogenesis [20, 146]. Other evidence comes from findings that CB2 receptors were found to promote neural progenitor cell proliferation via activation of mTORC1 signaling [147]. This suggests that CB2 receptor agonists might be promising targets for manipulation of neural progenitor proliferation and thereby neurogenesis (and it would avoid the potentially intoxicating effects of CB1 receptor activation) [147].

More recent research has demonstrated a close association between the actions of BDNF and cannabinoid receptor signaling. BDNF is an important modulator of SVZ and DG postnatal neurogenesis, and it has been demonstrated that its actions are under the control of cannabinoid receptors, whilst conversely, endogenous BDNF is critical for the cannabinoid-mediated effects on neurogenesis in the SVZ and DG. It thus seems that there are interactions between endocannabinoid and BDNF signaling which control neurogenesis at different levels. In other words, the effect of BDNF on SVZ neuronal differentiation depends on both CB1 and CB2 receptors, and the effects of CB1 and CB2 receptors are dependent on BDNF [145]. Such findings have important implications for many conditions where there is impaired neurogenesis (e.g., depression) or in conditions where there has been brain injury.

## Research Linking ECS Activity and Underlying Pathomechanisms Occurring in Depression

Several studies serve to link the neuroregulatory activity of the ECS with pathomechanisms of mood disorders such as depression. These also add to a growing evidence bank of how manipulation of the ECS might be able to assist in depression.

For example, in a recent study, adolescent rats were treated chronically with a FAAH inhibitor or a MAGL inhibitor—both reduced depressive-like behavior caused by maternal neglect, but only in males, demonstrating a sex difference. Such an effect depended on activation of CB1 receptors, and importantly, this was associated with increased BDNF in the hippocampus [123].

A systematic review of animal models of affective disorders concluded that in the presence of sub-chronic stress, CB1 activation can prevent the development of depressive-like behavior (as well as anxiety-like behavior), prevent neuroinflammation, and promote neurogenesis [92]. In an analysis of studies which used an inflammatory challenge like lipopolysaccharide (LPS) to induce depressive and anxiety-like behavior, animal studies suggest that in the presence of increased inflammation, endocannabinoid signaling activation has both an anti-inflammatory and antidepressant effect [92, 148, 149].

Here, in this aforementioned review [92], we see evidence linking the neuroregulatory role of the ECS, i.e., endocannabinoid signaling via brain CB1 receptors, and prevention of key pathomechanisms thought to be involved in depression such as impaired neurogenesis and neuroinflammation.

## Summary

It is important to realize that it is likely that many different pathophysiological changes are occurring in conditions such as depression. The findings of these various research findings and accompanying theories paint a very complex picture. The ECS is clearly present within those areas of the brain associated with emotional regulation, and there is clear evidence that there is dysregulation of the ECS in depression, in many different ways. The ECS is a neuromodulatory cell signaling system. It interacts with many other systems within the body, via cross-talk and communication with neurons, immune cells, and other types of cells. The actions and the dysregulation of the ECS and its components should not be considered in isolation from all other systems involved.

If we consider the various pathomechanisms of depression, and we understand the interrelationships between the ECS and other systems (e.g., its role in inflammation via the way in which it influences immune system functioning), we start to understand the critical role that the ECS plays in depression. We also begin to appreciate that the pharmaceutical approach that seeks to find the one "magic bullet" and one pathway to alter pharmaceutically is likely to be suboptimal at best. Humans are complex beings. A reductionist approach to understanding illness as well as health is unlikely to be successful.

## Scientific Evidence: CBD in the Treatment of Depression

CBD has been found to be anxiolytic; however, its potential for treating major depression has not been as well studied in humans. There is certainly some preclinical evidence that CBD may reduce depressive-like behaviors, and certainly such research has helped elucidate some of the potential mechanisms of action by which CBD may work. In contrast, there is limited clinical research of efficacy of CBD in treatment of depression at this point in time.

### Preclinical Research into CBD for Treatment of Depression

In preclinical research the "forced swim test" (FST) is often used as a model of depression. Mice are placed in a transparent tank of water, and their escape-related mobility behavior is measured. The rodents will swim, looking for an escape; however, when they give up, they will float. In the first 2 min, most mice will swim. In the next 4 min, there are likely to be periods of immobility, and the duration of immobility occurring in each minute is scored. When the mouse ceases struggling and floats while only making enough movements to keep its head above water, it is judged to be immobile [150]. It is somewhat depressing even thinking about the horror we humans put animals through for our potential benefit, in the name of science (there is always karma, however).

#### CBD Effects on the Serotonergic System

Several studies suggest that CBD's antidepressant effects might be mediated via its effects on the serotonergic system.

Models of depression, acute or chronic stress, and inescapable aversive stimuli often induce both depression- and anxiety-like symptoms and alter autonomic indices of stress [151]. Many animal studies have shown that CBD can reduce autonomic indices of stress and depression- and anxiety-like behaviors [152–158]. The effects of CBD are likely to be $5\text{-HT}_{1A}$-mediated [152, 158], potentially via enhancing both serotonergic and glutamate cortical signaling through a 5-HT1A receptor-dependent mechanism [155].

A study was conducted in rats where CBD, AEA, a 5HT1A agonist, or vehicle (control) was injected into the infralimbic and prelimbic subregions of the ventral medial prefrontal cortex (areas that receive dense serotonergic innervation and play a key role in the stress response) and then they were subjected to the FST or the open field test (OFT). Another CBD group were pretreated with either a 5-HT1A antagonist or a CB1 antagonist, and a further group was given the 5HT1A antagonist and then AEA in order to investigate potential mechanisms of action. CBD significantly reduced the immobility time in the FST (with no changes to locomotor activity in the OFT), indicating an antidepressant effect. This antidepressant effect of CBD was blocked by the CB1 receptor antagonist and the 5-HT1A antagonist (the latter also blocked the effect of AEA and the 5-HT1A agonist). The researchers concluded that administration of CBD into the ventrolateral PFC induced an antidepressant effect, and the likely mechanism was indirect activation of CB1 and 5-HT1A receptors [159].

In a mice experiment, CBD at doses of 10 mg/kg, a noradrenergic antidepressant desipramine (5 mg/kg), and a serotonergic antidepressant fluoxetine (10 mg/kg) induced antidepressant effects in mice subjected to the FST. Ineffective doses of CBD (7 mg/kg) when co-administered with ineffective doses of fluoxetine (5 mg/kg) or desipramine (2.5 mg/kg) resulted in significant antidepressant-like effects, suggesting an additive or synergistic effect. When they pretreated the mice with an inhibitor of serotonin synthesis, they found that it eliminated the CBD-induced behavioral effects seen in the FST, suggesting that CNS serotonergic mechanisms were involved in the antidepressant effect induced by CBD [157].

In an earlier mice study, mice were given CBD at various doses (3, 10, 30, and 100 mg/kg) or imipramine or "vehicle" (control) and, after 30 min, submitted to the FST or to an open field arena. An additional group was given a 5-HT1A antagonist prior to receiving 30 mg/kg CBD, and depressive activity was assessed via the FST. They also measured the BDNF protein levels in the hippocampus of another group of mice given 30 mg/kg CBD, before and after being submitted to the FST. They found that 30 mg/kg CBD reduced immobility time in the FST, meaning that it decreased depressive-like behavior but did not alter exploratory behavior in the open field test. Imipramine also had the same effect. Pretreatment with the 5-HT1A antagonist blocked the effect of treatment with 30 mg/kg CBD on the FST. CBD (30 mg/kg) did not alter BDNF levels in the hippocampi of mice. The conclusion was that CBD can induce an antidepressant effect comparable to that of imipramine, and the effects were probably mediated through 5-HT1A receptors [158].

In another mice model of depression (olfactory bulbectomy mouse model of depression), CBD was shown to promote fast and sustained antidepressant effects, evidenced by a reversal of the hyperactivity and anhedonia induced by the olfactory bulbectomy. CBD significantly increased serotonin and glutamate levels in the ventromedial PFC, an effect prevented by blockade of the 5-HT1A receptor (this blockade also prevented the antidepressant action). The authors concluded that CBD's antidepressant effects are mediated via enhancement of serotonergic and glutamate cortical signaling via a 5-HT1A receptor-dependent mechanism [155].

### CBD Reduces IDO-Mediated Degradation of Tryptophan

As discussed previously, the essential amino acid tryptophan is a precursor for serotonin production [52]. We learned earlier about the role of IDO, which can become activated by inflammatory cytokines [85]. IDO is one of the two key enzymes mediating the kynurenine pathway, one of the degradation pathways of tryptophan, the upregulation of which has been found to be associated with depression [84, 85]. Both CBD and THC have been found to suppress IDO-mediated degradation of tryptophan, and this may be an additional mechanism by which the anti-depressive effects of CBD and THC work, especially in those with diseases underpinned by inflammation [52]. We will discuss this again shortly when we explore CBD's role in reducing neuroinflammation.

## CBD May or May Not Reduce Depressive Symptoms Through Hippocampal Neurogenesis

CBD may also reduce depressive symptoms by stimulating hippocampal neurogenesis [160, 161]. This is supported by studies showing that repeated administration of CBD to mice exposed to chronic unpredictable stress reduced depressive- and anxiety-like behaviours and stimulated hippocampal progenitor proliferation and neurogenesis. These beneficial actions of CBD were prevented by the genetic ablation of proliferating progenitor cells. The mechanism whereby CBD stimulates neurogenesis is hypothesised to depend on the elevation of hippocampal AEA levels, as overexpression of FAAH inhibits CBD-induced cell proliferation [160].

Not all studies have found this, however. In a review of the effects of the ECS on inflammation and neurogenesis in animal models of affective disorders such as depression, two studies reported investigating the effects of CBD on depressive-like behavior [92], inflammation, and neurogenesis.

In one study, chronic CBD administration reduced behavioral despair in adult and adolescent rats; however, the effect was different in the adolescent rats compared with the adult rats. In adolescent rats, 10 mg/kg dose was effective at reducing despair, as observed up to 2 days posttreatment by the forced swim test, but not dosages of 3 mg/kg and 30 mg/kg [162]. When they assessed hippocampal neurogenesis markers in the adolescent rats, CBD administration at dosages of 3 mg/kg and 10 mg/kg was not associated with any changes in cell proliferation or early neuronal survival compared with control mice, as measured 2 days posttreatment which was the time when the antidepressant effect was noted. At 15 days posttreatment, 10 mg/kg CBD did not alter these markers either in the adolescent rats.

In adult mice, the 30 mg/kg dose (but not 3 mg/kg or 10 mg/kg doses) of CBD significantly reduced depressive-like behavior compared with control rats, an effect still apparent 21 days after treatment, thus demonstrating a sustained antidepressant effect of CBD. In adult rats, no changes were found in proliferation or early neuronal survival markers with CBD administration at 3 mg/kg and 10 mg/kg 2 days posttreatment, nor with a dose of 30 mg/kg when measured 28 days posttreatment (this was the dose at which the antidepressant effect was observed in the adult rats) [162]. Thus, it appears that CBD is not achieving the antidepressant effect by modulating hippocampal neurogenesis in either adolescent or adult rats, despite other studies indicating that CBD can induce hippocampal neurogenesis [162–164]. As stated by Bis-Humbert et al. [162], CBD may induce its antidepressant effects indirectly via increasing AEA levels (by inhibiting its uptake or metabolism) and/or activation of 5-HT1A receptors [34, 155, 162].

Another study also found single and repeated (chronic) CBD administration reduced behavioral despair in non-stressed adult mice (it had no effect on anxiety), with an effect comparable to imipramine (as measured by the tail suspension test). Repeated dosing of 3 mg/kg CBD was associated with increased cell proliferation and neurogenesis in the dentate gyrus and SVZ. However, with repeated dosing at the higher dose of 30 mg/kg, although the antidepressant effect was still evident, this was associated with decreased cell proliferation and neurogenesis in the dentate gyrus and SVZ [165]. This study also seems to indicate that the antidepressant effects of CBD occur independent of adult neurogenesis [165].

### CBD May Increase BDNF and Synaptic Plasticity

A study in mice demonstrated the rapid and sustained antidepressant effect of CBD. In male rodents, a single dose of CBD dose-dependently induced antidepressant-like effects (7–30 mg/kg) in the FST 30 min (acute) as well as 7 days (sustained) following treatment. In another strain of rats using a different depression model (learned helplessness paradigm), similar effects were found. They found that the acute antidepressant effects (30 min after treatment) were associated with increased levels of BDNF in the medial PFC and the hippocampus, as well as increased markers of synaptic plasticity (synaptophysin and PSD95) in the medial PFC. The CBD effect was blocked by injection of a TrkB receptor antagonist and an mTOR inhibitor. The study concluded that CBD is able to induce fast and sustained antidepressant-like effects in different animal models of depression and that this action may be associated with rapid changes in synaptic plasticity in the mPFC, mediated by activation of the BDNF-Trk signaling pathway [18].

Another study in mice demonstrated that the hippocampal BDNF-TrkB-mTOR pathway is critical for the antidepressant-like effects of CBD when administered locally, though the study authors acknowledged that other parts of the brain may also be involved in the case of systemic administration [166]. Remember that TrkB is the receptor for BDNF and reduced BDNF activity has been found in the brains of patients with MDD [75].

It is believed that the rapid antidepressant effects associated with acute CBD administration involve activation of the BDNF-TrkB-mTOR signaling pathway in the mPFC whilst the sustained effect may be associated with enhanced synaptic function in the mPFC [18].

### CBD Reduces Neuroinflammation

CBD is known to have anti-inflammatory effects, and as we have seen earlier, there is evidence that inflammation is involved in the pathogenesis of depression. Despite there being a link between inflammation and depression, there has been little research into the link between CBD's modulation of inflammation and its antidepressant effects using inflammatory animal models [167]. However, recently one such study has investigated this. A mice neuroinflammatory model was set up in which mice were systemically administered with LPS, which induced a depressive-like state, as demonstrated by increased behavioural despair and anhedonia. The administration of CBD was found to produce antidepressant-like effects (it reduced immobility time in the tail suspension test) and increased sucrose preference (in the sucrose preference test, used to measure anhedonia, mice are given a choice of water or sucrose solution), and this was associated with a reduction in the kynurenine pathway activation as well as reduction in IL-6 levels and NF-κB activation [167]. The researchers posit that CBD's antidepressant-like and hedonic-like effects on this LPS-induced neuroinflammatory model may be due to the reduction of brain IDO activity [167]. You will remember back to the section on pathogenesis of depression where we discussed the serotonin-kynurenine hypothesis of depression. The authors of this mice study explain that in animal models where neuroinflammation is induced with LPS, as well as in patients with depression, the neurotoxic component of the KYN pathway is increased, and the neuroprotective pathway is decreased, and this imbalance has been associated with depressive-like behaviour. They suggest that restoration of the neurotoxic/neuroprotective balance may be part of mechanism by which CBD's antidepressant-like effects may be operating [167].

### Other Targets of CBD

In addition to being a 5-HT1A agonist, CBD is able to modulate several pharmacological targets that may be involved in depression. CBD is an allosteric modulator of CB1 and CB2 receptors (though has low affinity for them), can inhibit AEA breakdown (inhibits FAAH) and uptake (thereby facilitating endocannabinoid signaling at CB1 and CB2 receptors and TRPV1), and it can bind directly at PPARϒ receptors. Other pharmacological targets of CBD include mu opioid receptors, adenosine, GABAA and others (see [89]).

Research has demonstrated antidepressant effects in relation to CB1 and CB2 receptor allosteric modulation, AEA uptake inhibition, FAAH inhibition, NF-κB inhibition, iNOS inhibition and mu opioid receptors, though mixed results have been found in relation to TRPV1 agonism, i.e. both antidepressant and depressant effects [89].

Despite the fact that CBD can modulate many pharmacological targets involved in the pathophysiology of depression, few have been investigated through in vivo research [89].

### CBD in the Treatment of Depression Comorbid with Diabetes

The prevalence rates of depression and anxiety are at least two times higher in diabetic patients, increasing morbidity and mortality. A study in rats provides evidence that CBD may be useful in treating psychiatric comorbidities of diabetes including depression. CBD treatment (only at the higher dose of 30 mg/kg) was found to reduce the exaggerated depressive- and anxiogenic-like behaviors of diabetic rats. The mechanisms of action may include altered 5-HT, noradrenaline, and dopamine levels observed in the PFC and hippocampus [168]. Treatment also induced a significant increase in weight gain and the insulin levels (and consequently reduced glycemia) in diabetic rats with possible regenerative effect on pancreatic beta cells. The authors suggest that CBD has potential to limit both the physiological and neurobehavioral deficits in diabetes [168].

### CBDA in Animal Models of Depression

The FST was used in two different genetic animal models of depression. The methyl ester of cannabidiolic acid (CBDA) (HU-580) was found (at a dose of 1 mg/kg) to reduce immobility and increase swimming in both rat strains compared with controls [169]. You will notice that the treatment dose with CBDA was considerably less than that of CBD studies above of 7–30 mg/kg.

## Human Research: CBD in the Treatment of Depression

There is much less clinical evidence available investigating CBD for treatment of depression, and this is clearly an area that could benefit with increased research. There are obviously some advantages of CBD over THC-containing medicines, should it be shown to be beneficial.

### Case Studies

A case study has been published of an adolescent (16 years old) with multiple substance abuse disorder (involving cannabis, MDMA, cocaine, and ecstasy) who also suffered severe depression, social anxiety and withdrawal, derealization, attention deficit, social phobia, and narcissistic personality disorder. He was using THC daily and consumed MDMA, cocaine, and ecstasy once a week. He had a history of psychiatric treatment over the past 2 years and had been treated with sertraline (100 mg orally once daily for 6 months). Since antidepressant medications were not successful, he was trialed on CBD (starting at 100 mg, titrating up to 600 mg over 3 weeks). CBD was found to be safe and well tolerated. He asked to discontinue sertraline after 3 weeks of CBD treatment. After cessation of the antidepressant medication and using CBD alone, his symptoms of anxiety and depression, as well as simple phobias and symptoms of paranoia and dissociation, continued to improve. There was no difference in mood and anxiety symptoms after abrupt cessation of the antidepressant medication. He also stopped using illegal drugs including THC without showing withdrawal symptoms [170]. This illustrates the possibility that CBD may assist in treatment of people with multiple substance abuse who have depression as well as other mental health problems. And at least for the SSRI drug class, abrupt discontinuation of antidepressants while using CBD may have no adverse effects.

Another case study published more informally on the Internet [171] was of a 49-year-old woman with depression, anxiety, and binge eating since early adulthood, treated with antidepressants previously but not within the last 15 years. She used medicinal cannabis oil containing 2.5 mg CBD once daily, increasing to twice daily after 2 weeks. She reported a 60–70% reduction in anxiety and depression symptoms. When she changed product brands, she noted feeling dark and depressed, symptoms which were alleviated by returning to the original product. She also noted better sleep and daytime energy, and no adverse effects were reported [171].

## Cannabis and THC: Evidence of Antidepressant Effects

In this section, we will examine some of the preclinical research into how THC might act in depression, as well as some of the research in humans.

## Preclinical Studies

Early studies began to piece together the mechanisms of action by which THC may act as an antidepressant which includes facilitation of effects of norepinephrine, as well as implicating effects on dopamine and serotonin transmission. Early studies in rats demonstrated that THC enhanced the uptake of several neurotransmitters (including dopamine, GABA, norepinephrine, and serotonin) into cortical synaptosomes, with the greatest effect on GABA and effects being greater in the cortex than striatum [172].

Studies of the effects of synthetic cannabinoid agonists [173] and FAAH inhibitors (which block anandamide hydrolysis) [118] have demonstrated 5-HT-augmenting mechanisms, whilst several studies have demonstrated antidepressant (and anxiolytic) effects in different animal models [174, 175].

### THC Effect on Dopaminergic System

Support for the role of the nigrostriatal dopaminergic system includes results from in vivo studies which have demonstrated an increase in extracellular dopamine levels following administration of THC via microdialysis into the nigrostriatal and mesolimbic regions of the brain [176, 177], as well as studies that have shown that THC can facilitate dopamine release in rat striatal slices [176]. In rats, the effect of THC on dopamine transmission was blocked by naloxone (general opioid antagonist) and naloxonazine ($\mu_1$-opioid receptor antagonist), infused into the ventral tegmentum, suggesting that THC and heroin both exerted effects on mesolimbic dopamine transmission through a common $\mu_1$-opioid receptor mechanism in the ventral mesencephalic tegmentum [177]. Another study in rats demonstrated that in vivo release of dopamine induced by THC was dependent on serotonin transmission [176].

### THC Effect on Serotonergic System

Animal research indicates that low-dose THC may produce antidepressant effects via effects on the serotonergic system. In a rat study, repeated (5 days) intraperitoneal treatment with 1 mg/kg THC produced antidepressant-like effects in a forced swim test. Electrophysiological investigation showed that THC modulated the 5-HT neuronal activity in the dorsal raphe via a CB1 receptor-dependent mechanism. Acute intravenous administration of 0.1–0.5 mg/kg THC produced variable effects on 5-HT neurons (excitatory, inhibitory, and inert responses). Repeated administration (but not single administration) of 1 mg/kg THC enhanced the tonic activity of hippocampal 5-HT1A receptors (this is a postsynaptic effect of standard pharmaceutical antidepressants). The results of this study suggest that THC may have antidepressant effects at low doses and may work in a way similar to SSRIs in modulating 5-HT transmission in the dorsal raphe and hippocampus [94].

### THC Use in Adolescent Animals Induced Depression

Not all studies in animals have been positive. In a study in rats, chronic administration with THC in adolescence actually induced depressive-like behavior, impaired short-term memory, and reduced social interactions and induced a persistent neuroinflammatory state within the adult PFC. This was evidenced by increased microglial activation and elevated expression of proinflammatory markers (TNF-α, iNOS, and COX-2) and reduced anti-inflammatory IL-10 [178]. This neuroinflammation was associated with downregulation of CB1 receptors on neuronal cells and upregulation of CB2 receptors on microglia. When the researchers blocked the microglia activation with the drug ibudilast during THC treatment, this significantly reduced the impairment of short-term memory in adulthood and prevented the increases in the proinflammatory markers and the upregulation of CB2 receptors on microglia, but it had no effect on the depressive-like behaviors [178].

The study authors concluded that their study supports a causal relationship between microglial activation and the development of longer-term cognitive changes associated with adolescent THC treatment [178]. They did point out, however, that the proinflammatory phenotype found in their study arises when healthy rats were exposed to THC and that in other studies utilizing models of particular neurological diseases, chronic THC administration reduces inflammatory events and the progression of disease. Nonetheless, their study findings are very interesting and tie with a later section where we discuss studies in humans that suggest that THC use in adolescents may be associated with later depression (see next section for this discussion).

## Human Studies: Cannabis, THC, and Depression

In relation to evidence that cannabis and THC may assist in depression, the results from a variety of types of studies are mixed. There is some evidence of a positive effect in altering depressive symptoms from cross-sectional surveys, a prospective cohort study, and a few case reports. In general, there is a real paucity of RCT data. Not all studies have been positive, with some associating cannabis use with depression, as we shall see shortly.

### Surveys of Cannabis Users

Epidemiological studies support the effectiveness of cannabis for depression, at least in some people. For example, a survey of 4500 people found fewer depressive symptoms in cannabis users compared with nonusers [179]. In a pilot study of 37 individuals who had smoked cannabis on at least 5000 separate occasions, 38% of these long-term, heavy cannabis users reported that it "frequently" relieved their depression. Only 3% said that it frequently caused depression [180].

Several surveys indicate people are self-medicating with cannabis to treat depressive symptoms. A systematic review and meta-analysis of empirical studies of patient-reported use of medicinal cannabis for pain, anxiety, and depression (13 studies) found that 34.7% cannabis users surveyed use medicinal cannabis for relief from depression symptoms whilst 51.7% use it for anxiety (and 67.2% for pain) [1]. In Australia, a survey of 1748 Australians who were using cannabis for medical reasons in 2016, prior to legalization of medical use, found that depression was a common reason for its medical use (49.3% of those surveyed) [181].

In the Washington State survey (cross-sectional survey of 1429 people identifying as medical cannabis users rather than recreational users, with respondents from 18 countries but predominantly from the USA), the most frequently reported conditions for cannabis use were pain (61% of respondents), anxiety (58%), and depression (50%). The mean effectiveness rating for depression was 3.76 (95% CI 3.66–3.85), and the mean effectiveness rating for anxiety was 3.53 (95% CI 3.44–3.63) on a scale of −5 to +5 (with 5 representing worsening symptoms, 0 representing no change in symptoms, and +5 representing improving symptoms) [182].

A recent longitudinal, cross-sectional web-based survey completed between 2016 and 2018 involved 1276 participants. These participants were either patients with a diagnosed health condition or caregivers of a patient with a diagnosed health condition registered with the Realm of Caring Foundation (not-for-profit organization). Participants were invited to participate in follow-up assessments every 3 months. A total of 33% of the participants completed one or more prospective follow-ups. The survey assessed patients on their medication use, pain, anxiety, depression, sleep, and quality of life (QoL). Statistical analysis was conducted on 808 cannabis users compared with 468 non-cannabis users (controls). Compared with nonusers, cannabis users self-reported significantly lower depression and lower anxiety (both $p < 0.001$), better quality of life ($p < 0.001$), greater health satisfaction ($p < 0.001$), as well as lower average pain severity ($p < 0.05$) and better sleep ($p < 0.01$ for children and for adults). In addition, compared with nonusers, cannabis users reported using 14% less prescription medications (rate ratio 0.86, 95% CI 0.77–0.96) and were significantly less likely to have a past-month hospital emergency department visit (RR = 0.61, 95% CI 0.44–0.84, i.e., a 39% reduction in likelihood) or hospital admission (RR 0.54, 95% CI 0.34–0.87, i.e., 46% less likely) [183].

This study also followed participants over time (longitudinal health symptoms) to evaluate changes in health symptoms on initiation, cessation, or maintenance of medicinal cannabis use. They found statistically significant within-person effects of medicinal cannabis, reflecting that initiation of medicinal cannabis use, on average, was associated with improved symptoms and cessation of use was associated with worsening of symptoms. This was found for anxiety ($p < 0.001$), depression ($p < 0.001$), quality of life ($p < 0.01$), health satisfaction ($p < 0.01$), past-month average pain ($p < 0.05$), and past-month worst pain ($p < 0.05$). The study also assessed what types of cannabis products were used by study participants and found that CBD-dominant products were found to be used at a higher rate than THC-dominant products. Mean dose of CBD was 79 mg/day (adjusted for body weight, 1.4 mg/kg; median 0.6 mg/kg; range 0.01–15.7 mg/kg), and mean dose of THC was 3 mg/day (adjusted for body weight, 0.05 mg/kg; median 0.02 mg/kg; range < 0.01–0.6 mg/kg) [183]. This study is important because it is not just looking for reduction of adverse symptoms, but is also examining quality of life and health satisfaction. More research needs to focus on health in a positive sense.

### Prospective Cohort Study

A study published in 2018 used an app to track changes in depression ($n$ = 561), anxiety ($n$ = 770), and stress ($n$ = 726) in medicinal cannabis users. The study focused only on inhalation methods (vaping, smoking, concentrates, dab bubbler, dab portable ($n$ = 13,687; 74.4% of data)). The study found that:

- Cannabis significantly reduced ratings of depression, anxiety, and stress (by 50%, 58%, and 58%, respectively).
- Women reported larger reductions in anxiety as a function of cannabis than men.
- Low THC (e.g., <5.5%)/high CBD (e.g., >9.5%) cannabis was best for reducing perceived symptoms of depression.
- High THC (e.g., >26.5%)/high CBD (e.g., >11%) cannabis was best for reducing perceived symptoms of stress.

The effects of dose on perceived changes were assessed for stress, anxiety, and depression. The results were as follows:

- Depression: no evidence for dose effects (i.e., 1 puff resulted in the same magnitude of change in ratings of depression as 10+ puffs).
- Stress: positive, linear relationship between dose and perceived changes in stress: 10+ puffs were associated with greatest change in ratings of stress.
- Anxiety: curvilinear relationship; follow-up tests—1 puff perceived as less effective than any other dose; however no other significant differences across any other doses (e.g., 2 puffs perceived as effective as 10+ puffs) [184].

However, the use of cannabis to treat depression appeared to exacerbate depression over time. Whilst baseline ratings of anxiety and stress remained fairly stable across tracked sessions, the baseline ratings of depression significantly increased over time and number of sessions. The authors of the paper felt that this was consistent with recent evidence indicating that using cannabis to cope with distress was associated with more cannabis-related problems and increased symptoms of depression [184].

### Prospective Study: Cannabis Flowers

An observational study of 1819 people was conducted between July 2016 and August 2019. Participants who self-administered with cannabis flowers to treat their depression rated their symptoms using the Releaf App™ which was an app where they could rate the symptom intensity as well as choose from a range of side effects (positive and negative).

On average, 95.8% of users reported symptom relief following cannabis consumption, with a mean symptom intensity reduction of −3.76 points (Std Dev 2.64, $p < 0.001$) on a visual analogue scale ranging from −10 to +10. There was no difference in symptom relief between plant phenotypes labelled "*C. indica*," "*C. sativa*," and "hybrid." There was no difference in symptom relief between combustion methods (i.e., joint, vape, pipe) though relative to joints, vaping was associated with less reporting of positive and context-specific side effects.

When they assessed cannabinoid levels, THC levels were the strongest independent predictor of symptom relief. CBD levels were generally not related to real-time changes in symptom intensity levels. In up to 20% of users, negative side effects that correspond to increased depression were found (e.g., feeling unmotivated); however, in up to 64% of users, positive side effects corresponding to decreased depression were found (e.g., feeling happy, optimistic, peaceful, or relaxed). The extent and magnitude of side effects varied with chemotype. Thus, the study authors concluded that cannabis flower appears to be an effective and fast-acting antidepressant, with the majority of patients using cannabis experiencing antidepressant effects, at least in the short term [185].

### Case Reports of Cannabis Use in Depression

In case reports of five people with depression, depression preceded cannabis use and cannabis use had some antidepressant effects [180]. All five people reported that cannabis was more effective in treating their depression than pharmaceutical medications (except for one patient who said this was true until he responded to venlafaxine). Three out of five patients reported that their mood deteriorated when they were not able to access cannabis and improved reliably on resumption [180].

### Randomized Controlled Trials of Cannabis and THC for Depression

The National Academies of Sciences, Engineering, and Medicine report on cannabis and cannabinoids, published in 2017, assessed evidence of efficacy from RCTs and systematic reviews in relation to several different medical conditions, including depression. They reported that there were no systematic reviews published which focused on depression as a primary outcome and no good-quality primary literature, that is, RCTs assessing the effect of medicinal cannabis on MDD [186].

A double-blind RCT, likely to have been published after the National Academies report, investigated the effects of THC on emotional responses to an acute psychosocial stress in 42 healthy volunteers. The volunteers took part in two experimental sessions, one with psychosocial stress (the Trier Social Stress Test, TSST) and one with a non-stressful task, following receiving 0 ($n$ = 13 participants), 7.5 mg ($n$ = 14), or 12.5 mg ($n$ = 15) of oral THC as capsules, 2.5 h prior to the tasks. When they assessed the effects of THC before the tasks, they found that 12.5 mg significantly increased depression, anxiety, and confusion compared with the placebo group, as measured by the POMS (Profile of Mood States). The higher dose of THC (12.5 mg) significantly increased ratings of subjective distress before the task compared with the low THC group (7.5 mg THC) or placebo group. When they assessed the effects of THC on task responses, they found that low doses (7.5 mg) of oral THC attenuated self-reported negative emotional effects of a psychosocial stressor (i.e., TSST-induced increases in subjective distress) but high doses of THC (12.5 mg) increased subjective distress, depression, and anxiety [187].

### RCTs Assessing Depression as Secondary Outcome Variables

Randomized controlled trials in patients with primary conditions including chronic pain, cancer, and multiple sclerosis found no significant effects of nabilone and dronabinol (both synthetic forms of THC) or nabiximols (THC and CBD in equal ratios) on secondary symptoms of depression and anxiety (e.g., [188–191]). In a study in fibromyalgia patients, nabilone (synthetic THC) significantly decreased anxiety but had no effects in depression [192]. These studies are assessing *synthetic* THC (dronabinol, nabilone) or a product (nabiximols) which is a combination of THC and CBD without other plant nutrients found in cannabis. These are not whole plant products which are likely to have quite different effects than isolated active constituents.

In an open label study of cannabis smoking in 28 patients with fibromyalgia compared with 28 nonusers with fibromyalgia (controls), visual analogue (VAS) scores indicated a significant reduction in pain and stiffness, enhancement of relaxation, increased feelings of well-being, and an increase in somnolence. The mental health component of the Quality of Life tool used (the SF-36) was significantly higher ($p < 0.05$) in cannabis users compared with nonusers [193].

## Palmitoylethanolamide (PEA) Supplementation for Depression

Research using animal models of depression have found that exogenous palmitoylethanolamide (PEA) has antidepressant effects [194–196]. Human studies also lend support to the idea that exogenous PEA might be a useful adjunct treatment for depression.

PEA is one of the N-acylethanolamines that make up the extended ECS and is an endogenous fatty acid amide with several targets including peroxisome proliferator-activated receptor alpha (PPAR-α) and NMDA receptors. Endogenous PEA exerts anti-inflammatory effects, principally via inhibiting the release of proinflammatory mediators from mast cells, monocytes, and macrophages [197]. It indirectly affects endocannabinoid signaling through activation of PPAR-α [195]: PEA was found to increase CB2 receptor mRNA through PPAR-α activation and induced morphological changes associated with a reactive microglia phenotype (increased migration and phagocytosis) suggesting that indirect regulation of microglial CB2 receptor expression is a potential mechanism of action of PEA [197].

PPAR-α agonists may help regulate mood disorders by regulating dopamine neuronal activity (and perhaps also serotonin) via nicotinic acetylcholine receptors. As we saw earlier, glutamate transmission is dysregulated in depression, and PEA can restore glutaminergic synapse proteins and amino acid release or homeostasis and in other research was found to protect against NMDA-induced neuronal death [195]. It has been posited that PEA may increase in depression as a compensatory mechanism, a hypothesis that is supported by findings that antidepressant drugs such as imipramine increase brain PEA levels [195].

### RCT: PEA Supplementation in Major Depressive Disorder

A randomized controlled trial (RCT) in 54 patients with MDD who were given either PEA or placebo as an adjunct to current therapy of citalopram for 6 weeks found evidence that PEA as an adjunct therapy effectively improved symptoms. At the end of week 2, those in the PEA group showed a significantly greater reduction in depression scores on the Hamilton Depression Rating Scale compared with the placebo group. Throughout the entire study, those in the PEA group showed significantly greater improvement in depressive symptoms and a greater response rate (defined as a 50% or more reduction in the HAM-D score) compared with the placebo group at the end of the 6 weeks (100% versus 74%, $p = 0.01$). There was no difference in frequency of side effects between groups [195].

## Can Cannabis Cause Depression?

### Studies of Associations Between Cannabis Use and Depression

Several studies have reported an association between cannabis use and depression [198–203] though other studies have not found an association [204, 205].

A meta-analysis of 14 longitudinal studies (total of 76,058 participants) found that the odds ratio for cannabis users developing depression compared with control is 1.17 (meaning there was a 17% increased risk, 95% CI 1.05–1.30) and there was a higher odds ratio (1.62, 95% CI 1.21–2.16) for heavy cannabis users developing depression compared with nonusers or light users [203]. Another meta-analysis (of prospective cohort or cross-sectional designs using non-institutionalized cases) found a significant association between comorbid anxiety and depression and cannabis use (OR 1.68, 95% CI 1.17–2.40, 5 studies) [202]. Interestingly, in this meta-analysis, cannabis use at baseline was significantly associated with increased odds of anxiety at follow-up in five studies (OR 1.28, 95% CI 1.06–1.54) [202].

A study was conducted in 1994–1996 which was a follow-up or reassessment of participants of the 1980 Baltimore Epidemiologic Catchment Area (ECA) study in the USA. In this follow-up study 1,920 of the participants enrolled in the 1980 study were interviewed. They found that in those with no baseline depressive symptoms (as assessed in the original study), those with a diagnosis of cannabis abuse at baseline were four times more likely to have depressive symptoms at follow-up (compared with those with no cannabis abuse diagnosis), and they were more likely to have experienced suicide ideation and anhedonia during the follow-up period [198].

Yet others have not found an association between cannabis use and depression. For example, the National Longitudinal Survey of Youth of 1979 is an ongoing longitudinal survey of 12,686 men and women in the USA that began in 1979. Analysis of data of 8759 adults (aged 29–37 years) interviewed in 1994 about past-year cannabis use and current depression found that past cannabis use was not a significant predictor of depression in adults when baseline differences between users and nonusers were controlled [204]. One large meta-analysis of studies on cannabis use and risk of affective mental health outcomes concluded that evidence that cannabis causes depression in humans is not convincing [205].

A major issue in trying to make sense of often conflicting results in the literature is the differences between studies in definitions of cannabis use and depression (and anxiety) and differences in numbers and types of confounders [206]. Many studies which initially found an apparent association between cannabis use and depression or anxiety found the association disappeared after adjusting for other potentially confounding factors [186, 205–207]. For example:

- In a longitudinal cohort study of 8598 Swedish men and women, at 3-year follow-up, once confounding factors were taken into account (alcohol and illicit drug use, education, family tension, place of upbringing, age, sex), no longitudinal associations were found between cannabis use and incidence of depression/anxiety or between depression/anxiety and later cannabis use [206].
- In a Swedish male cohort, there was an apparent increased risk of hospitalization from depression in men reporting heavy cannabis use in adolescence. This association disappeared after adjusting for conduct problems in childhood [207].

## Cannabis Use in Adolescence and Young Adulthood

There have been several studies that have linked heavy cannabis use in adolescence and development of depression later in life (e.g., [208–210]). For example, a longitudinal cohort study that spanned 30 years found that cannabis use in adolescence was associated with higher odds of depression (adjusted OR = 1.70, 95% CI = 1.24–2.32) and suicidality (adjusted OR = 1.65, 95% CI = 1.11–2.47) in adult life, with young age at first use and high frequency of use in adolescence particularly increasing the risk of depression in adulthood and suicidality [209].

A systematic review and meta-analysis that included 11 RCTs (23,317 individuals) found that the odds ratio of developing depression for cannabis users in young adulthood was 1.37 (95% CI 1.16–1.62) and the odds ratio for suicide ideation was 1.50 (95% CI 1.11–2.03) and suicide attempt was 3.46 (95% CI 1.5–7.84) though the odds ratio for anxiety was not statistically significant [208]. In contrast, the meta-analysis mentioned in the previous section which found greater odds of developing depression associated with cannabis use did not find any significant differences in effect based on age of participants [203].

In an Australian study which was a state-wide survey of 1601 secondary school students aged 14–15 who were followed for 7 years, they found that around 60% of participants had used cannabis by the time they were 20 and 7% were daily users. Daily use in young women was associated with a greater than fivefold increase in odds of reporting depression and anxiety (OR 5.6, 95% CI 2.6–12.0). Weekly or greater cannabis use in teenagers was associated with almost doubling of risk for later depression and anxiety (OR 1.9, 95% CI 1.1–3.3). However, depression and anxiety in teenagers did not predict later weekly or daily cannabis use [210].

We know that the ECS is particularly vulnerable in childhood and adolescence, a time of much neural change including synaptic pruning. Chronic use of cannabis to cope with symptoms of depression may increase susceptibility for depression by altering the ECS [184]. We learned earlier that in a study of healthy adolescent rats, THC administration in adolescent rats induced depressive-like behavior, impaired short-term memory, and reduced social interactions and induced a persistent neuroinflammatory state within the adult PFC, providing evidence of the underlying causal mechanism of action of the behavioral deficits in adult rats.

However, the ECS is malleable: alterations in CB1 receptor availability in chronic cannabis users are reversible after only a short (~2 day) period of abstinence, with no significant differences after 28 days of abstinence compared with healthy controls [211].

Most of this research focuses on the recreational use of cannabis. More research is needed in the context of medicinal use. Nonetheless, a prudent approach should be taken—adolescents should be steered away from recreational use of cannabis (as well as other illicit drugs and alcohol) given the potentially detrimental effects cannabis could have on the still-developing ECS.

## Legalization of Medicinal Cannabis Access and Suicide Reduction

It is worth noting that several studies have found an association between legal access to medicinal cannabis and reduction of suicide rates at the population level [212, 213]. The earlier of these studies found that legalization of medical cannabis was associated with a 10.8% (95% CI −17.1 to −3.7%) and 9.4% (95% CI = −16.1%, −2.4%) reduction in the suicide rate of men aged 20–29 years and 30–39 years, respectively [212], whilst the slightly later study of these studies found that California's 1996 legalization of recreational use resulted in statistically significant reductions in suicides and gun suicides, though only a non-statistically significant reduction in non-gun suicides [213]. This underscores the need for countries to consider the detrimental effect of criminalization of cannabis and the potential benefits which may include mental health benefits.

## What Is the Nature of the Association Between Cannabis Use and Depression?

There are at least three hypotheses that might explain an association between cannabis use and depression, examined by Harder et al. [204]. These are the self-medication hypothesis (i.e., depression causes cannabis use); the hypothesis that cannabis use causes depression; and the common factor hypothesis (there is a genetic or environmental cause for both depression and cannabis use) [204]. For a robust discussion, see Harder et al. [204].

There is support for the involvement of genetics and environmental factors: studies have found cannabis dependence and major depression arise from genetic as well as environmental vulnerabilities [214, 215]. Fu et al. [214] found that genetic factors associated with cannabis use and those associated with depression are moderately correlated. A study in twins where in each pair, one was cannabis-dependent and the other not, found that individuals who were cannabis dependent had significantly greater odds of suicide ideation and suicide attempt (OR 2.5 and 2.9, respectively) than their non-cannabis-dependent twin. Cannabis dependence was associated with elevated risks of major depressive disorder in dizygotic but not monozygotic twins. They found that those who started using cannabis before age 17 had increased rates of subsequent suicide attempts (OR 3.5, 95% CI 1.4–8.6) but not of major depressive disorder (MDD) or suicide ideation. The authors of this study concluded that the comorbidity between cannabis dependence and major depressive disorder was likely to arise through shared genetic and environmental vulnerabilities that predisposed to both outcomes [215].

## Dosing Guidelines for Treating Depression with Medicinal Cannabis

### When to Use Medicinal Cannabis

Medical cannabis treatment should be considered after a thorough clinical assessment and implementation of a comprehensive treatment plan including lifestyle modification, diet, and behavioral approaches. Anxiety or depression can be primary manifestations of several disease conditions that need to be addressed promptly. Medicinal cannabis treatment might also be considered after failure of usual drug therapy or in conjunction with diseases known to be associated with depression like diabetes, rheumatoid arthritis, and malignancy.

### Type of Product (Blends)

Ideal blends are high in CBD and low in THC but need to match the patient's age, level of sensitivity to cannabinoids or THC, urine drug testing requirements, body mass, and other associated symptoms. Several terpenes like caryophyllene may be a significant part of the product blend and combine well with hemp phytocannabinoids to complement the effects in both anxiety and depression as well as inflammatory conditions. These blends may represent variations of the "entourage" that enhance effectiveness and reduce adverse effects. This is in stark contrast with single component CBD or isolates that have shown a bell-shaped dose response with a narrow window of effectiveness compared with the linear dose response of plant-derived CBD.

Not only do plant-derived cannabinoids allow for lower amounts to achieve benefits; they also cause reduced adverse effects [216]. For example, in human anxiety studies, 300 mg to 600 mg of isolate was used to improve symptoms [170], whereas in a case study of 47 patients in a mental health facility, dosages of only 25–175 mg were needed to achieve significant improvements of anxiety symptoms in 79% of patients within 4 weeks with side benefits of sleep enhancement in 66% [217]. In another series of clinical cases with PTSD for which anxiety is a significant symptom, symptom control was achieved with average doses of 33–48 mg of plant-derived CBD within 3 weeks [218].

The benefits of CBD in the presence of other plant constituents are supported by some recent reports showing that CBD in a standardized cannabis extract is more potent or efficacious than pure CBD including the antiproliferative effect on tumor cells and the inhibitory effect on bladder contractility. The higher efficiency of plant extract might be explained by additive or synergistic interactions between CBD and minor phytocannabinoids or non-cannabinoids presented in the extracts. As mentioned in Chap. 4 (Overview of Medicinal Cannabis), a meta-analysis of observational studies of treatment of refractory epilepsy found significantly greater improvements in those treated with CBD-rich extracts than those treated with purified CBD, with significantly less mild and severe side effects, and those treated with CBD-rich extracts compared with purified CBD. The mean dose per day of those treated with CBD-rich extracts was significantly lower than in those treated with purified CBD [219].

Most research has characterized isolated single constituents of traditional herbal medicine. However, most data provide legitimation of whole plant extracts in contrast with synthetic drugs. The therapeutic synergy observed with plant extracts results in lesser dosing amounts with reduced adverse effects [216, 219].

THC content may be appropriate in some cases of depression to improve sleep, to address pain, and to reduce the need for larger amounts of CBD since higher THC blends tend to allow for decreased amounts of CBD.

## What Form of Product Should You Use?

The best form of product matches the patients' preferred lifestyle and tastes. Capsules have a longer duration of action, but tinctures sublingually often provide immediate relief of acute stressful situations. The treatment plan might include both approaches in some patients. Even capsules can be used sublingually if one does not mind the strong earthy flavor of less processed phytocannabinoids.

## Dosing

Age and body mass are only rough guides for the use of cannabinoids. Generally, standard serving sizes (doses) are appropriate for people 45 kg or greater and can be adjusted after first doses for response. Patients who are seniors 70 years or older should start with ½ usual servings. For individuals known to be sensitive to common medications like paracetamol or aspirin, consider starting with single drops of a liquid form or skin applications.

Typical response for depression is rapid using doses in the lower range of 25–50 mg of a CBD-dominant formulation either once or twice daily. Unlike SSRIs, often the effects are immediate lifting of mood within minutes or hours of the first dose.

## Titration and Follow-Up

Symptoms of depression respond very quickly to cannabinoids even on the first dose. If possible, have a staff member follow up the day of or day after first doses to guide or review the initial response and begin titration to optimize mood and performance or minimize rare adverse symptoms. If possible, have a family member or friend observe the patient for an independent response assessment, and don't rely entirely on the patient's statement alone. Practitioners might consider repeating of a standardized depression questionnaire.

Adjust the daily dose or frequency to best fit the patient's situation. Maintain that dose indefinitely or for 1 month and then consider reducing the dose by as much as half based on continuing need.

Often, as in the case of PTSD, patients can achieve remission. Others may decide the life-enhancing and transformative benefits of cannabinoids are too valuable to suspend and will make cannabinoids a part of their medical nutritional lifestyle.

## Other Tips to Enhance Therapeutic Action

Cannabinoids are best absorbed with food or fatty snack. Studies show that long-chain triglycerides (18 carbons or more) enhance absorption into the intestinal lymphatics bypassing hepatic first-pass effects providing increased concentrations of 250 times plasma levels [220]. This has important implications in those with inflammation needing immune modulation. In fact, cannabinoids ingested with triglycerides achieved higher concentrations (micromolar) in the intestinal lymphatics than could be obtained in general circulation effectively suppressing inflammatory cytokines-expressing T cells [220].

Sleep disorders are common in anxiety and depression. Most patients report improved depth and quality of sleep, but a few can feel activated mentally with an evening dose that can delay onset of sleep considerably. Until the patient has had some experience with daytime doses, avoid medicinal cannabis treatment within 2 h or more of bedtime. Practitioners can encourage the patient to use a smartphone sleep application to monitor their sleep patterns if they feel they are not getting adequate sleep. Often these software programs actually show a significant amount of deep sleep of which the patient was unaware. Characteristically patients may say they slept very little or not at all, but they do not report significant fatigue.

## Drug-Cannabis Interactions

Cannabinoids can interfere with drug metabolism based on modulation of the cytochrome 450 system specifically CYP2C and CYP3A classes of isozymes, in vitro and in animal models. However, the modulation is relative and dose-related, seen only with very large doses of CBD isolate, that is in large doses far exceeding customary medicinal cannabis treatment. As noted above CBD worked well in conjunction with SSRI medications and even allowed abrupt discontinuation of SSRI without loss of effectiveness or adverse effect. A frequent concern is serotonin syndrome when combining two medications that stimulate increased serotonin levels. Symptoms in mild cases include high blood pressure and a fast heart rate, usually without a fever. Symptoms in moderate cases include high body temperature, agitation, increased reflexes, tremor, sweating, dilated pupils, and diarrhea. However, no reports of serotonin syndrome have been documented or reported with the use of CBD or other natural phytocannabinoids, probably owing to the low dosing, lack of interference, and multiple positive mechanisms of action.

## Case Studies from Dr. Blair's Practice

### Case 1 Professional Male with Depression

The patient is a 53-year-old professional magician who was generally well until 5 years ago when he lost his job at a theme park in Los Angeles, gained weight, and developed prediabetes, hypertension, and subsequently depression. His pessimistic attitude seriously interferes with his profession and work opportunities. He denies suicidal thoughts or plans and does not own a "real" firearm. He has international travel work plans and worries that his depression will interfere. He reports swollen ankles and high blood pressure on medications. He also has chronic back pain that is poorly controlled on Tylenol and multiple other prescription pain medications "left over" from a broken ankle reconstruction surgery a few years ago. In the past he was somewhat successful with dieting, but deepening depression has prevented him from taking any action.

Blood pressure was 140/90 mmHg and weight 225 pounds (estimate, because he claimed he was too depressed to measure). A fasting blood glucose measured 6.2 mmol/l.

**Medications:** Losartan/HCTZ 100/12.5 mg, hydrocodone/acetaminophen 10 mg 4 per day. Fluoxetine 20 mg qd (duration 3 months).

#### Treatment

After reviewing his history and discussing benefits and risks of CBD, he underwent an initial trial of liposomal 1:20 CBD blend of 5 mg (i.e., 1:20 ratio THC to CBD). Within 10 min he reported decreased back pain and improved mood. In addition, he showed increased range of motion of the back with a toe touch maneuver, head turning, and trunk twisting of 15–20°. He had increased facial motion and was smiling with widening of the palpebral fissures. His pulse remained stable at 70 b.p.m.

Three days later he returned to demonstrate a "magic trick" his experience inspired. He used a clever device with four balls and a metal bar to metaphorically explain how CBD had worked for him connecting different body systems so that they would function more normally and restore his health.

One month later he reported CBD had completely "turned me around and now my attitude has completely changed." He also reported his back pain was improved and he was experiencing overall feelings of optimism and well-being. He was able to discontinue all pain medications.

At this point he had adjusted his dose to 20 mg three times per day. I suggested the client switch to a tincture with higher concentration for more cost-effective and practical approach.

Two months later he felt ready to "dive into a well monitored complete health program" with a dietitian. He also reported his blood pressure normalized to 120/80 mmHg and his fasting blood glucose dropped below 5.6 mmol/l. In addition, he insisted on introducing cannabinoid therapy to his wife and introducing his octogenarian parents to CBD (with guidance), and they also responded well for their pain symptoms. Later in the month, the patient performed an illusion of sawing a woman in half on the television show *Dancing with the Stars*.

## Case 2 Young Adult with Depression

The patient is an 18-year-old senior high school student in good general health except for depression since age 14. His symptoms included withdrawal from social activities and negative self-thoughts. Counseling produced no significant changes. Lexapro was prescribed and provided mood lifting and improved interactions but was associated with weight gain. After 2 years the medication no longer was felt to be effective. Lisdexamfetamine (a derivative of amphetamine) was added to treat attention-deficit hyperactivity disorder (ADHD) as well as moderate-to-severe binge-eating disorder.

His early childhood was associated with a parental divorce and abusive relationship with a stepfather.

Physical examination was normal, and no symptoms of flashbacks, panic, or night terrors were noted.

***Pathology Tests:*** Laboratory findings were normal range, and biochemical studies did not reveal any abnormalities.

***Medications:*** Lisdexamfetamine.

### Treatment

Broad spectrum, no THC product was recommended to avoid any long-term effects on brain function that might be related to THC. 25 mg liquid tincture twice daily along with supportive omega 3 and behavioral counselling support was recommended. Nutritional review was recommended for possible deficiencies and consideration of organic acid testing for indicators of metabolic enzyme disorders or toxin exposures.

After 2 weeks the patient's family reported increased interactions and more normal social activities. School work performance improved significantly with greater completion of assignments. His physical activity also increased and was associated with modest weight changes.

At 1 month the parents discontinued Lisdexamfetamine with no adverse change in school performance. A week later they also discontinued escitalopram without withdrawal or adverse symptoms. Organic acid testing suggested abnormal folate metabolism, and MTHFR C677T polymorphism was noted. Methylated folate was added to his regimen as he continued his improvement.

At 3 months the patient appeared to be interacting normally without further signs of withdrawal, sadness, or rumination. He joined a recreational sports team, lost significant weight, and participated in a school play. He was able to discontinue cannabinoid therapy without relapse and use sparingly for occasional acute symptoms such as pre-performance for school, competition, or stage acting.

## Conclusion

The pathogenesis of depression is complex and multifactorial. There are several lines of evidence to indicate that the endocannabinoid system is implicated in the pathophysiology of depression. Being a neuroregulatory system, one must consider whether changes in the endocannabinoid system are part of the etiology and pathogenesis of depression or simply a response by the body to try to regulate or correct imbalances in other systems, or both. There is preclinical research in animals and relatively limited research in humans in relation to the usefulness of CBD in treatment of depression. Preclinical research provides some support for efficacy of THC in alleviating depression. Results of human research investigating cannabis and THC for alleviation of depression are mixed, with some evidence of a positive effect in alleviating depression in some studies and other studies finding an association between cannabis use and depression. There is a serious paucity of RCT data.

It is important to remember that lifestyle factors, nutritional factors, environmental factors, and others (e.g., comorbidities, medications) may play very important roles in the etiology and pathogenesis of depression. Such factors will need to be considered and addressed in patients presenting with depression. An integrative approach to helping the patient heal is critical.

## References


1. Kosiba JD, Maisto SA, Ditre JW. Patient-reported use of medical cannabis for pain, anxiety, and depression symptoms : systematic review and meta-analysis. Soc Sci Med. 2019;233:181–92.
2. Arrow BA, Hunkeler EM, Blasey CM, et al. Comorbid depression, chronic pain and disability in primary care. Psychosom Med. 2006;68:262–8.
3. Coplan JD, Asronson CJ, Panthangi V, Kim Y. Treating comorbid anxiety and depression: psychosocial and pharmacological approaches. World J Psychiatry. 2015;5(4):366–78.
4. The Sacred Plant. The ultimate guide to CBD. US: TSP Publishing; 2020.

5. Mayo Clinic: Bipolar Disorder. Available at: https://www.mayoclinic.org/diseases-conditions/bipolar-disorder/symptoms-causes/syc-20355955. Accessed 25 June 2020.
6. American Psychiatric Association. What is depression. Available at: https://www.psychiatry.org/patients-families/depression/what-is-depression. Accessed 6 Jan 2021.
7. World Health Organization (WHO). Depression and other common mental disorders. Geneva: Global Health Estimates; 2017.
8. Williams HJ, Craddock N, Russo G, et al. Most genome-wide significant susceptibility loci for schizophrenia and bipolar disorder reported to date cross-traditional diagnostic boundaries. Hum Mol Genet. 2011;20:387–91.
9. Finan PH, Smith MT. The comorbidity of insomnia, chronic pain, and depression: dopamine as a putative mechanism. Sleep Med Rev. 2013;17(3):173–83. https://doi.org/10.1016/j.smrv.2012.03.003.
10. Demyttenaere K, Bruffaerts R, Lee S, et al. Mental disorders among persons with chronic back or neck pain: results from the world mental health surveys. Pain. 2007;129:332–42.
11. Kessler RC, Berglund P, Demler O, et al. The epidemiology of major depressive disorder: results from the National Comorbidity Survey Replication (NCS-R). JAMA. 2003;289:3095–105.
12. Hirschfeld RM. The comorbidity of major depression and anxiety disorders: recognition and management in primary care. Prim Care Companion J Clin Psychiatry. 2001;3(6):244–54.
13. Carter RM, Wittchen HU, Pfister H, Kessler RC. One-year prevalence of subthreshold and threshold DSM-IV generalized anxiety disorder in a nationally representative sample. Depress Anxiety. 2001;13(2):78–88.
14. Judd LL, Kessler RC, Paulus MP, et al. Comorbidity as a fundamental feature of generalized anxiety disorders: results from the National Comorbidity Study (NCS). Acta Psychiatr Scand Suppl. 1998;393:6–11.
15. Micale V, Tabiova K, Kucerova J, Drago F. Chapter 5. Role of the endocannabinoid system in depression: from preclinical to clinical evidence. In: Campolongo P, Fattore L, editors. Cannabinoids and modulation of emotion, memory, and motivation. New York: Springer Science + Business Media; 2015a. https://doi.org/10.1007/978-1-4939-2294-9_5.
16. Sansone RA, Sansone LA. Agometatine: a novel antidepressant. Innov Clin Neurosci. 2011;8:10–4.
17. Connolly KR, Thase ME. Emerging drugs for major depressive disorder. Expert Opin Emerg Drugs. 2012;17:105–26.
18. Sales AJ, Fogaca MV, Sartim AG, et al. Cannabidiol induces rapid and sustained antidepressant-like effects through increased BDNF signaling and synaptogenesis in the prefrontal cortex. Mol Neurobiol. 2019;56(2):1070–81.
19. Gotzsche PC. Deadly psychiatry and organised denial. Copenhagen: Peoples Press; 2015.
20. Boorman E, Zajkowska Z, Ahmed R, et al. Crosstalk between endocannabinoid and immune systems: a potential dysregulation in depression? Psychopharmacology (Berl). 2016;233(9):1591–604.
21. Savitz J, Frank MB, Victor T, et al. Inflammation and neurological disease-related genes are differentially expressed in depressed patients with mood disorders and correlate with morphometric and functional imaging abnormalities. Brain Behav Immun. 2013;31:161–71.
22. Miller BR, Hen R. The current state of the neurogenic theory of depression and anxiety. Curr Opin Neurobiol. 2015;30:51–8.
23. Chan SW, Harmer CJ, Norbury R, et al. Hippocampal volume in vulnerability and resilience to depression. J Affect Disord. 2016;189(1):199–202.
24. Liu W, Ge T, Leng Y, et al. The role of neural plasticity in depression: from hippocampus to prefrontal cortex. Neural Plasticity. 2017;2017:6871089. https://doi.org/10.1155/2017/6871089.
25. Sheline YI. Depression and the hippocampus: cause or effect? Biol Psychiatry. 2011;70(4):308–9.
26. Yi S. Depression and the hippocampus: cause or effect? Biol Psychiatry. 2011;70(4):308–9.
27. Drevets WC, Price JL, Simpson JR Jr, et al. Subgenual prefrontal cortex abnormalities in mood disorders. Nature. 1997;386(6627):824–7.

28. Drevets WC, Ongur D, Price DL. Neuroimaging abnormalities in the subgenual prefrontal cortex: implications for the pathophysiology of familial mood disorders. Mol Psychiatry. 1998;3(3):220–6.
29. Bora E, Harrison BJ, Davey CG, et al. Meta-analysis of volumetric abnormalities in cortico-striatal-pallidal-thalamic circuits in major depressive disorder. Psychol Med. 2012;42(4):671–81.
30. Kempton MJ, Salvador Z, Munafò MR, et al. Structural neuroimaging studies in major depressive disorder. Meta-analysis and comparison with bipolar disorder. Arch Gen Psychiatry. 2011;68(7):675–90.
31. Yu K, Cheung C, Leung M, et al. Are bipolar disorder and schizophrenia neuroanatomically distinct? An anatomical likelihood meta-analysis. Front Hum Neurosci. 2010;4:189.
32. Delgado PL. Depression: the case for a monoamine deficiency. J Clin Psychiatry. 2006;61(Suppl 6):7–11.
33. Ghasemi M, Phillips C, Trillo L, et al. The role of NMDA receptors in the pathophysiology and treatment of mood disorders. Neurosci Biobehav Rev. 2014;47:336–58.
34. Gorzalka BB, Hill MN. Putative role of endocannabinoid signaling in the etiology of depression and actions of antidepressants. Prog Neuro-Psychopharmacol Biol Psychiatry. 2011;35(7):1575–85.
35. Dantzer R, O'Connor JC, Freund GG, et al. From inflammation to sickness and depression: when the immune system subjugates the brain. Nat Rev Neurosci. 2008;9(1):46–56.
36. Felger JC. Role of inflammation in depression and treatment implications. Handb Exp Pharmacol. 2019;250:255–86.
37. Chen Y-H, Wang W-M, Li I-H, et al. Major depressive disorder increased risk of psoriasis: a propensity score matched cohort study. J Affect Disord. 2021;278:407–12.
38. Dalton EJ, Heinrichs RW. Depression in multiple sclerosis: a quantitative review of the evidence. Neuropsychology. 2005;19(2):152–8.
39. Figved N, Klevan G, Myhr KM, et al. Neuropsychiatric symptoms in patients with multiple sclerosis. Acta Psychiatr Scand. 2005;112(6):463–8.
40. Nouwen A, Winkley K, Twisk J, et al. European Depression in Diabetes (EDID) Research Consortium. Type 2 diabetes mellitus as a risk factor for the onset of depression: a systematic review and meta-analysis. Diabetologia. 2010;53(12):2480–6.
41. Van der Kooy K, van Hout H, Marwijk H, et al. Depression and the risk for cardiovascular diseases: systematic review and meta analysis. Int J Geriatr Psychiatry. 2007;22(7):613–26.
42. Lewinson RT, Vallerand IA, Lowerison MW, et al. Depression is associated with an increased risk of psoriatic arthritis among patients with psoriasis: a population-based study. J Invest Dermatol. 2017;137(4):828–35.
43. Howren MB, Lamkin DM, Suls J. Associations of depression with c-reactive protein, il-1, and il-6: a meta-analysis. Psychosom Med. 2009;71:171–86.
44. Dantzer R. Role of the kynurenine metabolism pathway in inflammation-induced depression: preclinical approaches. Curr Top Behav Neurosci. 2017;31:117–38.
45. Baraldi S, Hepgul N, Mondelli V, Pariante CM. Symptomatic treatment of interferon-α-induced depression in hepatitis C: a systematic review. J Clin Psychopharmacol. 2012;32(4):531–43.
46. Asnis GM, De La Garza R. Interferon-induced depression in chronic hepatitis c: a review of its prevalence, risk factors, biology, and treatment approaches. J Clin Gastroenterol. 2006;40(4):322–35.
47. Eisenberger NI, Inagaki TK, Rameson LT, et al. An fMRI study of cytokine-induced depressed mood and social pain: the role of sex differences. NeuroImage. 2009;47(3):881–90.
48. Harrison NA, Brydon L, Walker C, et al. Inflammation causes mood changes through alterations in subgenual cingulate activity and mesolimbic connectivity. Biol Psychiatry. 2009;66(5):407–14.
49. Müller N. COX-2 inhibitors, aspirin, and other potential anti-inflammatory treatments for psychiatric disorders. Front Psych. 2019;10:375.

50. De Berardis D, Conti CM, Serroni N, et al. The effect of newer serotonin-noradrenalin antidepressants on cytokine production: a review of the current literature. Int J Immunopathol Pharmacol. 2010;23(2):417–22.
51. Hannestad J, DellaGioia N, Gallezot J, et al. The neuroinflammation marker translocator protein is not elevated in individuals with mild-to-moderate depression: a [11C]PBR28 PET study. Brain Behav Immun. 2013;33:131–8.
52. Jenny M, Schrocksnadel S, Uberall F, Fuchs D. The potential role of cannabinoids in modulating serotonergic signaling by their influence on tryptophan metabolism. Pharmaceuticals (Basel). 2010;3:2647–60.
53. Bakunina N, Pariante CM, Zunszain PA. Immune mechanisms linked to depression via oxidative stress and neuroprogression. Immunology. 2015:144(3). https://doi.org/10.1111/imm.12443.
54. Suzuki H, Ohgidani M, Kuwano N, et al. Suicide and microglia: recent findings and future perspectives based on human studies. Front Cell Neurosci. 2019;13:31. https://doi.org/10.3389/fncel.2019.00031.
55. Louveau A, Smirnov I, Keyes TJ, et al. Structural and functional features of central nervous system lymphatic vessels. Nature. 2015;523(7560):337–41.
56. Pariante CM, Lightman SL. The HPA axis in major depression: classical theories and new developments. Trends Neurosci. 2008;31(9):464–8.
57. Hill MN, Gorzalka BB. Is there a role of the endocannabinoid system in the etiology and treatment of melancholic depression? Behav Pharmacol. 2005;16:333–52.
58. Krantz DS, Manuck SB. Acute psychophysiologic reactivity and risk of cardiovascular disease: A review and methodologic critique. Psychological Bulletin. 1984;96(3):435–64.
59. Larkin KT, Brown LA, Tiani AG. Chapter 5. The autonomic and neuroendocrine response to stress. In: Chantler PD, Larkin KT, editors. Cardiovascular implications of stress and depression. Academic Press; 2020. p. 87–110.
60. Herbert J. Cortisol and depression: three questions for psychiatry. Psychol Med. 2013;43(3):449–69.
61. Mausbach BT, Dimsdale JE, Ziegler MG, et al. epressive symptoms predict norepinephrine response to a psychological stressor task in Alzheimer's caregivers. Psychosom Med. 2005;67(4):638–42.
62. Whitaker AC, Batty GD, Gale CR, et al. Major depressive disorder, generalised anxiety disorder, and their comorbidity: associations with cortisol in the Vietnam experience study. Psychoneuroendocrinology. 2010;36(5):682–90.
63. Salomon K, Clift A, Karlsdóttir M, Rottenberg J. Major depressive disorder is associated with attenuated cardiovascular reactivity and impaired recovery among those free of cardiovascular disease. Health Psychol. 2009;28(2):157–65.
64. Burke HM, Davis MC, Otte C, Mohr DC. Depression and cortisol responses to psychological stress: a meta-analysis. Psychoneuroendocrinology. 2005;30(9):846–56.
65. Suzuki H, Belden AC, Spitznagel E, et al. Blunted stress cortisol reactivity and failure to acclimate to familiar stress in depressed and sub-syndromal children (article)(open access). Psychiatry Res. 2013;210(2):575–83.
66. Phillips A, Hunt K, Der G, Carroll D. Blunted cardiac reactions to acute psychological stress predict symptoms of depression five years later: evidence from a large community study. Psychophysiology. 2011;48:142–8.
67. Salomon K, Bylsma LM, White KE, et al. Is blunted cardiovascular reactivity in depression mood-state dependent? A comparison of major depressive disorder remitted depression and healthy controls. Int J Psychophysiol. 2013;90(1):50–7.
68. Carroll D, Phillips AC, Lovallo WR. Are large physiological reactions to acute psychological stress always bad for health? Soc Personal Compass (Health Section). 2009;3:725–43.
69. Weir GC, Bonner-Weir S. Five stages of evolving beta-cell dysfunction during progression to diabetes. Diabetes. 2005;53(Suppl 3):S16–21.
70. Figueiredo TC, de Oliveria JRM. Reconsidering the association between the major histocompatability complex and bipolar disorder. J Mol Neurosci. 2012;47:26–30.

71. Szabo ST, Nemeroff CB. Chapter 103 – Depression. In: Rosenberg RN, Pascual JM, editors. Rosenberg's molecular and genetic basis of neurological and psychiatric disease. 5th ed. Academic Press; 2015. p. 1253–74.
72. Masi G, Brovedani P. The Hippocampus, Neurotrophic Factors and Depression: Possible Implications for the Pharmacotherapy of Depression. CNS Drugs. 2011;25(11):913–31.
73. Liu B, Liu J, Wang M, et al. From serotonin to neuroplasticity: evolvement of theories for major depressive disorder. Front Cell Neurosci. 2017;11:305.
74. Xu L, Anwyl R, Rowan MJ. Behavioural stress facilitates the induction of long-term depression in the hippocampus. Nature. 1997;387(6632):497–500.
75. Lee BH, Kim YK. The roles of BDNF in the pathophysiology of major depression and in antidepressant treatment. Psychiatry Investig. 2010;7:231–5.
76. Dang Y-H, Ma X-C, Zhang J-C, et al. Targeting of NMDA receptors in the treatment of major depression. Curr Pharm Des. 2014;20(32):5151–9.
77. Inoshita M, Umehara H, Watanage S-Y, et al. Elevated peripheral blood glutamate levels in major depressive disorder. Neuropsychiatr Dis Treat. 2018;14:945–53.
78. Yüksel C, Öngür D. Magnetic resonance spectroscopy studies of glutamate-related abnormalities in mood disorders. Biol Psychiatry. 2010;68(9):785–94.
79. Levine J, Panchalingam K, Rapoport A, et al. Increased cerebrospinal fluid glutamine levels in depressed patients. Biol Psychiatry. 2000;47(7):586–93.
80. Hasler G, van der Veen JW, Tumonis T, et al. Reduced Prefrontal Glutamate/Glutamine and γ-Aminobutyric Acid Levels in Major Depression Determined Using Proton Magnetic Resonance Spectroscopy. Arch Gen Psychiatry. 2007;64(2):193–200.
81. Vostrikov VM, Uranova NA, Orlovskaya DD, et al. Deficit of perineuronal oligodendrocytes in the prefrontal cortex in schizophrenia and mood disorders. Schizophr Res. 2007;94:273–80.
82. Murr C, Widner B, Sperner-Unterweger B, et al. Immune reaction links disease progression in cancer patients with depression. Med Hypotheses. 2000;55(2):137–40.
83. Capuron L, Neurauter G, Musselman DL, et al. Interferon-alpha-induced changes in tryptophan metabolism. Relationship to depression and paroxetine treatment. Biol Psychiatry. 2003;54(9):906–14.
84. Oxenkrug GF. Serotonin – kynurenine hypothesis of depression: historical overview and recent developments. Curr Drug Targets. 2013;14(5):514–21.
85. Oxenkrug GF. Tryptophan–kynurenine metabolism as a common mediator of genetic and environmental impacts in major depressive disorder: the serotonin hypothesis revisited 40 years later. Isr J Psychiatry Relat Sci. 2010;47(1):56–63.
86. Müller N, Schwarz M. A psychoneuroimmunological perspective to Emil Kraepelins dichotomy: Schizophrenia and major depression as inflammatory CNS disorders. Eur Arch Psychiatry Clin Neurosci. 2008;258:97–106.
87. Ramirez LA, Perez-Padilla EA, Garcia-Oscos F, et al. A new theory of depression based on the serotonin/kynurenine relationship and the hypothalamic pituitary-adrenal axis. Biomedica. 2018;38(3):437–50.
88. Kwidzinski E, Bechmann I. IDO expression in the brain: a double-edged sword. J Mol Med (Berl). 2007;85(12):1351–9.
89. Silote GP, Sartima A, Sales A et al. Emerging evidence for the antidepressant effect of cannabidiol and the underlying molecular mechanisms. J Chem Neuroanatomy 2019; 98: 104–16.
90. Hill MN, Hillard CJ, Bambico FR, et al. The therapeutic potential of the endocannabinoid system for the development of a novel class of antidepressants. Trends Pharmacol Sci. 2009a;30(9):484–93.
91. World Health Organization (WHO). World Health Organization Expert Committee on drug dependence pre-review. Delta-9-Tetrahydrocannabinol. Geneva: World Health Organization; 2018.
92. Giacobbe J, Marrocu A, Di Genedetto MG, et al. A systematic, integrative review of the effects of the endocannabinoid system on inflammation and neurogenesis in animal models of affective disorders. Brain Behav Immun. 2021;93:353–67.

93. Micale V, Di Marzo V, Sulcova A, et al. Endocannabinoid system and mood disorders: priming a target for new therapies. Pharmacol Ther. 2015b;138:18–37.
94. Bambico FR, Hattan PR, Garant J-P, Gobbi G. Effect of delta-9-tetrahydrocannabinol on behavioral despair and on pre- and postsynaptic serotonergic transmission. Prog Neuro-Psychopharmacol Biol Psychiatry. 2012;38:88–96.
95. Aso E, Renoir T, Mengod G, et al. Lack of $CB_1$ receptor activity impairs serotonergic negative feedback. J Neurochemistry. 2009;109(3):935–44.
96. Beyer CE, Dwyer JM, Piesla MJ, et al. Depression-like phenotype following chronic CB1 receptor antagonism. Neurobiol Dis. 2012;39(2):148–55.
97. Marco EM, Garcia-Gutierrez MS, Bermudez-Silva F-J, et al. Endocannabinoid system and psychiatry: in search of a neurobiological basis for detrimental and potential therapeutic effects. Front Behav Neurosci. 2011;5:63. https://doi.org/10.3389/fnbeh.2011.00063.
98. Aso E, Ozaita A, Valdizan EM, et al. BDNF impairment in the hippocampus is related to enhanced despair behavior in CB1 knockout mice. J Neurochem. 2008;105:565–72.
99. Sanchis-Segura C, Cline BH, Marsicano G, et al. Reduced sensitivity to reward in CB1 knockout mice. Psychopharmacology. 2004;176:223–32.
100. Steiner MA, Wanisch K, Monory K, et al. Impaired cannabinoid receptor type 1 signaling interferes with stress-coping behavior in mice. Pharmacogenomics J. 2008;8:196–208.
101. Martin M, Ledent C, Parmentier M, et al. Involvement of CB1 cannabinoid receptors in emotional behaviour. Psychopharmacology. 2002;159(4):379–87.
102. Uriguen L, Perez-Rial S, Ledent C, et al. Impaired action of anxiolytic drugs in mice deficient in cannabinoid CB1 receptors. Neuropharmacology. 2004;46:966–73.
103. Christensen R, Kristensen PK, Bartels EM, et al. Efficacy and safety of the weight-loss drug rimonabant: a meta-analysis of randomised trials. Lancet. 2007;370(9600):1706–13.
104. Moreira FA, Crippa JA. The psychiatric side-effects of rimonabant. Braz J Psychiatry. 2009;31(2):145–53.
105. de Wit L, Luppino F, Van Straten A, et al. Depression and obesity: a meta-analysis of community-based studies. Psychiatry Res. 2010;178(2):230–5.
106. Suarez J, Rivera P, Rey AA, et al. Adipocyte cannabinoid CB1 receptor deficiency alleviates high fat diet-induced memory deficit, depressive-like behavior, neuroinflammation and impairment in adult neurogenesis. Psychoneuroendocrinology. 2019;110:104418.
107. Bahi A, Al Mansouri S, Al Memari E, et al. β-Caryophyllene, a $CB_2$ receptor agonist produces multiple behavioral changes relevant to anxiety and depression in mice. Phsyiol Behav. 2014;135:119–24.
108. Garcia-Gutierrez MS, Perez-Ortiz JM, Gutierrez-Adan A, Manzanares J. Depression-resistant endophenotype in mice overexpressing cannabinoid $CB_2$ receptors. Br J Pharmacol. 2010;160(7):1773–84.
109. Yu H, Chen ZY. The role of BDNF in depression on the basis of its location in the neural circuitry. Acta Pharmacol Sin. 2010;32:3–11.
110. Ortega-Alvaro A, Aracil-Fernandez A, García-Gutiérrez MS, et al. Deletion of CB2 cannabinoid receptor induces schizophrenia-related behaviors in mice. Neuropsychopharmacology. 2011;36:1489–504.
111. Onaivi ES, Ishiguro H, Gong JP, et al. Brain neuronal CB2 cannabinoid receptors in drug abuse and depression: from mice to human subjects. PLoS One. 2008;3:e1640.
112. Valverde O, Torrens M. CB1 receptor-deficient mice as a model for depression. Neuroscience. 2012;204:193–206.
113. Beyer CE, Dwyer JM, Piesla MJ et al. Depression-like phenotype following chronic CB1 receptor antagonism. Neurobiol Dis. 2010;39:148–155.
114. Wang W, Sun D, Pan B, et al. Deficiency in endocannabinoid signaling in the nucleus accumbens induced by chronic unpredictable stress. Neuropsychopharmacology. 2010;35(11):1149–2261.
115. Hill MN, Carrier EJ, McLaughlin RJ, et al. Regional alterations in the endocannabinoid system in an animal model of depression: effects of concurrent antidepressant treatment. J Neurochem. 2008a;106(6):2322–36.

116. Hill MN, Patel S, Carrier EJ, et al. Downregulation of endocannabinoid signaling in the hippocampus following chronic unpredictable stress. Neuropsychopharmacology. 2005;30:508–15.
117. Bortolato M, Mangieri RA, Fu J, et al. Anti-depressant-like activity of the fatty acid amide hydrolase inhibitor URB597 in a rat model of chronic mild stress. Biol Psychiatry. 2007;62(10):1103–10.
118. Gobbi G, Bambico FR, Mangieri R, et al. Anti-depressant like activity and modulation of brain monoaminergic transmission by blockade of anandamide hydrolysis. Proc Natl Acad Sci. 2005;103:18620–5.
119. Tejeda-Martínez AR, Viveros-Paredes JM, Hidalgo-Franco GV, et al. Chronic Inhibition of FAAH Reduces Depressive-Like Behavior and Improves Dentate Gyrus Proliferation after Chronic Unpredictable Stress Exposure. Behav Neurol. 2021;2021:6651492.
120. Jiang H-X, Ke B-W, Liu J, et al. Inhibition of Fatty Acid Amide Hydrolase Improves Depressive-Like Behaviors Independent of Its Peripheral Antinociceptive Effects in a Rat Model of Neuropathic Pain. Anesth Analg. 2019;129(2):587–97.
121. Patel S, Roelke CT, Rademacher DJ, et al. Inhibition of restraint stress-induced neural and behavioural activation by endogenous cannabinoid signalling. Eur J Neurosci. 2005;21(4):1057–69.
122. Navarria A, Tamburella A, Iannotti FA, et al. The dual blocker of FAAH/TRPV1 N-arachidonoylserotonin reverses the behaviour despair induced by stress in rats and modulates the HPA-axis. Pharmacol Res. 2014;87:151–9.
123. Alteba S, Zer-Aviv M, Tenenhaus A, et al. Antidepressant-like effects of URB597 and JZL184 in male and female rats exposed to early life stress. Eur Neuropsychopharmacol. 2020;39:70–86.
124. Adamczyk P, Golda A, McCreary AC, Filip M, Przegalinski E. Activation of endocannabinoid transmission induces antidepressant-like effects in rats. J Physiol Pharmacol. 2008;59:217–28.
125. Choi K, Le T, McGuire J, et al. Expression pattern of the cannabinoid receptor genes in the frontal cortex of mood disorder patients and mice selectively bred for high and low fear. J Psychiatr Res. 2012;46(7):882–9.
126. Hungund B, Vinod K, Kassir S, et al. Upregulation of CB 1 receptors and agonist-stimulated [35 S]GTPγS binding in the prefrontal cortex of depressed suicide victims. Molecular Psychiatry. 2004;9:184–90.
127. Koethe D, Llenos IC, Dulay JR, et al. Expression of CB1 cannabinoid receptor in the anterior cingulate cortex in schizophrenia, bipolar disorder, and major depression. J Neural Transm (Vienna). 2007;114(8):1055–63.
128. Topol EJ, Bousser MG, Fox KA, et al. Rimonabant for prevention of cardiovascular events (CRESCENDO): a randomised, multicentre, placebo-controlled trial. Lancet. 2010;376(9740):517–23.
129. Hill MN, Miller GE, Carrier EJ, et al. Circulating endocannabinoids and N-acyl ethanolamines are differentially regulated in major depression and following exposure to social stress. Psychoneuroendocrinology. 2009b;34(8):1257–62.
130. Barry A, O'Halloran KD, McKenna JP, et al. Plasma N-acylethanolamine and endocannabinoid levels in burning mouth syndrome: potential role in disease pathogenesis. J Oral Pathol Med. 2018;47(4):440–2.
131. Vinod KY, Arango V, Xie S, et al. Elevated levels of endocannabinoids and CB1 receptor-mediated G-protein signaling in the prefrontal cortex of alcoholic suicide victims. Biol Psychiatry. 2005;57:480–6.
132. Ho WS, Hill MN, Miller GE, et al. Serum contents of endocannabinoids are correlated with blood pressure in depressed women. Lipids Health Dis. 2012;11:32.
133. Hill MN, Miller GE, Ho WS, et al. Serum endocannabinoid content is altered in females with depressive disorders: a preliminary report. Pharmacopsychiatry. 2008b;41:48–53.
134. Paolucci EM, Loukov D, Bowdish DME, et al. Exercise reduces depression and inflammation but intensity matters. Biol Psychol. 2018;133:79–84.

135. Heyman E, Gamelin F-X, Goekint M, et al. Intense exercise increases circulating endocannabinoid and BDNF levels in humans—possible implications for reward and depression. Psychoneuroendocrinology. 2012;37(6):844–51.
136. Kong X, Miao Q, Lu X, et al. The association of endocannabinoid receptor genes (CNR1 and CNR2) polymorphisms with depression: a meta-analysis. Medicine (Baltimore). 2019;98(46):e17403.
137. Hillard CJ, Liu QS. Endocannabinoid signaling in the etiology and treatment of major depressive illness. Curr Pharm Des. 2014;20:3795–811.
138. Barrero FJ, Ampuero I, Morales B, et al. Depression in Parkinson's disease is related to a genetic polymorphism of the cannabinoid receptor gene (CNR1). Pharmacogenomics J. 2005;5:135–41.
139. Domschke K, Dannlowski U, Ohrmann P, et al. Cannabinoid receptor 1 (CNR1) gene: impact on antidepressant treatment response and emotion processing in major depression. Eur Neuropsychopharmacol. 2008;18:751–9.
140. Juhasz G, Chase D, Pegg E, et al. CNR1 gene is associated with high neuroticism and low agreeableness and interacts with recent negative life events to predict current depressive symptoms. Neuropsychopharmacology. 2009;34:2019–27.
141. Monteleone P, Bifulco M, Maina G, et al. Investigation of CNR1 and FAAH endocannabinoid gene polymorphisms in bipolar disorder and major depression. Pharmacol Res. 2010;61:400–4.
142. McPartland JM, Guy GW, Di Marzo V. Care and feeding of the endocannabinoid system: a systematic review of potential clinical interventions that upregulate the endocannabinoid system. PLoS One. 2014;9(3):e89566. https://doi.org/10.1371/journal.pone.0089566.
143. Hill MN, Ho WSV, Sinopoli KJ, et al. Involvement of the endocannabinoid system in the ability of long-term tricyclic antidepressant treatment to suppress stress-induced activation of the hypothalamic-pituitary-adrenal axis. Neuropsychopharmacology. 2006;31(12):2591–9.
144. Hill MN, Ho WSV, Hillard CJ, et al. Differential effects of the antidepressants tranylcypromine and fluoxetine on limbic cannabinoid receptor binding and endocannabinoid contents. J Neural Transm. 2008c;115(12):1673–9.
145. Ferreira FF, Ribeiro FF, Rodrigues RS, et al. Brain-derived neurotrophic factor (BDNF) role in cannabinoid-mediated neurogenesis. Front Cell Neurosci. 2018;12:441.
146. Wyrofsky R, McGonigle P, Van Bockstaele EJ. Drug discovery strategies that focus on the endocannabinoid signaling system in psychiatric disease. Expert Opin Drug Discov. 2015;10(1):17–36.
147. Palazuelos J, Ortega Z, Díaz-Alonso J, et al. CB2 cannabinoid receptors promote neural progenitor cell proliferation via mTORC1 signaling. J Biol Chem. 2012;287(2):1198–209.
148. Flannery LE, Kerr DM, Finn DP, Roche M. FAAH inhibition attenuates TLR3-mediated hyperthermia, nociceptive- and anxiety-like behaviour in female rats. Behav Brain Res. 2018;353:11–20.
149. Sayd A, Anton M, Alen F, et al. Systemic administration of oleoylethanolamide protects from neuroinflammation and anhedonia induced by LPS in rats. Int J Neuropsychopharmacol. 2015;18:1–14.
150. Petit-Demouliere B, Chenu F, Bourin M. Forced swimming test in mice a review of antidepressant activity. Psychopharmacology. 2005;177:245–55.
151. Zlebnik NE, Cheer JF. Beyond the CB1 receptor: is cannabidiol the answer for disorders of motivation? Annu Rev Neurosci. 2016;39:1–17.
152. Al-alfy AT, Ivey K, Robinson K, et al. Antidepressant-like effect of Δ 9 -tetrahydrocannabinol and other cannabinoids isolated from Cannabis sativa L. Pharmacol Biochem Behav. 2010;95:434–42.
153. Crippa JA, Guimaraes FS, Campos AC, Zuardi AW. Translational investigation of the therapeutic potential of cannabidiol (CBD): toward a new age. Front Immunol. 2018;9:2009.
154. Granjeiro EM, Gomes FV, Guimarães FS, et al. Effects of intracisternal administration of cannabidiol on the cardiovascular and behavioral responses to acute restraint stress. Pharmacol Biochem Behav. 2011;99:743–8.

155. Linge R, Jimenez-Sanches L, Campa L, et al. Cannabidiol induces rapid-acting antidepressant-like effects and enhances cortical 5-HT / glutamate neurotransmission: role of 5-HT 1A receptors. Neuropharmacology. 2016;103:16–26.
156. Resstel LB, Tavares RF, Lisboa SF, et al. 5-HT1A receptors are involved in the cannabidiol-induced attenuation of behavioral and cardiovascular responses to acute restraint stress in rats. Br J Pharmacol. 2009;156:181–8.
157. Sales AJ, Crestani CC, Guimaraes S, Joca SRL. Antidepressant-like effect induced by cannabidiol is dependent on brain serotonin levels. Prog Neuro-Psychopharmacol Biol Psychiatry. 2018;S0278-5846(18):30116–7.
158. Zanelati TV, Biojone C, Moreira FA, et al. Antidepressant-like effects of cannabidiol in mice: possible involvement of 5-HT1A receptors. Br J Pharmacol. 2010;159(1):122–8.
159. Sartim AG, Guimaraes FS, Joca SRL. Antidepressant-like effect of cannabidiol injection into the ventral medial prefrontal cortex-possible involvement of 5-HT1A and CB1 receptors. Brain Behav Res. 2016;303:218–27.
160. Campos AC, Ortega Z, Palazuelos J, et al. The anxiolytic effect of cannabidiol on chronically stressed mice depends on hippocampal neurogenesis: involvement of the endocannabinoid system. Int J Neuropsychopharmacol. 2013;16(6):1407–19.
161. David DJ, Wang J, Samuels BA, et al. Implications of the functional integration of adult-born hippocampal neurons in anxiety-depression disorders. Neuroscientist. 2010;16:578–91.
162. Bis-Humbert C, Garcia-Cabrerizo R, Garcia-Fuster MJ. Decreased sensitivity in adolescent versus adult rats to the antidepressant-like effects of cannabidiol. Psychopharmacology. 2020;237:1621–31.
163. Luján MÁ, Castro-Zavala A, Alegre-Zurano L, Valverde O. Repeated Cannabidiol treatment reduces cocaine intake and modulates neural proliferation and CB1R expression in the mouse hippocampus. Neuropharmacology. 2018;143:163–75.
164. Wolf SA, Bick-Sander A, Fabel K, et al. Cannabinoid receptor CB1 mediates baseline and activity-induced survival of new neurons in adult hippocampal neurogenesis. Cell Commun Signal. 2010;8:12.
165. Schiavon AP, Bonato JM, Milani H, et al. Influence of single and repeated cannabidiol administration on emotional behavior and markers of cell proliferation and neurogenesis in non-stressed mice. Prog Neuro-Psychopharmacol Biol Psychiatry. 2016;64:27–34.
166. Sartim AG, Sales AJ, Guimarães FS, Joca SR. Hippocampal mammalian target of rapamycin is implicated in stress-coping behavior induced by cannabidiol in the forced swim test. J Psychopharmacol. 2018;32(8):922–31.
167. Florensa-Zanuy E, Garro-Martinez E, Albert Adell A, et al. Cannabidiol antidepressant-like effect in the lipopolysaccharide model in mice: modulation of inflammatory pathways. Biochem Pharmacol. 2021;185:114433.
168. Chaves YC, Genaro K, Stern CA, et al. Two-weeks treatment with cannabidiol improves biophysical and behavioral deficits associated with experimental type-1 diabetes. Neurosci Lett. 2020;729:135020.
169. Hen-Shoval D, Amra S, Shbiro L, et al. Acute oral cannabidiolic acid methyl ester reduces depression-like behaviour in two genetic animal models of depression. Behav Brain Res. 2018;351:1–3.
170. Laczkovics C, Kothgassner OD, Felnhofer A, et al. Cannabidiol treatment in an adolescent with multiple substance abuse, social anxiety and depression. Neuropsychiatrie. 2021;35:31–4.
171. Shunney AG. CBD cases & clinical pearls: anxiety & depression. Botanical Medicine, Clinical Pearls, Mind/Body. Available at: https://ndnr.com/category/botanical-medicine/. Accessed 19 Mar 2021.
172. Hershkowitz M, Szechtman H. Pretreatment with delta9-tetrahydrocannabinol and psychoactive drugs: effects on uptake of biogenic amines and on behaviour. Eur J Pharmacol. 1979;59:267–76.

173. Bambico FR, Katz N, Debonnel G, Gobbi G. Cannabinoids elicit antidepressant-like behavior and activate serotonergic neurons through the medial prefrontal cortex. J Neurosci. 2007;27:11700–11.
174. Bambico FR, Gobbi G. The cannabinoid CB1 receptor and the endocannabinoid anandamide: possible antidepressant targets. Expert Opin Ther Targets. 2008;12(11):1347–66.
175. Bambico FR, Duranti A, Tontini A, Tarzia G, Gobbi G. Endocannabinoids in the treatment of mood disorders: evidence from animal models. Curr Pharm Des. 2009;15:1623–46.
176. Malone DT, Taylor DA. Modulation by fluoxetine of striatal dopamine release following delta-tetrahydrocannabinol: a microdialysis study in conscious rats. Br J Pharmacol. 1999;128:21–6.
177. Tanda G, Pontieri FE, Di Chiara G. Cannabinoid and heroin activation of mesolimbic dopamine transmission by a common mu1 opioid receptor mechanism. Science. 1997;276:2048–50.
178. Zamberletti E, Gabaglio M, Prini P, et al. Cortical neuroinflammation contributes to long-term cognitive dysfunction following adolescent delta-9-tetrahydrocannabinol treatment in female rats. Eur Neuropsychopharmacol. 2015;25:2404–15.
179. Denson TF, Earleywine M. Decreased depression in marijuana users. Addict Behav. 2006;31(4):738–42.
180. Gruber AJ, Pope HG, Brown ME. Do patients use marijuana as an antidepressant? Depression. 1996;4(2):77–80.
181. Lintzeris N, Driels J, Elias N, et al. Medicinal cannabis in Australia 2016: the Cannabis as medicine survey (CAMS-16). Med J Aust. 2018;209(5):211–6.
182. Sexton M, Cuttler C, Finnell JS, Mischley LK. A cross-section survey of medical cannabis users: patterns of use and perceived efficacy. Cannabis Cannabinoid Res. 2016;1(1):131–8.
183. Schlienz NJ, Scalsky R, Martin EL, et al. A cross-sectional and prospective comparison of medicinal cannabis users and controls on self-reported health. Cannabis Cannabinoid Res. 2020; https://doi.org/10.1089/can.2019.0096.
184. Cuttler C, et al. A naturalistic examination of the perceived effects of cannabis on negative affect. J Affect Disord. 2018;235:198–205.
185. Li X, Diviant JP, Stith SS, et al. The effectiveness of *cannabis* flower for immediate relief from symptoms of depression. Yale J Biol Med. 2020;93(2):251–64.
186. National Academies of Sciences, Engineering & Medicine. The health effects of cannabis and cannabinoids. National Academies of Sciences, Engineering & Medicine; 2017.
187. Childs E, Lutz AA, de Wit H. Dose-related effects of delta-9-THC on emotional responses to acute psychosocial stress. Drug Alcohol Depend. 2017;177:136–44.
188. Narang S, Gibson D, Wasan AD, et al. Efficacy of dronabinol as an adjuvant treatment for chronic pain patients on opioid therapy. J Pain. 2008;9(3):254–64.
189. Portenoy RK, Ganae-Motan ED, Allende S, et al. Nabiximols for opioid-treated cancer patients with poorly controlled chronic pain: a randomized, placebo-controlled, graded-dose trial. J Pain. 2012;13:438–49.
190. Rog DJ, Nurmikko TJ, Friede T, Young CA. Randomized, controlled trial of cannabis-based medicine in central pain in multiple sclerosis. Neurology. 2005;65(6):812–9.
191. Wade DT, Makela P, Robson P, et al. Do cannabis-based medicinal extracts have general or specific effects on symptoms in multiple sclerosis? A double-blind, randomized, placebo-controlled study on 160 patients. Mult Scler J. 2004;10(4):434–41.
192. Skrabek RQ, Galimova L, Ethans K, Perry D. Nabilone for the treatment of pain in fibromyalgia. J Pain. 2008;9(2):164–73.
193. Fiz J, Duran M, Capella D, et al. Cannabis use in patients with fibromyalgia: effect on symptoms relief and health-related quality of life. PLoS One. 2011;6(4):e18440.
194. Crupi R, Paterniti IA, Ahmad A, et al. Effects of palmitoylethanolamide and luteolin in an animal model of anxiety/depression. CNS Neurol Disord Drug Targets. 2013;12:989–1001.
195. Ghazizadeh-Hashemi M, Ghajar A, Shalbafan M-R, et al. Palmitoylethanolamide as adjunctive therapy in major depressive disorder: a double-blind, randomized and placebo-controlled trial. J Affect Disord. 2018;232:127–33.

196. Yu HL, Deng XQ, Li YJ, et al. N-palmitoylethanolamide, an endocannabinoid, exhibits antidepressant effects in the force swim test and the tail suspension test in mice. Pharmacol Rep. 2011;63:834–9.
197. Guida F, Luongo L, Boccella S, et al. Palmitoylethanolamide induces microglia changes associated with increased migration and phagocytic activity: involvement of the CB2 receptor. Sci Rep. 2017;7(1):375.
198. Bovasso G. Cannabis abuse as a risk factor for depressive symptoms. Am J Psychiatry. 2001;158:2033–7.
199. Chen CY, Wagner FA, Anthony JC. Marijuana use and the risk of major depressive episode. Epidemiological evidence from the United States National Comorbidity Survey. Soc Psychiatry Psychiatr Epidemiol. 2002;37:199–206.
200. Gorfinkel LR, Stohl M, Hasin D. Association of depression with past-month cannabis use among US adults aged 20 to 59 years, 2005 to 2016. JAMA. 2020;3(8):e2013802.
201. Grant BF, Hasin DS, Stinson FS, et al. Co-occurrence of 12-month mood and anxiety disorders and personality disorders in the US: results from the national epidemiologic survey on alcohol and related conditions. J Psychiatr Res. 2005;39:1–9.
202. Kedzior LL, Laeber T. A positive association between anxiety disorders and cannabis use or cannabis use disorders in the general population- a meta-analysis of 31 studies. BMC Psychiatry. 2014;14:136.
203. Lev-Ran S, Roerecke M, Le Foll B, et al. The association between cannabis use and depression: a systematic review and meta-analysis of longitudinal studies. Psychol Med. 2014;44:797–810.
204. Harder VS, Morral AR, Arkes J. Marijuana use and depression among adults: testing for causal associations. Addiction. 2006;101(10):1463–72.
205. Moore THM, Zammit S, Lingford-Hughes A, et al. Cannabis use and risk of psychotic or affective mental health outcomes: a systematic review. Lancet. 2007;370(9584):319–28.
206. Danielsson A-K, Lundin A, Agardh E, et al. Cannabis use, depression and anxiety: a 3-year prospective population based study. J Affect Disord. 2016;193:103–8.
207. Manrique-Garcia E, Zammit S, Dalman C, et al. Cannabis use and depression: a longitudinal study of a national cohort of Swedish conscripts. Psychiatry. 2012;12:112.
208. Gobbi G, Atkin T, Zytynski T, et al. Association of cannabis use in adolescence and risk of depression, anxiety, and suicidality in young adulthood: a systematic review and meta-analysis. JAMA Psychiat. 2019;76(4):426–34.
209. Hengartner MP, Angst J, Ajdacic-Gross V, et al. Cannabis use during adolescence and the occurrence of depression, suicidality and anxiety disorder across adulthood: findings from a longitudinal cohort study over 30 years. J Affect Disord. 2020;272:98–103.
210. Patton GC, Coffey C, Carlin J, et al. Cannabis use and mental health in young people: cohort study. BMJ. 2002;325:1195–8.
211. D'Souza CP, Cortes-Briones JA, Ranganathan M, et al. Rapid changes in CB1 receptor availability in cannabis dependent males after abstinence from cannabis. Biol Psychiatry Cogn Neurosci Neuroimaging. 2016;1(1):60–7.
212. Anderson DM, Rees DI, Sabia JJ. Medical marijuana laws and suicides by gender and age. Am J Public Health. 2014;104(12):2369–76.
213. Bartos BJ, Kubrin CE, Newark C. Medical marijuana laws and suicide. Arch Suicide Res. 2019;14:1–14.
214. Fu Q, Heath AC, Bucholz KK, et al. Shared genetic risk of major depression, alcohol dependence and marijuana dependence: contribution to antisocial personality disorder in men. Arch Gen Psychiatry. 2002;59:1125–32.
215. Lynskey MT, Glowinski AL, Todorov AA, et al. Major depressive disorder, suicidal ideation, and suicide attempt in twins discordant for cannabis dependence and early-onset cannabis use. Arch Gen Psychiatry. 2004;61(10):1026–32.
216. Gallily R, Yekhtin Z, Hanuš LO. Overcoming the Bell-Shaped Dose-Response of Cannabidiol by Using Cannabis Extract Enriched in Cannabidiol. Pharmacology & Pharmacy. 2015;6:75–85.

217. Shannon S, Lewis N, Lee H, Hughes S. Cannabidiol in anxiety and sleep: a large case series. Perm J. 2019;23:18–041.
218. Elms L, Shannon S, Hughes S, Lewis N. Cannabidiol in the treatment of Post-Traumatic Stress Disorder: a case series. J Altern Complement Med. 2019;25(4):392–7.
219. Pamplona FA, da Silva LR, Coan AC, et al. Potential clinical benefits of CBD-rich *cannabis* extracts over purified CBD in treatment-resistant epilepsy: observational data meta-analysis. Front Neurol. 2018;9:759.
220. Zgair A, Lee JB, Wong JCM, et al. Oral administration of cannabis with lipids leads to high levels of cannabinoids in the intestinal lymphatic system and prominent immunomodulation. Sci Rep. 2017;7(1):14542.

# Post-Traumatic Stress Disorder

# 7

## Introduction

Observational studies, in particular in war veterans, indicate that many people use cannabis to alleviate the symptoms associated with post-traumatic stress disorder (PTSD). Cross-sectional studies have found that PTSD patients reported using cannabis to cope with hyperarousal, coping, and sleep [1–3]. Other studies have found associations between PTSD, cannabis use, and cannabis use disorder [4]. Though we tend to associate PTSD with the armed forces, PTSD is not something just found in these men and women and other first responder occupations. In refugees, PTSD is the most frequently cited behavioral conditions, ranging from 15% to 80% prevalence [5]. It is unfortunately very common in women and children as a result of domestic violence and abuse, perhaps a more hidden demographic.

The pathophysiology of PTSD is, unsurprisingly, complex, and it has been described as an anxiety disorder, a disorder of dysregulation of fear and processing of stimuli associated with trauma, and a paradoxical disorder of memory. We have already seen how the endocannabinoid system (ECS) is intimately involved in regulation of our stress response, as well as in anxiety and depression, and these conditions are all intertwined with PTSD.

**This Chapter**
This chapter will examine what PTSD is, its prevalence, its pathophysiology, and how the endocannabinoid system may be involved, as through understanding its pathophysiology, we might then begin to understand how medicinal cannabis and some of its key constituents might assist in addressing the symptoms and underlying pathways involved. We examine the evidence associated with the use of medicinal cannabis to treat PTSD, including preclinical and human studies, and conclude with two case studies from Dr. Blair's practice.



K. O'Brien, P. Blair, *Medicinal Cannabis and CBD in Mental Healthcare*,
https://doi.org/10.1007/978-3-030-78559-8_7

## What Is PTSD?

PTSD is a debilitating mental illness with neurobiological abnormalities that can develop after exposure to a life-threatening or traumatic event. It is characterized by three main groups of symptoms:

1. Re-experiencing symptoms: persistent re-experiencing of the trauma(s), dreams and flashbacks (of the event), and intense physiological and psychological reactions to internal and external cues or stimuli
2. Avoidance symptoms: avoidance of trauma-related stimuli, avoidance of places that remind the person of the traumatic event, evasion of any thoughts or feelings of people that remind the person of the trauma, emotional numbing, and decreased interest in participating in activities
3. Hyperarousal symptoms: sleep disorders (difficulty falling asleep or staying asleep), anger, irritability, hypervigilance, and exaggerated startle reflex [6–8]

## PTSD as an Anxiety Disorder and a Paradoxical Disorder of Memory

PTSD is viewed as an anxiety disorder which is characterized by inappropriate persistent and uncontrolled retrieval of traumatic memories [9], as well as a paradoxical disorder of memory [10]. It has also been described as a disorder of dysregulation of fear and processing of stimuli associated with trauma [7]. Its description as a "paradoxical disorder of memory" is because there are intrusive memories or recollections of certain aspects of the trauma (flashbacks), as well as amnesia for other aspects [10–12]. Situations reflecting aspects of the traumatic event can trigger intrusive memories or flashbacks, and the trauma is re-experienced with a high level of arousal (emotion and sensory intensity), but there are also memory alterations, with difficulty in the recall of the corresponding contextual information and the chronological order of events [10, 11].

Much variability exists between individuals with respect to the types of symptoms experienced after trauma and duration and course of symptoms. Importantly, not everyone who experiences trauma will develop PTSD [13], and many who do will spontaneously recover [14]. Those who remit may relapse and those who remit are at high risk of recurrence of symptoms or full-blown PTSD [15, 16]. Several different factors contribute to the magnitude of PTSD symptoms, as well as determining someone's resilience to trauma. These include their early life experiences, genetic makeup and predisposition, and social support network [17].

## DSM-5 Definition

Post-traumatic stress disorder (PTSD) is defined under the *Diagnostic and Statistical Manual of Mental Disorders, fifth edition* (DSM-5) as a trauma- and stressor-related disorder [6]. According to the DSM-5, diagnosis is based on the individual being exposed to a traumatic event (Criteria A) and then meeting Criteria B (intrusive symptoms), C (avoidance), D (negative alterations in cognitions and/or mood), and E (alterations in arousal and reactivity), set out in more detail below (see Table 7.1). The duration of the disturbance (Criteria B, C, D, and E) must be more than 1 month, and the disturbance must cause clinically significant distress or impairment in social, occupational, or other important areas of functioning and may not be attributable to the physiological effects of a substance (e.g., medication or alcohol) or another medical condition [6].

**Table 7.1** DSM-5 diagnostic criteria PTSD: key points

| Criteria | Details |
| --- | --- |
| A. Exposure | Exposure to actual or threatened death, serious injury, or sexual violence in one or more of the following ways: (1) directly experiencing the event; (2) witnessing the event as it occurred to others; (3) learning that the traumatic event occurred to a close family member or friend, or (4) experiencing repeated or extreme exposure to aversive details of the traumatic event |
| B. Intrusion symptoms | Presence of one or more intrusion symptoms: recurrent, involuntary, and intrusive distressing memories of the event; recurrent distressing dreams; dissociative reactions (e.g., flashbacks); prolonged or intense psychological distress; marked physiological reactions to internal or external cues that symbolize or resemble an aspect of the event |
| C. Avoidance | Persistent avoidance of stimuli associated with the traumatic event(s), beginning after the traumatic event, evidenced by avoidance of or efforts to avoid stressing memories/thoughts/feelings associated with the event or avoidance of or efforts to avoid external reminders, e.g., people and places that arouse distressing memories or thoughts associated with the event |
| D. Negative alterations in cognitions and mood | Negative alterations in cognitions and mood associated with the traumatic event beginning or worsening after the event occurred, evidenced by two or more of the following: inability to remember an important aspect of the traumatic event(s) (typically dissociative amnesia and not to other factors such as head injury, alcohol, or drugs); persistent and exaggerated negative beliefs about oneself; and others (see DSM-5 for more information) |
| E. Marked alterations in arousal and reactivity | Marked alterations in arousal and reactivity associated with the traumatic event(s), beginning or worsening after the traumatic event occurred, as evidenced by one or more of the following including irritable behavior and angry outbursts with little or no provocation, hypervigilance, reckless or self-destructive behavior, and others (see DSM-5 for complete list) |

American Psychiatric Association [6]

There are two subtypes of PTSD under the DSM-5: PTSD preschool subtype (diagnosis in children under 6 years of age) and PTSD dissociative subtype which is used when a person has prominent dissociative symptoms (all other PTSD criteria must still be met) [6].

## Predisposing Factors and Epigenetics

An estimated 90% of people will experience a traumatic event in their life; however, most will recover and not go on to develop PTSD. Experiencing a traumatic event increases the risk of developing PTSD, with rates of 18–36% of PTSD occurring in patients exposed to trauma [7]. Various predisposing risks for PTSD include stress, depression, and trauma [7].

Epigenetics are very likely to play a key role in why some people develop PTSD and others don't [18]. Depression, stress, and trauma result in differential DNA methylation of endocrine genes, and it is possible that this could underpin different biological responses to trauma and therefore risk of developing PTSD [7, 18]. This will be discussed more later.

Adverse events of childhood occurrence appear to increase risk for PTSD. For example, 85% of veterans at a community-based mental health clinic within the US Department of Veterans Affairs reported experiencing at least one category of adverse childhood event before age 18 years, and 46% reported experiencing four or more categories [19].

## Comorbidities of PTSD

In more than 80% of cases of PTSD, there are comorbidities with other mental health and medical disorders [20]. The associated mood, physical, and dissociative symptoms can impair everyday functioning, including employment, relationships, and ability to look after oneself [20, 21].

Mental health comorbidities of PTSD include anxiety, depression, personality disorders, and substance abuse [20]. More than 50% of PTSD sufferers also have depression, and the comorbidity of PTSD and depression is a delayed phenomenon occurring later in the disease process [20]. This comorbidity can be associated with greater distress, symptomatology, occupational disability, global disability, and social impairment compared to either condition alone [20]. A review of studies published in 2012 concluded that there is strong support for the assertion that comorbidity of PTSD and depression modulates symptom severity across many different populations studied and that symptom severity is higher when both conditions are present than either alone [20].

There is evidence that PTSD sufferers engage in substance abuse in order to cope with these symptoms: rates of substance abuse are much higher in those with PTSD, and this relationship is partly mediated by sleep problems [22].

### Risk of Suicide

PTSD sufferers are at increased risk of suicide. A Danish study found that the odds ratio associating PTSD with suicide was 9.8 (95% CI 6.7–15). After controlling for psychiatric and demographic confounding factors, the odds ratio was 5.3 (95% CI 3.4–8.1). In addition, those with PTSD and depression had a greater suicide rate than expected based on their independent effects [23].

### Sleep Problems

Sleep disturbances (e.g., insomnia, daytime sleepiness, nightmares) are hallmark features of PTSD. Studies have shown that PTSD sufferers experience more stage 1 sleep and less slow-wave sleep (indicative of more shallow sleeping) and greater rapid eye movement density [24].

### Increased Risk of Diseases

PTSD sufferers are at increased risk for several different diseases which are associated with inflammation including cardiovascular disease, autoimmune disorders, metabolic disorders, and dementia [25, 26]. Associations in 1456 German veterans aged 60–85 years have been found between PTSD and angina/coronary artery disease, congestive heart failure, peripheral vascular disease, cardiovascular risk factors (hypertension, increased cholesterol), asthma, osteoporosis, back pain, cancer, stomach problems, hearing problems, and thyroid disorders [27]. A large study in 666,269 Afghanistan and Iraq veterans found that PTSD was associated with a twofold increase in the following diseases: autoimmune thyroiditis, inflammatory bowel disease, rheumatoid arthritis, multiple sclerosis, and lupus erythematosus [28]. This study found that being a female veteran was associated with a much higher risk of autoimmune disorders: 4.6% compared with 1.7% in male veterans [28].

## Prevalence of PTSD

PTSD's lifetime prevalence is higher than that of other anxiety disorders, including panic disorder, obsessive-compulsive disorder, and generalized anxiety disorder [29]. Any person experiencing trauma is at risk of developing PTSD. There are many first responder occupations which put individuals at risk of PTSD, and these can include members of the armed forces, police, ambulance officers, firefighters, emergency call dispatchers, and many others. We tend to think of PTSD in relation to the armed forces in particular; however, an important cohort which is not spoken about enough are those survivors of domestic violence, abuse, or neglect, and these tend to be women and children. Another important group are those living in or refugees from war-torn countries, and those living in abject poverty.

### General Population

Data from the National Comorbidity Survey Replication (2001–2003) indicates estimated 3.6% of US adults had PTSD in the past year, with the figure higher for women (5.2%) than men (1.8%). The lifetime prevalence of PTSD was 6.8% [30]. Of US adults who had PTSD in the past year, 30.2% were deemed mild, 33.1% moderate and 36.6% serious [31]. Data from the National Comorbidity Adolescent Supplement (NCS-A) indicates that an estimated 5.0% of adolescents aged 13–18 had PTSD, with higher prevalence again in females (8.0%) more than males (2.3%) [32].

Large community surveys in Australia and New Zealand show that 50–75% of people report at least one potentially traumatic event (PTE) in their lives, with most reporting two or more. PTEs are a risk factor for developing PTSD. It is also known that about 50% of PTSD will resolve within 12 months of the event [33]. The 12-month prevalence (those who have had PTSD in the previous 12 months) is estimated at 6.4% in Australia and 3.6% in the USA [30, 33]. Earlier (2011) figures put Australian prevalence rates for PTSD at 4.4% (12 month) and 7.2% (lifetime) [34], with higher rates after specific trauma. For example, interpersonal traumas such as rape and sexual assault other than rape are associated with greater probability of PTSD, of the order of 46.2% and 29.0%, respectively, in one study of 1698 young adults (mean age 21 years) in a mid-Atlantic city in the USA [35].

### Armed Forces

The prevalence of PTSD is particularly high in veterans from the armed forces. For example, a study of 1938 previously deployed armed service members who served in Afghanistan and Iraq found the prevalence of current PTSD was 13.8% [36]. A study conducted from 1995 to 1997 of 11,441 Gulf War veterans found a prevalence of current PTSD of 12.1% [37]. Further back in recent history, a study of Vietnam War veterans found an estimated lifetime prevalence of PTSD of 30.9% in men and 26.9% in women [38].

An estimated 8.3% of the Australian Defence Force (ADF) will have experienced PTSD in the past 12 months. ADF males report a greater rate of PTSD compared with males in the general population (8.1% vs 4.6% males). Deployment does not appear to influence rate: ADF members who have never been deployed experience PTSD at the same rate as those who have been deployed. Length of deployment is not a useful marker of risk; however, the number and type of traumas and roles while on deployment (e.g., combat, explosive ordinance roles) may be useful to identify "at-risk" persons. Experience of multiple traumas across lifetime including deployment is associated with greater risk of PTSD [39].

### Domestic Violence and Sexual Assault

PTSD can occur as a result of domestic violence (also known as intimate partner violence), which can involve both physical and mental abuse. Instead of occurring as a one-off event, domestic violence and emotional abuse tend to be chronic, occurring repeatedly over time, and this chronic exposure can lead to chronic PTSD [40]. Survivors of rape and other types of sexual assault have a higher risk of developing PTSD compared with survivors of other types of trauma. An estimated 94% of rape/

sexual assault survivors develop PTSD symptoms within 2 weeks after the event, with approximately 50% suffering long-term symptoms. This is even more so for child victims (PTSD UK, no date). A meta-analysis of intimate partner violence survivors indicated a mean prevalence of 64% for PTSD (48% for depression) [41].

A telephone interview study of 2181 people in the Detroit area (USA) aged 18–45 years found that the conditional risk of PTSD following exposure to trauma was 9.2%. It also found that the highest risk of PTSD was associated with assaultive violence (20.9%) and that the traumatic event most often reported as the precipitating event among people with PTSD was unexpected death of a loved one (31% of all PTSD cases), which was experienced by 60% of the sample and associated with a moderate risk of PTSD (14.3%). After controlling for type of trauma, women were at higher risk of PTSD than men [42]. A later epidemiological study in 1698 young adults (mean age 21 years) in a mid-Atlantic city in the USA also found that females had a higher risk of PTSD after assaultive violence, but not after other traumas, compared with men (OR 4.0, 95% CI 2.0–8.3) [35].

## Orthodox Treatment of PTSD

Treatment largely falls into two categories: psychological treatments and pharmaceutical treatments. There are drawbacks with both treatment strategies, and a need for other therapies that address the pathophysiology as well as the symptoms associated with PTSD.

### Psychological Treatments

Several types of psychological therapies for PTSD exist including:

- Trauma-focused cognitive behavioral therapy (TF-CBT): a variant of CBT which includes several techniques to help the person overcome a traumatic event. TF-CBT helps the person come to terms with a trauma through exposure to memories of the event. It combines cognitive therapy which aims to change the way a person thinks and behavioral therapy which aims to change the way a person acts [43].
- Eye movement desensitization and reprocessing (EMDR): aims to help a person reprocess memories of a traumatic event. In this therapy, trauma-related images, beliefs, and body sensations are brought to mind while the therapist guides eye movements from side to side. The aim is to identify more positive views with the aim of replacing the ones causing the problems [43].
- Exposure therapy: is a form of extinction learning; patients are repeatedly exposed to gradually increasing trauma-related stimuli to promote fear inhibition and tolerate the stimuli without suffering extreme fear [8].

The 2018 UK National Institute for Health and Care Excellence (NICE) Guidelines for PTSD recommend individual TF-CBT and, if they don't respond to that after TF-CBT, EMDR for children and young people aged 7–17 years as therapy, but do not recommend psychologically focused debriefing for prevention or treatment of PTSD (they actively recommend not offering it). For adults, other forms of therapy recommended include cognitive processing therapy, cognitive therapy for PTSD, narrative exposure therapy, prolonged exposure therapy, computerized TF-CBT, and EDMR [44].

A Cochrane systematic review of 70 studies (4761 people) found support for the efficacy of individual TF-CBT, EMDR, non-TF-CBT, and group TF-CBT in the treatment of chronic PTSD in adults, and also found that other non-trauma-focused psychological therapies did not reduce PTSD symptoms as significantly. The study found that individual TF-CBT, EMDR, and non-TF-CBT are equally effective immediately posttreatment in the treatment of PTSD, and some evidence that TF-CBT and EMDR are superior to non-TF-CBT between 1 and 4 months following treatment [43].

A major problem with therapy-based interventions is the high dropout rate (38.5% in one study of veterans) [45, 46].

## Pharmaceutical Interventions

According to the US 2010 Veterans Affairs (VA)/Department of Defense Guidelines, psychotherapy and pharmacotherapy with selective serotonin reuptake inhibitors (SSRIs) or serotonin and norepinephrine reuptake inhibitors are considered first-line treatment [21]. Other agents include venlafaxine, prazosin, monoamine oxidase inhibitors, tricyclic antidepressants, atypical antipsychotics, and anticonvulsants [47, 48].

The efficacy of recommended first- and second-line pharmaceutical agents used either alone or in combination to treat symptoms of PTSD, including nightmares, is often limited for many patients [29]. For example, to target the neurotransmitter imbalance, antidepressants are recommended to treat PTSD, but the number needed to treat (NNT) for a response is up to nine patients [21]. Remission rates with pharmacotherapy are 20–30% [21].

The 2009 American Psychiatric Association practice guidelines for the treatment of acute stress and PTSD note that pharmacotherapy is not as effective for combat-related trauma compared to civilian PTSD [49]. There is some evidence from a 2006 Cochrane Review that war veterans are more resistant to pharmacotherapy than other patient groups, with regard to reduction in symptom severity [50].

The UK NICE Clinical Guidelines for PTSD (2018) recommend not offering drug treatments including benzodiazepines to prevent PTSD in adults and suggest venlafaxine or a selective serotonin reuptake inhibitor (SSRI) should be considered in adults with PTSD if the person has a preference for drug treatment. It also suggests that antipsychotics such as risperidone in addition to psychological therapies should be considered for management of symptoms for adults with a diagnosis of

PTSD if they have disabling symptoms and signs, e.g., severe hyperarousal, or psychotic symptoms and their symptoms have not responded to other drug or psychological therapies [44].

Nonetheless, the Cochrane Review of pharmaceutical therapy for PTSD conducted in 2006 found support for some pharmaceuticals in the treatment of PTSD, though it was unable to demonstrate superior efficacy or acceptability for any particular drug class. The review included 35 short-term (14 weeks or less) RCTs (4597 participants). Symptom severity for 17 RCTs was significantly reduced in the medication groups compared to placebo (weighted mean difference –5.76, 95% CI –8.16 to −3.36, $n = 2507$ participants), and statistics for responder status ($n = 13$ RCTs) demonstrated overall superiority of a variety of pharmaceuticals over placebo (RR 1.49, 95% CI 1.28–1.73, NNT = 4.85, 95% CI 3.85 to 6.25, $n = 1272$) [50]. A later review published in 2012 stated that the largest body of evidence for short-term and long-term efficacy exists for SSRI, with venlafaxine (selective NA reuptake inhibitor) and risperidone (atypical antipsychotic) appearing promising, but that evidence for effectiveness of benzodiazepines was lacking despite their continued use. It also concluded that the α1-antagonist prazosin and the atypical antipsychotics demonstrate some efficacy for treatment-resistant PTSD [51].

The problem with pharmaceutical options is not just lack of efficacy for many patients but also the potential for side effects, some very serious. The negative impact of nightmares and side effects of psychotherapeutic medications may potentiate other symptoms of PTSD, such as those related to anxiety and depression, and other comorbid psychiatric conditions may also worsen [29]. SSRIs have been found to potentiate suicide ideation [52]. In addition, since PTSD patients are often prescribed more than one pharmaceutical, potential side effects associated with polypharmacy are also an issue [29].

Thus, given that neither psychological-based nor pharmaceutical therapies are particularly successful in treating PTSD, there is a need for other therapeutic options. Medicinal cannabis could, perhaps, be one of them.

## Pathophysiology of PTSD

The pathophysiology of PTSD can involve distinct genetic, endocrine, demographic, and environmental factors, and these are not all shared by all PTSD patients [53]. Chronic stress can interact with the pathophysiology of PTSD [54, 55], and anxiety is also a feature, so any discussion of pathophysiology must be inclusive of an understanding of the effects of chronic stress and anxiety on the individual.

As mentioned previously, PTSD is viewed as an anxiety disorder which is characterized by inappropriate persistent and uncontrolled retrieval of traumatic memories [9], as well as a paradoxical disorder of memory [10]. Its pathophysiology is complex and involves maladapted memory processes, including inability to extinguish learned fear responses and suppress episodic traumatic memory retrieval, as well as inability to acquire safety signals and/or dampen the over-consolidation process that occurs straight after re-experiencing of symptoms (e.g., as occurs in flashbacks) [56].

There are many neurophysiological disturbances involved in addition to disordered memory formation, including a dysregulated stress response and HPA-axis dysfunction, inflammation, brain morphological and functional changes in brain regions associated with emotion regulation and memory formation, and genetic and epigenetic factors. What follows is only some of the research in relation to these factors, so that the reader may gain an understanding of the complexity of its pathology.

## PTSD as a Disorder of Memory

PTSD is seen by many as a "paradoxical disorder" of memory since it involves intrusive memory recollection of some aspects as well as amnesia for other aspects of the traumatic event [10, 12]. There are several processes involved in memory occurring in PTSD, and these involve the acquisition, consolidation, retrieval, reconsolidation, and extinction of *aversive* fear memories [57].

Feeling afraid is a natural response to a threat. It triggers physiological changes in the body to defend oneself or get away from the perceived threat, the classic "fight or flight" response. Memories that are characterized by strong emotional salience or significance tend to be well-consolidated memories which are often retrieved from the brain and from an evolutionary perspective; this makes sense in terms of a survival instinct since you want to quickly remember a threat and be able to react. However, in PTSD, as we explain below, this process is maladapted [58].

Early research demonstrated that learned material is vulnerable to interference for some time after learning (termed "retroactive interference"). *Memory consolidation* is the process by which a temporary, unstable memory is transformed into a more stable, enduring memory [59]. The consolidation phase of memory appears to be particularly important in PTSD and may be amenable to therapeutic intervention [60].

In animal research into PTSD, the fear-conditioning paradigm has been used to understand the processes of acquisition, consolidation, retrieval, reconsolidation, and extinction of aversive memories. The expression of anxiety and fear in humans is approximated by the expression of *conditioned fear* in animals [57]. Animal research into PTSD and anxiety-related disorders is more easily translated into humans than for other mental health conditions because the neural circuitry modulating fear, which includes the key brain regions of the amygdala, prefrontal cortex, and hippocampus, is conserved across mammals [17].

In *contextual fear conditioning*, the term *acquisition* is the pairing of a shock and the context, while *consolidation* refers to the stabilization of the fear association into long-term memory [61].

*Retrieval* is the use of the fear memory and is dynamic in that it can trigger further rounds of processing. This processing can include *reconsolidation* and *extinction*, both of which rely on distinct signaling mechanisms and protein synthesis [61].

In the process of *reconsolidation*, retrieval activates a time interval during which the original memory becomes unstable and is restabilized, which preserves the memory for context [61]. *Extinction* is the process of learned inhibition of retrieval of previously acquired responses (a process initiated and maintained by interactions between the hippocampus, basolateral amygdala and ventromedial prefrontal cortex) [62].

*Fear extinction learning* is an active process by which a conditioned fear response gradually decreases over time as the individual learns to dissociate a response from the stimulus, thereby reducing contextual memory [61, 63, 64]. In fear extinction learning, the previously aversive stimulus/situation is learned to be no longer threatening, and it occurs through many experiences in which the stimulus or situation is not paired or linked with an aversive outcome [65]. In animal studies, the conditioned stimulus is presented alone for several trials until the conditioned response is reduced or eliminated [66, 67].

Extinction is an active learning process or a process of layering (but it is not accelerated forgetting or a process of unlearning) in which the original association is believed to remain only partially intact in PTSD [61, 65, 67]. Three different mechanisms of action have been proposed to explain the phenomenon of extinction: (1) a new inhibitory memory is formed, competing with the original fear memory (involves associative learning); (2) changes in synaptic efficacy induced during fear conditioning weaken the original fear memory (also involves associative learning); and (3) a nonassociative process in which responsiveness to the presentation of the non-reinforced conditioned stimulus becomes decreased by habituation [68].

*Fear extinction recall* is the retrieval and expression of the learned "extinction memory" after a delay [63]. It is the ability to retain *fear extinction learning* over a prolonged time period. If the fear memory resurfaces, the extinction memory has to be learned again [65]. Fear extinction recall is believed to aid recovery from a psychologically traumatic event [63].

## The Necessity of Sleep for Memory Processes

Sleep is important for memory formation. It is during sleep in particular that the unstable memory traces become reorganized into long-term storage (though it also occurs when an individual is awake). It seems that during sleep, hippocampal-cortical firing patterns representing the stored memory during waking states get played back to the cortex during sleep, and this strengthens the cortico-cortical associations, thereby integrating it into existing cortical memory circuits [60]. Therefore, if someone is not sleeping properly, one can understand some of the ramifications in terms of brain physiology. Insomnia or sleep disorders are very common in PTSD.

With respect to emotional memory, the process of memory consolidation helps to reduce the affective tone of the memory trace (i.e., depotentiate it) and integrate it into conceptualized networks, solidifying the factual aspect of the memory trace [69]. Certain stress hormones (e.g., cortisol) and neurotransmitters (e.g., norepinephrine) acting at the amygdala appear to modulate the hippocampal-cortical transfer and decouple emotion and memory [70].

Animal studies have shown that retention of emotionally aversive memories over neutral memories is regulated by glucocorticoids during memory consolidation, causing a gradual reorganization of emotional memory traces [70]. In human studies cortisol enhanced the difference between emotional and neutral consolidated memories, preferencing emotional memory consolidation, and reduced amygdala reactivity, supporting theories of emotional depotentiation following consolidation during normal sleep [70].

**Maladaptive Memory Processing in PTSD**

Three main types of symptoms are relevant to PTSD: persistent re-experiencing of the trauma, persistent symptoms of hyperarousal, and persistent avoidance of stimuli associated with the trauma, as well as forgetting important aspects of the trauma. Such symptoms are reflective of excessive retrieval of traumatic memories that become consolidated, solidifying the traumatic memory trace. The memory retains vividness and can evoke distress for many years [58].

This suggests that three phases of memory processing are maladaptive: *(1) consolidation, (2) extinction, and (3) retrieval.*

**Memory Consolidation Fails in PTSD**

Why is any of the previous information important to know? Van Marle [60] describes this in detail and what follows is a summary. It seems that in PTSD, the process of memory consolidation fails. The traumatic memory trace remains mainly in subcortical and primary perceptual areas rather than being integrated into cortical memory networks, and consequently stays linked/coupled to autonomic and perceptual markers. Then, when an individual is exposed to a (trauma) trigger, the result is an involuntary retrieved memory trace made up of mostly primary sensory information (e.g., images, sounds, aromas) that are linked to physiological fear symptoms [60, 71]. Since there is no autobiographical context, the memory is relived, with characteristic PTSD symptoms occurring (e.g., flashbacks, nightmares, hyperarousal, and so on). Fundamentally it appears that a lack of consolidation and emotional depotentiation of traumatic memories underpins PTSD and that successful transfer to preexistent, cortical memory circuits could reduce the symptoms [60].

**Fear Learning and Fear Conditioning in PTSD**

PTSD symptoms include persistent autonomic re-experiencing of the trauma, avoidance of trauma-related stimuli, and hyperarousal. These symptoms are believed partly to reflect a patient's inability to inhibit "conditioned fear," most notably during symptoms of re-experiencing [8].

PTSD involves learned fear which may persist for decades: abnormally high psychophysiological conditioned responses to reminders of traumatic events can persist up to 50 years after the traumatic event [63]. When fear is acquired during a traumatic event, *fear learning* occurs where an association between a fear stimulus and situation that occurs at the time of the trauma is maintained through a process of *associative learning*. In this process, a past trauma triggers fearful responses to what should be a benign stimulus or situation. This *fear learning* contributes to most of the symptoms associated with PTSD such as intrusive memories, hyperarousal, and avoidance behaviors [65].

**PTSD Is Associated with Deficits in Fear Extinction Learning and Fear Extinction Recall**

In PTSD, it is believed that there is a deficit in fear extinction learning and/or a deficit in retention of extinction learning (*fear extinction recall*) underlying the inability to recover from the effects of a trauma [63, 65, 66]. Those with PTSD show poorer fear extinction learning and fear extinction recall than healthy subjects [63, 66, 72]. Animal studies support this, indicating that repeated stress can enhance fear memories and impair recall of extinction [54, 55, 73].

Research was conducted in 14 pairs of Vietnam War veteran monozygotic twins, discordant for combat exposure (in 7 pairs, the combat-exposed twin had PTSD). When extinction retention was assessed, they found that skin conductance responses were higher in the PTSD combat veterans than in their co-twins and higher than in non-PTSD combat veterans and their co-twins. This demonstrated that retention of extinction is deficient in PTSD and supports the conclusion that this deficit is acquired as a result of combat stress leading to PTSD (rather than being a predisposing factor to PTSD development following stress encountered through combat) [66].

Reduced fear extinction learning prior to trauma exposure is correlated with severity of PTSD symptoms [74]. A study prospectively tested whether reduced capability of extinction learning might be a predictor for later development of PTSD. They tested 249 Dutch soldiers before a 4-month deployment to Afghanistan administering a conditioning task, then after returning home, PTSD level was measured. They found that reduced extinction learning *prior to deployment* predicted the PTSD severity, also suggesting that reduced extinction learning has a role in development of PTSD [74].

**Other Aspects of Memory Involved in PTSD**

There are several aspects of memory and cognitive processing that may play a role in the development or maintenance of PTSD including verbal memory deficits, over-general memory, suppression of memories, avoidance of memories, negative interpretation of memory symptoms and negative conceptual knowledge of self, integration of trauma with identity, impairment in retrieval of voluntary trauma memories, and increased flashbacks [71].

Many theories about PTSD suggest that those who develop the disorder have a greater propensity to consolidate or recall emotionally laden memories. Other deficits such as impaired physiological habituation and pathological sensitization may also contribute to delayed onset of PTSD which can lead to the re-experiencing of trauma via flashbacks and nightmares, and development of avoidance of situations that might trigger symptoms [75].

## Brain Morphological and Neurophysiological Functioning Changes in PTSD

There are several areas of the brain relevant to fear and memory that are implicated in PTSD which include the amygdala and hippocampus (both of which participate in early stages of memory formation and retrieval of inhibitory avoidance), and the prefrontal cortex (PFC) [76, 77] . Both posterior and anterior regions of the hippocampus are involved, with the posterior hippocampus playing an important role in memory retrieval and spatial cognition and the anterior hippocampus involved in emotional memory and reward-directed behaviour [77]. Compared with the posterior region, the anterior region of the hippocampus appears preferentially associated with the amygdala, the HPA axis, and the limbic prefrontal circuitry [77]. Other brain regions involved in PTSD include the bed nucleus of the stria terminalis (BNST) which provides an interface between the affective forebrain (amygdala, ventral hippocampus, medial PFC) and the hypothalamic and brainstem areas. This area has been implicated in neuroendocrine, autonomic, and behavioral responses to threats, both actual and anticipated [78].

The amygdala regulates learned fear, and the basolateral amygdala (BLA) is involved in the acquisition of extinction in particular [17, 79]. The PFC and hippocampus have dense connections to the amygdala, and these connections appear to be important for learned/conditioned fear as well as associative emotional learning. The PFC reactivates past emotional associations, while the hippocampus plays a role in explicit memories of trauma, facilitating learned responses to contextual cues and contextual modulation of extinction, and both these structures exert top-down control of the amygdala which may increase activation of the latter, something seen in PTSD sufferers [17, 80].

Other brain regions involved in PTSD include the anterior cingulate gyrus, orbitofrontal cortex, parahippocampal gyrus, sensorimotor cortex, and thalamus [17]. Recent research also suggests that a relatively unknown region of the brain, the zona incerta, might hold the key to understanding how we control our fear [81].

### Changes in Brain Morphology and Function in PTSD

Changes in brain structure and function have been found in key brain regions associated with PTSD, including increased activity in the amygdala (fear center of the brain), decreased volume in the PFC (executive function of the brain), and decreased volume in the hippocampus (memory center of the brain), which lead to an increase in fear response, generalized fear responses, increased stress sensitivity, impaired fear extinction, and the symptoms associated with PTSD [17, 21, 76]. Such changes in brain morphology are suggestive of long-term neuroplastic changes in these brain regions involved in emotional memory processing.

For example, compared with healthy youths, youths with PTSD symptoms (but not full-blown PTSD) had less total brain tissue and lower total cerebral gray matter volumes, with a particular decrease in left ventral inferior prefrontal areas [82]. Imaging studies have shown aberrant white matter integrity in the major neuronal tract that connects the ACC with the amygdala—the cingulum bundle—which may be responsible for impaired inhibitory interaction between the PFC and amygdala found in PTSD [83, 84].

These three brain regions (amygdala, ventral medial PFC (vmPFC), and hippocampus) are involved in fear extinction whereby fear extinction memories are formed through a neural circuit involving these three structures. The amygdala receives projections from the PFC and the hippocampus [17]. Inhibitory signals from the vmPFC attenuate signals from the amygdala. As we learned earlier, in the development of these new fear extinction memories, as with any memory, there is a gradual change from initial memory storage in the hippocampus to the neocortex. So, in extinction learning, the contextual information associated with fear learning that is stored in the hippocampus must be overridden [65]. Studies using MRIs indicate that fear extinction is greater with increased volume and activity of the vmPFC [63] and that cortisol and cortisol reactivity are also critical [85, 86]. Cortisol has been found to reduce fear recall at the beginning of extinction and facilitate consolidation of an extinction memory, exerting a critical effect on the amygdala-hippocampus-vmPFC network underlying fear and extinction memories [85]. The problem is that with PTSD, sufferers tend to have lower levels of cortisol and hypoactive vmPFCs (and hippocampi) [63], discussed in more detail in the next sections.

Table 7.2 sets out key brain areas and their functions, and some of the changes that may occur in PTSD.

**Table 7.2** Key brain regions involved in PTSD

| Brain region | Purpose/function | Changes in PTSD |
|---|---|---|
| Amygdala | Acquisition and extinction of conditioned fear; associative learning; detecting threats; role in fear learning, fear expression, and heightening memory for emotional events | Increased responsiveness to traumatic and emotional stimuli;<br>amygdala hyperfunction related to hypoactivity of the vmPFC; impaired inhibition of amygdala by the PFC during extinction learning |
| Prefrontal cortex (PFC) | Emotional regulation | Decreased gray and white matter density; decreased responsiveness to trauma and emotional stimuli; medial PFC is smaller in volume and hyporesponsive during symptomatic states; impaired inhibition of amygdala by PFC during extinction learning |
| Hippocampus | Conditioned fear, associative learning | Increased responsiveness to traumatic and emotional stimuli; smaller volumes and decreased neuronal and functional integrity of the hippocampus associated with PTSD |
| Parahippocampus | Important for memory encoding and retrieval | Shows stronger connectivity with medial PFC; decreased volume |
| Anterior cingulate gyrus | Autonomic functions, cognition | Decreased volume; higher resting metabolic activity |
| Thalamus | Sensory relay station | Decreased cerebral blood flow |
| Sensorimotor cortex | Coordination of sensory and motor functions | Symptom provocation results in increased activation |
| Orbitofrontal cortex | Executive function | Decreased volume |

Mahan and Ressler [17], Shin et al. [87], Hill et al. [75], Shin et al. [88], Pitman et al. [84]

**Prefrontal Cortex**

In PTSD, the medial PFC is smaller in volume and hyporesponsive during symptomatic states and during the performance of emotional cognitive tasks, and responsivity is inversely associated with PTSD severity [88]. Two subregions of the PFC are involved: the vmPFC and dorsal anterior cingulate cortex (dACC). The dACC appears *hyper*active in PTSD, while most (but not all) studies have shown the vmPFC to be *hypo*active in PTSD [63]. A promising finding, however, is that the hypoactivity of the PFC appears amenable to therapy: in an Australian study of civilian trauma victims, exposure-based therapy was associated with an increase in PFC activity and a decrease in amygdala activity [89].

**Amygdala**

The amygdala plays a key role in detecting threats as well as fear learning, fear expression, and heightening memory for emotional events [84]. In PTSD, there appears to be:

- Amygdala hyperfunction which is related to hypoactivity of the vmPFC
- Impaired inhibition of the amygdala by the PFC during extinction learning [75, 87]

The coupling of the amygdala and vmPFC, both structurally and functionally, is important for regulation of emotions, and impairment of this coupling is found in PTSD and anxiety [75, 90].

Human functional MRI studies indicate the amygdala plays an important role in acquisition and extinction of conditioned fear, with greater amygdala activation during acquisition of conditioned fear [84]. The vmPFC (subgenual anterior cingulate) plays a key role in retention of extinction learning [67]. Amygdala hyperfunction has been found in patients with PTSD [88], demonstrating exaggerated activity of the amygdala in response to trauma-related stimuli and generic stimuli compared to healthy controls [91, 92]. In a study of war veterans with PTSD, combat control subjects, and healthy normal controls, exposure to combat sounds led to activation for all groups in the anterior cingulate/middle prefrontal gyrus, but activation in the left amygdala/nucleus accumbens only occurred in the PTSD patients [92]. Other neuroimaging studies have demonstrated increased amygdala responsivity in PTSD patients during symptomatic states and processing of trauma-unrelated affective information, with responsivity positively associated with symptom severity [84, 88].

One of the neurobiological mechanisms underlying PTSD is impaired inhibition of the amygdala by the PFC during *extinction learning* [8]. MRI studies in PTSD sufferers have shown greater amygdala activation (fear center) in a PTSD group during extinction learning. During extinction recall, in the PTSD group, there was lesser activation in the hippocampus (memory center) and vmPFC, and greater activation in the dACC, supporting the idea that fear extinction is impaired in PTSD and that dysfunctional activation in various brain structures that mediate fear extinction and fear extinction recall underlie the impairment of fear extinction [63].

**Hippocampus**

Evidence points to smaller volumes and decreased neuronal and functional integrity of the hippocampus in PTSD [88]. Several studies have found smaller volumes in the hippocampus of veterans [93, 94], adult survivors of childhood abuse with PTSD [95], traumatized police officers [96] and women with a history of sexual abuse [97], with reductions in hippocampal volume ranging between 5% and 26% [94]. This suggests that structural changes in the hippocampus may be evidence of neuroanatomical changes associated with PTSD [98]. Other studies indicate that hippocampus activity is lower in PTSD sufferers than healthy normal people during extinction recall [63].

Not all studies in female survivors of domestic abuse with PTSD have shown such changes though. One study did not find smaller hippocampi; however, it did find lower volumes in the supratentorial cranial vaults, and lower frontal and occipital gray matter volumes compared with controls. The supratentorial cranial vault volume was inversely correlated with severity of childhood physical abuse but not with PTSD severity or intimate partner violence. The cerebral abnormalities were thought to be possibly reflective of the influence of early trauma on neurodevelopment or, alternatively, could reflect risk for psychosocial adversity [98].

There is a "chicken-and-egg" argument in the literature as to whether the smaller hippocampal volume is a risk factor for PTSD or a result of PTSD [84]. A study of identical twins discordant for combat exposure found that the combat-unexposed non-PTSD twin had hippocampal volumes that were similar to their co-twins with PTSD and these were lower than combat veterans without PTSD or their combat-unexposed co-twins, suggesting that smaller hippocampal volume may be a risk factor (pre-trauma) for later development of PTSD [99].

For a very deep dive into the neuroanatomical changes, see Pitman et al. [84].

**Locus Coeruleus**

Postmortem evidence also suggests there are noradrenergic abnormalities in the form of decreased cell numbers in the locus coeruleus (an area in the pons of the brainstem) associated with PTSD [100].

**A New Player on the Block: The Zona Incerta**

An area of the brain named the zona incerta (translation "unknown zone") is a small region located below the thalamus and above the brainstem and is hard to distinguish from surrounding brain regions. It contains many different types of neurons (including a group of dopamine-producing cells which may be relevant to Parkinson's disease, as an aside). This region is understood to be involved in learning, memory, and cognition, and recent research suggests it may play a critical role in how we learn to control fear, as it appears to be involved in how we learn to put stressful memories aside [81]. It receives input from the amygdala (where emotional memories such as fear are formed), and projects to areas involved in expression of fear including the periaqueductal gray region (in the midbrain), which suggests that the zona incerta might be involved in modulating whether a fear memory is expressed and causes a physical stress response, or whether it is inhibited or controlled. A study in mice using chemogenetics to control neurons in the zona incerta investigated how mice learned to suppress a fear that is no longer real. They found that by activating certain neurons, it was easier for the mice to suppress a learned fear and relearn and remember that the prior threat is now safe [81]. Research from this group at the University of Melbourne and the Florey Institute of Neuroscience and Mental Health will be one to watch.

## Dysregulation of the Stress Response, HPA-Axis Dysfunction, and Inflammation

The hypothalamic–pituitary–adrenal (HPA) axis and the sympathetic nervous system (SNS) are responsible for our response and adaptation to stress [101]. A dysregulation of neurotransmitters occurs in PTSD, resulting in failure of the stress response system to react, adapt, and recover from a situation. In addition to increased norepinephrine and increased corticotropin-releasing hormone, decreased serotonin and increased glutamate can also contribute to physical, mental, and emotional symptoms associated with PTSD [75, 102]. Hyperactivity of noradrenaline is known to contribute to the hyperarousal symptoms associated with the disorder [65, 84]. Animal and clinical studies implicate Neuropeptide Y (NPY) in the pathophysiology of PTSD. NPY a widely distributed neuropeptide in the brain, and is involved in many physiological functions. It is a stress regulatory transmitter of relevance to PTSD, being abundant in the forebrain limbic and brainstem areas that regulate stress and emotional behaviors [101]. Animals studies demonstrate that NPY plays roles in autonomic regulation, stress responses, fear and anxiety, whilst genetic studies suggest NPY polymorphisms are associated with stress coping. Studies have also found lower concentrations of NPY in cerebrospinal fluid of combat veterans with PTSD [101]. NPY is also involved in pain, depression, addiction, and metabolism, all of relevance to PTSD comorbidities [101]. There is evidence that NPY regulates the HPA axis and the sympathetic nervous system (SNS) [101].

PTSD symptoms are maintained by a combination of a dysregulated stress response and maladaptive memory processes due to the stress caused by a traumatic event [65]. During the trauma, excessive amounts of stress hormones including cortisol and noradrenaline are released, and this assigns emotional connection or importance to the traumatic event. Subsequently, this leads to an *over-consolidation of the trauma* and the context/environment in which it occurred, as emotional experiences are preferentially consolidated into long-term memory. However, as Ney et al. [65] explain, in PTSD this process is distorted and occurs at an extreme level, potentially due, at least in part, to the excessive hormones [84]. Over-consolidated trauma memories are poorly contextualized and fractured, and then return as intrusive memories, continuing to haunt the PTSD sufferer [65, 71, 84, 103].

For a good overview of the biological responses in PTSD, readers are referred to Ney et al. [65] and Pitman et al. [84].

### Sympathetic Nervous System Reactivity

The autonomic stress response (detailed in Chap. 3) has been shown to be altered in PTSD with associations between increased sympathetic nervous system (SNS) reactivity and increased trauma-associated arousal demonstrated, so much so that this association serves as part of the diagnostic criteria for PTSD [104]. Increased heart rate and blood pressure responses and greater decreases in heart rate variability (HRV) have been found in PTSD sufferers compared to healthy controls in response to exposure to various trauma stimuli in several studies [104–106].

### HPA-Axis Dysregulation

There is much evidence that the HPA axis is dysregulated in PTSD. During trauma, there is a cortisol surge followed by an HPA-axis dysfunction. Over time, this leads to a decreased baseline cortisol level, an increase in the negative feedback, and resultant hyperarousal and hypervigilance [21]. Chronic noradrenergic hyperactivity found in PTSD patients is also thought to contribute to the hyperarousal symptoms of PTSD [65]. There is evidence that Neuropeptide Y (mentioned previously) is involved in regulation of the HPA Axis. The NPY acts directly on the HPA axis, and also acts like a 'physiological brake' to counteract and regulate stress transmitters like norepinephrine (NE) and corticotropin releasing hormone (CRH), relevant to PTSD [101].

#### PTSD, Reduced Cortisol Levels, and Reduced Cortisol Reactivity to Stress

Studies have demonstrated that a significant percentage of PTSD sufferers have chronically depressed cortisol levels due to the negative feedback of the HPA axis [65, 107] and that decreased levels of cortisol are associated with greater risk of PTSD non-remission [53]. Thus, cortisol provides a predictive biomarker for PTSD [53].

A study in female survivors of domestic violence found that those with PTSD, regardless of whether there was comorbid depression or not, had significantly lower baseline cortisol levels at 9.00 am compared with healthy subjects or trauma survivors without PTSD. Women with PTSD demonstrated significantly greater cortisol suppression to dexamethasone challenge (this being used to assess HPA-axis functioning) compared with healthy subjects or those with PTSD plus depression, leading to the conclusion that HPA axis is severely dysregulated in PTSD [107]. However, while other studies of PTSD sufferers have also found lower 24-h urinary cortisol excretion, some have found higher cortisol excretion, and this could reflect the nature of the trauma, comorbidities, and gender [107]. Survivors of domestic violence tend to have repeated traumas which may be different to someone suffering a one-off traumatic event, for example.

PTSD sufferers have decreased cortisol reactivity to stress [107] which is problematic as cortisol reactivity is critical for fear extinction learning [86]. Evidence points to a possible association between alterations in glucocorticoid receptor sensitivity to cortisol and PTSD, with greater receptor sensitivity resulting in enhanced negative feedback and therefore reduced levels of circulating cortisol [108].

It is not known definitively if reduced glucocorticoids are a cause or effect of PTSD or whether they are reflective of early adverse experiences impacting HPA-axis function [75, 109]. Altered cortisol levels may reflect changes in regulatory components of the HPA axis, including FKBP5 which is a "chaperone protein" for the glucocorticoid receptor; polymorphisms of FKBP5 have been found to be associated with risk of PTSD [75, 110].

The primary malfunction may circle back to the ECS in that CB1 receptors and corticotropin-releasing factor (CRF)-containing afferents have been found co-located in the (noradrenergic) nucleus locus coeruleus (LC) (in both the core and peri-LC areas). CRF is critically involved in mediation of the stress-induced activation of noradrenergic neurons in the nucleus LC. The nucleus LC appears to be the stress switchboard of the brain linking pro-stress and anti-stress circuitry from the amygdala, PFC, stria terminalis, and the paraventricular nucleus of the hypothalamus. This includes CB1 receptors, CRF, and GABA synapses. The initial cortisol surge stimulates endocannabinoid production then activating CB1 receptors on presynaptic glutamatergic neurons in the paraventricular nucleus (PVN), thereby decreasing CRF release from the hypothalamus. However, chronic CB1 receptor activation might cause a disinhibition of GABAergic neurons in the bed nucleus of the stria terminalis (BNST). The stria terminalis then loops back to the PVN, ultimately sustaining a decreased CRF [111].

## Synaptic Plasticity in PTSD

Both animal models of PTSD and neuroimaging studies in humans support the proposition that dysregulated synaptic plasticity may underlie PTSD. Synaptic plasticity refers to changes occurring at a synapse with prolonged synaptic activity, and such changes can be morphological, functional/physiological, and molecular [17].

Research demonstrates that the BDNF-tyrosine kinase B (TrkB) pathway underlies synaptic plasticity and this has been implicated in PTSD. BDNF-TrkB signaling is required for different aspects of fear conditioning and extinction in the amygdala, the hippocampus, and the PFC. For example, BDNF signaling in the amygdala plays a key role in synaptic plasticity events involved in consolidation and persistence of fear memories, as well as being involved in different subregions of the PFC in retention and extinction of learned fear [17]. BDNF may mediate neural plasticity in two regions of the PFC with opposite effects—BDNF in the prelimbic region is required for fear memory formation and expression, and BDNF in the infralimbic region is needed for the inhibition/extinction of that fear. Experiments in mice where BDNF was removed from the hippocampus showed a marked decrease in extinction of conditioned fear (though no impairment of acquisition of fear conditioning) which indicates normal hippocampal plasticity is needed for context-dependent extinction of conditioned fear. Thus, it seems that BNDF signaling is important in regulation of fear and emotion and could be a therapeutic target for enhancing extinction in PTSD [17].

How the endocannabinoid system and indeed medicinal cannabis may potentially modify BDNF signaling and synaptic plasticity bears consideration.

## Dysregulation of Neurotransmitters in PTSD: GABA and Glutamate

Mahan and Ressler [17] describe the various actions of GABA and glutamate. GABAergic inhibitory microcircuits, in particular in the amygdala, appear to be involved in the regulation of acquisition, consolidation, expression, and extinction of fear conditioning. Various experiments have demonstrated that GABAergic inactivation of the amygdala, PFC, and parts of the striatum impairs aspects of conditioned fear, and inactivation of the infralimbic cortex, BLA, and ventral hippocampus impairs fear extinction. Fear conditioning causes a reduction in GABAergic signaling in the BLA, and experiments in which the a1 subunit of the GABAA receptor has been deleted resulted in enhanced auditory fear learning. In the amygdala, it was originally thought that the BLA was involved in associative learning and the central nucleus of the amygdala (CEA) involved in controlling expression of fear, but it is now known that the CEA plays a role in fear acquisition too, with two distinct inhibitory GABAergic microcircuits in the CEA.

GABAergic signaling tightly controls fear conditioning and extinction, and glutamate signaling also plays a role. Research in rats shows that glutamatergic cells in the BLA are activated after fear conditioning. Glutaminergic input to the BLA comes from the PFC, hippocampus, and sensory thalamic and cortical regions, and the BLA itself sends glutamatergic signals to the central nucleus of the amygdala (CEA) which is involved in regulating inhibitory GABAergic microcircuits. Glutamate acts on many ionotropic (e.g., NMDA, AMPA) and metabotropic receptors (mGlu 1–8) which are involved in fear conditioning. The ionotropic glutamate receptors mediate synaptic plasticity in long-term fear memories. Fear conditioning activates NMDA receptors which contribute to synaptic plasticity in the amygdala via various mechanisms. The mGlu receptors mediate synaptic plasticity in the brain via G-protein signal transduction and are important for consolidation of fear conditioning and extinction. Activation of mGlu receptor 1-containing receptors in the BLA enhances fear learning, while mGlu receptor antagonists impair consolidation and extinction of fear conditioning [17].

## Other Receptor-Ligand Systems Involved in PTSD

It is thought that many receptor-ligand systems are involved in modulation of fear conditioning, and these probably contribute to PTSD by modulating GABAergic and glutamatergic signaling. These include the endocannabinoid system (ECS), dopaminergic projections to the amygdala from the nucleus accumbens and ventral tegmental area, norepinephrine signaling (from the locus coeruleus), acetylcholine

(Ach), and nitric oxide synthase (NOS)-cGMP which all play roles in modulating synaptic plasticity and in consolidation and extinction of fear conditioning [17].

Mahan and Ressler conclude that the hope is that drugs may be able to be developed which can modulate such signaling pathways involved in fear conditioning and synaptic plasticity in the amygdala which could enhance extinction of inappropriate fear associations or perhaps even prevent development of these in the first place [17]. Given the role of the ECS as a retrograde neuromodulatory system, there seems potential for exploration of how medicinal cannabis and key phytocannabinoids might be able to impact on synaptic plasticity.

## Association Between PTSD and Inflammation

There is significant evidence in the literature that PTSD is associated with proinflammatory activation of the immune system. Veterans with PTSD suffer from diseases such as autoimmune diseases, cardiovascular diseases, dementia, and inflammation that may contribute to accelerated aging [25]. When the etiology and pathogenesis of such diseases are considered, they all involve inflammation in some way. Interesting, in his book *Lifespan* David Sinclair has described aging itself as a disease [112].

Several cross-sectional studies provide evidence that inflammation is involved in PTSD, set out well in Neylan and O'Donovan's review paper [25]. For example:

- A meta-analysis of 20 studies found that key inflammatory markers were raised and duration and severity of PTSD was positively associated with 1β-levels ($p < 0.001$) and IL-6 levels, respectively [113].
- A case-control study demonstrated a generalized proinflammatory pattern [114].
- A study in veterans found that increased inflammation was associated with current PTSD but not PTSD in remission [115].

However, the "chicken-and-egg" question arises here too: are inflammatory factors predisposing risk factors and therefore involved in the etiology of PTSD or are they are a result of PTSD or both? A study in nurses suggests that increased inflammation may be both a preexisting risk factor and effect of PTSD [25].

### Inflammation as Both a Pre-existing Risk Factor and a Result of PTSD

Nurses are another group of healthcare-workers who can suffer from PTSD [116]. Prevalence of PTSD in nurses was found to be 18% in a US study [117], but it was even greater in emergency department nurses (up to 82.96%) [118]. The Nurses' Health Study II found women with PTSD have elevated inflammatory markers including C-Reactive Protein (CRP), Intercellular Adhesion Molecule 1 (ICAM-1) and Soluble Tumor Necrosis Factor Receptor II (sTNF-RII) [119, 120]. A key finding was that women with new onset PTSD had increased levels of sTNF-RII and ICAM-1 *prior to trauma exposure* and development of PTSD [119] and also had greater increases in VCAM-1 between baseline and follow-up over 10–16 years

[120]. This suggests that increased inflammation may be *both a pre-existing risk factor and a consequence of PTSD* [25].

ICAM-1 and VCAM-1 play major roles maintaining intercellular barriers (tight junctions), but they also serve to bind leukocytes to endothelial cells and facilitate their transmigration into tissues. ICAM-1 is activated by the cytokines IL-1 and TNF-α [121]. Raised ICAM-1 is associated with several inflammatory and immune responses, including epithelial tumorigenesis in breast cancer [122], and raised levels of VCAM-1 and ICAM-1 have been found to be associated with several diseases including atherosclerotic cardiovascular disease and renal disease [123]. On the other hand, activation of the endocannabinoid system may downregulate ICAM-1 and associated pathology by reducing inflammatory cell attachment and migration [124].

### Relationship Between IL-6 and Noradrenergic Activity in PTSD

Since it is known that IL-6 secretion is suppressed by glucocorticoids and stimulated by catecholamines, and PTSD sufferers have decreased cortisol and increased catecholamine secretion, a small study was conducted in PTSD sufferers to investigate the relationship between interleukin-6 (IL-6) levels and HPA-axis and noradrenergic activity. Cerebrospinal fluid (CSF) was removed and blood taken from 11 combat veterans suffering PTSD and 8 age- and sex-matched healthy controls. Mean and median IL-6 concentrations in CSF were higher in PTSD patients than controls (mean 24.0 vs 14.6, $p = 0.05$ and median 26.7 vs 14.3, $p < 0.03$, respectively), but plasma IL-6 levels were no different between groups. Plasma IL-6 and norepinephrine were positively correlated in the PTSD group but not in the healthy controls [125].

## Genetic (and Epigenetic) Factors

It appears that genetic variations in certain genes may play a part in risk of PTSD development [126]. We have previously met brain-derived neurotrophic factor (BDNF) in the previous chapter. A common single-nucleotide polymorphism (SNP) in the human *BDNF* gene results in a Val66Met substitution in the BDNF prodomain region. This SNP is associated with alterations in memory and with enhanced risk to develop depression and anxiety disorders in humans [127]. Met/Met carriers show increased medial temporal lobe activation during episodic and encoding retrieval tasks and greater activity in the amygdala and PFC during memory formation and retrieval, as well as impaired extinction learning (correlated to altered activation of the amygdala, PFC, and hippocampus [17]).

Variations in the gene coding for serotonin transporter (SERT, which is involved in serotonin transport and reuptake) including both long and short alleles have been found to be associated with increased PTSD risk. However, it appears that the environment modifies this risk effect, with the short allele associated with decreased risk in a low-risk environment but increased risk in a high-risk environment [17].

In addition, polymorphisms in the FK506-binding protein, a glucocorticoid chaperone protein, may contribute to increased sensitivity of the amygdala/HPA-axis response to stress. Neuropsin, a serine protease, is vital for stress-related plasticity in the amygdala via regulation of EphB2-NDMA-receptor activation of FKBP5 expression [17].

Gene-specific methylation patterns may also potentially be associated with increased risk for as well as resilience to PTSD [128, 129]. Research provides some evidence to suggest that an external traumatic event can induce downstream changes in immune function by reducing methylation levels of immune-related genes, suggesting a biological model of etiology of PTSD [18].

## The Endocannabinoid System and PTSD

The endocannabinoid system (ECS) is involved in regulation of stress, emotions, memory, and inflammation, and thus it stands to reason that the ECS may be altered in PTSD [130]. Indeed, we know that the ECS plays an important role in the control of emotions, and its dysregulation has been implicated in several psychiatric disorders including anxiety and depression, as well as PTSD. When we consider PTSD, it is important to remember that it is a form of extreme, dysregulated anxiety, and depression is often comorbid with PTSD. Thus, what we learned in relation to anxiety and depression in previous chapters is also relevant in PTSD.

In addition to a key role maintaining emotional homeostasis [131, 132], the ECS plays an important role in regulating memory [10, 133–135]. CB1 receptors and endocannabinoids are found in memory-related brain areas and are involved in the modulation of memory [134, 135]. In particular, the ECS may modulate the consolidation, retrieval, and extinction of durable memory traces [10, 133], and as we saw previously, these memory processes are relevant to PTSD, a disorder of memory.

Studies of the ECS support its importance for many aspects of brain function including the following, all of which are relevant to PTSD symptomatology: modulation of the stress response and the HPA axis (stress response); regulation of mood, anxiety, and reward; and regulation of memory and extinction of fear learning [10, 65, 136]. The ECS plays a protective role under adverse conditions: increased endocannabinoid signaling which occurs during stress dampens development of anxiety and regulates encoding, retrieval, and extinction of traumatic memories [9]. Increasingly the literature demonstrates that there are alterations in ECS in patients with PTSD [9, 56, 137–140].

Activation of CB1 receptors in the amygdala can decrease anxiety, fear, and aversive memories, while activation of CB1 receptors in the PFC can increase serotonin (one of our "happy hormones") and reduce depression. Increased neurogenesis, mood and memory plus decreased hypervigilance, hyperarousal and intrusive memories, and cortisol normalization occur when CB1 receptors are agonized in the hippocampus. Meanwhile, stimulation of the limbic and paralimbic regions can result in amygdala and hypothalamus activity which may help regulate the HPA axis and cortisol, thereby reducing hypervigilance and hyperarousal [21].

## The Endocannabinoid System Modulation of Stress Response

As we saw in Chap. 3, the ECS is involved in regulation of stress, both acute and chronic. Hillard argues that chronic variable stress reduces CB1 signaling and the resultant deficiency in endocannabinoid signaling may contribute to associated negative health outcomes, but on the other hand, repeated exposure to the same stress can actually sensitize CB1 receptor signaling which can lead to a dampening of the stress response [141].

It has been argued that in PTSD, the stress response is maladaptive and, consequently, its symptoms including hyperarousal, poor sleep, and intrusive memories are facilitated by decreased endocannabinoid signaling [75]. AEA levels normally gate the stress response in a tonic manner via the HPA axis. Following acute stress, FAAH is activated and AEA levels rapidly decrease (remember FAAH hydrolyzes AEA), and the HPA-axis response is triggered. There is then an increase in glucocorticoids which mobilizes 2-AG, and this mediates a negative feedback loop, ending the stress response [65]. Disruption of endocannabinoid/CB1 signaling activates the HPA axis [142, 143].

Hillard argues that CB1 receptor signaling is stress responsive and that maintaining a healthy endocannabinoid/CB1 receptor signaling facilitates resilience against development of stress-related disorders [141]. Concentration of endocannabinoids and related N-acyl-ethanolamides (NAEs) in blood is higher in individuals who are more tolerant to stress, and lower in patients with depression [9, 144, 145]. Thus, nutritional approaches such as ensuring plenty of healthy omega-3 polyunsaturated fatty acids to support optimal functioning of the ECS, as well as a healthy diet that avoids proinflammatory foods including excessive amounts of omega-6 and omega-9 polyunsaturated fats, will be important.

Many preclinical and clinical studies support the role of the ECS in the modulation of the stress response, and the ECS has been suggested as a possible therapeutic target to treat the severe stress associated with PTSD as well as the associated emotional and cognitive dysfunctions [146]. For this reason, the ECS may be a potential therapeutic target which may address several elements involved in PTSD, namely, stress, anxiety, and memory [10].

### Chronic Mild Stress Alters Endocannabinoid-Mediated Neurotransmission

Chronic mild stress (CMS) is often used as an animal model of depression and leads to downregulation of CB1 receptors in male rat hippocampi [147]. In addition, it appears to sensitize CB1 function on GABAergic terminals and indirectly results in increased excitatory neurotransmission, rather than directly affecting glutaminergic neurotransmission [148], as described below.

CMS may not directly affect glutaminergic transmission but may sensitize CB1 function on GABAergic terminals, resulting in less inhibition and therefore increased excitatory neurotransmission [148]. A rat study was conducted to investigate how stress-induced change in CB1 receptors might affect endocannabinoid-mediated neurotransmission and found that CMS alters hippocampal endocannabinoid-mediated neurotransmission and synaptic plasticity. Rats were exposed to CMS for 21 days, and in vitro field potential recordings were used to measure the effects of CMS on endocannabinoid-modulated glutaminergic neurotransmission in the hippocampal CA1 region of the rat brain. Application of a CB1 agonist (WIN55,212-5) in rats exposed to CMS resulted in a 135% increase in excitatory (glutaminergic) neurotransmission, while CB1 activation in non-stressed rats leads to a 30% decrease in glutaminergic neurotransmission. Blockade of GABA transmission (GABA is an inhibitory neurotransmitter) was associated with a 35% decrease in glutaminergic neurotransmission in rats exposed to CMS [148].

## CB1 Signaling and the Amygdala Involved in Short- and Long-Term Fear Extinction

The ECS plays a key role in extinction of aversive memories (fear extinction), a process believed to be an active mnemonic process [135]. We gain information about the effects of CB1 receptor signaling in PTSD from animal experiments.

In one study, CB1-deficient (knockout) mice demonstrated impaired short- and long-term extinction in auditory fear-conditioning tests, but memory acquisition and consolidation were not affected. When normal (wild-type) mice were treated with a CB1 receptor antagonist, their behavior was similar to that of the CB1-deficient mice. The mice were trained to associate a tone with a foot shock (conditioning) and consequently froze when re-exposed to the tone; the response was an indicator of aversive memory, which is gradually reduced and eliminated on repeated tone exposures. This process is highly dependent on the amygdala and allows the different phases of memory formation to be examined (i.e., acquisition, consolidation, extinction). The study found that *acquisition* and *early consolidation* processes of memory did not involve CB1 receptors, and the endocannabinoids were found to have little role in memory acquisition, consolidation, and recall; however, they were found to selectively interfere with *extinction* of the freezing response to the tone. Tone presentation during extinction trials caused elevated levels of AEA and 2-AG in the basolateral amygdala complex (which controls extinction of aversive memories). In this brain region, endocannabinoids and CB1 receptors were involved in long-term depression of GABA-mediated inhibitory currents, leading the study authors to propose that endocannabinoids facilitate aversive memory extinction through inhibitory effects on local inhibitory (GABA) networks within the amygdala [135].

Other studies have also suggested that there may be unique pathways involved in fear extinction that are not involved in acquisition or consolidation of fear memories [135].

## CB1 Receptor mRNA Downregulation in Amygdaloid Complex and Frontal Cortex in PTSD

A rat study was conducted to investigate whether long-lasting behavioral effects of exposure to a predator (dummy or live cat, a traumatic event for a rat) were associated with changes in CB1 receptor and synaptophysin (SYP, a protein related to synaptic function which is used to indirectly evaluate the number of synapses and synaptic plastic change) in those areas of the brain related to PTSD (i.e., frontal cortex, hippocampus, amygdaloid complex). Single exposure to the predator produced long-lasting anxiogenic effects, and 7 days after exposure, CB1 mRNA expression was found to be downregulated in the frontal cortex and amygdaloid complex but not in the dorsal hippocampus. The study authors posited that since CB1 receptors modulate glutaminergic neurotransmission in the frontal cortex, downregulation may facilitate anxiety-like responses by increasing glutamate release in limbic areas like the amygdaloid complex [142]. Thus, the long-lasting anxiogenic effects appeared to be associated with hyperactivation of the amygdaloid complex and modulation of CB1 receptors in brain areas known to be related to PTSD.

What was also interesting in this study is that SYP was upregulated in the amygdaloid complex. Synaptic vesicle proteins are thought to be potentially involved in depression and schizophrenia pathophysiology, and there is evidence that PTSD is related to plastic changes also [142].

## Levels of Endocannabinoids Altered in PTSD

Hill and colleagues [75] suggest that a state of endocannabinoid deficiency or ECS tone may represent a stress susceptibility endophenotype which predisposes an individual to development of conditions like PTSD. Levels of endocannabinoids and related N-acyl-ethanolamides have been found to be significantly altered in PTSD suggesting involvement in its pathogenesis [9, 65, 130, 137]. However, the direction and nature of changes to the ECS as a result of chronic stress and trauma appears inconsistent. Some human studies have found decreased levels of endocannabinoids which might support the notion of an endocannabinoid deficiency, while others have found increased levels of endocannabinoids (described shortly). This may relate to when the traumatic event occurred.

### Age When Traumatic Event Occurred Affects ECS Changes

When a trauma occurs, it has an effect on the ECS changes. The effects of prolonged stress or trauma depend on the development age of the individual when they experience the traumatic event(s), its repetitiveness, and accumulative effects [149]. Animal models of childhood trauma suggest that if trauma occurs in childhood, it results in increased levels of endocannabinoids and decreased levels of CB1 receptors in childhood, decreased levels of endocannabinoids and increased levels of

CB1 receptors in adolescence, and, in adulthood, increased levels of endocannabinoids and decreased CB1 receptor levels [149].

A study in humans with a history of childhood trauma found increased levels of endocannabinoids, and another study in those with bipolar disease and PTSD with a history of childhood trauma found increased levels of AEA and 2-AG in those with bipolar disease and increased OEA levels in those with PTSD with a history of childhood trauma. There is thus evidence that suggests increased endocannabinoid and decreased CB1 receptor levels in adults with a history of childhood trauma and PTSD [149].

On the other hand, when a severe trauma occurs in adulthood, preclinical and clinical research supports the notion that it is associated with decreased levels of endocannabinoids and increased CB1 receptors [149].

This suggests that in PTSD research design, it is important to factor in when a traumatic event occurred into statistical modeling, as this could be a factor that could modify results, i.e., if you had a PTSD study population in which some had a trauma in childhood and others in adulthood, this could quite easily muddy the waters in making conclusions of data. Likewise, even if examining a cohort such as veterans who have been exposed to trauma in the line of duty as adults, it would also be prudent to factor in any potential childhood exposure to traumatic events as this could confound findings.

### Evidence of Altered Endocannabinoid Levels in Animal Models of PTSD

There are several animal models which have been used, typically on rats or mice, to probe aspects relevant to PTSD. These models include the chronic unpredictable stress model, single prolonged stress model, shock and reminder stress model, and the predator stress model. Results of several studies provide support that an ECS dysregulation is involved in PTSD pathogenesis, with several indicating reduced AEA levels, increased 2-AG levels, and CB1 downregulation in particular brain regions. Results of some of the experiments using such models are set out in Table 7.3.

Treatment of animals with FAAH inhibitors provides indirect evidence that reduced levels of endocannabinoids are associated with PTSD. Increased treatment raises levels of AEA, reduces PTSD symptoms, and promotes fear extinction [146, 157–160].

### Evidence of Altered Endocannabinoid Levels from Human Research

Studies indicate significant differences in plasma concentrations of endocannabinoids and related *N*-acyl-ethanolamides in PTSD sufferers compared with healthy controls and subjects who did not develop PTSD after trauma exposure [9]. The results are not always consistent with findings from animal studies or indeed other human studies, however. For example, survivors of the 9/11 World Trade Center attack in the USA who met the diagnostic criteria for PTSD had lower levels of circulating 2-AG though there was no significant difference between groups (i.e. those who met the criteria for PTSD compared with those who didn't) in AEA

**Table 7.3** Animal models of PTSD: effects of PTSD on ECS

| Model | Features | Results of studies demonstrated |
|---|---|---|
| *Chronic unpredictable stress (CUS) model* | Uses mild, unpredictable, and repetitive stressors to investigate the effects on the ECS [150] | Downregulation and deficiency of endocannabinoid/CB1-mediated responses in the nucleus accumbens [151]<br>Significantly decreased levels of AEA in several brain areas as well as reduced CB1 receptor binding density in the hippocampus, hypothalamus, and ventral striatum and increased CB1 receptor binding density in the prefrontal cortex [152]<br>CUS induces cognitive impairments in extinction and perservatory behavior (but does not affect acquisition of learning), and it also enhances hippocampal-dependent episodic fear memories, thereby increasing susceptibility to PTSD [150]. These conditions improve with CB1 receptor agonists: supports notion that PTSD is underpinned by ECS deficiency [147, 150] |
| *Single prolonged stress* | This model leads to enhanced conditioned avoidance, impaired extinction and increased acoustic startle response (ASR), negative feedback on HPA axis, and anxiety [146] | Lower levels of AEA in various brain regions including basolateral amygdala (BLA) and CA1 region [146] and nucleus accumbens [136] and decreased serum 2-AG (though no change in the BLA or CA1) [146]<br>CB1/CB2 receptor agonist WIN55,212-2 injected either systemically or into BLA at different time points: results suggest there may be an optimal time window for intervention treatment with cannabinoids following a traumatic event [153] |
| *Shock and reminder stress model* | Rats are exposed to a foot shock followed by exposure to situational reminders—this leads to long-term impairment of extinction and increased "startle response," and has also been shown to induce long-term impairment of fear extinction [154] | FAAH inhibitor URG597 was injected for 3 weeks in a group of rats exposed to the shock and reminders paradigm. Rats chronically treated with the FAAH inhibitor showed normalized startle response and normal extinction reactions; effect of the FAAH inhibitor was CB1 receptor dependent (effects were blocked by a CB1 receptor antagonist). URB597 normalized the shock/reminder-induced upregulation of CB1 receptors in the basolateral amygdala and CA1 region [154] |

(continued)

**Table 7.3** (continued)

| Model | Features | Results of studies demonstrated |
|---|---|---|
| *Life-threatening trauma model (predator stress model)* | One model: exposes to a chemical called 2,5-dihydro-2,4,5-trimethylthiazoline (TMT), a pheromone constituent of fox feces; produces anxiety-like behaviors and has been used as a model of post-traumatic long-term anxiety state [155] | Rats demonstrated increased levels of 2-AG in the amygdala following exposure to TMT. Administration of a FAAH inhibitor (URB597) increased brain AEA levels and prevented development of CB1-dependent post-traumatic anxiety-like behaviors [155]<br>Rats exposed to TMT exhibited a marked increase in 2-AG mobilization in the amygdala of traumatized rats with anxiety-like behaviors, which lasted at least 14 days after the stressful event. Systemic or local pharmacological inhibition of MAGL suppressed the anxiety-like behavior caused by exposure to TMT. The results suggest that a life-threatening trauma, in this case the threat of being eaten by a fox, triggers long-term changes in 2-AG-mediated cannabinoid signaling in the amygdala and may indicate a potential therapeutic target for treatment of trauma-initiated conditions [156] |

and cortisol levels [137]. AEA levels exhibited a negative relationship with the degree of intrusive symptoms, consistent with animal studies demonstrating that decreased AEA promotes retention of aversive memories. Given the role of 2-AG in regulation of the stress response, their findings support the contention that deficient endocannabinoid signaling may be part of the glucocorticoid dysregulation occurring in PTSD [137]. However, the findings here on cortisol do not accord with other studies which have found PTSD associated with chronic low levels of cortisol [53, 65, 161, 162].

A study used positron-emission tomography (PET) to investigate CB1 receptor availability in individuals with PTSD compared with those with lifetime histories of trauma (trauma controls [TC]) and healthy controls without such histories. They found that AEA levels were lower in the PTSD group compared with the TC group (53.1% lower) and HC group (58.2% lower). In addition, cortisol levels were lower in the PTSD group and TC group compared with the healthy controls [139].

Conversely, in another study of 10 patients with PTSD, 9 trauma-exposed individuals without evidence of PTSD ($n = 9$), and 29 healthy control subjects, PTSD was associated with significantly *higher* plasma levels of AEA, 2-AG, oleoylethanolamide (OEA), and stearoylethanolamine (SEA) and significantly lower levels of N-oleoyldopamine than healthy controls. Those with PTSD had significantly higher plasma levels of 2-AG and PEA than trauma-exposed individuals without PTSD [9]. This differs from other studies in which PTSD was associated with lower levels of endocannabinoids [137, 139] and PEA [130]. In the 19 individuals exposed to trauma (with and without PTSD), CAPS score positively correlated with plasma PEA levels ($r = 0.55$, $p = 0.02$) and negatively with plasma oleoyldopamine levels ($r = 20.68$, $p = 0.01$), and CAPS subscores for intrusions, avoidance, and hyperarousal were all negatively related to oleoyldopamine plasma concentrations. The individuals in this study had other comorbidities and heterogenicity in type and amount of trauma which might explain these seemingly contradictory results [9].

Wilker and colleagues [130] assessed concentrations of PEA, OEA, and SEA in hair samples of 38 rebel war survivors from Northern Uganda with PTSD and compared them with samples from 38 healthy rebel war survivors without current and lifetime PTSD. These three lesser studied endocannabinoids may provide an "entourage effect," themselves not acting on CB1 receptors but potentiating the effect of AEA [150]. PTSD sufferers had significantly lower levels of OEA, and there were strong negative associations between all three N-acyl-ethanolamides and severity of PTSD symptoms. They postulated the decreased levels might be responsible for the increased inflammatory state and failure to extinguish fear memories that are characteristic of PTSD [130].

In humans the variant FAAH 385A allele (which encodes a FAAH enzyme with decreased ability to hydrolyze AEA) was found to be dose-dependently associated with increased AEA levels and facilitated fear extinction and improved extinction recall. A-allele homozygotes were protected against stress-induced decreases in AEA and negative emotional consequences of stress, suggesting that AEA signaling can temper the stress response and inhibition of FAAH [160].

However, despite studies implicating lower AEA levels in PTSD (discussed earlier), research demonstrates mixed results of endocannabinoid effects on memory consolidation of traumatic events [56]. For example, researchers have speculated that the observed risk of PTSD linked to propofol use (anesthetic that inhibits FAAH) might be mediated by enhanced endocannabinoid transmission through *elevation* of AEA levels and thus by facilitation of traumatic memory consolidation [56]. In contrast with the research into memory consolidation, there is greater consensus in the areas of research of the effects of cannabinoids on memory retrieval, with most pointing to an impairing effect on (traumatic) memory retrieval of cannabinoid agonists [56].

## Levels of CB1 Receptors Altered in PTSD

CB1 receptors regulate the release of many neurotransmitters and are involved in plasticity within the CNS, including neurogenesis. It has been suggested that CB1 receptors may be involved in the modification of defensive behaviors and consolidation of aversive memories, and can modulate adaptation to stress (acute and chronic) via modulation of CB1-mediated neurotransmission, thereby disrupting the flow of synaptic information [142].

### Evidence of Altered CB1 Receptors in Animal Models of PTSD

CB1 receptors are critical in the process of extinguishing aversive memories [135]. This was demonstrated in a mice experiment in which CB1 receptors were blocked in previously fear-conditioned mice: this impaired short- and long-term extinction in fear-conditioning tests [135]. Animal experiments using various experimental fear and stress models indicate that CB1 receptors appear to be upregulated in the PFC [163, 164] and downregulated in the hippocampus [142, 165]. Chronic stress, involved in PTSD, has also been found to decrease CB1 receptor expression and binding within hippocampal areas [166]. See Table 7.3 for some studies.

#### Prefrontal Cortex CB1 Receptors: Upregulated

Several studies indicate the medial prefrontal cortex is an important site involved in stress responses, and research findings suggest that endocannabinoid-mediated neurotransmission in this brain area is involved [142]. Animal studies demonstrate that CB1 receptors are sensitive to stress, and animal models of a fear-conditioning paradigm have demonstrated upregulation of CB1 receptors in parts of the PFC [163, 164]. The ventral part of the medial prefrontal cortex appears involved in expression of contextual fear conditioning.

Male rats exposed to a contextual aversive conditioning session were re-exposed to this aversive context 48 h later. Their responses including freezing behavior and cardiovascular responses were measured. Intravenous administration of AEA or an AEA transport inhibitor prior to re-exposure to the aversive context attenuated the fear-condition responses, and this effect was blocked by a CB1 receptor antagonist. In a second experiment, CB1 receptor mRNA expression was found to be increased in the ventral portion of the medial prefrontal cortex 48 h after the conditioning session. Overall, the study concluded that facilitation of cannabinoid-mediated neurotransmission in the ventral portion of the medial PFC through activation of local CB1 receptors attenuates or decreases the expression of fear responses [164].

#### Hippocampal CB1 Receptors: Downregulated

In other animal experiments, chronic stress has also been associated with changes in hippocampal CB1 receptors [165, 167]. The CB1 receptor is normally abundant in the hippocampus, a neuroanatomical area of importance in depression [165, 168]. Here it is largely located on GABAergic interneurons [165].

Hippocampal CB1 receptors are understood to play an important role in maintenance of synaptic integrity and neuroplasticity in the hippocampus [169]. Chronic stress was found to downregulate CB1 expression and significantly decrease the amount of 2-AG in the hippocampus (but with no effect in the limbic forebrain), and this might contribute to problems in behavioral flexibility and contribute to development of ruminatory and perservatory behaviors that may be found in stress-related psychiatric disorders [142, 165]. In a study where rats were exposed to 21 days of restraint stress for 6 h, autoradiographical analysis was conducted to measure CB1 receptor binding site densities in specific regions of the hippocampus. Chronic stress was found to significantly reduce CB1 binding in the dentate gyrus while increasing it in the CA3 region of the hippocampus (with no effects found in CA1 or retrosplenial cortical gyrus and laterodorsal thalamus). The study authors suggested that stress-induced changes in CB1 receptor activity might contribute to stress-induced modulation of maintenance of synaptic integrity and neuroplasticity in the hippocampus (given the role of hippocampal CB1 receptors in these processes) [169].

### Evidence of Altered CB1 Receptor Levels from Human Research

PTSD patients demonstrate elevated brain CB1 receptor availability which may implicate deficient CB1 receptor-mediated AEA signaling in the etiology of PTSD [139]. Positron-emission tomography has demonstrated brain-wide increases in CB1 receptors in PTSD sufferers compared with healthy controls with a history of trauma and healthy (no trauma) controls without a history of trauma. AEA levels were reduced in the PTSD group compared with trauma-exposed group (53.1% lower) and healthy no-trauma group (58.2% lower), and cortisol levels were lower in the PTSD and trauma-exposed groups compared to the healthy controls. This is in accordance with other human studies which have found lower cortisol levels in association with PTSD [53, 161, 162].

This study also found a higher density of CB1 receptors under non-stress (basal) conditions in women compared with men. The authors postulate that this could potentially explain why there is a higher prevalence of PTSD in women than men. Three biomarkers assessed collectively AEA, cortisol, and CB1 receptor antagonist radiotracer [(11)C]OMAR (which measures the volume of distribution of CB1 receptors)—correctly classified almost 85% of PTSD cases. These results implicate abnormal CB1 receptor-mediated AEA signaling in PTSD etiology [139].

## Medicinal Cannabis and Cannabinoids for the Treatment of PTSD

There is potential for intervention in the processes of aversive memory formation that occur in PTSD. Bitencourt and Takahashi [57] suggest that intervention at the stage of aversive memory acquisition and consolidation is not very promising, as it would need to be implemented very soon after a traumatic event and at that point, it is not possible to know if PTSD will manifest or not. They believe that intervention in the retrieval, reconsolidation, and, in particular, the extinction processes is likely to be more fruitful. To recap, when reactivated by retrieval (re-exposure), the aversive memory becomes unstable again, and the original memory trace is either reconsolidated or extinguished. Therefore, it may be possible to block reconsolidation process or facilitate extinction. One treatment approach involves repeated exposure to the conditioned stimulus (smell or image) without the unconditioned stimulus (violence, trauma), leading to a new memory trace free of the unconditioned stimulus which overrides the old trace, in turn leading to a decrease in the physiological and behavioral responses to fear. Phytocannabinoids may amplify these mechanisms because extinguishing of aversive memories involves CB1 receptors [135].

We will look at some of the research into synthetic cannabinoids and then look at epidemiological studies that suggest many people with PTSD use cannabis to alleviate the symptoms. Then, we will look at how medicinal cannabis might work in alleviating PTSD symptoms, the possible mechanisms of action, and then at some of the clinical research into cannabis treatment of PTSD.

## Research into Synthetic Cannabinoids in PTSD

Research into synthetic cannabinoids (CB1 and CB2 receptor agonists) have provided insight into the potential mechanisms of action of cannabinoids. Synthetic agonists have been shown to improve fear extinction, reduce fear memories, improve neuroplasticity, and inhibit passive avoidance memory consolidation [65].

There are several potential mechanisms of action by which cannabinoids might help treat PTSD, supported by studies of synthetic cannabinoid agonists. Here are some of them:

- By administering immediately after the trauma, interfering with the memory consolidation process, thereby reducing the impact of the subsequent traumatic memory. This is thought to have less promising research support.
- Interfering with the memory recall or retrieval process (bringing stored information from long-term memory into consciousness). The theory is that once a memory trace is reactivated, it becomes unstable again and requires reconsolidation to be updated into long-term memory. A poorly retrieved memory will be less likely to be reconsolidated. Cannabinoid impairment of memory retrieval is well supported by animal studies.
- Enhancing extinction, in which a stimulus previously associated with a negative emotional experience that triggered anxiety and fear is transformed into non-threatening. This might be the most promising area [56].

### Animal Models of PTSD: Studies in Synthetic Cannabinoid Agonists

Pharmaceutical companies obviously have an interest in the development of synthetic drugs that might target the ECS and alleviate dysfunction in particular conditions, since these are patentable. Nonetheless, research using synthetic cannabinoid agonists can also provide some information about how THC itself might work since it is a CB1/CB2 partial agonist. Overall, animal studies support a strong enhancing effect of cannabinoid agonists on extinction processes which appears to be mediated by CB1 receptors, though evidence for effects in preclinical PTSD models is still lacking [56].

For example, WIN55,212-2 is a synthetic THC-like cannabinoid (CB1/CB2) receptor agonist drug which has been shown in other experiments to reduce anxiety and fear conditioning and facilitate fear extinction in rodents [153, 170, 171] as well as reduce fear memory retrieval [65, 172]. Potential mechanisms by which such agonists can impact memory are several and include improved neuroplasticity [65] and reduced inflammation.

### Cannabinoid Agonists Can Alter Neuroplastic Changes in Amygdala and Hippocampus

In an experiment using a shock and reminder model of PTSD, a traumatic memory was formed in rats after exposure to a severe foot shock, which was followed by exposure to trauma reminders. A glucocorticoid receptor (GR) antagonist RU486 and a CB1/CB2 receptor agonist WIN55,212-2 were injected into the basolateral amygdala (BLA), and these dampened the consolidation of the memory of the trauma as well as attenuating the increase in acoustic startle response in rats exposed to shock and reminders. In the CA1 region of the hippocampus, the CB1/CB2 agonist impaired consolidation of the traumatic memory and attenuated the increase in acoustic startle response, while the GR antagonist had no effect. Interestingly 1 month later, rats exposed to shock and reminders had increased CB1 receptor levels in the BLA and the CA1 region, and this increase was blocked by post-shock systemic administration of the CB1/CB2 agonist [172]. This suggests the BLA is a key brain region in which cannabinoids and glucocorticoids can act to modulate consolidation of traumatic memories [172]. It also suggests a potential role of cannabinoid agonists in altering neuroplastic changes in the amygdala and hippocampus that might occur as a result of PTSD.

### Cannabinoid Agonists Prevent BDNF Decreases in Brain Fear Circuits

The ECS and brain-derived neurotrophic factor (BDNF) are thought to be involved in both PTSD and depression. The protein BDNF promotes synaptic plasticity, neuronal survival, and neurogenesis, and has been shown to play a role in fear learning and extinction [173]. Studies indicate that decreased BDNF levels in the hippocampus, amygdala, and PFC were associated with impaired extinction learning [174] and downregulation of BDNF in the CA subregion of the hippocampus was associated with PTSD-like responses in rats [175]. BDNF interacts with the ECS in mediating synaptic plasticity and neuronal survival, and inhibition of CB1 receptors has been found to downregulate BDNF in the hippocampus [173, 176].

In a shock and reminder model of PTSD, CB1/CB2 receptor agonist WIN administered after the shock prevented depressive and PTSD-like behaviors in rats. It was able to prevent the shock and reminders-induced alterations in social recognition memory, passive coping, anxiety-like behavior, fear retrieval, fear extinction, and startle response. Significant negative correlations were found between depressive-like behaviors and BDNF levels in several brain regions. Administration of the CB1/CB2 receptor agonist WIN prevented the downregulation of BDNF in the CA1 region of the hippocampus and the prelimbic (PL) and infralimbic (IL) cortices of the rats [173]. This experiment suggests that CB1/CB2 receptor agonists may prevent depressive and PTSD-like symptoms following severe stress and implicates changes in BDNF levels in areas of the brain fear circuits [173].

### Cannabinoid Agonist Reverses Anxiety-Like Behavior and Reduces Inflammation in PTSD

Mice studies which use a repeated social defeat (RSD) paradigm are used to model the immune and behavioral responses to stress seen in humans. RSD causes anxiety-like behavior and release of inflammatory monocytes into circulation, and prolongs fear expression and impairs fear extinction recall, which was associated with increased IL-1β mRNA in the brain [171]. In this model, anxiety-like behavior is dependent on the recruitment of these monocytes to the brain.

In the first part of this study, mice subjected to RSD were injected pre-stress with CB1/CB2 agonist WIN55,212-2 that reversed the RSD-induced anxiety-like behavior and inflammatory response, e.g., decreased the accumulation of inflammatory monocytes in the brain and circulation, reduced the RSD-induced interleukin-1β mRNA expression in microglia/macrophages, and reduced the (ex vivo) reactivity of microglia/monocytes to lipopolysaccharides after RSD. In part two of the study, these same mice were subjected to contextual fear conditioning 7 days after RSD. RSD-exposed mice had prolonged and higher fear expression and impaired retention of fear extinction associated with increased IL-1β expression in the brain, deficits that were prevented by WIN [171].

This experiment demonstrates how activation of cannabinoid receptors by a cannabinoid agonist was able to limit immune and neuroinflammatory responses to RSD, as well as reverse the short- and long-term behavioral effects associated with this form of stress [171]. Thus, prophylactic cannabinoids were able to abort the PTSD pathophysiology.

What about post-trauma cannabinoid treatment? Indeed, a recent report showed that acute administration of WIN after exposing rats to a single prolonged stressor, a PTSD model, attenuated a stress-associated impairment of fear extinction [177].

### Synthetic Cannabinoids Promote Neurogenesis

In a rat model, synthetic cannabinoid HU210 was found to promote hippocampus neurogenesis and have both anxiolytic and antidepressant effects [178]. Since research has shown that the hippocampus is smaller in PTSD sufferers, this suggests an additional therapeutic action and role for cannabinoids in PTSD treatment [179].

### Cannabinoid Effects on Consolidation of Traumatic Experiences

The stage at which cannabinoids could be useful, immediately post-trauma (within hours) or later (days, weeks, years), has been examined by some researchers. There have been mixed results with respect to the potential effect of cannabinoids on consolidation of traumatic experiences. It is currently uncertain whether post-trauma administration of cannabinoids could be beneficial or even detrimental to later development of PTSD [56]. Not all people exposed to a traumatic event will go on to develop PTSD, and it is not easy to predict who will do so [56].

### Cannabinoid Agonists Impair Memory Retrieval

Berardi and colleagues believe a more promising research area is that focused on memory retrieval where there is consensus that cannabinoid agonists can impair memory retrieval [56]. Theoretically, by diminishing the retrieval of traumatic memories, it should be possible to reduce re-experiencing symptoms and thereby reduce the over-consolidation which characterizes PTSD, and therefore lessening the impact of those memories on anxiety and mood. Animal studies demonstrate that cannabinoid agonists can impair memory retrieval, though there are few studies in humans on traumatic memory retrieval and those that have been conducted were in marijuana smokers using memory tasks (e.g., lists of words or numbers, sematic knowledge). Such tasks have little in common with traumatic events in PTSD, limiting relevance [56].

### Problems with Synthetic Cannabinoid Agonists and Antagonists

With all such promising evidence about the potential effects of cannabinoid receptor agonists, why is it that we don't have a slew of drugs on the market to treat psychiatric illness? A key problem with them, like with THC (a partial CB1 receptor agonist), is that high doses can produce anxiety [65]. The synthetic CB1 antagonist rimonabant, marketed as a weight loss agent, was withdrawn from the market due to severe psychiatric side effects (including anxiety, depression, and suicide ideation) [180]. There have been other synthetic cannabinoids that became popular in the early 2000s, marketed as "designer drugs" under brand names such as Spice and K2. Synthetic cannabinoids are more potent (up to 100 times more potent) and have a greater likelihood of adverse effects than THC [181, 182] or indeed whole plant-derived cannabis medicines. Remember, the presence of CBD in sufficient amount is understood to be able to temper some of the more undesirable effects of THC. Mother nature wasn't stupid, but humans often are.

Another real problem with directly stimulating cannabinoid receptors, in particular CB1 receptors, is that it can produce potentially therapeutic effects in one brain region and detrimental effects in others [65]. For example, administration of THC to the medial PFC can reduce fear and anxiety responses, whereas administration in the nucleus accumbens potentiated fear reactivity [183, 184].

How do we make sense of such data? Are abnormal levels of endocannabinoids or receptors causative or compensation seeking homeostasis? This is a problem with applying a reductionistic and mechanistic way of looking at actions of cannabinoid agonists, that is, looking at their actions in various regions separately, rather than a systemic approach that considers how an agonist might act globally. In the end, research into mechanisms of action are useful, but the proof is generally in the pudding—is there clinical research that evidences a positive or negative effect of cannabinoids or not?

## Epidemiological Studies of Cannabis Use in Humans with PTSD

Epidemiological studies report positive associations between nonmedical cannabis use and PTSD [1, 4, 185, 186]. For example, Cougle and colleagues [186] found that PTSD diagnoses were associated with increased odds for lifetime history of cannabis use and past-year daily cannabis use.

In a cross-sectional survey using data from the 2012 Canadian Community Health Survey-Mental Health, among 24,089 eligible respondents, 420 (1.7%) reported a current clinical diagnosis of PTSD. A total of 106 (28.2%) of the latter group reported past-year cannabis use compared to 11.2% of those without PTSD, suggesting higher rates of self-treatment with cannabis. However, in cannabis users, PTSD was not significantly associated with either major depressive disorder or suicide ideation, but in non-cannabis users, PTSD *was* significantly associated with a recent major depressive episode (adjusted odds ratio = 7.18, 95% CI 4.32–11.91) and suicidal ideation (adjusted odds ratio = 4.76, 95% confidence interval: 2.39–9.47). This preliminary epidemiological evidence suggests that cannabis use might contribute to reducing the association between PTSD and severe depressive and suicidal states [187].

Cross-sectional studies have found high rates of nonmedical and medical use of cannabis to self-manage various symptoms associated with PTSD including coping, sleep, trauma-related re-experiencing, avoidance, and hyperarousal [1, 2, 185]. A cross-sectional study indicated that individuals with high levels of PTSD symptoms use medicinal cannabis for coping and sleep motives. This study also found that greater severity of PTSD was associated with more frequent medicinal cannabis use. In addition, sleep-motivated use, specifically, is associated with more frequent medicinal cannabis use [185].

Acute administration of cannabis appears to facilitate falling asleep and to increase stage 4 sleep while reducing REM sleep [3]. A cross-sectional study in New Mexico found that patients who used medicinal cannabis reported reductions of 75% in symptoms of trauma-related symptoms including re-experiencing, avoidance, and hyperarousal [188].

From these studies, it is clear that many people use cannabis to treat the symptoms of PTSD. To understand this better, we will examine the mechanisms of action of medicinal cannabis and two of its key constituents: CBD and THC.

## Potential Mechanisms of Action of Medicinal Cannabis in Alleviating PTSD Symptoms

There are several potential mechanisms by which medicinal cannabis may alleviate symptoms associated with PTSD including the following:

- Activating CB1 receptors in the amygdala can potentially decrease aversive memories, fear, and anxiety.
- Activating CB1 receptors in the prefrontal cortex can increase serotonin and therefore may reduce depression.
- When CB1 receptors are agonized in the hippocampus, an increase in neurogenesis, mood, and memory and a decrease in hypervigilance, hyperarousal, and intrusive memories and normalization of cortisol may occur.
- Stimulation of the receptors in the PFC, amygdala, and hippocampus may alleviate anxiety as well as cause sensitization of CB1 receptor-mediated G-protein signaling in the PFC, which may play a role in suicide and suicidal behavior.
- Stimulation of the limbic and paralimbic area may decrease activity in the amygdala and hypothalamus, which could assist in regulating the HPA axis and cortisol and, therefore, decrease hypervigilance and hyperarousal.

- Reducing inflammation.
- Stimulating neurogenesis, synaptogenesis, and neuritogenesis via effects on BDNF [21, 171, 173].

## CBD: Mechanisms of Action and Evidence of Efficacy from Animal Studies

There are several potential mechanisms by which CBD might address the underlying complex pathology associated with PTSD. We also know that CBD may be able to assist in treatment of stress, anxiety, and depression, as well as sleep disorders, all comorbidities of PTSD (see relevant chapters). We already know of CBD's anti-inflammatory effects, and we know that inflammation is associated with PTSD.

CBD is able to affect every stage of aversive conditioning, as well as reduce the cardiovascular responses and anxiogenic effects associated with stress [57, 189]. CBD reduces anxiety via 5-HT1A, and there is growing evidence from animal studies that it reduces learned fear in paradigms used to approximate PTSD. CBD reduces fear expression acutely and disrupts fear memory consolidation and facilitates fear extinction, and these can lead to a lasting decrease in fear memory recall [190].

The following describes some of the research into mechanisms of action of CBD by which it may address some of the memory aspects related to PTSD.

### CBD Disrupts the Acquisition of Fear Learning and Formation of Fear Memories

CBD has been found to disrupt the acquisition of fear learning. Acute systemic administration of CBD prior to fear conditioning attenuated fear expression during later memory retrieval testing in rats [191].

Contextual fear conditioning is an animal model used to study both anxiety and fear memory. Fear responses are evoked in the animals when they are re-exposed to a context previously paired with, for example, foot shocks. During the conditioned emotional response, the animals exhibit several behaviors including freezing behavior, vocalization, increased heart rate and blood pressure, and others [192].

Research in mice models of PTSD has found that CBD is able to disrupt 1- and 7-day-old fear memories when administered immediately after their retrieval for 3 min [193]. Fear memories disrupted by CBD treatment did not show reinstatement for the next 22 days without additional dosing, which hints at possible remission. Recent and older fear memories were found to be equally susceptible to disruption brought about by CBD through reconsolidation blockade, with a consequent long-lasting relief in contextual fear-generated freezing [193].

Administration of CBD into the nucleus accumbens shell region of rats inhibits the spontaneous firing rates and bursting levels of dopaminergic neurons in the ventral tegmental area, as well as blocking formation of aversive, fear-related associative memories [183, 194]. This is opposite what was found when THC was administered to this brain region in rats [183]. The ability of CBD administered to the shell region of the nucleus accumbens is dependent on GABAA/B receptor transmission within the ventral tegmental area [194].

However, results are conflicting when it comes to the potential effect of CBD on fear memory expression and fear learning. One study found that daily injections of CBD for 14 days prior to conditioning increased fear expression during retrieval testing, suggesting CBD actually facilitated fear learning, while another study in which CBD was administered for 21 days showed no effect on fear conditioning [190]. It appears that the effect of CBD may depend on the brain region involved, since infusion of CBD into the BSLT or the prelimbic cortex in rats reduced fear expression but infusion into the infralimbic cortex did the opposite, increasing the expression of learned fear [192].

Similarly, injection of CBD into the prelimbic PFC reduced the freezing response induced by re-exposure to the aversively conditioned context. But when injected into the infralimbic PFC, CBD increased the expression of contextual fear [192]. Other studies have found that prelimbic cortex region activation is required for the expression of learned memories [195].

### CBD Attenuates Fear Memory Reconsolidation

CBD has been found in animal models to block the process of reconsolidation [193]. In a rat model, CBD administration immediately after retrieval for 3 min disrupted 1- and 7-day-old memories (optimal dose 10 mg/kg) with this effect lasting at least 1 week. It was prevented if a CB1 receptor antagonist was administered. The study shows that recent and older fear memories are both able to be disrupted by CBD through reconsolidation blockade, with the rats consequently not displaying contextual fear-induced freezing. This CBD effect depended on memory reactivation in under 6 h, and results would suggest it was CB1 receptor dependent. Over the ensuing 22 days, the fear memories did not show reinstatement, which suggests the mechanism of action of CBD was via reconsolidation blockade, rather than facilitated extinction [193].

Since it has limited affinity for CB1 receptors, the CBD mechanism of action would appear to be indirect by influencing key enzymes or perhaps noncanonical docking sites for these receptors.

#### Attenuation of Fear Memory Reconsolidation: Whole Plant Versus Isolate

In another experiment, CBD as well as a combination of CBD and THC (but not THC alone) was found to significantly attenuate fear memory reconsolidation when administered immediately following recall, with the effect lasting at least 7 days. Rats were given foot shocks (contextual training) and then, 24 h later, re-exposed to the context (foot shocks). Immediately after memory retrieval (recall), they were given oral isolates of either (1) low-dose THC isolate, (2) high-dose THC isolate, (3) CBD isolate (4) CBD plus low THC (isolates), or (5) CBD plus high THC (isolates), and in another set of experiments, these were given with plant background material. Plant background material significantly attenuated reconsolidation of learned fear alone, and in combination with THC and CBD. THC was only able to attenuate reconsolidation when it was combined with CBD or plant background material [196].

This study would certainly seem to support the idea of an "entourage effect" whereby other phytochemicals are able to increase the therapeutic effect of a particular phytocannabinoid, in this case THC (and CBD). What was very interesting is that the plant background material had a therapeutic effect alone, though it is not clear what exact phytochemicals might specifically be responsible for this.

### CBD Enhances Extinction Learning and Retention

Formation of a fear memory following a traumatic event sets the stage for subsequent development of PTSD. Extinction learning diminishes PTSD. As explained previously, impaired extinction of fear memories is thought to contribute to the development and persistence of the persistent memories of the trauma and avoidance. Enhancing endocannabinoid signaling with phytocannabinoids has been shown to facilitate extinction in various studies [136].

Both CBD and THC may enhance extinction learning [157, 197, 198]. Studies in rats have shown that CBD is able to facilitate the extinction of contextual fear memory, and supports the role of CB1 receptors in contextual fear extinction, reinforcing findings of other studies demonstrating the involvement of the ECS in extinction of conditioned fear [157]. Animal research has demonstrated that CBD can enhance contextual fear-conditioning extinction when infused intracereboventricularly [157] and into the infralimbic area of the medial PFC [159].

### CBD Can Reduce Predator Anxiety

In a rat model of PTSD where the trauma was exposure to a predator cat, CBD treatment (5 mg/kg/day for 7 days) starting 1 h after exposure to the cat prevented anxiogenic effects in rats. The probable mechanism was by facilitating 5-HT1A receptor-mediated neurotransmission, and suggests a possible role for CBD in PTSD symptom treatment [142]. In another experiment using a mice model for progressive anxiety and repeated combination tests (RCT), it was found that the repeated combination tests induced an anxiogenic effect in the elevated plus maze and open-field tests, and caused PTSD-like sleep symptoms by decreasing non-REM sleep during the first hour after RCT and suppressing REM sleep during hours 4–10 after the repeated combination tests. When CBD was microinjected into the central nucleus of the amygdala, it had an anxiolytic effect (demonstrated in the elevated plus maze and open-field tests), and efficiently blocked anxiety-induced REM sleep suppression [199].

## THC: Mechanisms of Action and Evidence of Efficacy from Animal Studies

THC is a partial agonist with high affinity to both CB1 and CB2 receptors, and exerts most of its actions via these receptors [200]. As discussed in Chap. 4, THC exerts its effects by binding with CB1 receptors presynaptically, inhibiting the release of other neurotransmitters.

THC has been shown in several animal studies to have positive therapeutic effects relevant to PTSD including:

- Improving performance on fear and analogue emotional memory tasks
- Reducing the stress response and promoting antianxiety behaviors at mild-moderate doses
- Reducing anxiety produced by 2-AG inhibition
- Decreasing fearful behaviors to conditioned stimuli (mediated by CB1 receptor-dependent disruption of memory consolidation in the medial PFC)
- Reducing acquisition of fear learning [65]

THC administration was found to disrupt the reconsolidation of a contextual fear memory, evidenced by a reduced conditioned freezing behavior for more than 22 days. The effect was dependent on activation of CB1 receptors in the medial PFC and on memory retrieval/reactivation, and was not thought to be due to an anxiolytic effect [184]. CBD has been found to be less potent in mitigating fear memory through disruption of reconsolidation, so the researchers tested out a combination of subeffective doses of THC and CBD in a high CBD to low THC ratio. They found that this combination was also effective [184]. Since THC is a partial CB1 agonist and CBD can prevent AEA degradation and uptake, the additive effect appears to occur via direct and indirect potentiation of the CB1-mediated endocannabinoid signaling [184].

## Clinical Evidence of Efficacy of Treatment of PTSD with Medicinal Cannabis

There is some clinical evidence that medicinal cannabis can alleviate PTSD symptoms, including a case study, randomized controlled trials (RCTs), and systematic reviews. There are several measurement tools used in human studies of PTSD. One of the more popular ones is the Clinical Administered PTSD Scale (CAPS-5) which is a 30-item questionnaire, which corresponds to DSM-5 diagnostic criteria for PTSD. A 5-point ordinal rating scale is used to measure symptom severity (ranging from 0 = absent to 4 = extreme/incapacitating) on the 20 symptoms that correspond to PTSD diagnosis. The assessor combines information about frequency and intensity of an item into a single severity rating. The CAPS-5 Total Symptom Severity score is calculated by summing severity scores for the 20 *DSM-5* PTSD symptoms.

### Case Study of Cannabis in PTSD Treatment

There is a published case study involving a 19-year-old male with a history of sexual abuse who had severe PTSD symptoms including intense flashbacks, panic attacks, and self-mutilation. He had learned about smoking cannabis resin from other inpatients and found he could prevent the dissociative states by smoking cannabis when he first felt reactivation and intensification of traumatic memories that manifested as flashbacks. While he still had flashbacks, he found that smoking cannabis changed their intensity, and he felt he had increased ability to maintain cognitive control. While he still experienced traumatic images, he had less involvement with them, as smoking cannabis allowed him to view them on an "inner screen." He also had reduced urge to self-mutilate when he smoked straight after experiencing flashbacks. He also experienced less stress and a significant decrease in anxiety [201].

## Retrospective Study of Cannabis Use in PTSD

A study examined 404 medical cannabis users who self-identified as having PTSD who used a medical cannabis App to track changes in symptoms across time. The App was used 11,797 times over 31 months to track PTSD symptoms: intrusive thoughts, flashbacks, irritability, and/or anxiety, immediately before and after inhaling cannabis. The study found that all symptoms were decreased by more than 50% immediately after cannabis use. In their statistical modeling, higher doses of cannabis predicted larger reductions in anxiety and intrusive thoughts, and the dose used for anxiety increased over time, suggesting tolerance. Time predicted larger reductions in intrusions and irritability. The baseline severity of all symptoms was constant over time suggesting that cannabis did not appear to improve or worsen symptoms. They concluded that cannabis provides temporary relief from PTSD symptoms but may not be an effective long-term therapy [202].

## Qualitative Research in PTSD and Cannabis Use

Although qualitative research does not get the same airtime as randomized clinical trials, it is valuable to explore in depth many of the aspects, nuances, and patient experiences involved with illness and treatment. And so it is with cannabis use in PTSD sufferers. A focus group was organized among seven military veterans with chronic PTSD who were treated with medical cannabis. The study also included four partners who shared their perspectives on their partners. There were five key themes that were identified: (1) consideration, (2) initiation, (3) usage, (4) discontinuation, and (5) several general aspects of medical cannabis use. Key findings of the study were that patients used cannabis to manage their symptoms and not to "get high" [203].

The study reported that all ten participants mentioned negative experiences and side effects with other pharmaceutical medications taken during previous treatments. Side effects of orthodox pharmaceuticals mentioned included a hangover-like feeling, stomach pain, numbness, feeling of drunkenness, liver and kidney problems, and disorientation. The following quotes from their study exemplify the limitations of the pharmaceutical approach to treating PTSD, at least in the experience of these men:

- *Peter: "The problem with those regular medicines is if it doesn't work, then one more is added."*
- *Dave: "Or the dose is doubled!"*

- *Peter: "Or a different brand or name is prescribed. And then the dose is increased again. You feel dazed all day."*

The lack of therapeutic effect and/or side effects associated with orthodox pharmaceuticals was an important factor in patients' decisions to consider medical cannabis use. Participants also indicated they wished to reduce or stop the use of other medications and some had already done so. They strongly favored medical cannabis over many other medications they had used in terms of ratio of therapeutic benefits to side effects.

A variety of cannabis strains and dosages were used. Most used medical cannabis oil sublingually, and some used the inhalation route of delivery. Several therapeutic benefits were reported including increased quality of sleep and reduction in nightmares and flashbacks. Initiating cannabis use was perceived positively by all four partners who participated. Participants did not report many adverse effects of cannabis, with the main unpleasant effects associated with taking too much cannabis, and two participants stated that their nightmares returned when they stopped taking cannabis [203]. As you can see, understanding the lived experience of those with a condition, such as PTSD, including their experiences of therapies such as medicinal cannabis, is made possible by qualitative research designs.

### RCTs and Systematic Reviews

A systematic review of the efficacy of medicinal cannabis in the treatment of PTSD published in 2018 [21] included five studies [188, 204–207]. Three of the studies concluded cannabis might be a benefit, but two found a negative effect (worsening of PTSD symptoms, though the clinical significance is unclear) [21].

A systematic review conducted in 2019 reached a more promising conclusion that cannabis and synthetic cannabinoids may have potential to improve PTSD symptoms including anxiety, sleep disorders, and modulating memory-related processes, though they noted limited evidence in relation to safety and efficacy [208]. Yet another systematic review, this one published in 2020, included ten studies of which only one was a double-blind, placebo-controlled, crossover pilot study. They found that the studies were of low quality and with a medium to high risk of bias. They concluded that cannabinoids may decrease PTSD symptomatology, in particular global PTSD symptoms, sleep disturbances, and nightmares [209].

Table 7.4 sets out a selection of clinical studies in medicinal cannabis and PTSD. Table 7.5 sets out studies specific to THC.

### New Studies Examining Short-Term and Long-Term Effects of Cannabis with Different Ratios of THC/CBD

Two studies have examined the short-term and long-term (12 months) effects of cannabis with different THC/CBD ratios. In the short-term study, a double-blind crossover study, participants were randomized to receive 3 weeks of active treatment or placebo (stage 1 of the study, $n = 80$ participants) and, then after a 2-week washout period, re-randomized to receive 1 of the other 3 active treatments (stage 2, $n = 74$ participants). The active treatments were three active concentrations of

**Table 7.4** Human studies: medicinal cannabis and PTSD

| Reference | Study findings |
|---|---|
| Bonn-Miller et al. [204] | Study: longitudinal study of 260 male combat-exposed military veterans (mean 52.6 years) admitted to a Veterans Affairs residential rehabilitation program for PTSD between 2000 and 2008<br>Results: presence of a cannabis use disorder was significantly predictive of lower levels of change (between treatment intake and discharge) in PTSD severity and PTSD avoidance-numbing and hyperarousal symptom cluster severity |
| Bonn-Miller et al. [185] | Study: cross-sectional survey of 170 patients at a medical cannabis dispensary in California<br>Results: that those with high PTSD scores were more likely to use cannabis to improve sleep and in general to cope compared with those with low PTSD scores. Sleep improvement appeared to be the main motivator for coping-oriented use. Frequency of cannabis use was higher in those with high PTSD scores who used it for sleep promoting purposes compared with those with low PTSD scores or those who did not use it for sleep promoting purposes, providing empirical evidence that sleep-motivated use specifically is associated with more frequent cannabis use |
| Bonn-Miller et al. [210] | Study: a cross-sectional study involving 217 medical cannabis users in California (not specifically a study on PTSD)<br>Results: proportion of those surveyed who reported cannabis to be a primary benefit for various symptoms were as follows: stress (24.4%), anxiety (20,3%), depression (10.1%), insomnia (24.9%), and overall PTSD symptomatology (3.7%) |
| Greer et al. [188] | Study: retrospective study in New Mexico comparing pretreatment and posttreatment CAPS scores in 80 PTSD patients who took medical cannabis<br>Results: a greater than 75% reduction in CAPS symptom score in patients when they were using cannabis compared to when they were not using it; a significant reduction in the symptom clusters examined by the CAPS measurement tool including the total score, Criterion B (re-experiencing symptoms), Criterion C (avoidance), and Criterion C (hyperarousal) |
| Tull et al. [206] | Study: 202 patients with and without current PTSD consecutively admitted to a treatment facility<br>Results: current PTSD use was associated with greater emotional reactivity in those without cannabis dependence; however, in those who were cannabis dependent, there were no significant differences in emotional reactivity between those who did and didn't have PTSD. Cannabis-dependent patients (with and without PTSD) had less emotional reactivity than those with PTSD or patients without cannabis dependence. This suggests that patients with PTSD who are cannabis dependent may have altered emotional processing in response to a trauma, that is, a dampening of arousal |
| Wilkinson et al. [207] | Study: retrospective longitudinal observational study of 2276 veterans with severe PTSD admitted to intensive PTSD Veterans Affairs treatment programs from 1992 to 2011<br>Results: participants were categorized according to cannabis use before and after discharge (never users, stoppers, continuing users, and starters) and were assessed at baseline and 4 months after discharge. Starting cannabis was found to worsen PTSD symptoms by a moderate effect size of +0.34. Stopping cannabis use improved PTSD with a small effect size of −0.18. They found a significant association between days cannabis was used and change in PTSD symptoms, severity of violent behavior, alcohol use, and drug use as measured using validated scales. They also found that at follow-up, stoppers, and never users had lower levels of PTSD symptoms, while starters had the highest levels of violent behavior |

**Table 7.5** Clinical studies: THC and PTSD

| Reference | THC product | Study findings |
|---|---|---|
| Roitman et al. [205] | THC olive oil | Study: 3-week, open-label study in ten patients with chronic PTSD on stable medication (five were combat veterans). Patients were given 5 mg THC olive oil sublingually twice daily as an adjunct to their regular medication<br>Results: significant reduction in frequency of nightmares ($p < 0.04$), sleep quality ($p < 0.05$), and hyperarousal (CAPS, $p < 0.02$) and significant improvement in global symptom severity (CGI-5, $p < 0.02$). Mild adverse effects in 3/10 patients, and none of these led to discontinuation of the THC |
| Shalev et al. [211] | | Study: open-label study of ten patients with PTSD who received THC twice daily for 3 weeks<br>Results: significant improvement in arousal, sleep quality, and nightmares |
| Jetly et al. [212] | Nabilone (synthetic THC) | Study: double-blind, crossover RCT conducted in Canadian military personal with trauma-related nightmares despite standard treatment. Ten participants were randomized to either nabilone (synthetic THC, 0.5 mg titrated to daily max 3.0 mg) or placebo for 7 weeks and then 2-week washout period and then treated with opposite study medication for 7 weeks. Assessors assessed the effects on sleep, nightmares, and global clinical state<br>Results: participants self-reported sleep time & general well-being. The study found that nightmares, global clinical state, and general well-being improved significantly more with nabilone ($p < 0.05$), but there was no effect on sleep quality or quantity |
| Fraser et al. [29] | Nabilone (synthetic THC) | Study: open-label study was conducted in 47 PTSD patients with continuing treatment-resistant nightmares. Adjunctive treatment with nabilone (synthetic THC) was commenced, with a starting dose of 0.5 mg 1 h before bedtime, titrating up until effect, with doses kept below the maximum of 6 mg daily<br>Results: average effective dose was 0.5 mg 1 h before bedtime (range 0.2 mg–4.0 mg). The majority (72%) experienced cessation or a significant reduction in nightmare intensity, and some reported improvements in sleep time and quality of sleep and reduction of daytime flashbacks and night sweats. Discontinuation of medication was successful in four patients following 4–12 months of nabilone therapy with no more nightmares occuring thereafter, but the other patients experienced a recurrence of nightmares upon nabilone withdrawal (usually within the first two nights) which was alleviated on reinitiation of nabilone treatment. The study participants concomitantly received nabilone as well as one or more psychiatric medications they had been one for 2 or more years. Thirteen patients (28%) experienced mild-to-moderate side effects including light-headedness, forgetfulness, dizziness, and headache shortly after initiation of nabilone therapy, leading to its discontinuation. No tolerance to nabilone was observed. No tolerance to nabilone was observed among the patients. |

**Table 7.5** (continued)

| Reference | THC product | Study findings |
|---|---|---|
| Rabinak et al. [198] | Dronabinol (synthetic THC) | Study: double-blind, placebo-controlled RCT between-subjects designed study coupled a standard Pavlovian fear extinction paradigm and skin conductance response with challenge with oral dronabinol or placebo 2 h before extinction learning in healthy adults ($n$ = 14 THC, $n$ = 15 placebo), measuring extinction retention 24 h after extinction learning<br>Results: when extinction memory was tested 24 h after extinction learning, those who received THC showed a slowed skin conductance response to a previously extinguished conditioned stimulus (compared with placebo) which suggests THC prevented the recovery of fear. The study showed that THC only influenced the ability to successfully recall extinction memory (but did not affect the within-session extinction learning) which could suggest the effects of THC relate specifically to maintaining and/or successfully retrieving extinction memory |

smoked cannabis: high THC (approximately 12% THC and <0.05% CBD), high CBD (11% CBD and 0.50% THC), and THC + CBD (approximately 7.9% THC and 8.1% CBD), and the placebo contained less than 0.03% THC and less than 0.01% CBD. They did not find a significant difference in change in PTSD symptom severity between the active treatments and the placebo at the end of stage 1 of the study. All three active treatments (smoked cannabis) were well tolerated in general [213].

In the study on long-term use, the THC-dominant cannabis appeared associated with reduction in PTSD symptoms, primarily via reductions in hyperarousal symptoms, and a more than twofold reduction in likelihood of PTSD diagnosis at 12 months compared with nonusers [214].

## Clinical Studies of Efficacy of THC and Synthetic THC

In general, there is more data on synthetic versions of THC than THC from plant sources. Importantly, there is currently a lack of clinical data on the efficacy of CBD in treating PTSD, though there is research on its effects on stress and anxiety and sleep (covered in other chapters). This area should be pursued, as clinical research does support the involvement of the ECS in the pathology of PTSD and preclinical research indicates that CBD (and THC) are efficacious in addressing some aspects of the memory dysfunction occurring in PTSD.

Several of the published RCTs have been in nabilone, a synthetic form of THC, with fewer in whole plant medicinal cannabis products. A study used functional MRI using a double-blind, randomized, placebo-controlled between-subjects design study with 14 healthy participants in each group, coupled with a Pavlovian fear extinction paradigm to assess the effects of oral synthetic THC (dronabinol) on vmPFC and hippocampus activation 24 h after extinction learning. Those in the THC group showed increased activation in the vmPFC and hippocampus to a previously extinguished conditioned stimulus during extinction memory recall, in comparison with those in the placebo group. This was the first study to demonstrate that pre-extinction administration of THC is able to modulate the prefrontal-limbic circuits during fear extinction [159].

Clinical studies assessing THC and synthetic THC products are set out in Table 7.5.

## Clinical Studies of Efficacy of CBD

Despite promising preclinical evidence that CBD may be effective in treating symptoms of PTSD, there is a dearth of studies investigating the efficacy of CBD in treating symptoms of PTSD. There is one published case study and one clinical study which have focused specifically on PTSD.

### Case Studies

There is one published case that involved a 10-year old girl with a history of sexual abuse, diagnosed with PTSD. Her main problems were anxiety, insomnia, outbursts at school, suicidal ideation, and self-destructive behaviors. She was given CBD (25 mg, oral capsules) at bedtime, with 6 mg–12 mg of CBD sublingual spray used during the day on indication for anxiety. Her sleep quality and quantity gradually increased and her anxiety decreased. After 5 months, she could sleep in her own room most nights, and she was able to handle her new school. No side effects were experienced [215].

A case series from an outpatient psychiatry clinic reported retrospectively on 11 patients being followed for PTSD treated with CBD over 8 weeks [216]. PTSD was measured with the PCL-5 standard questionnaire, and the average full-spectrum hemp-derived CBD was 48 mg/day. 91% of patients experienced a decrease in PTSD symptom severity with an average symptom decrease of 28%. There are no dropouts and no significant side effects. Of particular note was the high rate of improvement in symptoms of nightmares and sleep disturbances (50% and 38%). This report supports a practical use approach that is sensitive to the patient lifestyle and adaptable to clinical situations in a high-volume outpatient setting.

### Clinical Study

Preliminary research in healthy volunteers supports the potential for CBD to impact on extinction processes. CBD was found to enhance consolidation of extinction learning when administered to healthy subjects after extinction learning. In a study of fear condition using brief electric shocks as unconditioned stimuli, participants were given 32 mg of CBD by inhalation prior to or immediately after the conditioned stimulus extinction procedure to investigate effect on acquisition or consolidation of extinction respectively. In a recall test performed 48 h after extinction, the group treated with CBD had reduced subjective shock expectancy ratings at the presentation of the extinguished conditioned stimulus. Also, when they reinstated the extinguished association through presenting another brief shock, there was a lower increase in the skin conductance responses in the CBD groups compared to placebo [197].

### Open-Label Pilot Study

Dr. Philip Blair conducted a pilot study in 2018 on 30 military veterans with self-reported PTSD over a 4-week period using self-directed medicinal cannabis (MC) without a control group. A total of 22 completed the biweekly PCL-5 questionnaires. Nine of the 22 participants included an exercise intervention in addition to the medicinal cannabis. Participants were male and female veterans of US Army, Navy, and Air Force services, with an age range of between 24 and 70 years of age. None had suicidal thoughts and a history of suicide attempts or felt they were at risk of suicide. All subjects were either using or failed medication. The medicinal cannabis formulation was a liposomal form of full-spectrum hemp extract, with enhanced bioavailability based on safety studies. A serving size of 5 mg of the liposomal oil was suggested to be 5–7 times greater potency than oil tincture. Patients were started on standard serving twice daily but allowed to titrate the dose to their symptom needs. The average self-adjusted dose of medicinal cannabis was 15 mg per day. The total average point values on the PCL-5 questionnaire pre-therapy were 46, the most severe 80, and the least severe 25. At the midpoint of the study (2-week data collection), the average score dropped to 37 (−20%). After 4 weeks of participation, the average score of the combined group was 21 (−54%), the most severe case scored 52, while the least severe score was 7. A total of 90% of the clients improved their scores. On average, symptom scores decreased 67%. The exercise group showed significantly better scores. Among the eight who failed to complete the study, there was one hospitalization that appeared unrelated to the study or CBD. The other seven took initial products but did not attend follow-up visits or questionnaires. Many of the clients reported sufficient resolution of symptoms to completely discontinue CBD. Others continued using the product as needed for stress-related symptoms.

This study is remarkable for the low dose and self-titration. The group had an initial meeting followed by shared questions and support in social media. Questionnaires were created in *Google Forms* and converted to spreadsheets for data collection. Unfortunately, the trial was brief, not blinded nor had a control group. Nevertheless, the high success rate did suggest a significant outcome that should be repeated in more carefully controlled studies [217].

## Safety Aspects of Use of Medicinal Cannabis in PTSD

Despite possible benefits, there is concern about development of cannabis use disorder (CUD) in people with PTSD. PTSD sufferers represent a vulnerable population in which substance use and addiction are common [21]. The prevalence of cannabis use in PTSD patients is high: a survey in the USA found that out of 5672 US adults, 65% with PTSD versus 41% without PTSD used cannabis [186]. In 2009, 30% of veterans within the VA with a PTSD diagnosis also had CUD though at this time, cannabis was not approved in any state for medical use, so presumably this related to smoking of marijuana [204].

## Heavy Cannabis Use and Impaired Fear Extinction

Heavy cannabis use has been associated with downregulation of endocannabinoid signaling and impaired fear extinction [218], as well as other side effects including depression, psychosis, and impaired cognition and memory [65, 219], and others (e.g., tachycardia, euphoria, and altered perceptions) [220]. Thus, while it is known that many PTSD sufferers use cannabis to deal with the symptoms of the illness, heavy use may be detrimental.

## THC May Distort Memories

THC can induce undesirable neuropsychiatric effects including psychosis, schizophrenia, impaired memory and learning, and distorted emotional salience, and this has been linked to its modulatory role on the mesolimbic dopaminergic transmission [183].

In a double-blind, placebo-controlled, within-subjects design, 23 healthy subjects viewed negative, neutral, and positive pictures (emotional memory task) and lists of semantically related words (false memory task). Forty-eight hours after, they were given either 15 mg THC or placebo and were given tasks to test their memories of the pictures and words. They found that THC increased false recollection of the emotional memory and false memory tasks, and this was found for neutral and emotional items. This suggests that THC adversely affects memory retrieval and can cause distortion of neutral and emotional memories [221]. This finding is supported by a rat study which demonstrated that THC modulated the salience of fear-related associative memory formation via direct effects in the nucleus accumbens. The mechanism of action seems to involve modulating the dopaminergic transmission in the ventral tegmental area and GABAergic signaling mechanisms. The study authors suggest that their findings might help explain the neurological mechanisms that link cannabis with potential psychiatric side effects [183].

## Medicinal Use Is Not Equivalent to Recreational Use

Recreational use of cannabis is not the same as its medicinal use in which the dose is individualized to the patient, titrating upward from a low dose slowly until a therapeutic effect is experienced. Nonetheless, there remains the possibility of addiction with THC-containing medicinal cannabis products. Medicinal cannabis products containing CBD without THC may be a safer option in this respect since CBD is not addictive [220].

## Guidelines for Treating PTSD with Medicinal Cannabis

### When to Use Medicinal Cannabis

Much of the attention has been focused on military veterans, but in fact 70% of PTSD occurs in nonmilitary and includes large numbers of women and children with 50% rates of occurrence in abuse and sexual assault (PTSD UK, no date). Clients with PTSD, even from the military, often indicate adverse events of childhood such as abuse, neglect, starvation, and violence that may cause deficiencies in the endocannabinoid system and predispose to PTSD. In fact, every one of my female clients with PTSD reports significant adverse childhood events. Remember too that all first responders are at risk including emergency telephone dispatchers.

As previously discussed, there are many symptoms of PTSD, but the most common ones are arousal, re-experiencing, avoidance, and negative moods and thoughts. These symptoms can be very disabling and too frequently lead to suicide. Experience suggests that this condition may manifest a spectrum of symptoms for which many clients may not meet all of the DSM-5 criteria. Or, the diagnosis may be confused by head trauma or blast injuries that can manifest similar symptoms. Regardless, patients with similar symptom complexes still have a high likelihood of positive response to medical cannabinoid therapy.

Phytocannabinoids are an excellent starting point for establishing patient-provider rapport with rapid improvements, but multiple modalities may be needed for some recalcitrant cases. Treatment programs for PTSD should encompass a comprehensive lifestyle approach that includes diet, exercise, psychological counseling, social assistance, sleep hygiene, and mindfulness/prayer/meditation. In an ideal situation, rehabilitation programs should be orchestrated by an interdisciplinary team, but this is rarely available. You perhaps can best assist the patients by advocating for and explaining the bigger picture of a treatment plan.

### Type of Product (Blends)

Full-spectrum medical cannabis with low THC is quite effective. Many patients will report self-treatment with cannabis with high THC content. This history suggests high THC treats symptoms temporarily but does not resolve persistent issues or the fear memory conditioning. In my experience full spectrum medicinal cannabis (MC) products with high concentrations of CBD and low THC may facilitate recovery. On the other hand, in some patients, a full-spectrum CBD predominant product containing THC may increase anxiety suggesting a sensitivity and paradoxical response to THC. In such cases micro-dosing such that the daily dose only delivers a few milligrams per day of THC may be considered, or consider trying a broad-spectrum MC without THC. Tinctures are a better choice when small adjustments may be needed.

## What Form of Product Should You Use?

All forms of low THC medicinal cannabis appear to be effective with capsules taken with fatty food showing extended duration of effects. Capsules also offer longer duration of effects that may be important for many sufferers. Oil tinctures deliver immediate benefits sublingually during exacerbations of anxiety or panic symptoms along with ease of titration. Topical CBD can be used with massage to amplify high-touch, interpersonal relaxation and communication especially with spouses or partners. Remember that high blood levels of CBD are not needed to modulate this condition which means that an occasional skipped dose is not a problem. My experience also showed sustained benefits of CBD even after CBD was discontinued. Vaping CBD (without vitamin E acetate or THC) has been used successfully for some, but I have found oral therapies more effective.

## Dosage Guidelines

The average dosage of medicinal cannabis in real-world clinical trials has been about 50 mg CBD oil (i.e. CBD dominant product, low THC) in divided doses, usually twice daily. Encourage clients to make adjustments within limits to respond to special situations or symptom variation. Half dosing is appropriate for young children and seniors. Rarely are PTSD patients particularly sensitive to cannabinoids, so a single serving in the range of 15–30 mg is an appropriate starting point.

## Titration and Follow-Up

Almost all of my clients showed some clinical signs of improvement with their first dose as sublingual. But if they showed no response, then I make an immediate increase. The common dictum is "start slow and go slow," but when you or one of your staff can guide the patient with their first dose, you can get immediate feedback, document response, and speed the treatment process. Typical responses are rapid so early follow-up gives providers an accurate picture of clinical progress or need for adjustments in the treatment program. On the other hand, remissions have been common even after the medical cannabis course is completed. But most patients do continue healthy self-medicating for their residual life stresses or for enhanced performance.

## Other Tips to Enhance Therapeutic Action

Cannabinoids are best absorbed with food or fatty snack. Studies show that long-chain triglycerides (18 carbons or more) enhance absorption into the intestinal lymphatics and reduced immediate liver deactivation.

Sleep disorders are common in PTSD with disturbing dreams. Medicinal cannabinoids can provide sedation for sleep and often stimulate vivid dreaming. These are not typically nightmares or reliving experiences and require only reassurance. Most patients report improved depth and quality of sleep, but a few can feel activated mentally. Most PTSD patients do well with an evening dose even immediately before bed.

Often sleep software programs actually show a significant amount of deep sleep of which the patient was unaware. Encourage the patient to use a smart phone sleep application to monitor their sleep patterns. This will be especially important in this condition for assessing sleep in follow-up interactions.

### Interactions with Other Drugs

PTSD clients are usually taking a variety of medications to control symptoms including antidepressants, benzodiazepines, and neurotransmission modulators with marginal improvement and host of adverse effects. It has been my experience that, fortunately, CBD rarely interacts so it can be added; however, it is always prudent to monitor for possible interactions. Other medication can be de-prescribed as symptoms are controlled and resolved. Occasionally, medications can cause withdrawal symptoms for which CBD can compensate with additional dosing as needed. Typical tapers of any medications start at about a one quarter (¼) reduction per week or slower, but in most cases patients accelerate the taper considerably completing the process in the second week.

Remarkably a significant number of PTSD patients achieve remission after 3–4 weeks of therapy and were able to discontinue CBD without recurrence of stress symptoms, and of course without withdrawal.

## Case Studies from Dr. Blair's Practice

### Case 1: Air Force Veteran with PTSD

A 33-year-old female US Air Force veteran requested medical cannabis treatment for PTSD because of lack of effective medical therapy from the Veteran Administration (VA). She was assigned to a combat aviation unit in Iraq and repeatedly witnessed pilots maimed and killed during her tour. She was also diagnosed with depression and panic disorder during her active duty. During a training mission, she was severely injured and underwent intensive therapy and discharged from the service. Medications provided caused significant side effects and did not resolve symptoms. She left the service with chronic pain, depression, anxiety, and panic attacks and was later diagnosed with PTSD. She uses NSAIDs, Zoloft, and clonazepam and participates in group counseling twice monthly. She complained that medications make her feel like zombie and she has not been able to maintain employment.

Initial PCL-5: 7/17 questions were rated with extremely severe symptoms.

### Initial Formulation and Dose

A full-spectrum (THC:CBD 1:20) liposomal product, 5 mg twice daily, was prescribed.

### Follow-Up

Follow-up questionnaire at 2 weeks showed all extreme severe symptoms were mitigated. At this point she revealed that she had been sexually abused by family member at age 7 that had only come to awareness 3 years ago and had deepened her depression.

At 4 weeks using 7 mg twice daily, she had 60% improvement in her symptoms and reports that her husband observed a major change in her behavior, mood, activity level, and overall performance. Her pain levels are significantly improved, and she is enthusiastic about her job with a car rental agency. She writes, "Is this feeling of relief really true?" And to other victims of assault and trauma, about medicinal cannabis, she said "you need to look into CBD because it can help you."

### Case Comment

This case is remarkable in the low dose and dramatic improvement across the full spectrum of symptoms along with the discontinuation of benzodiazepines to control anxiety. It also illustrates the common occurrences of adverse childhood events in clients with PTSD even if unreported.

## Case 2: Army Medic with PTSD

A 28-year-old US Army medic surgical assistant with a combat support hospital was stationed in Iraq during combat operations and experienced multiple roadside bombing and mortar attacks. In one episode he was briefly knocked unconscious. Shortly after he manifested symptoms of mental fog, anxiety, and depression and was diagnosed with PTSD. He was discharged in 2010 with Veteran Administration follow-up treatment with counseling and a list of medications which included Celexa, Zoloft, prazosin, Seroquel, Wellbutrin, Effexor, Adderall, nuvigil, and trazadone. All of these medications had failed to alleviate the symptoms, and many were often associated with adverse side effects. Despite multiple forms of therapy, he was unable to study, socially interact, or perform any meaningful work. He was chronically depressed with extreme moods and had considered suicide on some occasions.

His physical evaluation was normal and included multiple brain images that did not show objective signs of traumatic brain injury (TBI). He continued unsuccessful therapy for PTSD with multiple medications. He also tried a name brand medical cannabis 1:1 (THC/CBD) that caused him to feel very stoned and worsened his condition.

### Initial Dosing

He was assessed by teleconference and felt to have TBI with PTSD symptoms. A broad-spectrum CBD was recommended with very low THC (≤0.1%). His first dose was self-administered during a follow-up video conference. The dose was one quarter of a single serving, sublingually, which caused no adverse effect. A second application with one full single serving induced widening of the eyes, increased speech volume, a decrease in voice tone of about an octave, and improved enunciation. He also reported warmth over his face and chest. Visual perceptual changes include a sense of increased brightness, color perception, peripheral vision, and distance vision resolution. He reported improved clarity in thinking and processing. No anxiety or agitation was manifest. Twice daily dosing was recommended with additional doses as needed to control acute symptoms.

### Follow-Up

One week later he reported remarkable improvements in all areas on 30 mg/day. At 4 weeks he was interviewed by video conference. He reported 90% of his symptoms were resolved and he was planning to discontinue his other medications. He had formulated plans for returning to college and follow a career in psychology counseling. He also noted that his father who had been a helicopter crew chief in Vietnam had also benefited enormously with a brief trial of the same product.

### Case Comment

Blast injury can produce significant overlap in PTSD symptoms and potentiate neurodegenerative changes. Radiographic changes are subtle, often showing only volumetric changes. CBD has been effective in preclinical studies of TBI and should be effective in blast injuries as well. CBD may also stop neurodegenerative changes, improve blood brain barrier function, and reduce inflammation. The exact mechanism of improvement cannot be determined in this case. Another key observation is the adverse effects of THC that may be consistent with his sensitivity to other psychotropic medications. This suggests he may have some impaired metabolic pathways for drug processing and suggests initiating therapy with low doses of broad-spectrum medical cannabinoids.

## Case 3 War Photographer

The patient is a 66-year-old network news photographer and videographer with 35 years of experience covering war, violence, and disaster world events who developed progressive PTSD symptoms and impairment over the last 20 years that are now controlled with medicinal cannabis. After immigrating to Miami, he was subjected to ethnic-racial violence, abuse, and violence. His passion for photography abruptly extricated him into the news field with a penchant for covering violent situations unphased.

In 2001 he covered 9/11 World Trade Center attack at Ground Zero with exposure to massive destruction, human death, and toxic gases. He then took war assignments to Afghanistan for 6 years but was not exposed personally to blast or head injuries. In 2013 while filming in the Al-Shabaab Mall terrorist attack in Nairobi, Kenya, he noticed serious symptoms of anxiety, nightmares, cold sweats, and depression. In the past, faced with less difficult symptoms, he used alcohol and cannabis to control his symptoms and focus on his work.

On return home his marriage of 30 years dissolved, and he sought help at a California cannabis clinic. Cannabis improved some of his symptoms but failed to fully control them. While attending a cannabis exposition in Los Angeles, California, he sampled a high CBD low THC medical cannabis with substantial terpene beta-caryophyllene that was exceptionally effective for controlling his PTSD but without the anxiety symptoms related to THC. All of his symptoms were substantially improved using approximately 25 mg per day twice daily with supplementation during stressful periods. He optioned for less violent assignments in Washington DC and developed a deep loving relationship with a new partner. He made further improvements in PTSD symptom control using a medicinal cannabis blend with even higher amounts of beta-caryophyllene. He has chosen to retire but continues to take selective network coverage assignments while enhancing his fitness and resilience in a rural farm setting.

### Case Comment

This patient has several risk factors for PTSD including adverse childhood experiences, possible adolescent head trauma, exposure to repeated violence, and exposure to toxic chemicals known to be closely related to PTSD. He self-medicated with alcohol and cannabis, but this did not resolve symptoms, and these progressively worsened. A blend of low THC, high CBD with beta-caryophyllene is currently very effective for controlling his symptoms and improving overall performance and health.

## Conclusion

PTSD is a debilitating mental illness, variously described as an anxiety disorder, a disorder of dysregulation of fear and processing of stimuli associated with trauma, and a paradoxical disorder of memory. There is evidence that the endocannabinoid system is involved in the pathophysiology of PTSD, including findings that levels of endocannabinoids may be lower, and indications of changes in cannabinoid receptor levels in specific regions of the brain. Several lines of research indicate that medicinal cannabis may have a therapeutic role to play in alleviating some of the symptoms associated with PTSD. Animal research has helped elucidate potential mechanisms of action which two of its key constituents of cannabis, CBD and THC, may help address the pathophysiology of PTSD and reduce symptoms. Systematic review evidence suggests that cannabis and synthetic cannabinoids may have the potential to improve PTSD symptoms including anxiety, sleep disorders, and memory processes. In general, as with most clinical areas, more clinical research is needed into the efficacy of medicinal cannabis in alleviating symptoms of PTSD.

Although we have not discussed specific nutritional and lifestyle factors in this chapter, clinicians should address these factors, and perhaps others, in patients with PTSD to support the ECS, facilitate healing and prevent recurrence. Poor nutrition, for example, can enhance inflammation which may be part of the pathomechanism of PTSD, and can contribute to poor sleep and depression. Lack of physical activity is a risk factor for many illnesses, while there are clear benefits for physical and mental health of a range of exercise activities. Environmental toxins, workplace stress, home stresses, and many other factors can contribute to an unwell individual. Therefore, as always, we advise clinicians to take an integrative approach to address all the various factors that might be contributing to or exacerbating the condition of PTSD in their patient.

## Additional Reading

### Studies Evidencing Elevated Cytokines in Association with PTSD

| Reference | Study findings |
|---|---|
| Passos et al. [113] | Meta-analysis (20 studies) comparing individuals with PTSD and healthy subjects<br>Results: elevated levels of the following cytokines were associated with PTSD: interleukin-6 (IL-6), interleukin-1β (I1β), tumor necrosis factor-α (TNF-α), interferon-γ (IFN-γ)<br>Subgroup analysis of studies that excluded comorbid major depressive disorder: the three cytokines remained significantly elevated<br>Duration of PTSD was positively associated with 1β levels ($p < 0.001$), and severity was positively associated with IL-6 levels ($p = 0.042$) [113] |
| Hoge et al. [114] | Case-control study on peripheral blood markers for inflammation<br>Results: individuals with PTSD or panic disorder had significantly higher mean levels of 18 of 20 cytokines tested compared to matched healthy controls, including TNF-α, MIP-1α, GM-CSF, IFN-γ, IL-6, IL-1α, IL-1β, IL-2, IL-4, IL-7, IL-8, IL-10, IL12p40 and IL12p70, IL-13, IL-15, IP-10, and eotaxin (all $P < 0.0005$)<br>When a sub-analysis was conducted, for the PTSD group alone ($n = 28$), the following inflammatory markers were no longer significantly elevated compared with matched controls: GM-CSF ($P = 0.0071$) and IFN-γ ($P = 0.0072$) [114]<br>Study demonstrated a generalized proinflammatory pattern |
| O'Donovan et al. [115] | Study of 735 veterans<br>Results: increased inflammation was associated with current PTSD but not PTSD in remission, i.e., inflammatory markers for PTSD in remission were similar to veterans without PTSD<br>In patients with current PTSD, higher threat reactivity was independently associated with elevated inflammation, as evidenced by higher levels of hsCRP ($p = 0.01$) and higher WBC count ($p = 0.04$) |

## References

1. Bonn-Miller MO, Vujanovic AA, Drescher KD. Cannabis use among military veterans after residential treatment for posttraumatic stress disorder. Psychol Addict Behav. 2011;25(3):485–91.
2. Bremner JD, Southwick SM, Darnell A, Charney DS. Chronic PTSD in Vietnam combat veterans: course of illness and substance abuse. Am J Psychiatr. 1996;153:369–75.
3. Schierenbeck T, Riemann D, Berger M, Hornyak M. Effect of illicit recreational drugs upon sleep: cocaine, ecstasy and marijuana. Sleep Med Rev. 2008;12(5):381–9.
4. Kevorkian S, Bonn-Miller MO, Belendiuk K, et al. Associations among trauma, posttraumatic stress disorder, cannabis use, and cannabis use disorder in a nationally representative epidemiologic sample. Psychol Addict Behav. 2015;29:633–8.
5. Aoun J, Gerges E. Post-Traumatic Stress Disorder symptoms and associated risk factors: a cross-sectional study among Syrian refugees. BJMP. 2018;11(1):a1106.
6. American Psychiatric Association. Diagnostic and Statistical Manual 5 (DSM- 5). American Psychiatric Association; 2013. Available at: https://www.psychiatry.org/psychiatrists/practice/dsm. Accessed 20 Nov 2020.
7. Heinzelmann M, Gill J. Epigenetic mechanisms shape the biological response to trauma and risk for PTSD: a critical review. Nurs Res Pract. 2013;2013:417010.
8. Norrholm SD, Jovanovic T, Olin IW, et al. Fear extinction in traumatized civilians with posttraumatic stress disorder: relation to symptom severity. Biol Psychiatry. 2011;69:556–63.
9. Hauer D, Schelling G, Gola H, et al. Plasma concentrations of endocannabinoids and related primary fatty acid amides in patients with post-traumatic stress disorder. PLoS One. 2013;8:e62741.
10. Akirav I. Targeting the endocannabinoid system to treat haunting traumatic memories. Front Behav Neurosci. 2013;7:124. https://doi.org/10.3389/fnbeh.2013.00124.
11. Brewin CR. Re-experiencing traumatic events in PTSD: new avenues in research on intrusive memories and flashbacks. Eur J Psychotraumatol. 2015;6:27180.
12. Ehlers A, Hackmann A, Michael T. Intrusive reexperiencing in posttraumatic stress disorder: Phenomenology, theory, and therapy. Memory. 2004;12:403–15.
13. Perkonigg A, Kessler RC, Storz S, Wittchen H-U. Traumatic events and post-traumatic stress disorder in the community: prevalence, risk factors and comorbidity. Acta Psychiatr Scand. 2000;101(1):46–59.
14. Kessler RC, Sonnega A, Bromet E, et al. Posttraumatic stress disorder in the National Comorbidity Survey. Arch Gen Psychiatry. 1995;52(12):1048–60.
15. Solomon Z, Mikulincer M. Trajectories of PTSD: a 20-year longitudinal study. Am J Psychiatry. 2006;163(4):659–66.
16. Yehuda R, Bierer LM. The relevance of epigenetics to PTSD: implications for the DSM-V. J Trauma Stress. 2009;22(5):427–34.
17. Mahan AL, Ressler KJ. Fear conditioning, synaptic plasticity and the amygdala: implications for posttraumatic stress disorder. Trends Neurosci. 2012;35(1):24–35.
18. Uddin M, Aiello AE, Wildman DE, et al. Epigenetic and immune function profiles associated with posttraumatic stress disorder. Proc Natl Acad Sci (US). 2010;107(20):9470–5.
19. Laird CW, Alexander P. Prevalence of adverse childhood experiences among veterans. Clin Social Work J. 2019;47:384–93. https://doi.org/10.1007/s10615-019-00703-5.
20. Shah R, Shah A, Links P. Post-traumatic stress disorder and depression comorbidity: severity across different populations. Neuropsychiatry. 2012;2(6):521–9.
21. Shishko I, Oliveira R, Moore TA, Almedia K. A review of medical marijuana for the treatment of posttraumatic stress disorder: real symptom re-leaf or just high hopes? Ment Health Clin. 2018;8(2):86–94.
22. Vandrey R, Babson KA, Herrmann ES, Bonn-Miller MO. Interactions between disordered sleep, post-traumatic stress disorder, and substance use disorders. Int Rev Psychiatry. 2014;26(2):237–47.

23. Gradus JL, Qin P, Lincoln AK, et al. Posttraumatic stress disorder and completed suicide. Am J Epidemiol. 2010;171(6):721–7.
24. Kobayashi I, Boarts JM, Delahanty DL. Polysomnographically measured sleep abnormalities in PTSD: a meta-analytic review. Psychophysiology. 2007;44:660–9.
25. Neylan TC, O'Donovan O. Inflammation and PTSD. PTSD Res Q. 2019;29(4):1–4.
26. Roberts AL, Agnew JC, Blais D, et al. Posttraumatic stress disorder and incidence of type 2 diabetes mellitus in a sample of women: a 22-year longitudinal study. JAMA Psychiat. 2015;72(3):203–10.
27. Glaesmer H, Brahler E, Gundel H, Riedel-Heller SG. The association of traumatic experiences and posttraumatic stress disorder with physical morbidity in old age: a German population-based study. Psychosom Med. 2011;73(5):401–6.
28. O'Donovan A, Cohen BE, Seal KH, et al. Elevated risk for autoimmune disorders in Iraq and Afghanistan veterans with posttraumatic stress disorder. Biol Psychiatry. 2015;77:365–74.
29. Fraser GA. The use of a synthetic cannabinoid in the management of treatment-resistant nightmares in posttraumatic stress disorder (PTSD). CNS Neurosci Ther. 2009;15:84–8.
30. National Institutes of Health (NIH). Post-traumatic stress disorder. November 2017. Available at: https://www.nimh.nih.gov/health/statistics/post-traumatic-stress-disorder-ptsd. Accessed 23 July 2020.
31. Kessler RC, Chiu WT, Demler O, et al. Prevalence, severity, and comorbidity of 12-month DSM-IV disorders in the National Comorbidity Survey Replication. Arch Gen Psychiatry. 2005;62(6):617–27.
32. Merikangas KR, He JP, Burstein M, Swanson SA, Avenevoli S, Cui L, Benjet C, Georgiades K, Swendsen J. Lifetime prevalence of mental disorders in U.S. adolescents: results from the National Comorbidity Survey Replication–Adolescent Supplement (NCS-A). J Am Acad Child Adolesc Psychiatry. 2010;49(10):980–9.
33. AIPC Prevalence, Incidence, and Risk Factors for ASD and PTSD. Oct 27, 2015. Available at: https://www.aipc.net.au/articles/prevalence-incidence-and-risk-factors-for-asd-and-ptsd/. Accessed 27 Sept 2020.
34. McEvoy PM, Grove R, Slade T. Epidemiology of Anxiety Disorders in the Australian General Population: Findings of the 2007 Australian National Survey of Mental Health and Wellbeing Aust & NZ J Psychiatry. 2011; 2011;45(11):957–67.
35. Breslau N, Wilcox HC, Stor CL, et al. Trauma exposure and posttraumatic stress disorder: a study of youths in urban America. J Urgan Health. 2004;81(4):530–44.
36. Kulka RA, Schlenger WA, Fairbanks JA, et al. Trauma and the Vietnam War generation: report of findings from the National Vietnam Veterans Readjustment Study. New York: Brunner/Mazel, 1990. In: US Department of Veterans Affairs. PTSD: National Centre for PTSD. Available at: https://www.ptsd.va.gov/professional/treat/essentials/epidemiology.asp#three. Accessed 23 July 2020.
37. Kang HK, Natelson BH, Mahan CM, et al. Post-traumatic stress disorder and chronic fatigue syndrome-like illness among Gulf War veterans: a population-based survey of 30,000 veterans. Am J Epidemiol. 2003;157(2):141–8.
38. Tanielian T, Jaycox L, editors. Invisible wounds of war: psychological and cognitive injuries, their consequences, and services to assist recovery. Santa Monica, CA: RAND Corporation; 2008. In: US Department of Veterans Affairs. PTSD: National Centre for PTSD. Available at: https://www.ptsd.va.gov/professional/treat/essentials/epidemiology.asp#three. Accessed 23 July 2020.
39. Australian Government Department of Defence. Post-traumatic stress disorder. Available at: https://www1.defence.gov.au/adf-members-families/health-well-being/services-support-fighting-fit/mental-health-online/post-traumatic-stress-disorder.
40. Peterson T. PTSD from domestic violence, emotional abuse, childhood abuse. HealthyPlace. Available at: https://www.healthyplace.com/ptsd-and-stress-disorders/ptsd/ptsd-from-domestic-violence-emotional-abuse-childhood-abuse. Accessed 1 Oct 2020.

41. Golding JM. Intimate partner violence as a risk factor for mental disorders: a meta-analysis. J Fam Violence. 1999;14:99–132.
42. Breslau N, Kessler RC, Chilcoat HD, et al. Trauma and posttraumatic stress disorder in the community: the 1996 Detroit Area Survey of Trauma. Arch Gen Psychiatry. 1998;55(7):626–32.
43. Bisson JI, Roberts NP, Andrew M, et al. Psychological therapies for chronic post-traumatic stress disorder (PTSD) in adults. Cochrane Database Syst Rev. 2013;2013(12):CD003388.
44. NICE (National National Institute for Health and Care Excellence). Guidelines post-traumatic stress disorder. 2018. Available at: https://www.nice.org.uk/guidance/ng116/resources/posttraumatic-stress-disorder-pdf-66141601777861. Accessed 31 Mar 2021.
45. Kehle-Forbes FM, Meis LA, Spoont MR, Polusny MA. Treatment initiation and dropout from prolonged exposure and cognitive processing therapy in a VA outpatient clinic. Psychol Trauma. 2015;8:107–14.
46. Najavits LM. The problem of dropout from gold standard PTSD therapies. F1000Prime Rep. 2015;7:43.
47. Bernardy NC, Friedman MJ. Pharmacological management of posttraumatic stress disorder. Curr Opin Psychol. 2017;14:116–21.
48. Friedman MJ, Bernardy NC. Considering future pharmacotherapy for PTSD. Neurosci Lett. 2017;649:181–5.
49. Benedik DM, Friedman MJ, Zatzick Dm Ursano RJ. Guideline Watch (March 2009): practice guideline for the treatment of patients with acute stress disorder and posttraumatic stress disorder. American Psychiatric Association; 2009. Available at: https://psychiatryonline.org/pb/assets/raw/sitewide/practice_guidelines/guidelines/acutestressdisorderptsd-watch.pdf.
50. Stein DJ, Ipser JC, Seedat S, Sager C, Amos T. Pharmacotherapy for post traumatic stress disorder (PTSD). Cochrane Database Syst Rev. 2006;1:CD002795. https://doi.org/10.1002/14651858.CD002795.pub2.
51. Ipser JC, Stein DJ. Evidence-based pharmacotherapy of post-traumatic stress disorder (PTSD). Int J Neuropsychopharmacol. 2012;15(6):825–40.
52. Gotzsche PC. Deadly psychiatry and organized Denial. Copenhagen: People's Press; 2015.
53. Galatzer-Levy LR, Ma S, Stanikov A, et al. Utilization of machine learning for prediction of post-traumatic stress: a re-examination of cortisol in the prediction and pathways to non-remitting PTSD. Transl Pscyhiatry. 2017;7(3):e0.
54. Hoffman AN, Lorson NG, Sanabria F, et al. Chronic stress disrupts fear extinction and enhances amygdala and hippocampal Fos expression in an animal model of post-traumatic stress disorder. Neurobiol Learn Mem. 2014;112:139–47.
55. Miracle AD, Brace MF, Huyck KD, et al. Chronic stress impairs recall of extinction of conditioned fear. Neurobiol Learn Mem. 2006;85:213–8.
56. Berardi A, Schelling G, Campolongoa P. The endocannabinoid system and Post Traumatic Stress Disorder (PTSD): from preclinical findings to innovative therapeutic approaches in clinical settings. Pharmacol Res. 2016;111:668–78.
57. Bitencourt RM, Takahashi RN. Cannabidiol as a therapeutic alternative for post-traumatic stress disorder: from bench research to confirmation in human trials. Front Neurosci. 2018;12:502.
58. Trezza V, Campolongo P. The endocannabinoid system as a possible target to treat both the cognitive and emotional features of post-traumatic stress disorder (PTSD). Front Behav Neurosci. 2013;7:100. Available at: https://doi.org/10.3389/fnbeh.2013.00100.
59. Squire LR, Genzel L, Wixted JT, Morris RG. Memory consolidation. Cold Spring Harb Perspect Biol. 2015;7(8):a021766.
60. Van Marle H. PTSD as a memory disorder. Eur J Psychotraumaol. 2015;6:27633. https://doi.org/10.3402/ejpt.v6.27633.
61. Garelick MG, Storm DR. The relationship between memory retrieval and memory extinction. Proc Natl Acade Sci USA. 2005;102(26):9091–2.
62. Furini C, Myskiw J, Izquierdo I. The learning of fear extinction. Neuroscience & Biobehavioral Reviews 2014;47:670–83.

63. Milad MR, Pitman RK, Ellis CB, et al. Neurobiological basis of failure to recall extinction memory in posttraumatic stress disorder. Biol Psychiatry. 2009;66(12):1075–82.
64. Myers KM, Davis M. Behavioral and neural analysis of extinction. Neuron. 2002;36(4):567–84.
65. Ney LJ, Matthews A, Bruno R, Felmingham KL. Cannabinoid interventions for PTSD: where to next? Prog Neuro-Psychopharmacol Biol Psychiatry. 2019;93:124–40.
66. Milad MR, Orr SP, Lasko NB, et al. Presence and acquired origin of reduced recall for fear extinction in PTSD: results of a twin study. J Psychiatr Res. 2008;42:515–20.
67. Phelps EA, Delgado MR, Nearing K, Le Doux JE. Extinction Learning in Humans: role of the Amygdala and vmPFC. Neuron. 2004;43(6):897–905.
68. Ruehle S, Rey AA, Remmers F, Lutz B. The endocannabinoid system in anxiety, fear memory and habituation. J Psychopharmacol. 2012;26(1):23–39.
69. Walker MP, van der Helm E. Overnight therapy? The role of sleep in emotional brain processing. Psychol Bull. 2009;135:731–48.
70. Van Marle HJ, Hermans EJ, Qin S, et al. The effect of exogenous cortisol during sleep on the behavioral and neural correlates of emotional memory consolidation in humans. Psychoneuroendocrinology. 2013;38(9):1639–49.
71. Brewin CR. The nature and significance of memory disturbance in posttraumatic stress disorder. Annu Rev Clin Psychol. 2011;7:203–27.
72. Zuj DV, Palmer MA, Hsu CK, et al. Impaired fear extinction associated with PTSD increases with hours-since-waking. Depress Anxiety. 2016;33(3):203–10.
73. Suvrathan A, Bennur S, Ghosh S, et al. Stress enhances fear by forming new synapses with greater capacity for long-term potentiation in the amygdala. Philos Trans R Soc Lond B Biol Sci. 2014;369:151–9.
74. Lommen MJ, Engelhard IM, Sijbrandij M, et al. Pre-trauma individual differences in extinction learning predict posttraumatic stress. Behav Res Ther. 2013;51(2):63–7.
75. Hill MN, Campolongo P, Yehuda R, Patel S. Integrating endocannabinoid signaling and cannabinoids into the biology and treatment of posttraumatic stress disorder. Neuropsychopharmacology. 2018;43:80–102.
76. Heim C, Nemeroff CB. Neurobiology of posttraumatic stress disorder. CNS Spectr. 2009;14:13–24.
77. Malivoire BL, Girard TA, Patel R, Monson CM. Functional connectivity of hippocampal subregions in PTSD: relations with symptoms. BMC Psychiatry 2018;18(1):129.
78. Goode TD, Maren S. Role of the bed nucleus of the stria terminalis in aversive learning and memory. Learning & Memory 2017;24:480–91.
79. Berlau DJ, McGaugh JL. Enhancement of extinction memory consolidation: the role of the noradrenergic and GABAergic systems within the basolateral amygdala. Learn Mem. 2006;86:123–32.
80. Ji J, Maren S. Hippocampal involvement in contextual modulation of fear extinction. Hippocampus. 2007;17:749–58.
81. Perry C, Lawrence A. Fear, memory and brain exploration. University of Melbourne, 18 January 2021. Available at: https://pursuit.unimelb.edu.au/articles/fear-memory-and-brain-exploration. Accessed 21 Jan 2021.
82. Carrion VG, Weems CF, Richert K, et al. Decreased prefrontal cortical volume associated with increased bedtime cortisol in traumatized youth. Biol Psychiatry. 2010;68:491–3.
83. Kim SJ, Jeong DU, Sim ME, et al. Asymmetrically altered integrity of cingulum bundle in posttraumatic stress disorder. Neuropsychobiology. 2006;54:120–5.
84. Pitman RK, Rasmusson AM, Koenen KC, et al. Biological studies of post-traumatic stress disorder. Nat Rev Neurosci. 2012;13(11):769–87.
85. Merz CJ, Hamacher-Dang TC, Stark R, et al. Neural underpinnings of cortisol effects on fear extinction. Neuropsychopharmacology. 2018;43(2):384–92.
86. Rodrigues SM, LeDoux JE, Sapolsky RM. The influence of stress hormones on fear circuitry. Ann Rev Neurosci. 2009;32:289–313.
87. Shin LM, Shin PS, Heckers S, et al. Hippocampal function in posttraumatic stress disorder. Hippocampus. 2004;14(3):292–300.

88. Shin LM, Rauch SL, Pitman RK. Amygdala, medial prefrontal cortex, and hippocampal function in PTSD. Ann NY Acad Sci. 2006;1071:67–79.
89. Felmingham K, Kemp A, Williams L, et al. Changes in anterior cingulate and amygdala after cognitive behavior therapy of posttraumatic stress disorder. Psychol Sci. 2007;18(2):127–9.
90. Kim MJ, Loucks RA, Palmer AL, et al. The structural and functional connectivity of the amygdala: from normal emotion to pathological anxiety. Behav Brain Res. 2011;223:403–10.
91. Etkin A, Wager TD. Functional neuroimaging of anxiety: a meta-analysis of emotional processing in PTSD, social anxiety disorder, and specific phobia. Am J Psychiatry. 2007;164:1476–88.
92. Liberzon I, Taylor SF, Admur R, et al. Brain activation in PTSD in response to trauma-related stimuli. Biol Psychiatry. 1999;45:817–26.
93. Bremner JD, Randall PR, Scott TM, et al. MRI-based measurement of hippocampal volume in posttraumatic stress disorder. American Journal of Psychiatry. 1995;152:973–81.
94. Pavic L, Gregurekb R, RAdos M et al. Smaller right hippocampus in war veterans with posttraumatic stress disorder. Psychiatry Research: Neuroimaging 2007; 154:191–198.
95. Bremner JD, Randall P, Vermetten E. Magnetic resonance imaging-based measurement of hippocampal volume in posttraumatic stress disorder related to childhood physical and sexual abuse- a preliminary report. Biol Psychiatry. 1997;41:23–32.
96. Lindauer RJL, Vlieger EJ, Jalinka M et al. Smaller hippocampal volume in Dutch police officers with posttraumatic stress disorder. Biological Psychiatry 2004; 56: 356–363.
97. Stein MB, Koverola C, Hanna C, et al. Hippocampal volume in women victimised by childhood sexual abuse. Psychol Med. 1997;27:951–9.
98. Fennema-Notestine C, Stein MB, Kennedy CM, et al. Brain morphometry in female victims of intimate partner violence with and without posttraumatic stress disorder. Biol Psychiatry. 2002;52(11):1089–101.
99. Gilbertson MW, Shenton ME, Ciszewski A, et al. Smaller hippocampal volume predicts pathologic vulnerability to psychological trauma. Nat Neurosci. 2002;5:1242–7.
100. Bracha HS, Garcia-Rill E, Mrak RE, Skinner R. Postmortem locus coeruleus neuron count in three American veterans with probable or possible war-related PTSD. J Neuropsychiatry Clin Neurosci. 2005;17:503–9.
101. Schmeltzer SN, James P. Herman JP, Sah R. Neuropeptide Y (NPY) and posttraumatic stress disorder (PTSD): A translational update. Experimental Neurology. 2016;284(Part B): 196–210.
102. Ravindran LN, Stein MB. Pharmacotherapy of post-traumatic stress disorder. Curr Top Behav Neurosci. 2010;2:505–25.
103. Brewin CR. Coherence, Disorganization, and Fragmentation in Traumatic Memory Reconsidered: A Response to Rubin et al. (2016). J Abnormal Psychology. 2016;125(7): 1011–17.
104. Larkin KT, Brown LA, Tiani AG. Chapter 5. The autonomic and neuroendocrine response to stress. In: Chantler PD, Larkin KT, editors. Cardiovascular implications of stress and depression. Academic Press; 2020. p. 87–110.
105. Nachar N, Lavoie ME, Marchand A, et al. The effect of talking about psychological trauma with a significant other on heart rate reactivity in individuals with posttraumatic stress disorder. Psychiatry Res. 2014;19:171–6.
106. Pole N. The psychophysiology of posttraumatic stress disorder: a meta-analysis. Psychol Bull. 2007;33(5):725–46.
107. Griffin MG, Resick PA, Yehuda R. Enhanced cortisol suppression following dexamethasone administration in domestic violence survivors. Am J Psychiatry. 2005;162(6):1192–9.
108. Binder EB. The role of FKBP5, a co-chaperone of the glucocorticoid receptor in the pathogenesis and therapy of affective and anxiety disorders. Psychoneuroendocrinology. 2009;34(Suppl 1):S186–95.
109. Daskalakis NP, Lehrner A, Yehuda R. Endocrine aspects of post-traumatic stress disorder and implications for diagnosis and treatment. Endocrinol. Metab. Clin. N. Am. 2013;42:503–13.

110. Binder EB, Bradley RG, Liu W, et al. Association of FKBP5 polymorphisms and childhood abuse with risk of posttraumatic stress disorder symptoms in adults. JAMA. 2008;299:1291–305.
111. Wyrofsky R, Reyes BAS, Van Bockstaele EJ. Co-localization of the cannabinoid type 1 receptor with corticotropin-releasing factor-containing afferents in the noradrenergic nucleus locus coeruleus: implications for the cognitive limb of the stress response. Brain Struct Funct. 2017;222(7):3007–23.
112. Sinclair DA. Lifespan. Why we Age and Why We Don't Have To. US: Atria Books, 2019.
113. Passos IC, Vasconcelos-Moreno MP, Costa LG, et al. Inflammatory markers in post-traumatic stress disorder: a systematic review, meta-analysis, and meta-regression. Lancet Psychiatry. 2015;2:1002–12.
114. Hoge EA, Brandstetter K, Moshier S, et al. Broad spectrum of cytokine abnormalities in panic disorder and posttraumatic stress disorder. Depress Anxiety. 2009;6:447–55.
115. O'Donovan A, Ahmadian AJ, Neylan TC, et al. Current posttraumatic stress disorder and exaggerated threat sensitivity associated with elevated inflammation in the Mind Your Heart Study. Brain Behav Immun. 2017;60:198–205.
116. Schuster M, Fwyer PA. Post-traumatic stress disorder in nurses: An integrative review. J Clin Nursing 2020;29(15–16):2769–87.
117. Mealer M, Burnham EL, Goode C, et al. The prevalence and impact of post traumatic stress disorder and burnout syndrome in nurses. Depress Anxiety. 2009;26(12):1118–26.
118. Hosseininejad SM, Jahanian F, Elyasi F, et al. The prevalence of post-traumatic stress disorder among emergency nurses: a cross sectional study in northern Iran. Biomedicine (Taipei). 2019;9(3):19.
119. Sumner JA, Chen Q, Roberts AL, et al. Cross-sectional and longitudinal associations of chronic posttraumatic stress disorder with inflammatory and endothelial function markers in women. Biol Psychiatry. 2017;82:875–84.
120. Sumner JA, Chen Q, Roberts AL, et al. Posttraumatic stress disorder onset and inflammatory and endothelial function biomarkers in women. Brain Behav Immun. 2018;9:203–9.
121. Bella J, Kolatkar PR, Marlor CW, et al. The structure of the two amino-terminal domains of human ICAM-1 suggests how it functions as a rhinovirus receptor and as an LFA-1 integrin ligand. Proc Natl Acad Sci U S A. 1998;95(8):4140–5.
122. Rosette C, Roth RB, Oeth P, et al. Role of ICAM1 in invasion of human breast cancer cells. Carcinogenesis. 2005;26(5):943–50.
123. Papyianni A, Alexopoulos E, Giamalis P, et al. Circulating levels of ICAM-1, VCAM-1, and MCP-1 are increased in haemodialysis patients: association with inflammation, dyslipidaemia, and vascular events. Nephrol Dial Transplant. 2002;17(3):435–41.
124. Ramirez SH, Hasko J, Skuba A, et al. Activation of cannabinoid receptor 2 attenuates leukocyte-endothelial cell interactions and blood-brain-barrier dysfunction under inflammatory conditions. J Neurosci. 2012;32(12):4004–16.
125. Baker DG, Ekhator NN, Kasckow JW, et al. Plasma and cerebrospinal fluid interleukin-6concentrations in Posttraumatic Stress Disorder. Neuroimmunomodulation. 2001;9:209–17.
126. Koenen KC, Nugent NR, Amstadter AB. Gene-environment interaction in PTSD: Review, strategy and new directions for future research. Eur Arch Psychiatry Clin Neurosci. 2008;258(2):82–96.
127. Anastasia A, Deinhardt K, Chao MV, et al. Val66Met polymorphism of BDNF alters prodomain structure to induce neuronal growth cone retraction. Nat Commun. 2013;4:2490.
128. Koenen KC, Uddin M, Chang SC, et al. SLC6A4 methylation modifies the effect of the number of traumatic events on risk for posttraumatic stress disorder. Depress Anxiety. 2011;28(8):639–47.
129. Uddin M, Galea S, Chang SC, et al. Gene expression and methylation signatures of MAN2C1 are associated with PTSD. Dis Markers. 2011;30(2–3):111–21.
130. Wilker S, Pfeiffer A, Albert T, et al. Endocannabinoid concentrations in hair are associated with PTSD severity. Psychoneuroendocrinology. 2016;67:198–206.

131. Hill MN, Gorzalka BB. The endocannabinoid system and the treatment of mood and anxiety disorders. CNS Neurol Disord Drug Targets. 2009;8:451–8.
132. Parolaro D, Realini N, Vigano D, et al. The endocannabinoid system and psychiatric disorders. Exp Neurol. 2010;224:3–14.
133. Campolongo P, Morena M, Scaccianoce S, et al. Novelty-induced emotional arousal modulates cannabinoid effects on recognition memory and adrenocortical activity. Neuropsychopharmacology. 2013;38:1276–86.
134. Hampson RE, Deadwyler SA. Role of cannabinoid receptors in memory storage. Neurobiol Dis. 1998;5:474–82.
135. Marsicano G, Wotjak CT, Azad SC, et al. The endogenous cannabinoid system controls extinction of aversive memories. Nature. 2002;418:530–4.
136. Korem N, Zer-Aviv TM, Ganon-Elazar E, et al. Targeting the endocannabinoid system to treat anxiety-related disorders. J Basic Clin Physiol Pharmacol. 2016;27(3):193–202.
137. Hill MN, Bierer LM, Makotkine I, et al. Reductions in circulating endocannabinoid levels in individuals with post-traumatic stress disorder following exposure to the World Trade Center attacks. Psychoneuro. 2013;38:2952–61.
138. Morena M, Patel S, Bains JS, Hill MN. Neurobiological interactions between stress and the endocannabinoid system. Neuropsychopharmacology. 2016;41:80–102.
139. Neumeister A, Normandin MD, Pietrzak RH, et al. Elevated brain cannabinoid CB1 receptor availability in post-traumatic stress disorder: a positron emission tomography study. Mol Psychiatry. 2013;18:1034–40.
140. Neumeister A, Seidel J, Ragen BJ, Pietrzak RH. Translational evidence for a role of endocannabinoids in the etiology and treatment of post-traumatic stress disorder. Psychoneuroendocrinology. 2015;51:577–84.
141. Hillard CJ. Stress regulates endocannabinoid -CB1 receptor signaling. Semin Immunol. 2014:380–8.
142. Campos AC, Ferreira FR, da Silva WA, Guimaraes FS. Predator threat stress promotes long-lasting anxiety-like behaviours and modulates synaptophysin and CB1 receptors in brain areas associated with PTSD symptoms. Neurosci Lett. 2013;533:34–8.
143. Steiner MA, Wotjak CT. Role of the endocannabinoid system in regulation of the hypothalamic-pituitary-adrenocortical axis. Prog Brain Res. 2008;170:397–432.
144. Chouker A, Kaufmann I, Kreth S, Hauer D, Feuerecker M, et al. Motion sickness, stress and the endocannabinoid system. PLoS One. 2010;5:e10752.
145. Hill MN, Miller GE, Ho WS, Gorzalka BB, Hillard CJ. Serum endocannabinoid content is altered in females with depressive disorders: a preliminary report. Pharmacopsychiatry. 2008a;41:48–53.
146. Fidelman S, Zer-Aviv TM, Lange R, et al. Chronic treatment with URB597 ameliorates post-stress symptoms in a rat model of PTSD. Eur Neuropsychopharmacol. 2018;28(5):630–42.
147. Reich CG, Iskander AN, Weiss MS. Cannabinoid modulation of chronic mild stress-induced selective enhancement of trace fear conditioning in adolescent rats. J Psychopharmacol. 2013a;27(10):947–55.
148. Reich CG, Mihalik GR, Iskander AN, et al. Adolescent chronic mild stress alters hippocampal CB1 receptor-mediated excitatory neurotransmission and plasticity. Neuroscience. 2013b;253:444–54.
149. Bassir NA, Ricci B, Harpaz-Rotem I. Endocannabinoid system alterations in posttraumatic stress disorder: a review of developmental and accumulative effects of trauma. Chronic Stress (Thousand Oaks). 2019;3:2470547019864096. http://dx.doi.org.ezproxy.uws.edu.au/10.1177/2470547019864096.
150. Nia AB, Bender R, Harpaz-Rotem I. Endocannabinoid system alterations in posttraumatic stress disorder: a review of developmental and accumulative effects of trauma. Chronic Stress (Thousand Oaks). 2019;3:1–17.
151. Wang W, Sun D, Pan B, et al. Deficiency in endocannabinoid signaling in the nucleus accumbens induced by chronic unpredictable stress. Neuropsychopharmacology. 2010;35(11):2249–61.

152. Hill MN, Carrier EJ, McLaughlin RJ, et al. Regional alterations in the endocannabinoid system in an animal model of depression: effects of concurrent antidepressant treatment. J Neurochem. 2008b;106:2322–36.
153. Ganon-Elazar E, Akirav I. Cannabinoids prevent the development of behavioral and endocrine alterations in a rat model of intense stress. Neuropsychopharmacology. 2012;37:456–66.
154. Gunduz-Cinar O, MacPherson KP, Cinar R, et al. Convergent translational evidence of a role for anandamide in amygdala-mediated fear extinction, threat processing and stress-reactivity. Mol Psychiatry. 2013;18(7):813–23.
155. Danandeh A, Vozella V, Lim J, et al. Effects of fatty acid amide hydrolase inhibitor URB597 in a rat model of trauma-induced long-term anxiety. Psychopharmacology. 2018;235(11):3211–21.
156. Lim J, Igarashi M, Jung KM, et al. Endocannabinoid modulation of predator stress-induced long-term anxiety in rats. Neuropsychopharmacology. 2016;41(5):1329–39.
157. Bitencourt RM, Pamplona FA, Takahashi RN. Facilitation of contextual fear memory extinction and anti-anxiogenic effects of AM404 and cannabidiol in conditioned rats. Eur Neuropsychopharmacol. 2008;18(12):849–59.
158. Chhatwal JP, Davis M, Maguschak KA, Ressler KJ. Enhancing cannabinoid neurotransmission augments the extinction of conditioned fear. Neuropsychopharmacology. 2005;30:516–24.
159. Do Monte FH, Souza RR, Beitencourt RM, et al. Infusion of cannabidiol into infralimbic cortex facilitates fear extinction via CB1 receptors. Behav Brain Res. 2013;250:23–7.
160. Mayo LM, Asratian A, Linde J, et al. Protective effects of elevated anandamide on stress and fear-related behaviors: translational evidence from humans and mice. Mol Psychiatry. 2020;25(5):993–1005.
161. Yehuda R, Bierer LM, Schmeidler J et al. Cortisol metabolic predictors of response to psychotherapy for PTSD in survivors of the World Trade Center attacks on September 11, 2001. Psychoneuroendocrinology. 2009;34(9):1304–13.
162. Yehuda R, Southwick SM, Nussbaum G, Wahby V, Giller EL Jr, Mason JW. Low urinary cortisol excretion in patients with posttraumatic stress disorder. J. Nerv. Ment. Dis. 1990; 178(6):366–69.
163. Choi K, Le T, McGuire J, et al. Expression pattern of cannabinoid receptor genes in the frontal cortex of mood disorder patients and mice selectively bred for high and low fear. J Psychiatr Res. 2012;46(7):882–9.
164. Lisboa SF, Reis DG, da Silva AL, et al. Cannabinoid CB1 receptors in the medial prefrontal cortex modulate the expression of contextual fear conditioning. J Psychiatr Res. 2012;46(7):882–9.
165. Hill MN, Patel S, Carrier EJ, et al. Downregulation of endocannabinoid signaling in the hippocampus following chronic unpredictable stress. Neuropsychopharmacology. 2005;30(3):508–15.
166. Hill MN, McEwen BS. Endocannabinoids: the silent partner of glucocorticoids in the synapse. Proc Natl Acad Sci U S A. 2009;106:4579–80.
167. Scarante FF, Vila-Verde C, Detoni V et al. Cannabinoid modulation of the stressed hippocampus. Front Mol Neurosci 2017;10:411.
168. MacQueen G, Frodl T. The hippocampus in major depression: evidence for the convergence of the bench and bedside in psychiatric research? Mol Psychiatry. 2011;16:252–64.
169. Hill MN, Hunter RG, McEwen BS. Chronic stress differentially regulates cannabinoid CB1 receptor binding in distinct hippocampal subfields. Eur J Pharmacol. 2009;614:66–9.
170. Lisboa SF, Gomes FV, Terzian AL, Aguiar DC, Moreira FA, Resstel LB, et al. The endocannabinoid system and anxiety. Vitam Horm. 2017;103:193–279.
171. Lisboa SF, Niraula A, Resstel LB, et al. Repeated social defeat-induced neuroinflammation, anxiety0like behaviour and resistance to fear extinction were attenuated by the cannabinoid receptor agonist WIN55,212-2. Neuropsychopharmacology. 2018;43(9):1924–33.
172. Shosan N, Akirav I. The effects of cannabinoid receptors activation and glucocorticoid receptors deactivation in the amygdala and hippocampus on the consolidation of a traumatic event. Neurobiol Learn Mem. 2017;144:248–58.

173. Burstein OR, Shoshan N, Dorona R, Akirav I. Cannabinoids prevent depressive-like symptoms and alterations in BDNF expression in a rat model of PTSD. Prog Neuropsychopharmacol Biol Psychiatry. 2018;84(Part A):129–39.
174. Psotta L, Lessmann V, Endres T. Impaired fear extinction learning in adult heterozygous BDNF knock-out mice. Neurobiol Learn Mem. 2013;103:34–8.
175. Kozlovsky N, Matar MA, Kaplan Z, et al. Long-term down-regulation of BDNF mRNA in rat hippocampal CA1 subregion correlates with PTSD-like behavioural stress response. Int J Neuropsychopharmacol. 2007;10(6):741–58. https://doi.org/10.1017/S1461145707007560.
176. Ferreira-Vieira TH, Bastos CP, Pereira GS, et al. A role for the endocannabinoid system in exercise-induced spatial memory enhancement in mice. Hippocampus. 2014;24:79–88.
177. Ganon-Elazar E, Akirav I. Cannabinoids and traumatic stress modulation of contextual fear extinction and GR expression in the amygdala-hippocampal-prefrontal circuit. Psychoneuroendocrinology. 2013;38:1675–87.
178. Jiang W, Zhang Y, Xiao L, et al. Cannabinoids promote embryonic and adult hippocampus neurogenesis and produce anxiolytic- and antidepressant-like effects. J Clin Invest. 2005;115(11):3104–16.
179. Cameron C, Watson D, Robinson J. Use of a synthetic cannabinoid in a correctional population for posttraumatic stress disorder-related insomnia and nightmares, chronic pain, harm reduction and other indications: a retrospective evaluation. J Clin Psychopharmacol. 2014;34(5):559–64.
180. Stapelton JA. Trial comes too late as psychiatric side effects end hope for rimonabant. Addiction. 2009;104(2):277–8.
181. Castaneto MS, Gorelick DA, Desrosiers NA, et al. Synthetic cannabinoids: epidemiology, pharmacodynamics, and clinical implications. Drug Alcohol Depend. 2014;144:12–41.
182. Spaderna M, Addy PH, D'Souza DC. Spicing things up: synthetic cannabinoids. Psychopharmacology. 2013;228(4):525–40.
183. Fitoussi A, Zunder J, Tan H, Laviolette SR. Delta-9-tetrhydrocannabinol potentiates fear memory salience through functional modulation of mesolimbic dopaminergic states. Eur Neuropsychopharmacol. 2018;47(11):1385–400.
184. Stern CA, Gazarini L, Vanvossen AC, et al. Delta9-tetrahydrocannabinol alone and combined with cannabidiol mitigate fear memory through reconsolidation disruption. Eur Neuropsychopharmacol. 2015;25(6):958–65.
185. Bonn-Miller MO, Babson KA, Vandrey R. Using cannabis to help you sleep: heightened frequency of medical cannabis use among those with PTSD. Drug Alcohol Depend. 2014a;136:162–5.
186. Cougle JR, Bonn-Miller MO, Vujanovic AA, et al. Posttraumatic stress disorder and cannabis use in a nationally representative sample. Psychol Addict Behav. 2011;25(3):554–8.
187. Lake S, Kerr T, Buxton J, et al. Does cannabis use modify the effect of post-traumatic stress disorder on severe depression and suicidal ideation? Evidence from a population-based cross-sectional study of Canadians. J Psychopharmacol. 2019;34(2):181–8.
188. Greer GR, Grob CS, Halberstadt AL. PTSD symptom reports of patients evaluated for the New Mexico Medical Cannabis Program. J Psychoactive Drugs. 2014;46:73–7.
189. Resstel LB, Joca SR, Moreira FA, et al. Effects of cannabidiol and diazepam on behavioral and cardiovascular responses induced by contextual conditioned fear in rats. Behav Brain Res. 2006;172(2):294–8.
190. Lee JLC, Bertoglio LJ, Guimaraes FS, Stevenson CW. Cannabidiol regulation of emotion and emotional memory processing: relevance for treating anxiety-related and substance abuse disorders. Br J Pharmacol. 2017;174(19):3242–56.
191. Levin R, Almeida V, Peres FF, Calzavara MB, da Silva ND, Suiama MA, et al. Antipsychotic profile of cannabidiol and rimonabant in an animal model of emotional context processing in schizophrenia. Curr Pharm Des. 2012b;18:4960–5.
192. Lemos JI, Resstel LB, Guimaraes FS. Involvement of the prelimbic prefrontal cortex on cannabidiol-induced attenuation of contextual conditioned fear in rats. Behav Brain Res. 2010;207:105–11.

193. Stern CA, Gazarini L, Takahashi RN, et al. On disruption of fear memory by reconsolidation blockade: evidence from cannabidiol treatment. Neuropsychopharmacology. 2012;37(9):2132–42.
194. Norris C, Loureiro M, Kramar C, et al. Cannabidiol modulates fear memory formation through interactions with serotonergic transmission in the mesolimbic system. Neuropsychopharmacology. 2016;41:2839–50.
195. Corcoran KA, Quirk GJ. Activity in prelimbic cortex is necessary for the expression of learned, but not innate, fears. J Neurosci. 2007;27:840–4.
196. Murkar A, Kent P, Cayer C, et al. Cannabidiol and the remainder of the plant extract modulate the effects of δ9-tetrahydrocannabinol on fear memory reconsolidation. Front Behav Neurosci. 2019;13:174. https://doi.org/10.3389/fnbeh.2019.00174.
197. Das RK, Kamboj SK, Ramadas M, et al. Cannabidiol enhances consolidation of explicit fear extinction in humans. Psychopharmacology. 2013;226:781–92.
198. Rabinak CA, Angstadt M, Sripada CS, et al. Cannabinoid facilitation of fear extinction memory recall in humans. Neuropharmacology. 2013;64:396–402.
199. Hsiao YT, Yi PL, Li CL, Chang FC. Effect of cannabidiol on sleep disruption induced by the repeated combination tests consisting of open field and elevated plus-maze in rats. Neuropharmacology. 2012;62(1):373–84.
200. Ligresti A, De Petrocellis L, Di Marzo V. From phytocannabinoids to cannabinoid receptors and endocannabinoids: pleiotropic physiological and pathological roles through complex pharmacology. Physiol Rev. 2016;96(4):1593–659.
201. Passie T, Emrich HM, Karst M, et al. Mitigation of post-traumatic stress symptoms by Cannabis resin: a review of the clinical and neurobiological evidence. Drug Test Anal. 2012;4(7–8):649–59.
202. LaFrance EM, Glodosky NC, Bonn-Miller M, Cuttler C. Short and long-term effects of cannabis on symptoms of Post-Traumatic Stress Disorder. J Affect Disord. 2020;274:298–304.
203. Krediet E, Janssen DGA, Heerdink ER, et al. Experiences with medical cannabis in the treatment of veterans with PTSD: results from a focus group discussion. Eur Neuropsychopharmacol. 2020;36:244–54.
204. Bonn-Miller MO, Boden MT, Vujanovic AA, Drescher KD. Prospective investigation of the impact of cannabis use disorders on posttraumatic stress disorder symptoms among veterans in residential treatment. Psychol Trauma. 2013;5(2):193–200.
205. Roitman P, Mechoulam R, Cooper-Kazaz R, Shalev A. Preliminary, open-label pilot study of add-on oral Δ9-tetrahydrocannabinol in chronic post-traumatic stress disorder. Clin Drug Invest. 2014;34:587–91.
206. Tull MT, McDermott MJ, Gratz KL, et al. Marijuana dependence moderates the effect of posttraumatic stress disorder on trauma cue reactivity in substance dependent patients. Drug Alcohol Depend. 2016;159:219–26.
207. Wilkinson ST, Stefanovics E, Rosenheck RA. Marijuana use is associated with worse outcomes in symptom severity and violent behavior in patients with posttraumatic stress disorder. J Clin Psychiatry. 2015;76(9):1174–80.
208. Orsolini L, Chiappini S, Volpe U, et al. Use of medicinal cannabis and synthetic cannabinoids in post-traumatic stress disorder (ptsd): a systematic review. Medicina (Kaunas). 2019;55(9):525.
209. Hindocha C, Cousijn Rall JM, Bloomfield MAP. The effectiveness of cannabinoids in the treatment of Posttraumatic Stress Disorder (PTSD): a systematic review. J Dual Diagn. 2020;16(1):120–39.
210. Bonn-Miller MO, Boden MT, Bucossi MM, Babson KA. Self-reported cannabis use characteristics, patterns and helpfulness among medical cannabis users. Am J Drug Alcohol Abuse. 2014b;40:23–30.
211. Shalev A, Roitman P, Mechoulam R. Pilot open label trial on oral absorbable Δ-9 THC for chronic PTSD. Israel Soc Biological Psychiatry Abstract Book, Hagoshrim, Israel, 2013.

212. Jetly R, Heber A, Fraser G, Boisvert D. The efficacy of nabilone, a synthetic cannabinoid, in the treatment of PTSD-associated nightmares: a preliminary randomized, double blind, placebo-controlled cross-over design. Psychoneuro. 2015;51:585–8.
213. Bonn-Miller MO, Sisley S, Riggs P, et al. The short-term impact of 3 smoked cannabis preparations versus placebo on PTSD symptoms: a randomized cross-over clinical trial. PLoS One. 2021;16(3):e0246990. https://doi-org.ezproxy.uws.edu.au/10.1371/journal.pone.0246990.
214. Bonn-Miller MO, Brunstetter M, Simonian A, et al. The long-term, prospective, therapeutic impact of cannabis on PTSD. Cannabis Cannabinoid Res. 2020;274:298–304.
215. Shannon S, Opila-Lehman J. Effectiveness of cannabidiol oil for pediatric anxiety and insomnia as part of posttraumatic stress disorder: a case report. Perm J. 2016;20:108–11.
216. Elms L, Shannon S, Hughes S, Lewis N. Cannabidiol in the treatment of Post-Traumatic Stress Disorder: a case series. J Altern Complement Med. 2019;25(4):392–7.
217. Blair P. Pilot study: using CBD as a natural intervention for PTSD symptoms of post-service veterans. Poster Session. Integrative Healthcare Symposium, 2018, NYC.
218. Papini S, Ruglass LM, Lopez-Castro T, et al. Chronic cannabis use is associated with impaired fear extinction in humans. J Abnorm Psychol. 2017;126(1):117–24.
219. Calabrese EJ, Rubio-Casillas A. Biphasic effects of THC in memory and cognition. Eur J Clin Investig. 2018;48(5):e12920. https://doi.org/10.1111/eci.12920.
220. World Health Organization (WHO). World Health Organization Expert Committee on Drug Dependence. Cannabidiol (CBD) Critical Review Report. Expert Committee on Drug Dependence Fortieth Meeting Geneva, 4–7 June 2018. World Health Organization (WHO), 2018. Available at: https://www.who.int/medicines/access/controlled-substances/CannabidiolCriticalReview.pdf.
221. Doss MK, Weafer J, Gallo DA, de Wit H. Δ9-tetrahydrocannabinol at retrieval drives false recollection of neutral and emotional memories. Biol Psychiatry. 2018; https://doi.org/10.1016/j.biopsych.2018.04.020.

# Insomnia

# 8

## Introduction

Good sleep is vital for good health. Sleep is something we often take for granted, until we don't sleep well. Poor sleep can affect most, if not all, of us now and then, but for some, poor sleep can be chronic. When poor sleep becomes chronic, it can begin to affect health seriously. It is estimated that sleep disorders could contribute to up to 70% of diseases [1]. Sleep loss impairs cognitive performance; induces sleepiness, fatigue, and mood changes; and, in simulated driving, reduces performance [2]. Sleep disorders are common, with 13–33% of the Australian adult population have regular difficulty either getting to sleep or staying asleep [3]. In the USA in 2014, the prevalence of short sleep duration (<7 h) was 35.2% [4].

Sleep disorders are some of the more common reasons why people self-medicate with cannabis [5, 6]. Medicinal cannabis has, in fact, a long history of use in treating sleep disorders. Research indicates that the endocannabinoid system plays an important role in the regulation of sleep.

**This Chapter**

In this chapter, we will discuss the most common sleep disorder, insomnia, and examine how medicinal cannabis might be of use in its treatment. We will firstly examine why sleep is important, types of sleep disorders, our sleep-regulatory mechanisms, what insomnia is, and how it is treated. We will then explore how the endocannabinoid system is involved in our sleep, and what is happening in the ECS in insomnia. Then, we will examine the preclinical and clinical evidence for the use of medicinal cannabis, cannabidiol (CBD), and tetrahydrocannabinol (THC) in the treatment of these conditions. Finally, Dr. Blair will share some case studies from his practice.



K. O'Brien, P. Blair, *Medicinal Cannabis and CBD in Mental Healthcare*,
https://doi.org/10.1007/978-3-030-78559-8_8

## Sleep and Sleep Health

Sleep is a complex, reversible state in which the individual is perceptually disengaged and unresponsive to their environment [7, 8]. Sleep has a particular architecture or pattern, and the sleep-wake cycle is controlled by two main mechanisms which we will examine shortly.

Sleep health is defined as *"a multidimensional pattern of sleep-wakefulness adapted to individual, social and environmental demands, which promotes physical and mental wellbeing"* [7, 9].

What typifies good sleep health? Factors such as satisfaction, adequate length (not too short, not too long), appropriate timing, and high efficiency and sustained alertness during the waking hours are characteristics of good sleep health [7, 9].

## Why Do We Need Sleep?

Sleep is an integral part of our biological rhythm, is essential for health, and provides cyclical times in which the body can perform complex hormonal and neurochemical processes that keep us healthy. During sleep, our bodies repair DNA, build and repair muscles and tissues, and regulate weight and mood chemicals [10].

Some of the processes regulated by sleep include:

- Processing of memories and newly learned tasks
- Ability to perform complex and abstract tasks using higher cortical functions
- Hunger and appetite (via hormones leptin and ghrelin)
- Regulation of hormone levels (e.g., involved in normalization of blood sugar)
- Regeneration of cells (including muscles and tissues, liver regeneration)
- DNA repair
- Weight regulation
- Regulation of mood and behavior [10]

### Sleep and the Immune and Endocrine Systems

Sleep is restorative for the immune and endocrine systems. It assists recovery from the various influences and effects on our nervous system and metabolism during the waking state [7]. For example, sleep, particularly the N3 phase of non-rapid eye movement sleep (explained more later), promotes the release of prolactin [7]. When we are deprived of sleep, it adversely impacts on neuroendocrine function and glucose metabolism, and this can then impact on carbohydrate metabolism, as well as appetite, energy intake, and protein synthesis [7].

Acute sleep deprivation and disturbed sleep have been found to impair adaptive immunity, and this is thought to be due to decreased release of growth hormone during deep sleep plus increased sympathetic output [11]. The downstream effects of this are an increased susceptibility to infectious diseases and poorer response to vaccines [11].

## Sleep and Emotional Well-Being

Sleep is vital for our emotional well-being, and critical for regulating emotions as well as recovery from stress [12, 13]. Sleep deprivation makes people more sensitive to emotional and stressful situations and stimuli [13]. Rapid eye movement (REM) sleep particularly affects next day moods and emotions [13], and changes in sleep are likely to affect both physical and mental health, in particular if disease is also present [14].

Experiments have shown that sleep deprivation is associated with a more than 60% increase in emotional reactivity, demonstrated in brain scans of the amygdala. Why might this be the case? Walker explains that it appears that it has to do with the relationship between the prefrontal cortex (the area associated with rational thought and decision-making, which exerts top-down control on the amygdala) and the amygdala (key area associated with emotions). He explains that after a full night's sleep, there is a balanced relationship between these two brain regions, but when the person is sleep deprived, the prefrontal cortex is unable to regulate or control the amygdala sufficiently. Also, in the sleep deprived individual, the prefrontal cortex is unable to control the striatum (associated with impulsivity and reward) which becomes hyperactive in response to pleasurable experiences. Human experiments have demonstrated that sleep deprivation is associated with swinging between positive and negative extremes of emotional valence, and this could even explain the link between sleep disruption and suicide ideation and attempts found in adolescents [15].

## Sleep and Memory Formation

Sleep is important in our formation of memories. During sleep, unstable memory traces become re-organized into long-term storage (though this also occurs when an individual is awake). When we sleep, hippocampal-cortical firing patterns representing the stored memory during waking states get played back to the cortex, and this strengthens the cortico-cortical associations, thereby integrating it into existing cortical memory circuits [16]. Performance in abstract and complex tasks involving higher brain functions decreases more strongly following sleep deprivation than performance in simple memory tasks [17]. Total sleep deprivation impairs attention, working memory, decision-making, and long-term memory, while partial sleep deprivation influences attention, especially vigilance [18].

Sleeping after learning plays a vitally important role in enhancing remembering and avoiding forgetting. Experiments have shown that after a night's sleep, you regain access to memories that you were not able to retrieve before sleep [15]. Research has also shown the benefits of a nap on a task in which subjects were shown a list of words, with some tagged to remember and others tagged to forget. Half the subjects were allowed a 90-min nap and the other half remained awake. At the end of that period, they were asked to recall as many words as possible regardless of whether they had been tagged to remember or discard. They found that the more sleep spindles occurred (we will learn about these shortly), the greater the efficiency with which items tagged for someone to remember were strengthened, and those designated for forgetting were eliminated [15]. This experiment, and others described by Walker in *Why We Sleep* [15], brings home the fact that sleep is not something that is a random act of nature and that it is very much of intelligent design.

### Synaptogenesis

We need sleep for brain development. Synaptogenesis is the formation of new neural synapses. Sleep is involved in synaptogenesis and neural plasticity [15], and such sleep-dependent plasticity may be important in recovery from sleep conditions such as sleep apnea [19]. In the developing fetus, the growth of neuronal pathways and connections (synaptogenesis) occurs during REM sleep [15]. If infant rats are deprived of rapid eye movement (REM) sleep, it leads to disrupted development of the cerebral cortex [15].

In adolescence, synaptic pruning occurs in particular during deep non-rapid eye movement sleep (NREM sleep). Using electrical recordings of the brains of a cohort of children over the span of childhood, sleep researcher Irwin Feinberg found that during mid- and late childhood, children had moderate amounts of deep sleep during the times when the last neural growth spurts were occurring. When the brain switched from growing connections to pruning them, he found there was a sharp rise in deep sleep intensity (i.e., deep NREM sleep). Then, once pruning was nearly complete, the electrical recordings showed a decreased deep NREM sleep intensity [15].

Changes in deep NREM sleep have been shown to occur several weeks or months before cognitive and developmental milestones in the brain, suggesting that deep sleep drives brain maturation [15]. Animal studies support these findings in humans. Experiments have demonstrated that depriving animals of deep sleep blocked or delayed the maturational refinement of synaptic connectivity and development of social activity, plus other measures of self-motivated learning [20, 21].

## Sleep Needs Over Our Life Cycle

Generally speaking, we need at least 7 h of good-quality sleep per night. When people get 6 or less hours of sleep each night, there is evidence of increased vigilance objectively, even if they only subjectively experience minimal sleepiness [22].

Sleep needs change over our lifetime. Newborns enter active sleep (REM sleep) before quiet sleep (NREM) and have a shorter sleep cycle of around 50 min. At birth REM sleep constitutes about 50% total sleep, and by age 2, REM only constitutes 20–25% of total sleep. Newborns don't have NREM slow waves: these develop in the first 2 years of life. Slow-wave sleep (stage N3 of NREM sleep) decreases across adolescence by 40% from preteen years and continues to decrease thereafter, albeit at a slower rate, through to old age [23].

### Teenagers

Walker [15] points out in his book *Why We Sleep* that adolescent teenagers have a different circadian rhythm to younger children and that during puberty, the timing of the suprachiasmic nucleus shifts progressively forward. Thus, peak wakefulness will be around 9 pm at a time when parents of said teenagers are themselves starting to get tired. He advises that as parents, we should accept that teenagers are wired to obtain sleep at a different time. The good news is that when the teenager grows into young and middle adulthood, their circadian rhythm gradually slides back to an earlier schedule. He also points out that in teenagers, there is a need for a longer period of sleep. Thus, expecting them to get out of bed in time for school at 7 am alert and in a good mood is akin to asking yourself to get out of bed at 4 am [15]. For those who don't get up early to meditate, see how that works for you!

Walker also points out that sleep can be more problematic in older adults, and this may be related to health conditions and pharmaceutical medications. He says that the idea that older adults need less sleep is not true: older adults require as much sleep as they did in middle age [15].

### As We Age

The stabilization of deep NREM sleep that occurs in the early twenties does not remain stable for long. For the most part, REM sleep stays stable in midlife; however, deep NREM sleep starts to decline in our late twenties and early thirties. This means we get fewer hours of deep sleep, and the deep NREM brainwaves become fewer in number, and smaller and less powerful. By the mid- to late forties, we have lost 60–70% of the deep sleep we had as teenagers, and by age 70, we have lost 80–90% [15].

As we age, sleep also becomes more fragmented, which means we wake more during the night, and again this can be due to medications, illnesses, and in particular a weak bladder. Because of this fragmented sleep, there is decreased sleep efficiency. In teenagers, sleep efficiency is around 95%, whereas when in our eighties, it is often less than 70–80%. In comparison, sleep efficiency of 90% or higher is considered characteristic of good-quality sleep [15]. The problem with lower sleep efficiency is that it is associated with higher mortality risk, lower energy, and lower cognitive function, demonstrated particularly by forgetfulness [24]. Walker [15] cautions that there can be a failure to connect the deterioration in health in older people with the degradation in quality and quantity of deep sleep.

For more information and a very good read on why we need sleep, read Matthew Walker's *Why We Sleep* (US: Allen Lane, 2017). Another very good read is *ABC of Sleep* by Paul Reading (UK: BMJ Books, 2013).

## The Mechanism of Sleep

In this section we will look at the architecture of the sleep cycle, and what internal mechanisms operate within us to control sleep: sleep-wake homeostasis and our circadian rhythms.

## Architecture of Sleep

There are two states of normal sleep that alternate through night:

1. Non-rapid eye movement (NREM) sleep (75–80% of sleep time)
2. REM sleep (remaining 20–25%) [23]

Normally in young people, there are 4–5 cycles of REM/NREM per night. Deep NREM sleep dominates the first third of the night, and REM sleep dominates the last third [22]. This will have important ramifications as we will see later.

### NREM Sleep

NREM sleep was classically subcategorized into four stages (1–4), but this has since been revised to three stages, stages N1, N2, and N3 (combines stages 3 and 4), which parallel the depth of sleep (though we note many publications still refer to N4). Arousal thresholds are lowest in stage N1, with N3 (known as slow-wave sleep) being the deepest level of sleep.

Sleep normally begins in NREM and progresses through stages N1, N2, and N3 (deepest); then, the first REM sleep occurs. NREM and REM cycle every 90 min, but with the ratio of NREM to REM sleep within each 90-min cycle changes across the night. In the first half of the night, the majority of our 90-min cycles are made up of deep NREM sleep (stage N3 of NREM or slow-wave sleep), while in the second half of the night, most of the time is consumed by REM sleep with little, if any, deep NREM sleep [15, 23]. Walker explains that there is a reason for this difference in length of the NREM and REM cycles over the course of the night's sleep. It is related to the function of deep NREM sleep which is to "weed out" and remove unnecessary neural connections, while the REM state is involved in strengthening neural connections, in a sense a refining task. However, as a consequence of this skewing of REM/NREM sleep in the different halves of the night, if you wake up early at say 6 am instead of 8 am (having gone to sleep at 12.00 am), you are going to lose 25% of your total sleep time, but 60–90% of your REM sleep (as that is concentrated in the second half of the night). If you go to bed at 2 am instead of, say, midnight, and wake up at 8 am, you are losing a significant percentage of your NREM sleep [15]. Both these scenarios will have consequences for learning and memory formation.

NREM sleep is promoted in the anterior hypothalamus (medial and ventrolateral preoptic region) and GABA, adenosine, and PGD2 participate in regulation [25]. During NREM sleep, there is usually minimal or fragmented mental activity, low muscle activity, and minimal physiological activity, and there may be some dreaming [23, 25] though some authors state there is no dreaming in this phase [15].

When we fall asleep, the thalamus acts as a sensory gate to block the transfer of perceptual signals from our senses (e.g., sound, touch, sight) to the cortex, and the cortex enters a default mode of operation, that of slow-wave sleep (deep NREM sleep) [15]. During NREM sleep, our body temperature drops, heart rate and breathing slow, and the deepest stage of NREM produces physiological changes that increase immune system functioning [26].

### Memory

One of the major processes that occurs during NREM, particularly during stage N3, is consolidation of declarative memory [27]. NREM is responsible for making fact-based memories permanent—it is during slow-wave NREM sleep that memory packets of recent experiences are transferred from the short-term storage region (hippocampus, where memories are relatively unstable) to the more permanent and stable long-term storage site of the cortex [15].

### Sleep Spindles

Another thing that happens during NREM is the phenomenon of "sleep spindles." Sleep spindles are a burst of brainwave activity that occur during both lighter and deeper stages of NREM sleep. Spindles are involved in a repetitive pattern of activity between the hippocampus (memory storage) and the frontal lobe (the region programming the decision of intentionality, i.e., deciding this is important or this is not important). The cycling between these two areas of the brain occurs 10–15 times per second during sleep spindles and is a way of the brain ultimately deciding and selecting what to keep and what to discard [15].

## REM Sleep

In contrast, during REM sleep, there are characteristic episodic bursts of rapid eye movements (hence the name) and muscle atonia/paralysis (spinal motor neurons are inhibited by the brainstem, suppressing muscle tonus), and heart and respiratory rates are variable [7, 23]. REM sleep is associated with cognitive activity and EEG activation [7]. During REM sleep is when the most vivid dreaming occurs [15]. For these reasons, REM sleep has been described *"an activated brain in a paralysed body"* [23, p. 16].

REM sleep is promoted mostly by nuclei in the brainstem including the peduncle pontine tegmental, laterodorsal tegmental, and pontis oralis nuclei. The neurotransmitters involved include acetylcholine and glutamate and melanin-concentrating hormone [25].

REM sleep is vital to health, and many sleep disorders, including lack of sleep, are problematic due to the impact on REM cycle sleep [23]. Research on REM sleep indicates a role in memory consolidation, and it is likely that processing of emotional memories is an important function [22]. During REM, contextual memory and creativity is facilitated [27, 28].

In REM sleep there is a strong activation in the visual, motor, emotional, and autobiographical areas of the brain, with deactivation occurring in those areas controlling rational thought processes [15]. The emotional areas of the brain are around 30% more active during REM sleep compared to when we are awake. The areas that increase in activity during dreaming are the visual spatial regions of the brain (occipital cortex), the motor cortex, the hippocampus and surrounding areas (which supports autobiographical memory), and the amygdala and cingulate cortex (emotional areas of the brain) [15]. During REM there is a deactivation of the prefrontal cortex (which controls rational thought and exerts top-down control over emotional areas of the brain). During the dreaming state of REM, the sensory gate of the thalamus once again opens, but instead of allowing outside perceptions (e.g., sound, touch, etc.) to enter and travel to the cortex, this time it allows signals from emotions, memories, and motivations to enter the visual, auditory, and kinesthetic sensory cortices [15].

Reading [22] points out several interesting facts about REM sleep including the fact that there is no thermoregulation during REM, and therefore if a room is too hot or cold, arousals during REM sleep are likely. Depressed patients enter REM sleep more quickly, and most of the antidepressant pharmaceuticals delay or suppress REM sleep. Many drugs including alcohol also suppress REM sleep, and withdrawal of medications can cause rebound symptoms such as vivid dreaming. In rat experiments, preventing REM sleep for about 4 weeks was associated with fatal consequences for the rats [22].

Walker describes the role of the waking state as reception of the outside sensory world, deep NREM as a state of reflection that fosters the transfer of information and distillation of memories, and REM sleep as integration, whereby past experiences are connected with new ones [15].

## Our Internal Biological Mechanisms Regulating Sleep

The sleep-wake cycle is a complex and involves many complex neurobiological networks [29]. In the waking state, there are different levels of alertness, depending on activity, and several cognitive processes occur (such as attention and learning) [25].

We have two internal biological mechanisms which work together to regulate our sleep-wake cycle. These are our:

1. Processes of sleep-wake homeostasis (sleep homeostat; sleep pressure or urge to sleep accumulating in wakefulness; a function of sleep and waking)
2. Circadian rhythms (endogenous timing system, controlled by a circadian oscillator)

These two systems operate completely independent of each other although they are usually aligned [15].

### Sleep-Wake Homeostasis

Sleep-wake homeostasis, or sleep pressure (also known as process S), describes our innate drive or need for sleep, and this is a function of time since the last adequate sleep [30]. Normal sleep is an innate drive state, one which builds with prolonged wakefulness and is only satisfied by sleep [22]. Sleep-wake homeostasis keeps track of our need for sleep, and this homeostatic sleep drive reminds the body to sleep after a certain time and regulates sleep intensity. Sleep debt increases during waking and decreases during sleep *"within a range that oscillates within a period that is normally entrained to day and night"* by the circadian process (see below) [7].

### Role of Adenosine in Sleep Pressure

Adenosine accumulation in the brain plays a key role in regulation of sleep pressure. Essentially, adenosine builds up while we are awake, and as a consequence of increasing adenosine in the brain, there is an increasing pressure to sleep [15]. Adenosine promotes sleep and can inhibit arousal by blocking the orexin system (involved in wakefulness and arousal) [31]. During sleep, adenosine is broken down, and this is efficient if we have a full night's sleep. The problem with not getting enough sleep, however, is that adenosine concentrations remain too high, causing sleepiness into your day [15].

Adenosine agonists have been shown to inhibit cholinergic neurons, so it is thought that decreasing activity in the cholinergic, glutaminergic, and GABAergic cells in the mesopontine tegmentum region could facilitate sleep. Adenosine agonists inhibit the wake-active hypocretin/orexin neurons in the hypothalamus and disinhibit or excite the sleep-active neurons in the preoptic/anterior hypothalamic area and the ventrolateral preoptic area, while in the basal forebrain, they inhibit wake-on neurons [32].

## Circadian Rhythms

The second process involved in sleep regulation is the circadian rhythm, our 24-h internal biological clock (also known as process C). Unlike the homeostatic process of sleep, the circadian process is independent of sleep and waking and receives cues from the external environment [7]. Such cues include light and darkness, or other external cues such as food, temperature changes, exercise, and even regularly timed social interactions [7, 15]. Circadian rhythms are superimposed on the homeostatic sleep drive and confer different levels of sleepiness at different times of the day such as a decrease in alertness between 3.00 and 4.00 pm that occurs regardless of level of sleep [7].

### Control of Circadian Rhythms

Our 24-h biological rhythmicity is regulated by specific internal clock genes. The part of the brain primarily responsible for regulating our circadian rhythms (or chronobiology) is the suprachiasmic nucleus (part of the anterior hypothalamus), comprised of around 25,000 neurons [22, 33], though secondary clock systems have been identified in other parts of the brain and body [7, 34, 35]. All cells contain a core internal clock [30]. There have been several "core circadian clock genes" identified which are involved in regulation of circadian rhythmicity. These include CLOCK, BMAL1, PER1 (period circadian clock 1), PER2 (period circadian clock 2), CRY1 (cryptochrome circadian clock 1), and CRY2 (cryptochrome circadian clock 2) [36]. For the most part, autoregulatory genetic feedback loops driven by the transcription factors CLOCK and BMAL1 generate circadian rhythms [35]. As described by Lafaye and colleagues [33], BMAL1 becomes heterodimerized with the CLOCK (or NPAS2) protein which activates translation of other particular genes, PER and CRY, whose mRNA builds up in the cell nucleus in the morning, while in the afternoon, the PER and CRY proteins become heterodimerized in the cytoplasm and then phosphorylated by casein kinase 1. This then inhibits activity of the BMAL-CLOCK heteromer in the evening [33, 36].

The circadian rhythm is a little over 24 h: 24 h and 15 min approximately [15]. The brain uses cues called zeitgebers, environmental factors such as light, temperature, availability of food, and social interactions, to reset the circadian clock to 24 h. Photosensitive retinal ganglion cells in the eye carry information from light to the suprachiasmic nucleus via the retinohypothalamic tract. There are other inputs including afferents from the intergeniculate leaflet of the thalamus (integration of light and non-light information) and serotonergic projections from the raphe nuclei which are able to entrain the clock in a non-photic way, as well as affecting light input [37].

Circadian rhythms direct many different body functions, not just daily fluctuations in wakefulness, including body temperature, metabolism, and release of hormones. Circadian rhythms control the timing of sleep, causing us to become sleepy at night and wake up in the morning, synchronizing environmental cues (e.g., light, temperature), but they continue even in the absence of such cues [38].

**Role of Melatonin in Circadian Rhythms and Sleep Pressure**

Melatonin impacts on both aspects of regulation of the sleep-wake cycle, i.e., the circadian rhythm (process C) and the homeostatic drive to sleep (process S). It promotes sleep onset and continuity in a "hypnotic" manner by increasing process S and entrains and shifts the circadian rhythm [39].

The suprachiasmic nucleus instructs the pineal gland to release melatonin into the bloodstream, and this is the chemical messenger that signals that darkness is occurring to the body. In this way it regulates the timing of when sleep occurs; however, it does not influence the generation of sleep per se to any great extent [15]. Melatonin is produced from a pathway that includes serotonin and tryptophan. Melatonin is secreted at twilight, increasing to a maximum in the middle of the night [7]. Once sleep occurs, melatonin levels slowly decrease. When sunlight appears the next day, melatonin production from the pineal gland is suppressed, and the absence of circulating melatonin signals the brain and body that sleep is over [7, 15]. Most of melatonin's chronobiotic and hypnotic effects are mediated by MT1 and MT2 receptors which are located in the suprachiasmic nucleus in high density, and also in other areas of the brain and body [39]. Factors including light, medication, and behavior may alter melatonin levels [39].

**Chronotypes and Circadian Rhythmicity**

There is only a small range of variability in circadian rhythms in humans; however, there are differences between humans in terms of *chronotype*—the behavioral manifestation of our individual circadian rhythmicity [7]. Chronotypes are categorized into morning (14%), intermediate (70%), and evening (16%) types [40, 41], the first group being the "fowls" (those who are naturally early morning risers) and the last group being the "owls" (those who naturally like to go to sleep late). A person's chronotype is partly genetically determined, but there are cultural and environmental factors involved [41].

Because of this phenomenon of chronotypes, rigidity in work hours and school start times, to name but a few, can be quite problematic. For example, if you are an evening type, you will naturally go to sleep at a later time of the evening, but to get a good night's sleep, you will need to get at least 8-h sleep. Getting up at 6 am for work will cut that time short and, as we also know, cut down the amount of REM sleep you are getting substantially. Greater detrimental health effects occur in those with evening chronotype including higher rates of depression, anxiety, cardiovascular disease, and cancer [15].

Core body temperature and melatonin levels are markers for circadian processes [7]. Melatonin and adenosine are key chemicals involved regulating the sleep-wake cycle [30], though as we will see later, the endocannabinoid system is also involved.

## Regulation of the Sleep-Wake State

There have been various explanations for how the sleep-wake state is regulated. The two-process model for sleep regulation describes this interaction between the circadian system and the sleep-wake homeostasis (sleep pressure) system. Essentially sleep-wake homeostasis (process S) increases during waking and decreases during sleep, interacting with the circadian processes (process C) which are independent of sleep and wake states and instead receives environmental cues, e.g., from light and other external cues [7]. However, a three-step model of sleep regulation has also been proposed [42] in which sleepiness and alertness are stimulated by three factors, the homeostatic process, the circadian process, and a sleep inertia process which takes into account additional factors such as sleep onset latency, length, and performance [7].

### The Flip-Flop Switch Model of Sleep-Wake Cycle

The sleep-promoting and arousal systems are mutually inhibitory. A sleep switch model, also termed "flip-flop" model, has been proposed to explain the sleep-wake cycle. Essentially the brain has electrical circuits that switch on and off to promote the states of wakefulness and sleep, and these systems are mutually inhibitory (hence the name "flip-flop model") [7]. Activation of arousal systems inhibits sleep-promoting neurons, thereby facilitating wakefulness. Conversely, when sleep-promoting neurons are activated, this inhibits the arousal-promoting neurons, facilitating sleep.

- **Awake state**: orexin neurons promote the activity of monoaminergic nuclei. The monoaminergic cells (in the raphe nuclei, locus coeruleus, and tuberomammillary nucleus) directly stimulate wakefulness, and the monoaminergic nuclei also inhibit sleep-promoting neurons in the ventrolateral preoptic nucleus (which then relieves the inhibition of orexin neurons and monoaminergic cells).
- **Sleep state**: ventrolateral preoptic nucleus neurons promote sleep. Disinhibition of the ventrolateral preoptic nucleus neurons inhibits orexin neurons which then prevent activation of monoaminergic nuclei. The ventrolateral preoptic nucleus neurons inhibit the monoaminergic neurons and thereby relieve their own inhibition (which occurs in the wake state) [30].

### Brain Pathways, Neurotransmitters, and Hormones Involved in the Sleep-Wake Cycle

There are several brain areas thought to be involved in sleep control including the mesopontine tegmentum (part of the cholinergic arousal system), hypothalamus, basal forebrain, and reticular activating system [30, 32].

- Brain pathways involved in wakefulness include: the ascending reticular activating system in the brainstem (which contains monoaminergic, cholinergic, histaminergic, and glycinergic neurons). These project to several brain regions including the thalamus, basal forebrain, and cerebral cortex [30]. The state of waking is modulated predominantly by neurons in the lateral and posterior hypothalamus (synthesizing neurotransmitters such as orexins/hypocretins and histamine) and in the brainstem (synthesizing noradrenaline [locus coeruleus], serotonin [dorsal raphe nucleus], and acetylcholine [peduncle pontine tegmental nucleus]) [25].
- Brain pathways involved in sleep promotion include the ventrolateral and medial preoptic nucleus which inhibits the ascending reticular activating system [30].

### Neurotransmitters and Hormones Involved in Sleep-Wake Cycle Regulation

Several different neurotransmitters are involved in regulation of the sleep-wake cycle. These include serotonin, GABA, orexin, melanin-concentrating hormone, noradrenaline, cholinergic, galanin, and histamine [8]. Endogenous neurotransmitters categorized as primarily wake-promoting and sleep-suppressing include catecholamines, orexin, and histamine. Those which are primarily sleep-promoting and wake-suppressing include GABA, adenosine, serotonin, melatonin, and prostaglandin D2 [43]. These sleep-regulatory molecules interact in complex ways, and their effects are often dependent on the brain milieu or state [43].

An example of one of the key neurotransmitters is serotonin. Once considered the key neurotransmitter responsible for sleep, it is now known to be associated with both wakefulness and sleep, depending on the brain region and receptor type involved as well as the current behavioral state of the individual. Essentially higher levels of serotonin are linked to wakefulness and lower levels with sleep. During sleep, serotonin levels are lowest during REM sleep. Brain acetylcholine (ACh) levels rise when serotonin levels decrease. Some antidepressants such as selective serotonin reuptake inhibitors (SSRIs) inhibit REM sleep, supporting its role in modulating REM [44].

We will talk about the involvement of these neurotransmitters in chronic insomnia shortly.

### Factors Affecting the Sleep-Wake Cycle

Factors affecting our sleep-wake cycle needs include the following: exposure to light (greatest influence), stress, medical conditions, medications, sleep environment, and nutritional factors and diet. Blue light, eating, physical activity, and social activity are considered *zeitgebers* or time-givers, able to influence our endogenous rhythms [30]. Night shift workers can have trouble falling asleep when they go to bed and have trouble staying awake at work as their natural circadian rhythm and sleep-wake cycle are disrupted [38].

## Types of Sleep Disorders

There are several different types of sleep disorders. While many of these are associated with sleep loss, excessive sleep can also be problematic (as occurs in hypersomnolence disorder). Sleep can be examined from the perspective of quantity of sleep (duration) and quality of sleep [45]. Insomnia is the most common cause of sleep loss; however, there are several other causes including "chronic sleep restriction," defined as habitual sleep durations that are less than 7 h, but more than 4 h per night [46]. Chronic sleep restriction can occur due to work, medical conditions, or lifestyle [2]. Sleep loss can also be due to total sleep deprivation, as can occur in shift work, and it can occur in sleep disorders such as restless legs syndrome and sleep apnea [2].

A cross-sectional, population survey conducted in the USA between 2004 and 2007 found that 28.3% of adults sleep 6 or fewer hours (chronic sleep restriction), 8.5% sleep 9 or more hours, and only 63.3% sleep 7 or 8 h [47]. In Australia, around 16.6% and 13.9% of middle-aged Australians reported short and long sleep, respectively [48].

While much is understood about the detrimental effects of insomnia and shortened sleep, excess sleep also can adversely impact on health: long duration of sleep has been found to be associated with a significantly greater risk of developing or dying of coronary heart disease (RR 1.38), stroke (RR 1.65), and total cardiovascular disease (RR 1.41) [49]. In men, the European EGIT-RISC Study found that too little or too much sleep was associated with increased risk of diabetes or impaired glucose metabolism [50].

Common types of sleep disorders are set out in Table 8.1.

## What Is Insomnia?

The *Diagnostic and Statistical Manual of Mental Disorders, 5th Edition* (DSM-5) defines insomnia as difficulty getting to sleep, staying asleep, or having nonrestorative sleep despite having adequate opportunity to sleep, together with associated impairment of daytime functioning, with symptoms being present for at least 4 weeks [51]. Insomnia is characterized by an inability to initiate or maintain sleep

**Table 8.1** Types of sleep disorders

| Sleep disorders | |
|---|---|
| Insomnia | Nightmare disorder |
| Hypersomnolence disorder | Non-REM movement sleep arousal disorders |
| Narcolepsy | Rapid eye movement sleep behavior disorder |
| Breathing-related sleep disorders (obstructive sleep apnea) | Substance-/medication-induced sleep disorder |
| Restless legs syndrome | |
| Circadian rhythm sleep-wake disorders | |

American Psychiatric Association [51]

and can also include *early morning awakening* where the individual wakes up several hours early and cannot fall back to sleep. Insomnia often manifests as *excessive daytime sleepiness*, which can result in functional impairment throughout the day [52]. Insomnia is either transient, acute, or chronic:

1. **Transient insomnia** is a few insomniac episodes before or during a stressful experience [29].
2. **Acute insomnia** is generally triggered by a precipitating event, and occurs over a duration of less than 4 weeks. Once the event passes, normal sleep returns [3, 51].
3. **Chronic insomnia** is insomnia continuing for more than 4 weeks [51], and it tends to form a pattern of relapse and remission rather than resolving [53]. Chronic insomnia has a genetic component, with hereditary coefficients of 42–57%, and it is more prevalent in women (female to male ratio of 1.4: 1 which increases to 1.7:1 over the age of 45 years) [54]. An estimated 50% of insomnia cases are due to psychological factors including stress, anxiety, and depression [55].

Defining chronic insomnia is not necessarily easy due to the heterogeneous nature of the complaint. Broadly speaking, it includes any aspect of sleep including initiation, duration, consolidation, and quality [22]. Authorities consider that more than 30 min trying to fall asleep or a similar time spent awake after falling asleep constitutes significant insomnia, and it needs to be present for most weeknights for over a month and be associated with significant daytime impairment. This can include malaise, lethargy, and cognitive blunting, in particular on tasks requiring attention, and in severe cases, can dominate the patient's life [22].

## Subtypes of Insomnia

There are several subtypes of insomnia (all of which have been reported in association with aging) including:

- Sleep-onset insomnia: persistent difficulty in falling asleep
- Sleep maintenance insomnia: difficulty staying asleep
- Early morning insomnia: identified by early morning awakenings
- Psychophysiological insomnia: characterized by cognitive and behavioral elements, stress, attention bias, and intrusive thoughts [29]

### Insomnia as Primary and Secondary Phenomena

Insomnia may be a primary phenomenon, that is, reflecting an intrinsic sleep disorder, or it may be related to extrinsic factors including a medical condition, medications, environment, and other factors. Secondary insomnia is common in nearly all significant neurodegenerative and psychiatric conditions [22]. Some medical conditions which can be causes of secondary insomnia include asthma, esophageal reflux, nocturia and hyperplasia of the prostate, pain syndromes (including neuropathic pain, fibromyalgia, nocturnal headaches), and neurological conditions including restless legs syndrome and epilepsy [22].

## Prevalence of Insomnia

Insomnia is the most common sleep disorder, and chronic insomnia affects 9–15% of the general population worldwide, with a prevalence of approximately 6% in countries of high income [56].

The prevalence of short sleep in the USA, defined as less than 7-h sleep per night, is 35.2%, with much variability across races. The age-adjusted prevalence of short sleep duration was higher in Native Hawaiians/Pacific Islanders (46.3%), non-Hispanic blacks (45.8%), multiracial non-Hispanics (44.3%), and American Indians/Alaska Natives (40.4%) compared with non-Hispanic whites (33.4%), Hispanics (34.5%), and Asians (37.5%) [4].

## Insomnia Can Be Persistent

Insomnia is common and persistent in many, with older persons particularly vulnerable to persistent symptoms. A survey conducted in the UK for 2363 participants found that 37% had insomnia and 63% didn't at the start of the study. Of those without insomnia at baseline, the incidence of insomnia 12 months later was 15% and found to be significantly associated with anxiety, depression, and pain at baseline. Of those who had insomnia at baseline, 67% still had insomnia 12 months later, and persistence was significantly associated with increased age. Insomnia at baseline was found to be significantly associated with pain, anxiety, and depression at 12-month follow-up. This study demonstrates that pain, insomnia, and psychological distress are often comorbid [57], something that will be discussed in more detail later.

## Insomnia in the Aging Population

What is often overlooked is the fact that sleep becomes aberrant as we age [29]. Insomnia and excessive daytime sleepiness or hypersomnolence are common sleep complaints within the aged population [29]. Chronic insomnia has been found to affect 57% of the US elderly population [29, 58].

## Risk Factors for Short Sleep

There are several risk factors for shortened as well as long sleep duration. The 2004–2007 National Health Interview Survey Sample Adult Files in the USA which provided nationally representative data for 110,441 US adults 18 years and over found that the following were associated with both short and long sleep duration:

- Being older
- Being non-Hispanic black
- Being a smoker or former smoker
- Lower level of education
- Lower income level or few income sources
- Consuming few or numerous alcoholic drinks per week
- Reporting cardiovascular disease, diabetes, depression, underweight, or activity limitations [47]

Other variables associated with short sleep duration included living with young children, being unmarried, working long hours, and more frequent binge drinking [47]. Insomnia is more prevalent in women than men [60]. Other factors that can contribute to insomnia are an excessively sedentary lifestyle and very irregular sleep-wake scheduling during the week and on weekends [22].

## Comorbidities of Insomnia

Insomnia interacts with several different medical conditions. Comorbidities of sleep disorders include:

- Chronic pain [61].
- Neurological illness, e.g., >80% of MS patients suffer from debilitating fatigue symptoms and complain of significant sleep disturbance [61].
- Obesity (risk factor for cancer, cardiovascular disease, and others) [10].
- Altered moods, anxiety, and depression [62, 63].
- MS may also be associated with sleep apnea (which has been shown to respond favorably to treatment with THC in an animal model) [64].

Sleep loss causes impairment in cognitive performance, and it induces fatigue, sleepiness, and mood changes and has been shown to impair driving performance in simulated driving experiments [2]. In fact, lack of sleep has been found to be as dangerous as alcohol with respect to driving [2]. It has also been associated with motor vehicle and industrial accidents and increased all-cause mortality [48, 65, 66].

Partial sleep deprivation has been found to impact on glucose metabolism and neuroendocrine function which can lead to alterations in carbohydrate metabolism, protein synthesis, appetite, food intake, and protein synthesis [7, 8]. Of course, these factors are important in all people, but can be particularly relevant in athletes [8].

## Insomnia and Cardiovascular Disease

Insomnia has been found to be associated with a range of cardiovascular diseases (CVD) [49, 65, 67] and risk factors including hypertension [62, 68–70], diabetes [71], and obesity [72, 73]. Lack of sleep and shortened sleep duration result in decreased insulin sensitivity, increased cortisol levels in the evening, increased ghrelin (hormone that increases appetite and promotes fat storage), and decreased leptin (hormone that promotes satiation) [74, 75]. An Italian study conducted over 6 years found that each additional hour of sleep decreased the incidence of obesity by 30% [74].

Evidence from a systematic review demonstrates that shortened sleep duration is associated with a significantly greater risk of developing or dying of coronary heart disease (i.e., a 48% increased risk, with a relative risk of RR 1.48), and also an increased risk of stroke (RR 1.15) [49].

## Sleep and Obesity and Diabetes

Too little and too much sleep has been found to be associated with a higher risk of diabetes [71]. In a large US study conducted between 1982 and 1992, the odds ratio of incident diabetes over the follow-up period for individuals with sleep durations of 5 h or less was 1.47 (95% CI 1.03–2.09) and for those with sleep durations of 9 h or more, 1.52 (95% CI 1.06–2.18) [71].

Chronic sleep restriction may increase risk of diabetes and obesity through several different mechanisms of action. These include adverse impacts on glucose homeostasis, dysregulation of the neuroendocrine control of appetite, and reduction in energy expenditure [76].

Studies in healthy participants indicate that sleep restriction has an adverse effect on glucose homeostasis, associated with a rapid, marked decrease in insulin sensitivity (which is not compensated for by pancreatic beta cells), thereby increasing risk of diabetes [76]. Many studies indicate shortened sleep increases the risk of developing or having diabetes type 2 and impaired glucose tolerance [76–79]. This link between shortened sleep (as well as poor sleep) and diabetes risk is supported by prospective epidemiological studies in several populations [76, 77, 80, 81].

Multiple lines of evidence also link shortened sleep with obesity [76, 82], and of course, it is known that obesity is a risk factor for diabetes and other cardiovascular diseases, as well as cancer. This evidence includes cross-sectional studies in several different countries which have found statistically significant associations between shortened sleep and obesity in adults [82–85] and in children (e.g., Chaput et al. [86]; Seicean et al. [87]), as well as prospective epidemiological studies in adults and children (see Knutson and Van Cauter [76]). A meta-analysis of cross-sectional studies (over 600,000 adults) found an odds ratio for short sleep duration and obesity of 1.55 [82].

The pathomechanisms by which sleep deprivation negatively impacts on metabolism include upregulation of orexin neurons, increased sympathetic nervous system activity, increased evening cortisol levels, and increased daytime growth hormone levels which can all lead to increased insulin resistance and decreased glucose tolerance, thereby increasing diabetes risk [76].

Studies have demonstrated that the neuroendocrine control of appetite becomes dysregulated when sleep is restricted [76]. Sleep restriction impacts on two key hormones involved in appetite regulation, leptin (signals satiety) and ghrelin (signals hunger). A study of healthy men who were deprived of sleep (sleeping 4 h a night for two nights) found an 18% decrease in leptin, a 28% increase in the hormone ghrelin, and a 24% increase in appetite, with an increased urge for sweets, salty foods, and starchy foods (e.g., pasta, bread) [88]. Acute loss of sleep has been found to be associated with increased food intake and portion sizes [89, 90] as well as increased hedonic response to food and impaired ability to inhibit prepotent responses to rewarding food stimuli [91–93].

Less sleeping time can also mean more time to eat. Lack of sleep and associated daytime fatigue may result in less energy being expended, and this may occur through less physical activity as well as decreased non-exercise activity thermogenesis (NEAT). This reduction in energy expenditure could also link short sleep to increased risk of overweight and obesity (NEAT) [76].

### Insomnia and Anxiety, Depression, and Pain

Insomnia has been found to be associated with depression [59, 62, 63], anxiety [59], cognitive decline [94], cortical atrophy [95], and decreased immune functioning [96]. Epidemiological, cross-sectional, and prospective studies indicate that insomnia, chronic pain, and depression are mutually interacting, each increasing risk for emergence and/or exacerbation of the other [97].

Adolescent insomnia has been found to be a risk factor for early adult depression and substance abuse [2]. Night shift workers triple their risk of a mental health illness [1].

The presence of insomnia in anxiety disorders is associated with increased morbidity. For example, in PTSD, insomnia is associated with a greater likelihood of suicidal behavior, depression, and substance abuse [98]. The relationship between insomnia and anxiety disorders is also affected by comorbid depressive disorder [99]. Insomnia is a common side effect of antidepressants, so it is important to check the potential side effects of antidepressants in patients who are taking these and reporting insomnia [100].

A study in the UK found that patients with musculoskeletal pain had a significantly higher prevalence of insomnia (difference 25.5%, $p < 0.0001$), anxiety (difference 24.3%, $p < 0.0001$), and depressive symptoms (difference 11%, $p < 0.0001$) compared with those without such pain. Patients with both musculoskeletal pain and insomnia had significantly higher levels of anxiety and symptoms of depression compared with patients who had musculoskeletal pain but not insomnia ($p < 0.0001$), and these remained significant after controlling for age, sex, and body mass index in statistical analysis [101].

Sleep monitoring of patients with advanced cancers demonstrated opioid treatment, and pain disrupted nocturnal sleep, prolonged sleep latency, and limited attainment of stages 3 and 4 NREM sleep as well as REM sleep [102]. Such sleep disturbances were found to be due to opioid treatment itself, which contributed to depression and enhanced pain [103]. Therefore, there is a need for new approaches to the management of chronic pain and resultant sleep disorders [61].

### Insomnia and PTSD

As we saw in the last chapter, sleep disturbances (e.g., insomnia, daytime sleepiness, nightmares) are hallmark features of PTSD [51, 104, 105]. Studies have shown that PTSD sufferers experience more stage 1 sleep and less slow-wave sleep (NREM sleep, indicative of more shallow sleeping) and greater rapid eye movement density [106]. There is evidence that PTSD sufferers engage in substance abuse in order to cope with these symptoms: rates of substance abuse are much higher in those with PTSD, and this relationship is partly mediated by sleep problems [107].

### Insomnia and Cognition

It is generally agreed that insufficient sleep leads to slower response speed and greater performance variability for simple measures of alertness, attention, and vigilance [108]. There is less agreement in the literature, however, about the effect of lack of sleep on higher-order cognitive functions (e.g., perception, memory, and executive functions), in particular if it affects cognitive abilities globally or whether it affects some aspects more specifically [108].

Neuroimaging studies suggest the prefrontal cortex may be affected by sleep deprivation, but executive function tasks that assess prefrontal functioning have not found consistent results. It seems that some aspects of higher-level cortical function remain degraded after sleep deprivation, even when alertness and vigilance have been restored. Increasingly, evidence indicates a lack of sleep may affect cognitive systems that rely in particular on emotional data or information [108].

### Insomnia and Cancer

Insomnia occurs at a much higher rate (three times) in cancer patients than the general population [109], affecting up to 50% of cancer patients [110, 111]. There are many factors that might lead to disruption of sleep in cancer patients, including anxiety and cancer-related pain, for example, as well as treatments such as chemotherapy, radiotherapy, use of corticosteroids (e.g., dexamethasone), use of antiepileptics (in treatment of brain tumors), and psychoactive medications. In those with brain tumors, damage to the brain parenchyma from the tumor or its surgical treatment might also be involved [111]. In patients with recurrent glial tumors, for example, 46.8% of patients reported insomnia, with around 20% using sleep medication. In this study, corticosterone use was significantly associated with insomnia [111].

Looking at it from the other direction, though, there is some evidence that disruption and sleep loss are associated with increased risk of prostate cancer [112] and longer sleep duration with colorectal cancer [113].

## Inflammation, Immune Function, and Sleep

How poor sleep affects the body at the cellular level is complex. Sleep disturbance including short sleep is a risk factor for inflammation [45], and as it is well known, inflammation underpins many (if not all) chronic illnesses such as cardiovascular disease and cancer.

Research indicates that sleep is involved in the regulation of inflammatory cytokines and hormones. Sleep is involved in the nocturnal regulation of interleukin-6 (IL-6) as well as growth hormone: analysis of sleep stages in healthy males showed that there was a nocturnal increase in IL-6 associated with stage 1–2 sleep and REM sleep (though levels during slow-wave sleep were no different from those while awake), and growth hormone showed a similar pattern. In contrast, melatonin and cortisol levels showed no concordance with sleep [114]. The authors of this study posited that given the association between increases in IL-6 and REM sleep, disturbances in sleep architecture could interfere with sleep-associated IL-6 release. They suggest that in depression as well as aging where REM sleep is increased at the expense of slow-wave sleep, abnormal elevations in IL-6 might occur, with consequent implications for inflammatory disease risk [114].

Loss of sleep can induce a functional alteration of the monocyte proinflammatory response and the molecular processes controlling cellular immune activation and inducing inflammatory cytokines. IL-6 plays an important part in the function and regulation of the immune system's peripheral blood mononuclear cells. It is an inflammatory cytokine which causes fatigue and somnolence and activation of the HPA axis [115], and is under the tonic negative control of glucocorticoids [116]. It is secreted during stress and is positively controlled by catecholamines. IL-6 stimulates secretion of growth hormone, as well as inhibiting thyroid-stimulating hormone secretion and decreasing serum lipid concentrations [116].

IL-6 may be involved in sleep mediation and may be influenced by circadian and homeostatic processes [115]. Circulating levels of IL-6 are low during the day and higher at night under normal circumstances. A night of total sleep loss in healthy young men was associated with a significant shift in the circadian secretion of IL-6, with undersecretion of IL-6 at nighttime and a significant increase in circulating IL-6 levels the following day along with increased sleepiness, and fatigue [115]. Levels of IL-6 during the day were negatively related to the amount of nocturnal sleep. The daytime oversecretion of IL-6 may be responsible for the fatigue and somnolence experienced during the day. This study suggests that having a good night's sleep is associated with lower daytime secretion of IL-6 and therefore decreased exposure to the proinflammatory effects of this cytokine [115].

In another study, sleep loss was found to induce a significantly greater monocyte production of IL-6 and TNF-$\alpha$, and a three- and twofold increase in transcription of IL mRNA and TNF-$\alpha$ mRNA, respectively [117]. Sleep loss was also found to be associated with changes in NF-$\kappa$B in a small study of 14 healthy volunteers (7 women, 7 men): there was a significantly greater level of mononuclear cell NF-$\kappa$B activation the morning after a night of sleep loss compared with morning levels after uninterrupted baseline sleep in women though not in men [118]. The authors of this study concluded that NF-κB activation may be a molecular pathway by which disturbed sleep might impact on leukocyte inflammatory gene expression and risk of inflammation-associated illness [118].

Sleep restriction of young healthy adults to 6 h per night for 1 week was associated with significantly increased sleepiness, impaired psychomotor performance, and increased secretion of proinflammatory cytokines, evidenced by an increase in the 24-h secretory profile of IL-6 (both genders), an increase in TNF-α (men), and lower peak cortisol secretion (compared to baseline) [119]. Another study showed that sleep restriction to 4 h/day for 6 days was associated with significant impairment of glucose metabolism [120].

### Meta-analysis

A meta-analysis of 72 studies found that sleep disturbance was associated with statistically significant increases in levels of two markers of systemic inflammation, C-reactive protein (CRP) and IL-6 [121]. You will recall that CRP is an acute-phase protein of hepatic origin that increases following IL-6 secretion by macrophages and T cells that targets lysophosphatidylcholine on the surface of dead or dying cells (and some types of bacteria) in order to activate the complement system [122]. An interesting fact reported in this systematic review was that it appears women may be more susceptible to the ill effects of sleep disturbance than men, as individual studies showed greater increases in CRP and IL-6, greater increase in NF-κB, and greater increase in toll-like receptor 4 (TLR-4) simulated monocyte production of inflammatory cytokines (see Irwin et al. [121] for individual studies).

## Treatment of Insomnia

There are a variety of treatment options for insomnia including sleep hygiene recommendations, acupuncture, psychological therapies such as cognitive behavioral therapy, hypnotherapy, pharmaceutical approaches, and more. Changes such as sleeping on a regular schedule, exercising, avoiding caffeine, reducing stress, and avoiding daytime naps can be all help [123].

### Cognitive Behavioral Therapy

Cognitive behavioral therapy (CBT) is usually the first-line therapy for treatment of insomnia [54, 123] with research indicating that it can be equally or more effective than pharmaceutical medication for chronic insomnia [124, 125] (Mayo Clinic). In CBT, the patient works with a therapist who guides them to identify beliefs, thoughts, and behaviors that contribute to poor sleep and replace them with those that contribute to good sleep. CBTY techniques include sleep restriction, relaxation training, stimulus control therapy, remaining passively awake, and light therapy [123].

### Pharmaceutical Approaches

Pharmaceutical approaches to treatment of insomnia include hypnotics and benzodiazepines, benzodiazepine receptor agonists, antidepressants, dopamine-blocking agents, antiepilepsy drugs, analgesics, antihistamines (e.g., medicines containing diphenhydramine), and melatonin [22, 126]. Hypnotics are the most common class of drugs used to treat insomnia; however, there are concerns about tolerance, morning side effects, and, in some cases, addiction [22].

In general, the problem with pharmaceuticals used to treat insomnia is that many are associated with side effects, some can be addictive, and many don't work well. For example, many drugs including benzodiazepines and most antidepressants produce drowsiness but often do not improve quality of sleep, and rarely do hypnotic or sedative drugs increase or improve deeper NREM sleep states [22].

## Pathophysiology of Insomnia

There are several models of insomnia that have been developed to explain its pathogenesis. These include the hyperarousal theory, the local sleep theory, the neurocognitive model, the REM sleep instability model, the psychologic inhibition model, and the cognitive model [43]. Other factors that may be involved in the pathophysiology of insomnia include genetics, neuroanatomical changes in particular brain regions, and alterations in hormones and neurotransmitters involved in sleep regulation. We will discuss these briefly. Readers are referred to Levenson et al. [43] for an in-depth discussion of these.

### Hyperarousal Theory of Insomnia

Insomnia is considered a disorder of hyperarousal of both central and peripheral nervous systems, i.e., cortical and autonomic. The term hyperarousal may also refer to hyperarousal of emotional and cognitive processes. Hyperarousal has been conceptualized as *"heightened physiologic, affective or cognitive activity, which interferes with the natural 'disengagement from […] the environment' and decreases the likelihood of sleep"* [43]. Hyperarousal may be detected by objective markers such as increased cortisol levels, EEG, and heart rate variability, and it may also be reported by the individual subjectively, for example, the experience of not being able to switch off. Cognitive and affective hyperarousal at bedtime has been hypothesized to contribute to acute and chronic insomnia [43].

However, according to Levenson et al. [43], despite evidence in support of the hyperarousal theory, for example, changes in various markers of physiologic arousal (cortisol, adrenocorticotropic hormone) recorded in insomniacs, there are some as-yet unresolved issues including whether hyperarousal is a cause or effect of insomnia. They also state that therapies that address hyperarousal such as relaxation training are often not as effective as therapies targeting enhancement of sleep processes like sleep restriction. Finally, they point out that physiologic markers of hyperarousal could just as easily be seen as insufficient inhibition of arousal by sleep-promoting processes [43].

## Other Models of Insomnia

Other theories of insomnia such as the local sleep theory center on the idea that synchronous firing in cortical columns locally propagates slow-wave activity in surrounding regions, leading to a global sleep state. Another theory is based on the two-process model described earlier, in which insufficient sleep propensity occurs due to dysfunction of the S or C (sleep pressure or circadian) processes. Yet another theory posits that the overriding of the flip-flop switch (described earlier) underlies insomnia and that chronic coactivation of sleep and wake circuits during the desired sleep period is the underlying problem. Others have suggested that in insomnia, individuals transition rapidly in and out of sleep-wake states (like a flickering switch) [43].

The neurocognitive model of insomnia suggests that acute insomnia is the result of maladaptive coping strategies and may develop into chronic insomnia due to conditioned arousal. The REM sleep instability model suggests that insomnia is related to decreased percentage of REM sleep and increased REM EEG arousals. The "3P model" describes predisposing, precipitating, and perpetuating factors that contribute to insomnia development and maintenance. Examples of perpetuating factors are behaviors and beliefs which serve to maintain insomnia including the idea of "catch-up sleep" [43].

In the cognitive model of insomnia, it is argued that insomniacs are prone to excessive worry and intrusive thoughts, in particular about getting enough sleep, which can develop into sleep-related anxiety and increased vigilance leading to an exaggeration of sleep disruption. A related theory is the psychologic inhibition model where sleep is seen as automatic and insomnia a failure of automatic sleep [43].

## Genetics and Insomnia

Genetics are understood to play a role in the pathophysiology of insomnia, with several gene variants associated with insomnia. In a 2017 study of 113,006 individuals, researchers found 7 genes associated with insomnia, and the one gene most strongly associated with insomnia complaints (MEIS1) was also associated with restless legs syndrome. Significant correlations were found between insomnia complaints and ten other traits, with strong positive genetic correlations found with anxiety, depressive symptoms, neuroticism, and major depressive disorder, and positive but weaker correlations with metabolic traits including diabetes type 2, waist circumference, waist-to-hip ratio, and body mass index. There were also substantial negative genetic correlations between insomnia complaints and subjective well-being and educational attainment [127].

## Neuroanatomical and Functional Brain Changes in Insomnia

Studies of the brains of animals and humans have identified brain regions that are linked with insomnia. For example, patients with insomnia have been found to have gray matter volume changes in the cerebellum and the lingual, precentral, and postcentral gyri compared with controls [128]. Interestingly, these areas were also found to show a similar pattern in migraine sufferers [128].

Other studies in humans have found reduced gray matter volume in several brain areas including left orbitofrontal, prefrontal, precuneus, and temporal cortices in insomniacs, and in animal studies, lesions in various areas including the thalamus, raphe nucleus, and mediobasal preoptic area have been found to result in insomnia [43]. An activation likelihood estimation meta-analysis for multimodal neuroimaging in insomnia indicated that insomnia patients showed significant gray matter reductions in the right middle frontal gyrus compared with healthy controls [129]. In positron-emission tomography studies, analysis indicated reduced relative cerebral glucose metabolism in the right amygdala, right anterior cingulate cortex, and right posterior cingulate gyrus in insomniacs compared with healthy controls. When this study examined diffusion tensor imaging studies, insomnia sufferers showed reduced fractional anisotropy values in the left putamen and right caudate body, and reduced regional homogeneity in several brain regions, compared with healthy controls [129].

## Neurotransmitter and Hormone Involvement in Insomnia

We have seen that there are many different neurotransmitters and hormones involved in regulation of the sleep-wake cycle. If we look at the effects of particular drugs used to treat insomnia, we see a range of neurotransmitters targeted. For example, benzodiazepine receptor agonists promote sleep by enhancing the inhibitory action of GABA, while the sedative effects of drugs like doxepin (tricyclic) and trazodone are achieved by targeting the histaminergic arousal system, and new drugs such as suvorexant are orexin receptor antagonists [43].

According to Levenson et al. [43], there has been no consistent pattern which emerges from the studies into the role of wake- and sleep-promoting molecules in insomnia. While a few molecular studies have been carried out in insomnia (e.g., investigating levels of calcium, GABA, melatonin, noradrenaline, corticotropin-releasing hormone, adrenocorticotropic hormone, and cortisol in insomniacs versus controls), findings have been mixed, though attempts have been made to explain findings within the context of the hyperarousal hypothesis. The complicating issue is the complexity with which sleep-regulatory molecules interact with each other and effects often depend on the brain milieu, so it is unlikely that changes in one type of molecule will be the key to explaining all cases of insomnia—it appears far more complex than that. Levenson et al. [43] suggest that a better way of thinking about it may be that chronic insomnia is due to a breakdown of the alternating rhythms of wake- and sleep-regulatory molecules in the brain.

Now let us have a look at how the endocannabinoid system might be involved in sleep regulation, as well as what happens in insomnia.

## The Endocannabinoid System and Regulation of Sleep

The endocannabinoid system (ECS) is involved in the circadian sleep-wake cycle, including maintenance and promotion of sleep, and the ECS may provide the link between the circadian regulation systems (suprachiasmic nucleus) and the physiological process of sleep [37, 130]. Support for the role of the ECS in circadian rhythms comes from research that has found that plasma concentration of the endocannabinoid AEA demonstrates a circadian rhythm, that lack of normal sleep causes ECS dysregulation, and that elevation of cannabinoid receptors is involved in the homeostatic recovery of sleep following non-normal sleep [37, 130].

Both the endocannabinoids and other non-endocannabinoid *N*-acylethanolamines (NAEs) are involved in the sleep-wake cycle. Two such members of the NAE family are oleoylethanolamide (OEA) and palmitoylethanolamide (PEA) which are active endogenous lipids which bind to PPAR-$\alpha$ (but not CB1 receptors) [25]. Oleamide is another endocannabinoid amide involved with sleep that is synthesized in neuroendocrine cells from oleic acid and glycine similar to endogenous neurotransmitter compounds.

Rodents have been used extensively to study the sleep-wake cycle as they have similar neurocircuitry and neurochemistry to humans, though there are key differences: mice and rats are polyphasic sleepers and have shorter and more frequent bouts of slow-wave sleep (akin to NREM sleep) and paradoxical sleep (akin to REM sleep) than humans, and they spend more time sleeping than humans (12–15 h compared with our 7–8 h) [131]. Another difference is that mice and rats are more nocturnally active whereas humans are diurnal, and we are active during the day and sleep at night [131]. In rat studies, rats are subjected to periods of lights-on and lights-off (i.e., light-dark phases): during the light phase, rats spend more time sleeping, while the dark phase corresponds to increased arousal and wake activities [131]. Much of what we understand about the endocannabinoid system and sleep is gleaned from rodent research.

In summary, the following effects of components of the ECS in relation to the sleep-wake cycle are supported in the literature [25, 131]:

- Endocannabinoids:
  - AEA fluctuates diurnally in several brain regions (in opposite direction to 2-AG): higher during dark phase of light-dark cycle (rats).

  - 2-AG fluctuates diurnally in several brain regions (in opposite direction to AEA): higher during light phase of light-dark cycle (rats).
  - Oleamide: involved in sleep modulation and promotes sleep.
- Cannabinoid receptors:
  - CB1 receptors fluctuate diurnally.
  - CB2 receptors don't fluctuate diurnally.
- NAEs:
  - Oleoylethanolamide (OEA) promotes waking.
  - Palmitoylethanolamide (PEA) promotes waking.

## Cannabinoid Receptors and Sleep

CB1 receptors are involved in sleep, demonstrated in rat experiments in which antagonism of CB1 receptors blocked the sleep-promoting effects of CB1 agonists and acute elevation of endocannabinoids [132]. AEA and 2-AG promote sleep through the activation of CB1 receptors [29]. CB1 receptor inverse agonists were shown to decrease REM sleep, implicating CB1 receptors in promoting deep sleep (including when there was no pharmacological enhancement of 2-AG and AEA signaling) [131, 132]. Blockade of CB1 receptors increases wakefulness and reduces sleep [25].

As explained by Kesner and Lovinger [131], the intracellular mechanisms proximal to CB1 activation are probably the first steps in sleep regulation, in which the $G\alpha_{i/0}$ subunit liberated then inhibits adenyl cyclase. This enzyme catalyzes production of cAMP, and cAMP signaling is highly controlled in sleep regulation. The mechanism from this point on is complex (readers are referred to Kesner and Lovinger [131]); however, it seems that the presynaptic CB1 receptor may reduce the release of various neurotransmitters via different mechanisms, not dissimilar to hypnogenic pharmaceuticals such as benzodiazepines and non-benzodiazepine-type hypnogenics (which reduce neuronal activity by blocking excitatory tone or increasing inhibitory tone). Another way in which CB1 receptors may be involved in sleep regulation is via altering intracellular signaling in glia, implicated in research demonstrating that neurons in the suprachiasmic nucleus release endocannabinoids which activate astrocyte signaling which then impacts on circadian timing [131].

### Diurnal Fluctuations of CB1 Receptors

Levels of CB1 receptors but not CB2 receptors fluctuate diurnally [133]. Rat experiments indicate that CB1 receptor protein expression in the pons (an area of the brainstem involved in sleep-wake regulation and REM sleep generation) fluctuates diurnally, peaking during the lights-on period (which is the time when mice are generally sleeping) [134]. In contrast, CB1 receptor protein expression was highest in the rat cerebral cortex during the dark phase (lights-off) [133]. There are also diurnal fluctuation in the genes coding for CB1 receptors, with CB1 mRNA highest during the dark phase (no fluctuations in CB2 mRNA), while the CB1 receptor protein expression was greater during the light phase [133].

As discussed earlier, there are two mechanisms involved in sleep regulation: the homeostatic drive (sleep pressure—involving adenosine) and the circadian rhythm processes. Research in mice indicates that the ECS plays a role in regulating sleep stability rather than mediating sleep homeostatic drive [131]. For example, in mice experiments blocking of CB1 receptors did not affect overall sleep time or amount of sleep following sleep deprivation [131] contrary to expectations in homeostasis. Instead, individual bouts of sleep architecture were modified for, perhaps, efficiency. Polysomnography experiments in mice support the contention that endocannabinoid signaling via CB1 receptors is necessary for NREM stability but not necessarily for sleep homeostasis and that homeostatic regulation of sleep remains intact in the absence of CB1 receptor signaling [132].

### CB1 Receptors and Orexins/Hypocretins and Melanin-Concentrating Hormone Neurons

Orexins/hypocretins (OX) neurons and melanin-concentrating hormone (MCH) neurons in the lateral hypothalamus modulate different stages of the sleep-wake cycle. OX neurons are wake-active and promote wakefulness, and MCH neurons are REM sleep active and promote REM sleep [135]. In vitro studies indicate that activation of CB1 receptors in the lateral hypothalamus of rats excites MCH neurons and inhibits OX neurons, thereby promoting sleep overall [136]. In a rat experiment, 2-AG was found to increase REM sleep via activation of CB1 receptors in MCH neurons [136].

## Endocannabinoids and Sleep

Evidence indicates involvement of the ECS in circadian components of the sleep-wake cycle [131]. Research evidence suggests that both endocannabinoids and NAEs are under circadian control [25]. AEA and 2-AG promote sleep by activating CB1 receptors, while NAEs promote waking [25, 29]. Endocannabinoids promote REM sleep by interacting with melanin-concentrating hormone neurons in the lateral hypothalamus and also promote NREM [25].

### Endocannabinoids Fluctuate and Follow Circadian Rhythmicity

Endocannabinoids exhibit diurnal fluctuations in neural tissue and follow circadian rhythmicity [37], and animal research suggests CB1 receptor signaling is involved in circadian rhythmicity [137].

Rat studies indicate that AEA and 2-AG fluctuate diurnally in several brain regions including the hippocampus, PFC, hypothalamus, striatum, pons, and nucleus accumbens and also in cerebrospinal fluid, with differences in peak activity depending on region [25, 29, 131]. For example, in the PFC, striatum, nucleus accumbens, and hippocampus (areas involved in learning, memory, and sensorimotor functions), AEA and 2-AG have opposite diurnal rhythms; levels of AEA are higher and FAAH significantly lower during the dark phase, and 2-AG is higher during the light phase [138, 139]. In the pons (area of the brainstem involved in sleep-wake regulation and generation of REM sleep), AEA levels are lower during the light phase and maximal during the dark phase [138]. Diurnal fluctuations have also been found in activity of the ECS enzymes (FAAH, MAGL, DAGL) [139], potentially related to light-dark cycle fluctuations in their encoding genes [25].

There is less consistency in human studies. One study in healthy humans found that plasma concentrations of AEA exhibit a circadian rhythm, with concentrations three times higher on awakening than just before sleep [37]. After 24 h of sleep deprivation, there was an increase in AEA, in particular in the evening after sleep deprivation [37]. The significance of this is unclear; it may indicate that AEA promotes sleep or that the higher concentration was facilitating wakefulness [25]. Diurnal variations in 2-AG have also been found in human studies, with the lowest levels in the middle of sleep (e.g., around 2–4 am) and highest levels in the early afternoon [140, 141] suggesting involvement in promoting wakefulness [25].

**Animal Studies: AEA**

Animal studies suggest AEA (and 2-AG) promotes sleep (NREM, REM) and reduces wakefulness [136, 142, 143]:

- Intracerebroventricular administration of AEA increased slow-wave sleep and REM sleep at the expense of wakefulness, as well as deteriorating memory consolidation and increasing locomotor activity [144].
- Injection of AEA increased adenosine levels with peak levels 2–3 h after injection, and a significant increase in slow-wave sleep occurred during the third hour also. Sleep induction and adenosine increase were blocked by a CB1 receptor antagonist, indicating this effect was mediated by CB1 receptors [143].
- FAAH knockout mice (FAAH gene is disrupted, leading to increased endogenous AEA levels and reduced hydrolysis rates for AEA and oleamide) showed higher values and more intense episodes of slow-wave sleep than control mice, supporting the role of AEA and oleamide as modulators of sleep [145].
- Inhibition of AEA membrane transporter function has also been found to enhance sleep [146].

However, there have been some inconsistencies. Some experiments have shown that inhibition of FAAH activity (which should increase the amount of AEA available) promotes wakefulness [148, 147], and one study found that an FAAH inhibitor decreased NREM sleep [132]. The apparent lack of consistency in study findings probably relates to different administration routes and dosing, including timing of dosing in the light-dark cycle of the rodents [131].

**Animal Studies: 2-AG**

The effect of 2-AG appears to depend on brain region and may be sleep-promoting in some and wake-promoting in others [131]. When an MAGL inhibitor was given to rats systemically to increase 2-AG tone, slow-wave sleep was significantly augmented (slight reduction in paradoxical sleeping) when administered just before the dark phase. However, it had a different effect when it was given just before the light phase: the effect on paradoxical sleep was stronger, with a modest effect on slow-wave sleep [132]. These findings support the contention that 2-AG promotes sleep. However, in another experiment, injection of a MAGL inhibitor into the lateral hypothalamus had the opposite effect, promoting wakefulness (see Kesner and Lovinger [131]).

**Oleamide**

Oleamide is a fatty amide lipid molecule that is (like AEA) degraded by FAAH. Research suggests it promotes NREM sleep [25, 149]. How it does so is uncertain: some evidence suggests the serotonergic system is involved [150]; however, an alternative view is that oleamide interferes with degradation of AEA and therefore AEA is responsible for sleep promotion [25, 151]. Oleamide induced significant hypomotility in rats and decreased sleep latency, with an effect comparable to neurosteroid and benzodiazepine hypnotics. Levels of oleamide in cerebrospinal fluid increased after 6 h of sleep deprivation which the study authors posited might be sufficient to increase serotonergic or GABAergic transmission and therefore might be the pathway through which oleamide might induce sleep. Because the actions of oleamide were not blocked by a CB1 receptor antagonist, this suggests its sleep-inducing action is independent of CB1 receptors [142].

**N-Acyl-Ethanolamines: Oleoylethanolamide (OEA) and Palmitoylethanolamide (PEA)**

The N-acyl-ethanolamines (NAEs) oleoylethanolamide (OEA; an endogenous PPAR-α agonist) and palmitoylethanolamide (PEA; an endogenous ligand to PPAR-α, GPR-55, and GPR-199) appear to play a role in promoting waking, since in brain regions of rats including the pons, hypothalamus, and hippocampus, their levels peak during the dark phase of lights-on/off cycle (in rat studies, the dark phase is associated with increased arousal and wake activity) [25].

Human studies support the contention that OEA promotes wakefulness where it was found to be increased in volunteers following 24 h of sleep deprivation [25, 152]. Little is known about the effect of PEA on sleep in humans.

## How Do Changes in the Endocannabinoid System and Age Contribute to Sleep Disorders in the Elderly?

Comparatively little is yet understood about how the ECS changes with age and how that might contribute, potentially, to sleep disorders that become prevalent in the elderly. Rat experiments demonstrate that the CB1 receptor is decreased with aging [153], whereas other research has demonstrated that MAGL levels (the key enzyme which breaks down 2-AG) are elevated during aging [154]. Somewhat is known about AEA changes with conditions such as Alzheimer's disease, although the relevance of this to normal aging without dementia is undetermined. Knowledge is limited about the effect of aging on anandamide membrane transporter (AMT)

[29], only that CB1 receptor knockout mice (bred without CB1 receptors) had higher levels of AMT with age compared to control mice [155]. This will be an important area to understand in the future, not only in relation to sleep disorders.

The effects of the ECS on sleep homeostasis and circadian rhythms are very complex. Two good review papers are recommended for those who would like to explore this further: Kesner and Lovinger [131] and Prospero-Garcia et al. [25].

## The Involvement of the ECS in Insomnia

There is evidence that the ECS is involved in the pathogenesis of insomnia. Again, rodent studies assist in helping us understand.

### Animal Studies

One rat model of insomnia is a maternal care deprivation model in which pups separated from their mothers have been shown to have disturbed sleep-wake cycles, particularly reduction in sleep in general and in particular less REM sleep, as well as suffering from anxiety and depression [25]. When such insomniac rats were given systemic oleamide, it restored the REM and NREM sleep. When these insomniac rats were given systemic AM251 (a CB1 receptor inverse agonist), it worsened the insomnia [156]. This study also suggests an association between modification of CB1 receptor expression and sleep: decreased levels of CB1 receptors in the PFC and hippocampus were demonstrated in rats subjected to maternal care deprivation [156]. In another study using the maternal care deprivation model of insomnia, rats who had 2-AG injected into the lateral hypothalamus showed a significant increase in REM sleep which was blocked by the CB1 receptor inverse agonist AM251 [157], which suggests that both types of sleep are facilitated via CB1 receptor activation.

These two animal studies provide a level of support for a role of the endocannabinoids and lateral hypothalamus in promoting REM sleep [25].

### Human Studies

There are a small number of studies in humans which have linked changes in endocannabinoids, albeit contradictory, with acute sleep loss [37, 93, 141, 152]. In one study [152], sleep deprivation did not result in any significant changes in plasma AEA concentrations, whereas in another small study [37], sleep deprivation was associated with a significant dysregulation of circulating AEA.

Another study investigated the impact of sleep deprivation on 2-AG [141]. A randomized crossover trial in 14 healthy young adults examined the 24-h profile of

2-AG under the conditions of 4 nights of restricted sleep (4.5 h/night) and 4 nights of normal sleep (8.5 h/night). The study also measured hunger, appetite, and food intake. They found a daily variation in 2-AG concentration, with the lowest levels around the middle of the sleep/overnight fast, and then a continuous increase culminating midafternoon. This occurred in both normal sleep and sleep-restricted conditions; however, in the case of sleep restriction, this pattern was amplified with delayed and extended maximum values. For example, under conditions of sleep restriction, the amplitude of the 24-h profile of 2-AG was increased by an average of 33%, due to an increase in the peak 2-AG level by an average of 22%, and the time of peak occurred around 2 h later than under the normal sleep conditions. Of note was the fact that neither the nadir concentration (lowest level of 2-AG) nor its timing was affected by sleep duration. Also, the mean 24-h 2-AG concentration was the same for a given individual under both experimental conditions (remember, this was a crossover study) even though the experimental sessions were separated by at least 1 month. At the same time as the elevation of 2-AG, when sleep was restricted, participants reported higher hunger, desire to eat, appetite, and quantity of food that could be eaten, which led the study authors to hypothesize that increases in peripheral endocannabinoid levels might be the mechanism by which chronic sleep restriction results in excessive food intake, particularly snacks [141].

Another study, this one investigating the impact of sleep restriction on 16 healthy men, found that concentrations of 2-AG were 80% higher 1.5 h after awakening under conditions of sleep deprivation (3 nights of short sleep) compared with normal sleep ($p < 0.05$), which coincided with 25% higher hunger ratings compared with normal sleep ($p < 0.05$) [93]. This contrasts with Hanlon and colleagues' study [141] which found circulating levels of 2-AG to be higher midafternoon following 4 nights of sleep restriction, though this might have been due to differences in experimental conditions [93]. Also, in Cedernae and colleagues' study, on day 4, while there was a difference in plasma concentration at 8.30 am (between sleep restricted and normal sleep conditions), this appeared to be transient as it disappeared at 10 am (i.e., there was no significant difference). There was no apparent effect of sleep deprivation on circulating levels of AEA, PEA, or OEA found in their study either [93].

## Cannabis in the Treatment of Insomnia

Evidence of efficacy of medicinal cannabis and cannabinoids in the treatment of sleep disorders comes from cross-sectional surveys as well as randomized controlled trials and systematic reviews. There have been many early studies in the 1970s which have suggested that acute exposure to cannabis or THC was associated with decreased sleep onset latency, less waking after sleep onset, increased slow-wave (NREM) sleep, and decreased REM sleep [158–161]. These will be discussed later in the section on Human Studies on THC and Sleep.

## Historical Use

We don't have to look far back into history to realize that cannabis has been used for sleep disorders for quite a long time. Cannabis has a long history of use in Ayurveda, one of the main Indian traditional forms of medicine, and one of the indications from ancient times to date was for treating insomnia [162]. The Swedish taxonomist Linnaeus recognized cannabis as *narcotica* and *anodyna* in his Materia Medica in the eighteenth century [61].

Journal articles in the 1800s reported the sleep-promoting effects of cannabis [131]. The Irish physician, Sir William B. O'Shaughnessy, reintroduced cannabis to western medicine from India in the nineteenth century, with benefits found for sleep problems as well as pain reduction in rheumatism sufferers, as well as many other conditions [61, 163].

Dr. Jacques-Joseph Moreau de Tours, French psychiatrist, learned about cannabis while traveling through the Middle East in the 1830s, and brought hashish back to Paris. He noted back there that cannabis use improved the sleep of some hospitalized insomniacs and seemed to improve depression also [163]. One of the gods of medicine in the UK, Sir John Russell Reynolds, personal physician to Queen Victoria recommended cannabis for insomnia and also prescribed hemp tincture for menstrual cramps [163].

The beneficial effects of cannabis on sleep were noted in relation to various pain states throughout the nineteenth and early twentieth century, prior to prohibition [163]. In recent history, the Californian physician Dr. Mollie Fry was arrested in 2001 and thrown into jail for violating the US Federal Controlled Substances Act. Her crime? Recommending to several patients that they use cannabis for sleep disorders [163].

## Epidemiological Studies

Several surveys have found that people are using cannabis to address sleep problems [164–168]. Cross-sectional studies have found nonmedical and medical use of cannabis to cope with various symptoms associated with PTSD including sleep problems, as well as others (coping, sleep, trauma-related re-experiencing, avoidance, and hyperarousal) [169–171]. Not all studies have found that cannabis use is associated with positive effects on sleep.

Whether age is a factor in the use of cannabis for treatment of insomnia is not known definitively. However, one survey conducted in medical cannabis patients grouped into three different age groups (18–30, 31–50, 51–72 years) found that middle-aged adults were more likely to report using medical cannabis for insomnia, while older adults were more likely to report using it for chronic diseases including cancer, glaucoma, and HIV/AIDS [166].

Let us have a look at some of the studies.

## Positive Effects of Cannabis Use on Sleep

Here are some results of studies that have found positive effects of cannabis use on sleep:

- A 1991 survey of Indian cannabis users in Varanasi found that 90% of participants reported cannabis effective for sleep [100].
- A survey was conducted of 1000 adult-use customers of two dispensaries in Colorado (USA), 74% of which reported taking cannabis to promote sleep and 65% of whom reported taking it to relieve pain. Among those taking it for sleep, 84% reported that it was very helpful or extremely helpful, and most taking over-the-counter sleep medications (87%) or prescription sleep medications (83%) reported reducing or ceasing use of such medications [164].
- A qualitative study in Norway that investigated the medical motives of 100 cannabis users (who did not have legal access to medical cannabis) found that cannabis was used for quality of life aspects including quality of sleep, relaxation, and well-being as well as for medical conditions such as multiple sclerosis, ADHD, and rheumatism [168].
- A cross-sectional survey of 170 patients at a medical cannabis dispensary in California found that those with high PTSD scores were more likely to use cannabis to improve sleep and in general to cope compared with those with low PTSD scores. Sleep improvement appeared to be the main motivator for coping-oriented use. Frequency of cannabis use was higher in those with high PTSD scores who used it for sleep-promoting purposes compared with those with low PTSD scores or those who did not use it for sleep-promoting purposes, providing evidence that sleep-motivated use specifically is associated with more frequent cannabis use [170].
- A survey of cannabis users in Australia in 2016, conducted just before medical cannabis use was legalized, surveyed 1748 cannabis users who were using cannabis for medicinal reasons. Mean length of use was 9.8 years. The most frequent reasons for medical cannabis use were anxiety (50.7%), back pain (50.0%), depression (49.3%), and sleep problems (43.9%) [167].
- A 2017 survey of 1513 patients at a New England medical cannabis dispensary found that 65.2% of respondents had decreased use of sleep medications subsequent to medical cannabis use [172].

Not all epidemiological studies have shown positive results in relation to cannabis use and sleep. A survey of problematic alcohol and cannabis users found that cannabis use was associated with poor sleep quality [173].

## Surveys Indicating Preference for CBD-Dominant Products

In a survey of 163 cannabis users, 49.7% were using it to treat insomnia and 8.5% to reduce nightmares. Those with current insomnia and greater sleep latency were significantly more likely to report strains of cannabis with higher concentrations of

CBD. Those who reported at least weekly use of hypnotic medications used cannabis with lower THC concentrations compared to those using sleep medications less than weekly [5].

A longitudinal, cross-sectional survey of patients and caregivers of patients with diagnosed health condition registered with the Realm of Caring Foundation assessed patients on their medication use, pain, anxiety, depression, sleep, and quality of life. Statistical analysis was conducted in 108 cannabis users compared with 468 controls (non-cannabis users). Cannabis users were found to have significantly better sleep ($p < 0.01$ children, $p < 0.01$ for adults), lower anxiety and depression (both $p < 0.001$), better quality of life ($p < 0.001$), greater health satisfaction ($p < 0.001$), and lower average pain severity ($p < 0.05$) compared with nonusers. They also found that cannabis users used 14% less prescription medications (rate ratio 0.86, 95% CI 0.77–0.96) compared with nonusers. Like in the previous survey, this survey found that cannabis users preferentially used CBD-dominant products compared with THC-dominant products. Mean dose of CBD was 79 mg/day (1.4 mg/kg, with a median of 0.6 mg/kg and range 0.01–15.7 mg/kg). Mean dose of THC was 3 mg/day (0.05 mg/kg; median 0.02 mg/kg; range <0.01–0.6 mg/kg) [174].

### Cannabis Use and Expectations of Better Sleep

Expectations of a positive effect of cannabis on sleep might be expected to influence outcomes. This was tested out in a study of 152 moderate cannabis users (mean age 31.45, age range 21–70, mean days of cannabis use in prior 2 weeks 5.5) which used the Pittsburgh Quality Sleep Index (PSQI) to examine the potential influence of cannabis use and expectations of cannabis being a sleep aid on actual sleep outcomes. The study found that greater number of days of cannabis use and endorsing cannabis use were associated with increased expectations that cannabis use would improve sleep. However, they found that endorsing cannabis use was associated with significantly worse subjective quality of sleep [175]. This finding is clearly contrary to what one might expect.

## Observational Study in Insomniacs

In a study of 409 people with insomnia, participants completed 1056 medical cannabis administration sessions using a phone app which recorded real-time ratings of self-perceived insomnia severity levels and any side effects. The study found an average symptom severity reduction of – 4.5 points (std dev 2.5, $p < 0.001$) on a 0–10-point visual analogue scale (VAS; participants are asked to indicate where along a straight line the severity of their symptoms lies, with 0 being least in terms of severity and 10 the worst). The use of pipes and vaporizers was associated with greater symptom relief and more positive and context-specific side effects compared with *joints*. Vaporization was associated with lower negative effects. CBD was found to be associated with greater statistically significant insomnia relief than THC, though there was no difference in side effects [176].

## RCTs and Systematic Reviews

A 2017 report on cannabis and cannabinoids conducted by the National Academies of Sciences, Engineering, and Medicine found: *"Moderate evidence that cannabis or cannabinoids are effective for improving short-term sleep outcomes in individuals with sleep disturbance associated with: obstructive sleep apnea syndrome; fibromyalgia; chronic pain, and multiple sclerosis (cannabinoids, primarily nabiximols)"* [177]. Nabiximols is a combination of THC and CBD in an almost 1:1 ratio. This report used only evidence from systematic reviews and randomized controlled trials (RCTs). The conclusion was based on a meta-analysis by Whiting et al. [178] which found greater improvements with cannabinoids in sleep quality among eight RCTs and sleep disturbance among three RCTs (results relate primarily to nabiximols). The National Academies review did not identify any clinical trials that evaluated effects of cannabinoids on patients with primary chronic insomnia.

A systematic review analyzed 11 studies that investigated the impact of *recreational* cannabis use on sleep (total of 203 participants) [179]. All were conducted in the USA or Canada. The overall quality of the studies was poor, and there was a lack of control for confounding factors in many, such as age, gender, and preexisting sleep problems. As known, prevalence of insomnia increases with age and is greater in females. There was substantial variation between studies in cannabis dose and dosing duration. Six of these studies used objective measures (electroencephalogram, EEG). There was little consistency in results, with one study reporting an increase in slow-wave sleep, three reporting a decrease, and one study finding no change, while for REM sleep, one study found it increased, another found it decreased, and four studies found no effect. Stage 2 sleep was found to increase in two studies and four studies reported no effect. Sleep latency increased in one study and decreased in another with high THC dose, and two studies found no effect. Cannabis was not found to significantly impact on overall sleep time or time spent in stage 1 sleep.

Five studies used subjective measures of sleep, often the Pittsburgh Sleep Quality Index. In three of these studies, cannabis was found to decrease sleep latency (time to fall asleep), while it had no effect in one study and wasn't measured in another. No study showed any significant effect on the number of awakenings during the night which was assessed in four studies, and no studies found any effect on daytime behavior (assessed in three studies). Results varied in respect to overall sleep time. Three studies assessed effects of dose, and only one found that higher doses improved sleep while the other two found no effect of dose [179].

## Some Negative Results: Cannabis Use and Disturbances to Sleep

Not all studies have found beneficial effects of cannabis on sleep. Several studies have, in fact, found that cannabis use has been associated with sleep problems including poorer sleep quality, with many of these studies in children or adolescents [173, 175, 180–184].

A survey of 248 alcohol or cannabis users (mean age 26 years) found that sleep quality problems were more commonly reported than excessive daytime sleepiness and that poor sleep quality was associated with comorbid alcohol and cannabis use (with women reporting problem alcohol and cannabis use demonstrating poorer sleep outcomes than men) [173]. A study in 152 moderate cannabis users found that increased frequency of cannabis edible consumption was associated with significantly worse subjective sleep efficiency, decreased sleep duration, and higher global Pittsburgh Sleep Quality Index (PSQI) scores indicating worse overall sleep [175].

### Adolescents and Children at Risk

Adolescents seem particularly at risk, and several studies point to an association between poorer sleep and cannabis use. For example, adolescents with insomnia have been found to be 1.8 times more likely to report cannabis use than adolescents without insomnia [183]. Another study in adolescents found that adolescents reporting using any illicit drug, most often cannabis, were 2.6 times more likely to report problematic sleep than those who did not use drugs [180]. Insufficient sleep was found to be associated with an age-adjusted odds ratio of 1.52 (95%CI 1.31–1.76) of using cannabis in an analysis of the 2007 US national Youth Risk Behaviour Survey (12, 154 high school students) [181]. A study that followed a cohort of 12-year-old children through to the age of 18 found that recent cannabis use at age 18 years was associated with poor sleep quality [182].

Disturbingly, sleep problems in young children have been found to predict later use of cannabis. In a prospective longitudinal study of 292 boys and 94 girls from a community sample of high-risk families and controls, sleep problems at ages 3–8 have been found to predict the onset of cannabis, alcohol, and cigarette use among boys (and onset of alcohol use in girls) [184].

### Cofounding Factors in Research

However, the devil is sometimes in the detail. In Conroy and colleagues' study, 98 participants with a mean age of 22.3 years were stratified as daily users ($n$ = 29), non-daily users ($n$ = 49), and nonuser controls ($n$ = 20) [185]. Four sleep measurement tools were used. They found that the Pittsburgh Sleep Quality Index (PSQI) scores in daily users were higher than in non-daily and nonusers (7.0+/−3.8 vs 4.9+/−3.2 vs 5.0+/−3.7, respectively, $p = 0.02$) and that the Insomnia Severity Index scores in daily users were higher in daily users than in non-daily users and nonusers (7.9+/− 6.6 vs 5.1 +/−4.3 vs 4.3 +/−4.8, respectively, $p = 0.01$). Covariate-adjusted regression analysis showed that the mean PSQI and Insomnia Severity Index scores were significantly higher in daily users compared to non-daily users and nonusers; however, when they adjusted for anxiety and depression (i.e., statistically took these factors into account in their statistical modeling), these associations were no longer statistically significant [185]. Essentially this means that anxiety and depression may have been the reason for the difference between daily users and the other two groups in the PSQI and Insomnia Severity Index scores, rather than frequency of cannabis use. The study also found that there was no significant difference between all three groups in the Epworth Sleepiness Scale or the Morningness Eveningness Questionnaire, though daily users endorsed more sleep disturbance compared with non-daily users [185].

## Chronic Use and Tolerance

There is some evidence that chronic or repeated exposure to cannabis and THC can produce tolerance to its actions, including those on sleep, thus requiring greater dosages to obtain sleep-promoting effects [131, 186]. For example, in one study of 13 male cannabis smokers who smoked a mean of 5.5+/− 3.9, joint-equivalents daily were administered oral THC (20 mg) around the clock for 7 days (40–120 mg daily). Participants completed a sleep questionnaire, and changes in sleep characteristics over time and associations between sleep characteristics and plasma cannabinoid concentrations were assessed. They found that higher evening THC and its metabolite 11-OH-THC were significantly associated with shorter sleep latency, less difficulty falling asleep, and increased daytime sleep the next day; however, the duration of both self-reported and calculated nighttime sleep decreased significantly (of the order of 5.34 and 3.54 min per night, respectively) which suggests that tolerance to the somnolent effects of THC may have occurred [186].

## Sleep Disruption in Cannabis Withdrawal

Cannabis use withdrawal from chronic cannabis use is commonly associated with sleep disturbances including sleep disruption, vivid dreams, and reduced stage 4 NREM sleep [130, 159, 187–190], and disturbed sleep can last up to 45 days post-cessation [191]. Sleep problem experienced is one of the more consistent and problematic factors found associated with cannabis withdrawal, and there is some evidence to suggest it can contribute to relapse [131, 192, 193]. In fact, one of the most severe symptoms of cannabis withdrawal found in laboratory sleep studies is sleep difficulty [193].

A systematic review of 36 publications concluded that sleep was frequently interrupted during cannabis withdrawal, though the mechanisms of action are not clear [189]. A study of 17 heavy cannabis users discontinuing cannabis use and 14 drug-free controls (age 18–30 years) found that discontinuation of cannabis use was associated with polysomnographic measures of sleep disturbance compared with nonusers including lower total sleep time, less NREM, worse sleep efficiency, longer sleep onset, and shorter REM latency [187]. These findings are supported by other studies of heavy cannabis users investigating abrupt cannabis discontinuation [188, 190]. In another study of regular cannabis users, short-term abstinence (3 days) from cannabis use was associated with reduced sleep efficiency, total sleep time, percentage time spent in stage 1 and stage 2 NREM sleep, REM latency, and subjective sleep quality and increased sleep latency and time spent in REM sleep compared to when they were using cannabis [190]. An early sleep study found that on withdrawal from THC (regime was 3 nights under initial dosage of 70 mg/day, the last 3 nights of a 2-wk period of 210 mg/day), there was a significant reduction in stage 4 NREM sleep though the change was only marked on the first of night of withdrawal [159].

## Evidence of Efficacy of CBD for Sleep Disorders

### Preclinical Studies: CBD and Sleep

In the early 1970s, research findings began to suggest that CBD had a sedative action, based on observations that CBD reduced ambulation in rats [194] and with higher doses, it affected the operant behavior of rats and pigeons [195].

However, since then, preclinical studies demonstrate somewhat contradictory results, with some animal studies suggesting that CBD promotes wakefulness or is alerting [196–200], and others suggesting that CBD promotes sleep [201, 202].

For example, microdialysis perfusion of CBD (30, 60, 90 nM) into the lateral hypothalamus of rats increased alertness and suppressed sleep, an effect that was associated with an increase in extracellular dopamine collected from the nucleus accumbens. Perfusion of CBD into the lateral hypothalamus following total sleep deprivation prevented sleep rebound effect [200].

In contrast, a study in rats was conducted in which the rats were injected intraperitoneally with CBD at three different doses (2.5 mg/kg, 10 mg/kg, 40 mg/kg) or vehicle/placebo ($n = 7$ rats per group). Sleep recordings were conducted during light and dark periods over 4 days (with baseline recordings conducted on days 1 and 2, day 3 being the test day and day 4 being the post-test day). On the test day (day of administration), during the light period, total percentage sleep significantly increased in rats in the 10 mg/kg and 40 mg/kg groups compared with placebo, and in the 40 mg/kg group, sleep latency was also significantly increased (and there was also a nonsignificant increase in time of slow-wave sleep). On the post-test day, rats treated with 10 mg/kg had significantly decreased REM sleep latency also [202].

There is some evidence that the effect of CBD on sleep quality might work via its anxiolytic effects [130]. For example, in a mice model of PTSD, repeated combination tests (RCT) using an elevated plus maze and open-field tests over 4 days were used to induce anxiety. This resulted in decreased NREM sleep during the first hour after RCT and suppression of REM sleep during hours 4–10 after the RCT in the mice. When CBD was microinjected into the central nucleus of the amygdala, it had an anxiolytic effect (demonstrated in the elevated plus maze and open-field tests). It also efficiently blocked anxiety-induced REM sleep suppression, but had no effect on non-REM sleep, leading the researchers to conclude that CBD can block anxiety-induced REM sleep alteration via an anxiolytic effect, rather than via sleep regulation [203].

It is possible that the different findings of these animal studies, that is, sleep-promoting or alerting effects, are related to the experimental conditions used, in particular those parts of the brain being injected with CBD. Results from studies injecting parts of the brain are likely to be different from those using systemic administration. At the end of the day, the point of animal research is to seek to understand how CBD might affect humans and we don't take CBD by injecting it into a particular part of our brains. Taking a mechanistic approach to understanding how a complex plant such as cannabis, or even a CBD isolate, works in the body has limitations. We should also remember when interpreting data from animal studies that pure CBD isolate is generally being tested (not whole plant products).

## Effect of Chronic CBD Use in Adolescent Rats on Adult Rat Sleep Patterns

A recent study in juvenile (adolescent) rats was conducted to investigate the effects on sleep in adulthood after long-term administration of CBD in adolescence. Juvenile rats were treated with 5 or 30 mg/kg CBD daily (injection, i.p.), from postnatal day 30 for 2 weeks. At postnatal day 80, sleep-wake cycle and expression of NeuN were assessed [204]. NeuN is an antibody derived from rodents inoculated with purified neuronal nuclei and is specific to an unknown nuclear protein expressed by most neurons (but not glia). It allows neurons to be visualized separately from glia [205].

The study found that systemic administration of CBD in adolescence was associated with the following changes in adulthood:

- Increased wakefulness and decreased REM sleep during the lights-on period (this is normally when rats would be less active and would sleep)
- Decreased wakefulness and enhanced slow-wave sleep during the lights-off period (this is the time when rodents are normally more active, i.e., at night) [204]

In addition, CBD administration in the rats affected the NeuN expression in the suprachiasmic nucleus [204]. Thus, in rats, chronic administration of CBD during adolescence was associated with changes in neuronal development in a key brain region involved in sleep, and the implication is that this has affected the sleep-wake patterns in adulthood. The relevance of these findings to humans is, as yet, unknown.

## Cell Research: Effect of CBD on Circadian Clock Genes

We know that many physiological functions of the body are regulated by our circadian rhythm. In an experiment in mice microglial cells that investigated the effect of CBD and THC on clock gene expression, CBD was found to induce deregulation of circadian core genes: CBD, downregulated CLOCK, and upregulated ARNTL, CRY2, and PER1. CBD also deregulated (i.e., either upregulated or downregulated) circadian rhythm in other nuclear molecules in microglial cells including RORA and RXRA (nuclear receptors), RevErba, RORB, CREBBP, activating transcription factor 4 (AFT4), AFT5, and NFIL3 (nuclear factor, interleukin-3 regulated). The receptor 1B of melatonin, Mtmr1b (myotubularin-related protein 1), was downregulated by CBD, as were some of the dopamine receptors Drd2 (dopamine receptor D2) and Drd4 (dopamine receptor D4) [33].

THC did not have this deregulatory effect on circadian rhythmicity in microglial cells that CBD displayed. Interestingly, the effect of CBD was tested under inflammatory (LPS induced) and noninflammatory conditions, and there was no difference in effect, suggesting the mechanism of action of CBD may be independent of the neuroinflammatory state and cannabinoid receptors in microglial BV cells. The results of this mice cell study suggest that CBD is able to block cells in a waking state via its effects on the expression of the main clock genes in BV-2 microglial cells [33]. Clinically we might see this effect in the rapid adaptation to new time zones or shift work.

## Human Studies: CBD and Sleep

A few studies including case reports [206], case series [207], and randomized controlled trials [201, 208] indicate that CBD may be efficacious in promoting sleep. Some studies suggest CBD has a stimulating or alerting effect [209, 210], others suggest CBD has a sedating effect [201, 208], and one found no effect in terms of sleepiness [211]. See Table 8.2 for details.

CBD used as an adjunct therapy (to usual care and medications) has also been found in an open-label retrospective case series of 11 PTSD patients of an outpatient psychiatric clinic to reduce nightmares in a subset of patients experiencing frequent nightmares, as well as reduce PTSD symptom severity [212].

### Sedating or Alerting: Which Is It?

These potentially different effects, i.e., sedating or alerting, might be related to dose. It has been thought that low-dose CBD may be more alerting and higher-dose CBD sedating, and there is some animal data to support this. However, the human research evidence is mixed.

For example, in a clinical study in insomniacs, 15 participants were given 40 mg, 80 mg, and 160 mg oral doses of CBD as a hypnotic (in gel capsules). The control medications were nitrazepam (5 mg) and placebo. None of the CBD doses was associated with any improvements in sleep induction, sleep fragmentation, and reports of good sleep compared with placebo. In comparison with placebo, only the high dose of CBD (160 mg) increased duration of sleep significantly. All three doses of CBD reduced dream recall compared with placebo [201]. This study would seem to support the contention that higher doses of CBD might be needed for a sedative effect.

In Nicholson and colleagues' study [209], 5 mg CBD and 15 mg CBD were both associated decreased stage 3 NREM sleep, and the 15 mg CBD/15 mg THC combination was associated with increased alertness. This might support the contention that low-dose CBD may be alerting; however, in Zuardi and colleagues' study [208], 1 mg/kg CBD was found to be alerting and that is not a particularly low dose, and in another (retrospective) study, doses of 25 mg/day were effective in improving sleep for the majority of patients [207].

Thus, based on the current evidence, it is still unclear what doses are alerting or sedating. Further studies are needed to ascertain the effects of different CBD doses,

**Table 8.2** Human studies of sedative and stimulating effects of CBD

| CBD promotes wakefulness | CBD promotes sleep | CBD has no effect on sleep |
|---|---|---|
| **Nicholson et al.** [209]: effects of cannabis extracts (15 mg THC; 5 mg THC + 5 mg CBD; 15 mg THC + 15 mg CBD, placebo; oromucosal spray given 30 min from 10 pm)[f] on nocturnal sleep, early morning performance, memory, and sleepiness studied in 8 *healthy volunteers* (4 males, 4 females, 21–34 years); double-blind, placebo-controlled, 4-way crossover design<br>*Results:* no effects of 15 mg THC on sleep. Both doses of THC/CBD combination associated with decrease in stage 3 sleep; higher CBD/THC dose (15 mg each) combination increased wakefulness<br>The following day: 15 mg THC associated with impaired memory, reduced sleep latency, and increased sleepiness and mood changes<br>With the lower-dose (5 mg) CBD/THC combination, recall time was faster on digital recall task. With the higher-dose (15 mg) CBD/THC combination, participants reported increased sleepiness and mood changes. 15 mg THC appears to be sedative and 15 mg<br>*Conclusion:* CBD appears to have alerting properties as it increased awake activity during sleep and counteracted sedative activity of 15 mg THC | **Shannon & Opila-Lehman** [206]: **Case report,** 27-year-old male with bipolar disorder and cannabis addiction. CBD oil added to current medications (CannaVest CBD oil[a] was used). Initial dosage 24 mg CBD oil, 6 sprays PRN and 2 sprays QHS, with dosage gradually decreased to 18 mg/day, with no sprays during the day and 6 sprays at bedtime). Over a period of 4 months, patient able to stop use of cannabis and anxiety reduced and able to maintain regular sleep pattern<br>**Zuardi et al.** [208]: *11 healthy participants* received placebo or CBD[b] at doses of 300 mg ($n = 7$) or 600 mg ($n = 4$) in a double-blind manner in two experimental sessions separated by at least 1 week. CBD was found to have a sedative effect<br>**Carlini & Cunha** [201]: double-blind RCT; *15 insomniac participants* were given 40 mg, 80 mg, and 160 mg oral doses of CBD[c] and placebo and 5 mg nitrazepam; each week each participant received a different medication, over 5 weeks Dosing was once a week, 30 min before bed; then the following morning participants completed a questionnaire<br>*Results*<br>Sleep induction: The effect of all 3 doses of CBD and nitrazepam on sleep induction was not significantly different to placebo. There was no difference in quality of sleep induction between the groups<br>Sleep quality: The 160 mg CBD was associated with significantly increased sleep duration compared with placebo. There was no difference between the CBD 40 mg and CBD 80 mg groups and placebo group for sleep duration. There was no difference between any of the CBD groups and placebo for sleep fragmentation and reports of good sleep | **Spindle et al.** [211]: 18 *healthy adults* ($n = 9$ men, $n = 9$ women) completed four double-blind, double-dummy drug administration sessions that were separated by at least 1 week. Study medications: oral CBD (100 mg), vaporized pure CBD (synthetic crystalline form) (100 mg), vaporized CBD-dominant cannabis (100 mg CBD, 3.7 mg THC), and placebo cannabis[h]<br>Participants completed a Drug Effect Questionnaire at each session<br>*Results:* no significant difference between placebo, oral CBD, and vaporized pure (synthetic) CBD (100 mg) in terms of sleepiness |

(continued)

**Table 8.2** (continued)

| CBD promotes wakefulness | CBD promotes sleep | CBD has no effect on sleep |
|---|---|---|
| **Zuardi et al.** [210]: *8 healthy volunteers* dosed with 0.5 mg/kg THC, or 1 mg/kg CBD, or mixture of 0.5 mg/kg THC & 1 mg/kg CBD[g], or placebo or diazepam (10 mg) (the last two controls) in double-blind procedure (each participant participated in 5 experimental sessions separated by a week). Dosing with CBD was associated with a significant increase in "clear minded" & "quick-witted" feelings compared with THC (0.5 mg/Kg) which induced an increase in "muzzy" feelings | Dreams: Participants reported significantly less dream recall with all 3 doses of CBD compared with placebo<br>**Shannon et al.** [207]: **retrospective case series**, 72 *adults from an outpatient psychiatric clinic* with primary concerns of poor sleep ($n = 25$) or anxiety ($n = 47$). Most were given CBD 25 mg/day in capsule form (small no. given 50 mg/day or 75 mg/day, and one patient received CBD that was increased gradually to 175 mg/day)[d]. If anxiety complaints predominated, dosing was after breakfast and if sleep complaints predominated, dosing was after dinner<br>*Results*: on average sleep and anxiety improved for most patients and this was sustained over time<br>First month follow-up: 79.2% (57/72) and 66.7% (48/72) experienced an improvement in anxiety and sleep, respectively; 15.3% (11/72) and 25.0% (18/72) experienced worsening anxiety and sleep, respectively<br>Two-month follow-up: 78.1% (32/41) and 56.1% (23/41) reported improvement in anxiety and sleep, respectively, compared with the prior monthly visit; 19.5% (8/41) and 26.8% (11/41) reported worsening anxiety and sleep as compared with prior month<br>In group whose main complaint was poor sleep: PSQI changed from 13.08 (std dev 3.03) at baseline to 10.64 (std dev 3.89) at 1-month follow-up, 9.39 (std dev 3.81) at 2-month follow-up, and 9.33 (std dev 4.63) at 3-month follow-up[e]. Suggests no real improvement past the first month; no statistical analysis was conducted on the change from baseline to follow-up visits to ascertain if this was statistically significant | Vaporized CBD-dominant cannabis was associated with significant increase in sleepiness relative to vaporized pure CBD only (but not compared with placebo or oral CBD) [211] |

[a]From their website, CannaVest CBD oil appears to be a full-spectrum CBD product
[b]Little information is provided about the CBD except that it was sourced from Dr. R Mechoulam (Israel), mixed with alcohol and placed inside chocolate candies (same was done for placebo)
[c]Little information is provided about the CBD except that it was crystalized form, supplied by the US National Institutes of Health (NIH) and placed in gelatin capsules
[d]No information provided as to the actual CBD product used
[e]Pittsburgh Sleep Quality Index (PSQI): score of 0–21, higher number indicates more sleep-related problems [score >5 indicates a poor sleeper]
[f]CBD and THC provided by GW Pharmaceuticals plc. THC and the THC/CBD combinations were formulated in 50:50 ethanol to propylene glycol
[g]Little information is provided about the CBD except that it was sourced from Israel and prepared by mixing with 99% ethanol

[h]The vaporized CBD was a synthetic crystalline CBD; the CBD-dominant cannabis contained 10.5% CBD, 0.39% THC, 0.02% Δ8THC, and 0.05% cannabinol (CBN); the placebo cannabis contained 0.001% THC, 0.003% CBD, and 0.005% CBN; no Δ8 THC detected; the oral CBD had three formulations to assess pharmacokinetics: first six participants ingested CBD in a gelcap filled with cellulose; next six ingested 1 ml Epidiolex; last six ingested CBD in 10 ml pharmacy-grade cherry-flavored syrup. The study results collapsed data from all three into one as there was no difference across these subgroups

and what is considered a low or high dose needs to be better defined. It is more than possible that the effects of CBD in relation to sleep, i.e., potentially alerting or sedating at various doses, will vary between individuals depending on the relative state of their ECS (their "ECS tone"). In Dr. Blair's clinical experience, low doses (15–30 mg ~0.5 mg/kg) can be both alerting or sedating depending on context. In a wakeful environment of work or travel, CBD has alerting effects, whereas in a sleep or resting situation, the same CBD dose can be sedating. This might also be a function of the neurotransmitters and hormones (e.g., melatonin) circulating at that particular time and their interactions with CBD. This suggests that CBD may well be an *adaptogenic* herb which responds to the body's requirements in particular states.

Another key issue with research to date is that many of the studies have been conducted in healthy people [208–211] with few studies in people suffering from insomnia (e.g., Carlini & Cunha et al. [201]). More studies are needed in people suffering from actual insomnia since the state of the ECS is likely to be different in an insomniac compared with someone regularly getting adequate or good sleep. The ECS is, after all, a homeostatic regulator of sorts. Better attention to potentially confounding factors will also be needed in studies. In addition, new studies should include more objective parameters of sleep versus subjective surveys.

Importantly, the results of studies of CBD isolates are likely to differ from whole plant CBD oil with the additional terpenes and other phytonutrients present. Remember that terpenes also have their own therapeutic effects and some terpenes have sedative actions.

### CBD and Parasomnias

REM sleep behavior disorder is a parasomnia characterized by the loss of muscle atonia during REM sleep, associated with nightmares and active physical behavior during dreaming. The underlying cause is not well understood, but it occurs in synucleinopathies. Brainstem circuits that control atonia during REM sleep are damaged leading to random limb movements that are sometimes violent. In a case series of four patients with Parkinson's disease, treatment with CBD was associated with a prompt and substantial reduction in frequency of REM sleep behavior disorder events without side effects [213].

### Restless Legs Syndrome

Restless legs syndrome is a sleep-related movement disorder associated with a number of conditions including iron deficiency, Parkinson's disease, diabetes mellitus, and antidepressants to name a few. The syndrome is an irritating sensation in the lower extremities that stimulates limb movement and may disturb sleep. The cause may be genetically primary or secondary to drugs, mineral deficiencies, or dopamine dysregulation. Treatment for most is elimination of drugs, correction of deficiencies, or lifestyle modification. A case study of six patients with severe RLS unresponsive to opioids, benzodiazepines, gabapentin, or dopamine agonists achieved 100% relief with occasional recreational cannabis or CBD [214]. Oddly enough no other studies with cannabinoids have been completed for this condition.

## Efficacy of THC in Sleep Disorders

There is both preclinical and clinical research that supports a role of THC in modulating sleep. One of the effects of THC is sedation, and there are two potential mechanisms of action that may explain this [215]. The first is that endocannabinoids have been found to increase adenosine levels (which promotes sleep), and the second is that CB1 receptors are expressed in lateral hypothalamus neurons involved in arousal system regulation, resulting in inhibition of the arousal systems [215].

### Animal Studies: THC and Sleep

Preclinical research demonstrated that low and high doses of THC were associated with significantly increased brain temperature compared to control rats and that circadian rhythms were less pronounced. When THC was discontinued, circadian rhythms became inverted, i.e., the brain temperature at night of both low- and high-dose groups was that of the control rats during the day, leading the researchers to speculate that the circadian clock in the suprachiasmic nucleus might be affected by THC in an opposing manner [216].

A study found that 10 mg/kg of THC administered intravenously to mice potentiated the sleep inducing effect of pentobarbital, prolonging phenobarbital-induced sleep by 3.3-fold and that this effect that was attenuated by co-administration of CB1 receptor antagonists [217]. This finding supported a previous study which found that THC prolonged phenobarbital-induced sleeping time [218].

The acute effects of various doses of a specific strain of cannabis (11.5% THC, negligible amounts of other cannabinoids) administered by vaporization were investigated in rats. Polysomnographic recordings were taken in rats treated with 0 mg (control), 40 mg, 80 mg, and 200 mg of cannabis immediately prior to recordings. They found that 200 mg dosage increased NREM sleep time during the light phase but only during the first hour of recording and that no changes in sleep were found in the dark phase (active phase for rats) or with lower doses (40 mg, 80 mg). This was accompanied by EEG power reductions in different cortices, mainly in high-frequency bands during W and REM sleep and only during the light phase, as well as a decrease in sleep spindles intra-hemispheric coherence during NREM sleep during the dark phase [219].

**Table 8.3** Studies of the effects of THC on sleep

| Reference | Study features | Key results |
| --- | --- | --- |
| Pivik et al. [161] | Effects of THC on both undisturbed and experimentally altered (by REM deprivation) sleep patterns investigated in young adult male volunteers<br>Study 1 (normative experiments): 4 participants received THC in doses ranging from 61 to 258 μg per kilogram shortly before sleep onset<br>Study 2 (deprivation experiments): $n = 2$ received either THC (244 μg per kilogram and 259 μg per kilogram) or synhexl (semisynthetic THC, 733 μg per kilogram and 777 μg per kilogram) the morning after the second of two consecutive nights of REM deprivation | Both experiments indicated THC was associated with increased increments in stage 4 sleep and decrements in REM sleep<br>Normative experiments: a reduction in stage 1 and the time awake after sleep onset was observed with the highest THC dose level |
| Hosko et al. [220] | $N = 7$ subjects were administered oral THC at doses of 0.2 mg/kg and 0.3 mg/kg for 1 night each | Subjects appeared to show REM suppression and increases above baseline on withdrawal, but these were not statistically significant |
| Cousens and DiMascio [158] | **Participants: $n = 9$ healthy insomniacs**<br>Participants tested once a week for a 6-week period to investigate the effects of THC in altering usual sleep patterns<br>**Study medication: oral route**<br>THC was 95% THC in dehydrated alcohol in a drink composed of Fresca, bitter lemon, and cherry juice plus a few drops of almond extract. Placebo was the same minus the THC<br>**Doses**: the three doses of THC were 10 mg, 20 mg, and 30 mg<br>Participants received the THC or placebo 1.5 h before the average bedtime of the group<br>Each participant received all three doses of the THC and the placebo, with the sequence of administration in accordance with an incomplete Latin square design | All three doses of THC significantly decreased time to fall asleep (sleep latency) compared with placebo<br>Once asleep, interruptions (no. of awakenings during the night) were not significantly different for any of the THC doses compared with placebo<br>However, when they analyzed the data in 4-h blocks, for the time between midnight and 4 am, THC tended to be associated fewer awakenings and less time awake afterward, and the higher the dose of THC, the higher the trend (but it wasn't statistically significant). A nonsignificant trend was found for the second half of the night (4–8 am) in which increasingly more time was spent awake with higher doses of THC<br>The main side effects at all dose levels in presleep phase were temporal disorganization and changes in mood. The intensity of side effects and no. of subjects affected increased with increasing dosage of THC. The main side effect the following day was a "hangover" phenomenon, a continued "high" with some temporal disorganization and the intensity and duration of this increased with increasing dosage. This led the authors to conclude that this hangover effect was severe enough to limit consideration of 30 mg as a hypnotic |

| | | |
|---|---|---|
| Barratt et al. [221] | $N = 8$ subjects smoked 2 cannabis cigarettes per night (equivalent to 0.2 mg/kg THC) for 10 nights | Increase in delta sleep (combined stages 3 & 4) during the first 4 nights and then a decrease thereafter. No significant effect on REM time or eye movement activity |
| Freemon [222] | $N = 5$ subjects<br>20 mg THC given for 4 nights before sleep | REM time lower on THC compared with baseline<br>No tendency to rebound on withdrawal<br>Found one instance of early REM onset on withdrawal |
| Feinberg et al. [159] | **Participants**: $n = 7$ subjects who were experienced cannabis users (mean age 25 years). $N = 4$ were studied for 3 baseline nights, 3 nights under an initial dose of 70 mg THC/day and last 3 nights of a 2-week period of 210 mg/day THC plus first 3 nights of withdrawal. $N = 3$ additional subjects studied during the last 3 nights of a 2-week period of 210 mg/day THC plus first 3 nights of withdrawal. Participants lived in the hospital during the study<br>**Study medication**: THC administered orally as capsules containing 30 mg THC in sesame oil. Placebo capsules contained only sesame oil<br>**Dosages**: 70 mg/day and 210 mg/day (see schedule above)<br>For the 210 mg/day condition, capsules were administered at 8 am, 12.00 pm, 6.00 pm, 9.00 pm, and 4 am, with 60 mg given prior to sleep (10–11 pm)<br>For the 70 mg condition, 10 mg was administered at each of these time points with 20 mg administered prior to sleep<br>EEG readings and eye movements investigated | Subjects were lethargic and sedated with the high dose of THC initially, but by 5–6 days of the 210 mg dose, tolerance was apparent. The drug withdrawal phase was associated with alertness and irritability<br>THC significantly reduced eye movement activity during REM sleep and, to a lesser extent, reduced the duration of REM itself (this was significant statistically though). The disproportionate reduction in eye movements compared with REM duration (EM density) resembled effects of sedative/hypnotics such as benzodiazepines and barbiturates. Withdrawal led to increases above baseline in both measures, but the "rebound" effect was greater for eye movement<br>There was a nonsignificant increase in stage 4 sleep associated with THC. On withdrawal, stage 4 sleep decreased significantly, but this was only marked on the first night |

(continued)

**Table 8.3** (continued)

| Reference | Study features | Key results |
|---|---|---|
| Feinberg et al. [160] | **Participants**: $n = 4$ paid participants, all experienced cannabis users (mean age 25.6 years)<br>**Study medication**: crude ethanolic cannabis extract containing 29% THC, 1.5% CBD) Doses of 10 mg and 30 mg THC content were given in gelatin capsules with the cannabis extract dissolved in 0.4 ml of ethanol. Placebo capsules contained only the 0.4 ml ethanol<br>**Dosage**: low dose (70 mg/day) compared with high dose (210 mg/day)<br>Dosing schedule: 2 subjects started on an initial dose of 70 mg/day for 3 days and 2 subjects started on a high dose (210 mg) for 3 nights. Then, the 4 participants all took the high dose for the next 3 nights. Then withdrawal was measured for all 4 over the next 4 nights, and then finally for 2 participants, withdrawal was tracked for an additional 3 nights<br>Sleep data of the four participants in this study were compared with that obtained from seven participants in a previous study who had received pure THC (96% THC, though it was acknowledged that other phytocannabinoids were present)<br>Sleep study methods: EEG recordings | *REM sleep:* both extract and pure THC reduced eye movement density with some tolerance developing to this effect. Stage 4 tended to increase with drug administration Initial intake of 70 mg THC (either pure or extract) reduced REM time and to a greater extent suppressed EM. Increasing the dose to 210 mg THC after 3 days of 70 mg produced some increase in these effects, but increments were relatively small which suggests tolerance had developed<br>Abrupt withdrawal led to very high densities of rapid eye movement, increased REM durations, and sharp and transient fall in stage 4 to baseline levels<br>*NREM sleep*: total NREM sleep increased as REM decreased during drug administration and significantly decreased during the REM sleep rebound in withdrawal. Distribution of NREM sleep among stages 2, 3, and 4 showed little change. Architecture of NREM sleep was essentially normal under high-dose (210 mg) pure THC and extract and after abrupt withdrawal<br>*Sleep latency* (time from lights-out to onset of sleep) was not significantly altered by THC except during immediate withdrawal when it nearly doubled. This increase in sleep latency with time in bed and time awake after sleep onset constant produced a significant reduction in total sleep time. There was no increase in amount or % time awake after sleep onset in the withdrawal condition |

| | | |
|---|---|---|
| Tassarini et al. [223] | **Participants**: two groups of volunteers (21–25 years)<br>**Study medication and dosing:**<br>Group A: $n = 7$ young volunteers (21–25 years old) who had never used cannabis before; all received one single **oral dose** of THC in alcoholic solution in dosages of 0.7 mg/kg to 1 mg/kg THC<br>Group B: 4 young subjects (21–25 years old), $n = 2$ given 10 g hashish in sachets taken **orally** (doses corresponded to 1 and 1.4 mg/kg) and $n = 2$ given THC in oily solution in **oral** dosages of 0.7 mg/kg and 0.9 mg/kg<br>Polygraphic recordings taken | Group A: THC was associated with significant changes in nocturnal sleep with disappearance of REM stages and a decrease of slow sleep (stages 3 and 4)<br>Group B: sleep EEG was recorded in one subject who had hashish at the equivalent of 1.4 mg/kg. He slept only in stage 2 sleep and no REM or slow sleep stages were recorded.<br>Heavy (0.7–1 mg/kg) single oral doses of THC in alcohol or in oily solution led to effects similar to oral doses of hashish containing a similar amount of THC |
| Freemon [224] | **Participants**: $n = 2$ subjects, brothers in their 20s. Slept in laboratory for 27 consecutive nights and then after 4 nights at home, for another 4 nights<br>**Study medication and dosing:**<br>One subject received placebo for 4 baseline nights, 30 mg THC for the next 14 nights, and placebo during the 4 withdrawal nights<br>The other subject received the placebo during the study period | During the first 2 nights of placebo (after 14 consecutive drug nights), subjects had difficulty falling and staying asleep. This was not accompanied by an increase in REM sleep (which can occur on withdrawal from other drugs)<br>After about 1 week of THC administration and continuing for a week after discontinuation of the drug, there was a marked decrease in slow-wave sleep, NREM sleep (stages 3 & 4) |
| Zuardi et al. [210] | **Participants:** *8 healthy volunteers*<br>**Study medication**: participants dosed with 0.5 mg/kg THC, or 1 mg/kg CBD, or mixture of 0.5 mg/kg THC & 1 mg/kg CBD, or placebo or diazepam (10 mg) (the last two controls) in double-blind procedure (each participant participated in five experimental sessions separated by a week) | Dosing with CBD was associated with a significant increase in "clear minded" & "quick-witted" feelings compared with THC (0.5 mg/kg) which induced an increase in "muzzy" feelings |

(continued)

**Table 8.3** (continued)

| Reference | Study features | Key results |
|---|---|---|
| Chait [225] | **Participants**: $n = 12$ regular cannabis smokers (who smoked cannabis 1–2 times per week)<br>Study investigated potential side effects of cannabis smoking<br>**Study medication:**<br>Pre-rolled cannabis cigarettes weighing between 800 and 900 mg were supplied by the National Institute on Drug Abuse. THC content of cigarettes was 0.0% (placebo) or 2.1% (active). Cigarettes were smoked through a plastic cigarette holder<br>Each participant assessed for 2 weekends: during one weekend they received placebo cannabis (0% THC) and the other weekend active cannabis (2.1% THC). Each weekend, participants received 40 standardized puffs of cannabis smoke, administered during 5 separate smoking sessions in the late afternoon and evenings. Participants were told not to smoke cannabis outside the laboratory during the 24 h before scheduled sessions<br>The next morning after smoking, participants completed a series of questionnaires to evaluate sleep (Leeds Sleep Evaluation Questionnaire [LSEQ]) and mood, and performed tests of psychomotor and cognitive function. The LSEQ measures four aspects of sleep: getting to sleep, quality of sleep, awakening from sleep, and behavior following wakefulness | Leeds Sleep Evaluation Questionnaire: Mean score on LSEQ was not significantly different between groups (group mean scores after placebo and active marijuana were 42.3 and 54.4, respectively [0–100 scale]). Subanalysis showed a statistically significant difference between groups for "getting to sleep" indicating THC was associated with greater ease of getting to sleep compared with placebo<br>The study found no indication of residual intoxication after the active cannabis |
| Neff et al. [226] | Case report: three patients with intractable pruritus associated with cholestatic liver disease given dronabinol<br>Medication: all patients started on 5 mg dronabinol at bedtime | All patients reported decreased pruritus and marked improvement in sleep and were eventually able to return to work. Depression was resolved in two patients<br>Side effects included one patient experiencing disturbance in coordination, with resolution of this when dosage was decreased to 2.5 mg<br>Duration of antipruritic effect: approximately 4–6 h (suggests more frequent dosing needed) |

| | | |
|---|---|---|
| Nicholson et al. [209] | Effects of oromucosal high THC extract product (**active constituent dronabinol**) and a THC/CBD extract (using doses of 5 mg and 15 mg THC equivalent) was assessed in eight participants in a double-blind, four-way crossover study | THC 15 mg alone: had little effect on sleep architecture, sleep latency reduced, memory impaired, residual sleepiness, and mood changes<br>Both dose levels of combined THC/CBD: associated with decreased stage 3 sleep (compared with placebo) and the 15 mg dose was associated with increased wakefulness compared with 5 mg dose<br>5 mg CBD/THC dose: produced faster reaction times on digit recall test compared with placebo<br>15 mg THC alone: impaired memory the next day while there were no such effects for 15 mg CBD/15 mg THC combination (nabiximols)<br>*Conclusion:* THC was sedative, and the presence of CBD was alerting and tended to counteract the THC-associated adverse effects on cognition and impairment of wakefulness |
| Gorelick et al. [186] | *N* = 13 male chronic daily cannabis smokers (mean age 24.6 years +/−3.7) who smoked 5.5 +/−5.9 joint-equivalents per day; 10 of these reported no sleep problems prior to admission into the study<br>**Study medication**: oral synthetic THC (dronabinol) in 20 mg capsules<br>**Doses**: administered around the clock for 7 days; day 1 40 mg; day 2–4100 mg; day 5, 6120 mg (40 mg–120 mg/day) starting the afternoon after admission<br>Measurements included St. Mary's Hospital Sleep Questionnaire (completed each morning) and plasma THC and 11-OH-THC (active metabolite) concentrations | Higher evening THC and 11-OH-THC concentrations were significantly associated with shorter sleep latency, lower self-rated difficulty falling asleep, and greater hours of daytime sleep the following day<br>Duration of calculated and self-reported nighttime sleep decreased slightly (3.54 and 5.34 min per night, respectively, statistically significant)<br>Note: 1 withdrew from the study after 1 day for personal reasons; 2 were discharged on day 4 (one due to premature ventricular contractions, another due to psychological reaction) |
| Farabi et al. [227] | **Participants**: *n* = 15 patients with obstructive sleep apnea<br>**Study medication**: dronabinol | Dronabinol is associated with change in delta and theta frequencies and an increase in ultradian rhythms which correlated with improvement in apneas and decrease in sleepiness |

## Human Studies: THC and Sleep

Research indicates that THC is associated with a sedative effect [130], though one review [215] reported that three studies found high doses of THC were associated with an alerting effect reflected in increased latency to sleep onset.

A summary of the findings of several studies from the early 1970s to current times is included in Table 8.3. Most of these studies assess the effects of acute dosing of THC.

Few studies have assessed the effect of chronic consumption of THC on sleep. There are some studies on longer-term cannabis use, for example, Halikas et al. [228], a longitudinal study. Their findings suggest some individuals may develop tolerance to the sleep-enhancing effects of cannabis and that the positive effect on self-reported sleep quality is less frequent among long-term cannabis users [228].

More targeted studies including longer-term studies (e.g., over weeks or months of use) are required to assess the effects of various doses of THC on various aspects of sleep.

A review of the effects of cannabis and THC on sleep in 2008 concluded that smoked cannabis and oral THC reduce REM sleep and that acute administration of cannabis seems to facilitate falling asleep as well as increased stage 4 sleep. It also reported that difficulty sleep and strange dreams were commonly reported symptoms of acute and subacute cannabis withdrawal and that longer sleep onset latency, reduced slow-wave sleep, and an REM rebound were also observed [229].

### Cannabis, THC, and Sleep as a Secondary Outcome Measure

Impact on sleep is often measured in studies as a secondary outcome variable to some other outcome which is the main focus of the study (the "primary outcome variable"). In one double-blind, randomized, placebo-controlled study of 15 healthy men (who had used cannabis 15 times or less during their lives), functional magnetic resonance imaging was used while they viewed faces that elicited different levels of anxiety. Participants were given either 10 mg THC, 600 mg CBD, or placebo prior to scanning session. THC increased anxiety and levels of sedation, intoxication, and psychotic symptoms. There was a trend of reduction in anxiety after administration of CBD [230].

In a systematic review of medicinal cannabis in sleep, 28 studies with a total of 3658 participants included a measure of sleep as a treatment outcome for various illnesses. Such illnesses included pain, MS, anorexia, cancer, and immune deficiency. Study medications included synthetic THC analogues of dronabinol and nabilone (14 studies), synthetic CBD analogues (4 studies), and nabiximols (1:1 ratio of THC: CBD). Most of the studies did not include a validated measure of sleep; however, most reported a significant and positive impact on sleep with 17 studies showing improvement in sleep and 1 showing a decrease in bad dreams [179].

### Nabiximols and Insomnia

Nabiximols is a product which contains plant-derived THC and CBD (no terpenes) in a ratio of approximately 1:1 (2.7 mg THC: 2.5 mg CBD with each spray). Its onset of activity is around 15–40 min. A 2007 review of nabiximols concluded it was highly effective in treating pain-induced insomnia in 13 different studies. The review summarized the findings associated with numerous phase I–III studies (2000 participants with 1000 patient years of exposure) as follows:

- Marked improvement in subjective sleep parameters in patients with a wide variety of pain conditions including multiple sclerosis, peripheral neuropathic pain, intractable cancer pain, and rheumatoid arthritis
- Acceptable adverse event profile
- No tolerance its benefit on pain or sleep, nor need for dosage increases noted in safety extension studies of up to 4 years
- 40–50% of subjects attained good or very good sleep quality [231]

## Studies of THC in Treatment of Sleep Disorders Associated with PTSD

Several studies, many open-label in nature, have investigated the efficacy of THC in alleviating sleep problems associated with PTSD, including nightmares. In general, they support the use of THC for reducing nightmares and improving sleep quality. Studies are set out in Table 8.4.

**Table 8.4** Studies of THC treatment of PTSD sufferers with sleep problems

| Reference | Study design | Results |
|---|---|---|
| Fraser [232] | Open-label study<br>**Participants**: $n = 47$ PTSD patients with continuing treatment-resistant nightmares<br>**Study medication**: adjunctive treatment with nabilone<br>**Dosing**: doses of 0.5 mg 1 h prior to bedtime; titration indicated if medication well tolerated and if symptom control of nightmares not achieved. All were kept below maximum 6 mg/day. Average effective dose was 0.5 mg 1 h before bedtime, with a range of 0.2 mg to 4.0 mg nightly | Cessation or a significant reduction in nightmare intensity in 72% of participants; some reported improvements in sleep time, quality of sleep, and reduction of daytime flashbacks and night sweats<br>Discontinuation of medication success for four patients after 4–12 months of nabilone therapy (nightmares did not return or returned at a reduced level, not needing further medication control) Other patients experienced a recurrence of nightmares upon nabilone withdrawal (usually within the first two nights) and regained control once nabilone reinitiated |
| Shalev et al. [233] | Open-label study of ten patients with PTSD who received THC twice daily for 3 weeks | Significant improvement in arousal, sleep quality, and nightmares |
| Roitman et al. [234] | Three-week, open-label study was conducted in ten patients with chronic PTSD on stable medication (five were combat veterans). Patients were given 5 mg THC olive oil sublingually twice daily as an adjunct to their regular medication | Significant reduction in frequency of nightmares ($p < 0.04$), sleep quality ($p < 0.05$), as well as hyperarousal (CAPS, $p < 0.02$) and significant improvement in global symptom severity (CGI-5, $p < 0.02$) |

(continued)

**Table 8.4** (continued)

| Reference | Study design | Results |
|---|---|---|
| Cameron et al. [235] | Retrospective study (chart review)<br>**Participants**: 104 male inmates with serious mental illness, mean age 32.7 years (range, 19–55 years)<br>**Doses**: mean initial dose 1.4 mg daily (0.5–2.0 mg), mean final dose of nabilone was 4.0 mg (range 0.5–6.0 mg). Mean length on nabilone 11.2 weeks (range 1 day to 36 weeks)<br>Patients with hepatitis C had a mean final dose of 4.2 mg; cannabis-naive individuals had a mean final dose of 3.2 mg | Nabilone (synthetic THC) targeted a mean 3.5 indications per patient; most common were insomnia ($n = 101$, 97.1%), nightmares ($n = 90$, 86.5%), and chronic pain ($n = 68$, 65.4%)<br>Significant reductions in PTSD-associated insomnia and nightmares as well as other symptoms. Medications with greater risk of adverse effects/abuse were often able to be discontinued with initiation of nabilone (typically antipsychotics and sedative/hypnotics) |
| Jetly et al. [236] | Double-blind, crossover RCT conducted in Canadian military personal with trauma-related nightmares $N = 10$ participants randomized to either nabilone (0.5 mg titrated to daily max 3.0 mg) or placebo for 7 weeks, followed by a 2-week washout period and then treated with opposite study medication for 7 weeks | Significant improvement in nightmares but no effect on sleep quality or quantity |

## Other Phytocannabinoids and Terpenes in the Treatment of Insomnia

Other phytocannabinoids and terpenes may also be useful in the treatment of insomnia. Cannabinol (CBN) is one such phytocannabinoid which appears to have sedative properties, though the evidence is largely anecdotal at this point.

### Cannabinol (CBN)

A study in mice assessed eight halogenated derivatives of CBN by intracerebroventricular injection (50 micrograms/mouse). In one experiment investigating interaction with pentobarbital, two of the derivatives of CBN exhibited a significant prolongation of sleeping time, but the other derivatives did not [237].

A study conducted in 1975 which assessed the effects of THC, CBN, and a combination of the two on various paraments in five male volunteers. Study medications were placebo, 50 mg CBN, 25 mg THC, 12.5 mg THC + 25 mg CBD, and 25 mg

THC + 50 mg CBN (orally), with administration spaced a week apart. THC produced an increase in heart rate, CBN did not, and the combination did not alter the effect of THC alone. On a 66-item drug reaction scale, participants reported feeling drugged, drunk, dizzy, and drowsy after THC ingestion but not after CBD ingestion, but the combination elicited reports of feeling more drugged/drunk/dizzy/drowsy [238]. Thus, this might be some evidence of a synergistic effect of CBN on the sedative effect of THC; however, the study has low numbers of participants. It certainly doesn't provide direct evidence of a sedative effect of CBN alone.

### Terpenes

Several of the terpenes are known to have sedative effects. These include myrcene and linalool [239, 240]. High myrcene varieties of cannabis that produce linalool are noted for their effectiveness in sleep disorders as these terpenes are calming and lightly sedative [100].

These terpenes found in cannabis are also found in other foods and plants. Myrcene is contained in mango, for example. Therefore, consuming a mango a few hours prior to bedtime might potentially enhance the effect of a cannabis medicine, in a similar way to which myrcene within the cannabis plant provides an entourage effect. The use of lavender oil in infusers or sleep pillows is another example of using a terpene such as linalool from another source to provide an entourage effect.

## Nutritional Factors Impacting Sleep Quality

Our diet can play a very important role in our sleep quality. It is known, for example, that carbohydrates and fats regulate sleep quality by affecting duration of REM and NREM sleep, and research indicates that those with short sleep duration take in more energy from carbohydrates and fats [45]. Consumption of protein has a positive correlation with sleep duration; those with normal sleep duration had higher protein intake than insomniacs [241], and those on high-protein diets were found to have fewer wake times compared to those on a control diet [242]. The amino acid tryptophan found in proteins is the precursor to melatonin and serotonin and plays a key role in sleep quality [45]. The timing and macronutrient content of diet both impact on sleep, and food eaten before bedtime has a strong impact on how we sleep and has been found to be associated with sleep disorders [45, 243, 244].

Habitual short sleep increases appetite and plasma ghrelin levels and decreases leptin levels [45]. Ghrelin, the hormone that increases appetite, promotes sleep by stimulating slow-wave sleep and growth hormone released at night. Ghrelin levels are high during sleep and start to decrease a few hours after breakfast. The effect of short sleep on leptin may occur via several mechanisms. Leptin secretion is inhibited by sympathetic nervous system activity, and this could be a mechanism by which leptin levels are lowered during chronic partial sleep loss, or it may be that the decrease in leptin after sleep restriction is simply a normal adaptation to the increased energy required to stay awake for a longer period of time [45]. Orexin-containing neurons in the hypothalamus are believed to provide the molecular basis for interactions between nutrition and sleep [45].

Epidemiological studies indicate that an unhealthy diet is associated with irregular sleep patterns and shorter sleep [45, 245–247]. Research indicates that those with poor sleep have irregular or poor nutritional habits including consuming energy-dense foods, eating more fat and refined carbohydrates and snacks, and consuming less fruit and vegetables [45, 248, 246].

A discussion of dietary factors is beyond the scope of this book; however, the point we want to make is that when assessing factors that might be impacting on sleep, you should certainly consider diet and nutrition as well as many other factors that might also be impacting on sleep. If nutritional medicine is not your forte, refer the patient for a nutritional assessment to a nutritional medicine practitioner.

For a good summary of the effect of diet on sleep see Sanlier and Sabuncular [45].

## Obstructive Sleep Apnea

Obstructive sleep apnea (OSA) is also a prevalent form of sleep-disordered breathing affecting approximately 9% of adults in the USA [249]. In OSA, the individual repeatedly stops and starts breathing during sleep. Sufferers characteristically make gasping or snorting sounds during which sleep is disrupted [52]. Symptoms and signs associated with OSA include excessive sleepiness or fatigue, morning headache, poor concentration, cognitive dysfunction, sore throat, lower libido, erectile dysfunction, poor work performance, personality change, snoring, choking, restless sleep, nocturia, sweating, acid reflux, dry mouth during the night, and sleep maintenance insomnia [22].

The US National Health and Nutrition Study 2005–2008 found that 6% of men and 3.1% of women reported physician-diagnosed sleep apnea [250]. This study found that frequent snorting and stopping breathing were associated with probable major depression [250]. Obstructive sleep apnea is a strong, independent risk factor for later development of cardiovascular disease and stroke [251]. Other consequences of OSA include hypertension, impaired inflammatory response, hormonal changes, increased risk of cancer, and brain atrophy [22]. OSA is also very underdiagnosed: in most western countries, less than a quarter of the potential sleep apneic population are diagnosed [251].

Those who are particularly at risk of OSA are males who are overweight with central obesity. Apart from obesity, other risk factors for OSA are tobacco smoking, hormonal factors (including hypothyroidism), upper airway lesions, lying in a supine position, sedative drugs, and anesthetics [22].

## Cannabinoids in the Treatment of Obstructive Sleep Apnea (OSA)

The ECS appears to be involved in obstructive sleep apnea (OSA) with higher concentrations of the endocannabinoid oleoylethanolamide (OEA) but not AEA or 2-AG found in patients with OSA which were associated with difficulty breathing [252].

### Animal Research

Animal experiments suggest that THC may be useful in reducing sleep apnea and shed light on potential mechanisms of action. In a rat study, the exogenous (phyto) cannabinoid THC and the endogenous endocannabinoid (fatty acid amide) oleamide reduced apneic events, providing initial evidence that the ECS may function to suppress serotonin-mediated symptoms of obstructive sleep apnea [64]. In that study, intraperitoneal injections were given of various doses of THC, oleamide, and serotonin, alone and in combination to 11 male rats, and polysomnographic measurements taken. They found that THC and oleamide each stabilized respiration during all sleep stages, with significant reductions in the apnea sleep index of 42% and 58% in NREM and REM sleep, respectively. Oleamide produced a similar suppression of apnea, and both oleamide and THC were able to block serotonin-induced exacerbation of sleep apnea. The authors concluded that their results suggest that endocannabinoids play an important role in maintaining autonomic stability during sleep [64].

In another experiment in rats, results suggested that dronabinol (THC) stabilized respiratory pattern, modulated upper airway muscles responsible for regulating breathing during sleep, and reduced 5-HT-induced reflex apneas by acting at the nodose ganglia [253]. While injection of dronabinol into the nodose ganglia of rats attenuated reflex apnea and increased genioglossus activity, an effect blocked by pre-systemic treatment of CB1 and/or CB2 receptor antagonists suggesting that dronabinol's effects were facilitated via cannabinoid receptors), no effect was found on 5-HT-induced apneas or genioglossus activity when dronabinol was injected intracerebrovascularly [254]. Thus, efficacy of dronabinol in suppressing apneas appears to be facilitated by peripheral rather than central nervous system activity, via suppression of vagal nerve activity [254].

### Human Research

Human research supports the potential therapeutic role of THC in treatment of OSA. For example, in a study on the effects of dronabinol on objective measures of sleep process in adults, dronabinol was associated with changes in delta and theta frequencies and an increase in ultradian rhythms which correlated with improvement in apneas and decrease in sleepiness [227].

In an RCT comprised of 73 adults with moderate or severe obstructive sleep apnea, 25 participants received placebo, 21 participants received 2.5 mg dronabinol, and 27 participants received 10 mg dronabinol (synthetic THC) daily, an hour before bedtime, for up to 6 weeks [255].

The results were as follows:

- Compared with placebo, dronabinol dose-dependently reduced apnea-hypopnea index (AHI):
  - 2.5 mg/day: reduction of 10.7 ± 4.4 events/hour ($p = 0.02$)
  - 10 mg/day: reduction of 12.9 ± 4.3 events/hour ($p = 0.003$)
- Participants on 10 mg/day of dronabinol:
  - Had highest overall satisfaction with treatment ($p = 0.04$)
  - Had reductions in the Epworth Sleepiness Scale (ESS) score by −3.8 ± 0.8 points from baseline ($p < 0.0001$) and by −2.3 ± 1.2 points compared with placebo ($p = 0.05$)
- Maintenance of Wakefulness Test (MWT) sleep latencies, gross sleep architecture, and overnight oxygenation parameters were unchanged from baseline in any treatment group [255].

## Guidelines for Treating Insomnia with Medicinal Cannabis

Treatment of sleep disorders such as insomnia with medicinal cannabis should be within the context of an integrative medicine approach to health which considers the role of stress (and stress reduction), nutrition, exercise, vitamin D, and other lifestyle factors. Remember that insomnia can be a side effect of several pharmaceutical medications including antidepressants, so it is important to review the patient's medications and supplements.

Sleep hygiene is one of the first things to consider. Since sleep disorders, anxiety, depression, and pain are often comorbid, it is important to take a thorough case history and address these issues if they are present. Medicinal cannabis has the advantage that you can address several symptoms/signs simultaneously.

### When to Use Medicinal Cannabis

Consider the use of cannabinoids in patients after a thorough history, prescription review, and general examination. Sleep disorders can be the result or cause of many chronic medical conditions and therefore should almost always be addressed. Most frequently another provider has already done so by prescribing a sedative/hypnotic either temporarily or indefinitely. Some patients realize the danger of hypnotics by seeking cannabis consultation to ease the transition often from dependence and challenging withdrawal symptoms. Patients must appreciate that the sleep effects of phytocannabinoids are highly individualized but generally positive by improving sleep latency, duration, depth, circadian adjustments, and overall quality.

Potential candidates for the use of medicinal cannabis include:

- Patients who want to improve the quality of their lives through sleep and reduce inflammatory risks of shift work schedules
- Travelers who wish to optimize rest, recover, and time-zone adaptation quickly during extended travel

- Those who have not had success using other medications including herbal medicines
- Those at risk of addiction, drug interactions, and adverse effects from conventional pharmaceuticals
- Those with established sleep disorders like restless legs syndrome, sleep apnea, narcolepsy, and REM sleep behavior disorder [213]
- Patients facing end of life care issues wanting to maintain maximal cognitive awareness

### Comprehensive Treatment Plan

Medicinal cannabis can be used primarily or secondarily for insomnia as part of a comprehensive treatment plan. The insomnia component should include all relevant therapies including cannabinoids that could be effective. The plan can function as a checklist, patient log, and guide for the clinician in follow-up appointments. It should include self-assessment sleep parameters and a simple, perhaps five-level scoring rather than "better, worse, or about the same" (e.g., "On a scale of 1–5, 1 being the worst, 5 being best, how would you rate your sleep?"). It should also include a notes section in which a patient can flag some events or associations as well as subjective associations. This treatment plan or log should include the primary symptom target(s), e.g., anxiety, pain, etc., since insomnia is often a secondary issue in most consultations. As soon as possible the patient and healthcare practitioner should set the benchmark from which to measure success.

Sleep-sensing devices and phone apps can be a valuable part of sleep assessment and tracking. The apps usually provide sleep times, durations, and levels for confirming sleep patterns and tweaking treatment programs. Apps with wearable devices can track heart rates and variability that can be used to assess general health improvements [256]. Patients can engage in the process of looking for comprehensive solutions rather than just a sleeping potion.

## Type of Product (Blends)

The following recommendations are made by Backes [100]:

- Anxiety and rumination can interfere with restful sleep; THC is effective for anxiety and rumination at 1–5 mg sublingually (or swallowed for a more potent and soporific effect).
- THC taken orally is recommended for sleep: 5–7.5 mg 1 hour before bed or when bed rest needed. Vaporized cannabis is also effective for insomnia when taken 1 hour before bedtime, for waking during the night.
- Day timc use of CBD may be useful: CBD's anti-anxiety effects help in calming so that patients can sleep better (he cautions that observational reports suggest CBD may make sleep-deprived patients sleepy but it becomes wake-promoting if it is taken after 5pm or once the patient has caught up on rest).
- High-myrcene 'Purple' varieties or cultivars of cannabis (e.g. Grape Apes, Purps) that produce linalool are noted for effectiveness in sleep disorders as these

terpenes are calming and lightly sedative. Kush varieties also contain lmyrcene (eg. Bubba Kush, Hindu Kush) [100].

Clearly the usual recommendations with respect to dosing with THC (start at a low dose and titrate up slowly) apply. Cannabis expert Dr. Daniel Stein recommends cannabis medicines with THC plus terpenes linalool and myrcene for treatment of sleep disorders like insomnia. He suggests a starting dose of THC of 2–4 mg/day. Dr. Stein also recommends that CBD may also be used to treat insomnia however cautions that small doses (5–10 mg) for new users may be alerting and that they may need to increase the dosage up to 25–30 mg to get a sedative effect [257]. Some sources also recommend that indica-dominant strains of cannabis are advisable for night-time use as they are believed to be more sedating (rather than sativa-dominant strains which are believed to be more alerting).

Dr. Blair has found full-spectrum CBD (with low THC) to be effective in the higher dosage range above. As mentioned above, CBD products can be immediately activating for some but sedating for others.

## What Form of Product Should You Use?

The best formulation matches the patients preferred lifestyle and tastes. Capsules have a longer duration of action, but sublingual tinctures may be faster acting. Topical dosing can avoid some of the activating features of cannabis bypassing the liver and the mouth after brushing the teeth and mouthwash. Topical can be quite effective applied to any areas of the body but particularly thin skin or covered areas that will not stain the bedding.

## Dosing Guidelines

The optimum dose of medicinal cannabis allows for rapid sleep onset, healthy sleep stages, minimal awakenings, 6–8 h of duration, and refreshment upon waking. Usually, average doses of medicinal cannabis typically used for other minor issues also improve sleep experience (i.e., in the range of 25–50 mg per day for a full spectrum CBD dominant oil). With respect to timing, because of the variability in response, dosing 2 h before sleep time seems to allow the mind time to relax and set the stage for normal sleep. Other patients have found the most effective timing is immediately before sleep or after an early morning awakening. Note that as always, particularly in the case of cannabis naive patients and where products contain THC, the general guideline of 'start low and go slow' applies (i.e., start at a low dose, titrate up slowly until there is a therapeutic effect). Having an adverse effect due to taking a dose of THC that is too high could serve to put the patient off medicinal cannabis.

## Titration and Follow-Up

Cannabis does not cause respiratory depression, so patients can titrate their use to optimize their sleep. A sleep app gives them better feedback as to what actually happened during the night to better guide them. Most patients perceive the greatest improvements associated with duration and percentage of deep sleep. Sleep apps can be shared and reviewed by the healthcare practitioner for better objective decision-making. Performance, mood, and activity in addition to the primary symptom(s) can all be indicators of improved sleep changes. A week or longer will establish a clear pattern for interpretation and guide possible dose changes if needed.

## Other Tips to Enhance Therapeutic Action

Cannabis works well with other therapies so feel free to add tried and true approaches like melatonin, magnesium, or Epsom salt soaks (magnesium). A more recent finding is regarding zinc as a sleep modulator. The mechanism of action is undetermined but focuses on Zn2+-containing presynaptic vesicles to be co-released with glutamate. In addition, Zn2+ is also found in some inhibitory glycinergic terminals of the cerebellum and in the spinal cord [258]. Interestingly CBD affects the expression of genes involved in zinc homeostasis in microglial cells, modulating zinc transporters regulating intracellular zinc concentration imperative for cytokine release, oxidative stress, and immunoreactivity [259]. Zinc doses have ranged between 25 and 50 mg elemental zinc before sleep.

On the other hand, patients dependent on benzodiazepines can taper those agents safely, controlling some of the anxiety and irritability associated with withdrawal. A slow taper is recommended, but most often patients find that once they establish confidence in cannabinoids, they stop the offending drug completely within a few weeks. Liberal use of cannabis will mitigate withdrawal symptoms and maintain activities of daily living and work performance.

Travelers are a special category that can greatly benefit for broad-spectrum cannabis to maintain their waking, sleeping, and time-zone transitions no matter what the range traversed. CBD has the unique property of allowing alertness and facilitating sleep during the appropriate diurnal phases. Furthermore, CBD appears to allow the circadian regulators to "float" to allow for rapid and immediate reset to current location [33]. Consistent with clinical observations of the use of therapeutic cannabis to treat insomnia, circadian rhythm is deregulated in microglial cells by CBD to allow for time-zone adaption (but this does not occur with THC) [33].

## Case Studies from Dr. Blair's Practice

### Case 1

International business consultant traveling California to Colorado for 2 days, then Jordan for 6 days and returning to California. A 68-year-old man in average health and fitness requested aid to manage physical and cognitive demands while traveling. He had several high-level meetings and presentations in both locations and did not have the luxury of layovers and time-zone adjustments.

His only medications were T4 thyroid and he used a number of supplements. Capsules were recommended of broad-spectrum CBD to avoid issues in countries with cannabis restrictions. In addition, capsules could be easily carried and available on demand when symptoms occurred. A dose of four capsules per day of travel was anticipated and placed in two containers to avoid loss or inability to access. Aspirin 80 mg was also included to augment cannabinoid effects if needed along with capsules of omega-3.

Travel to Colorado was uneventful and supported with maintenance of 25 mg CBD twice daily. An additional capsule was used midday sublingual before a scheduled presentation because of noted afternoon fatigue. Alertness was enhanced and anxiety was reduced. Two days later he departed on 19-h travel to Jordan through Chicago in coach class. While traveling he used additional capsules for fatigue and restless legs symptoms during the 11 h first Jordan leg and 13 h return leg. Sleep was limited to a few hours at a time before being disturbed or uncomfortable.

Upon arrival at midday, he again used sublingual capsules to manage alertness and an early evening dose to facilitate sleep. An early morning awakening was also supplemented with a capsule. In the morning he was alert and rested and attended all business meetings and presentations as well as extensive travel around the city to key locations. Capsule supplements were taken as needed for fatigue, preparation for presentation and sleep adjustments. He adapted to the new time zone quickly without impairment. The same strategy was used on return travel and after arriving home to California. Again, time-zone adjustment occurred rapidly within 2 days without the need for additional rest periods.

A total of 48 capsules were provided, counting 2 days travel on either end for a total of 12 days, but only 32 capsules were needed. Aspirin was used on four occasions to enhance effects of the cannabinoid.

In this case broad-spectrum CBD was able to manage usual travel stress and symptoms while improving sleep quality and allowed for rapid time-zone adaptation. This allowed peak performance and cognitive function without impairment or lasting residual ill effects. Long haul and extensive travel is not fun, but medicinal cannabis can help regulate the discomfort and sleep disturbances.

## Case 2: Insomnia Secondary to Restless Legs Syndrome

A 66-year-old woman developed restless legs syndrome (RLS) 3 months prior to consultation. She had suffered work-related physical and stress injuries and was disabled and on workers' compensation. She had recently been treated for adhesive capsulitis (related to repetitive moving and computer issues), bilateral otitis externa, abscess-related tooth extraction 9 months ago, and COVID-19 postinfection depression and fatigue. She had a few episodes of RLS when she was younger which had been successfully treated with Elavil. She also had major depressive disorder requiring the following medications including Cymbalta, Wellbutrin, and Trazodone for sleep. A neurologist also prescribed ropinirole, a dopamine agonist indicated for Parkinson symptoms and restless legs syndrome (RLS), but she experienced disturbing side effects of nausea, diarrhea, and difficulty remembering or concentrating. Because of these side effects, she discontinued this drug. She was following a plant-based diet and has been using a variety of supplements including a blend of ginger, cayenne, and black pepper; elderberry capsules with zinc; Vit C 500 mg; Vit D3 2000 IU; Vit B12; and probiotics. After 3 months she sought consultation for medicinal cannabis.

RLS has been associated with several abnormalities including dopamine levels, iron metabolism, and REM sleep motor disinhibition. Cannabis has been shown to modulate all of these mechanisms [198]. In REM sleep disturbances, CBD can modify this natural cycle to improve sleep quality. CBD is well established as a neurotransmitter modulator for maintaining natural balance including dopamine pathways [198]. Another problem frequently seen in RLS is elevated hypoxic-inducible factor 1-alpha related to disordered iron metabolism for which the cause is undetermined. Two studies found hypoxia in the leg muscles of RLS patients without any evidence of actual hypoxia [260]. CBD has been shown to reduce levels of this signaling factor [261].

L-DOPA is commonly used as a temporary treatment for RLS with some good effects temporarily but not without ill effects. CBD protects dopamine cells and increases dopamine receptors in the brain. It has been effective in Parkinson's disease for quality of life and in my clinical experience resolving motor dysfunction [262].

For this patient a high potency, full-spectrum tincture (1:20 THC/CBD) was prescribed at a starting dose of 25 mg in early evening for RLS but suggested twice daily in consideration of other post-COVID-19 symptoms and capsulitis. The evening dose was 2 h before sleep time. Remarkably all RLS symptoms resolved on first dose. Sleep duration and quality improved as well as improved mental concentration and physical performance. She was able to successfully rehabilitate her shoulder with physical therapy. She was also able to discontinue most other medications and her depressive symptoms resolved. She was able to reduce the daily dose by half after 2 months and maintain her symptom-free condition with a single nightly dose of 25 mg of CBD at bedtime. However, she ran out of product and her RLS has returned. An alternate local cannabis product with 1:1 THC/CBD ¼ mL has given no symptom relief. She plans to reorder the original full-spectrum CBD product immediately.

## Conclusion

Sleep disorders are common and important reasons why people self-medicate with cannabis. Insomnia is associated with a range of poor health outcomes. There are several models of insomnia that have been developed to explain its pathogenesis, and other factors including genetics, brain neuroanatomical changes, and altered neurotransmitters are also likely to be involved. There is evidence that the endocannabinoid system is involved in the circadian sleep-wake cycle and may provide the link between the circadian regulation systems and the physiological process of sleep. Preclinical and clinical evidence indicate that cannabidiol and tetrahydrocannabinol may have a role to play in the treatment of sleep disorders.

Chronic or severe sleep disorders including insomnia should be evaluated and treated in an integrative manner not merely substituting a phytocannabinoid as an alternative for a benzodiazepine hypnotic. Cannabinoids should certainly be considered early in the clinical relationship because of the excellent safety profile, immediate results, and side benefits as an anti-inflammatory agent. And, cannabinoids may be good first step in establishing rapport and a comprehensive program. Sleep hygiene recommendations are something that clinicians can readily advise on. Referrals to other colleagues may be necessary to address some of the etiological factors that may be involved, for example, anxiety and stress. Optimal nutrition and diet will help support not only a well-functioning ECS but a well-functioning human, period. While we have not addressed nutritional and dietary factors nor environmental factors in this chapter, suffice to say that clinicians should consider these potential contributing factors carefully as well. The root cause of the insomnia must be addressed.

## References

1. Samvat R, Osiecki H. Sleep, health and consciousness- a physician's guide. Queensland: Bio Concepts Publishing; 2009.
2. Reynolds AC, Banks S. Total sleep deprivation, chronic sleep restriction and sleep disruption. Prog Brain Res. 2010;185:91–103.
3. Cunnington D, Junge MF, Fernando AT. Insomnia: prevalence, consequences and effective treatment. Med J Aust. 2013;199(8):36–40.
4. CDC (Centers for Disease Control and Prevention). Short sleep duration among US adults. Centre for Disease Control and Prevention, 2017. Available at: https://www.cdc.gov/sleep/data_statistics.html. Accessed 14 Sept 2020.
5. Belenduik KA, Babson KA, Vandrey R, Bonn-Miller MO. Cannabis species and cannabinoid concentration preference among sleep-disturbed medicinal cannabis users. Addict Behav. 2015;50:178.
6. Tringale R, Jensen C. Cannabis and insomnia. Depression. 2011;4(12):68.
7. Doherty R, Madigan S, Warrington G, Ellis J. Sleep and nutrition interactions: implications for athletes. Nutrients. 2019;11(4):822.
8. Halson SL. Sleep in elite athletes and nutritional interventions to enhance sleep. Sports Med. 2014;44:13–23.
9. Buysse DJ. Sleep health: can we define it? Does it matter? Sleep. 2014;37:9–17.
10. O'Brien K, Sali A. A Clinician's guide to integrative oncology. What you should be talking about with cancer patients and why. US: Springer; 2017.
11. Irwin MR. Why sleep is important for health: a psychoneuroimmunology perspective. Annu Rev Psychol. 2015;66:143–72.
12. Racine C, Kalra K, Ceide M, et al. Sleep duration, insomnia symptoms and emotion regulation among black women. J Sleep Dis Ther. 2013;2(122):pii 1000122.
13. Vandekerckhove M, Cluydts R. The emotional brain and sleep: an intimate relationship. Sleep Med Rev. 2010;14(4):219–26.
14. Aghayev E, Sprott H, Bohler D, et al. Sleep quality, the neglected outcome variable in clinical studies focusing on locomotor system; a construct validation study. BMC Musculoskelet Disord. 2010;11:224. https://doi.org/10.1186/1471-2474-11-224.

15. Walker M. Why we sleep. Allen Lane: UK; 2017.
16. Van Marle H. PTSD as a memory disorder. Eur J Psychotraumaol. 2015;6:27633. https://doi.org/10.3402/ejpt.v6.27633.
17. Kopasz M, Loessl M, Hornyak M, et al. Sleep and memory in healthy children and adolescents - a critical review. Sleep Med Rev. 2010;14(3):167–77.
18. Alhola P, Polo-Kantola P. Sleep deprivation: impact on cognitive performance. Neuropsychiatr Dis Treat. 2007;3(5):553–67.
19. Gorgoni M, D'Atri A, Lauri G, et al. Is sleep essential for neural plasticity in humans, and how does it affect motor and cognitive recover? Neural Plasticity. 2013; Article ID 103949. https://doi.org/10.1155/2013/103949. Accessed 16 Jan 2017.
20. Frank MG, Issa NP, Stryker MP. Sleep enhances plasticity in the developing visual cortex. Neuron. 2001;30(1):275–87.
21. Olini N, Kurth S, Huber R. The effects of caffeine on sleep and maturational markers in the rat. PLoS One. 2013;8(9):e72539.
22. Reading P. ABC of sleep medicine. UK: BMJ Books; 2013.
23. Carskadon MA, Dement WC. Monitoring and staging human sleep. In: Kryger MH, Roth R, Dement WC, editors. Principles and practice of sleep medicine. 5th ed. Philadelphia: Elsevier; 2011. p. 16–26.
24. Foley DJ, Monjan AA, Brown SL, et al. Sleep complaints among elderly persons: an epidemiological study of three communities. Sleep. 1995;6:425–32.
25. Prospero-Garcia O, Amancio-Belmont O, Becerril Melendez AL, et al. Endocannabinoids and sleep. Neurosci Behav Rev. 2016;71:671–9.
26. Harvard Health Publications. Sleep and mental health. 2009. Available at: http://www.health.harvard.edu/newsletter_article/Sleep-and-mental-health. Accessed 2 Oct 2020.
27. Stickgold R. Parsing the role of sleep in memory processing. Curr Opin Neurobiol. 2013;23:847–53.
28. Boyce R, Glasgow SD, Williams S, Adamantidis A. Causal evidence for the role of REM sleep theta rhythm in contextual memory consolidation. Science. 2016;352:812–6.
29. Murillo-Rodriguez E, Budde H, Barciela Veras A, et al. The endocannabinoid system may modulate sleep disorders in aging. Curr Neuropharmacol. 2020;18:97–108.
30. Cunningham D. Insomnia- neurobiology, pathophysiology, assessment and management. PsychSceneHub, 27 Sept 2020. Available at: https://psychscenehub.com/psychinsights/insomnia-assessment-management/. Accessed 15 Oct 2020.
31. Liu ZW, Gao XB. Adenosine inhibits activity of hypocretin/orexin neurons by the A1 receptor in the lateral hypothalamus: a possible sleep-promoting effect. J Neurophysiol. 2007;97:837–48.
32. Bjorness TE, Greene RW. Adenosine and sleep. Curr Neuropharmacol. 2009;7(3):238–45.
33. Lafaye G, Desterke C, Marulaz L, Benyamina A. Cannabidiol affects circadian clock core complex and its regulation in microglia cells. Addict Biol. 2019;24(5):921–34.
34. Borbély AA, Daan S, Wirz-Justice A, Deboer T. The two-process model of sleep regulation: a reappraisal. J Sleep Res. 2016;25:131–43.
35. Geoffray MM, Nicolas A, Speranza M, et al. Are circadian rhythms new pathways to understand Autism Spectrum Disorder? J Physiol-Paris. 2016;110(4, Part B):434–8.
36. Takahashi JS. Molecular components of the circadian clock in mammals. Diabetes Obes Metab. 2015;17(Suppl 1):6–11.
37. Vaughn LK, Denning G, Stuhr KL, et al. Endocannabinoid signalling: has it got rhythm? Br J Pharmacol. 2010;160(3):530–43.
38. National Institute Neurological Disorders & Stroke. 2019. https://www.ninds.nih.gov/Disorders/Patient-Caregiver-Education/understanding-Sleep.
39. Khullar A. The role of melatonin in the circadian rhythm sleep-wake cycle. Psychiatric Times. 2012;29(7):26.
40. Rosenthal L, Day R, Gerhardstein R, et al. Sleepiness/alertness among healthy evening and morning type individuals. Sleep Med. 2001;2:243–8.

41. Vitale JA, Weydahl A. Chronotype, physical activity, and sport performance: a systematic review. Sports Med. 2017;47:1859–68.
42. Åkerstedt T, Folkard S. The three-process model of alertness and its extension to performance, sleep latency, and sleep length. Chronobiol Int. 1997;14:115–23.
43. Levenson JC, Kay DB, Buysse DJ. The pathophysiology of insomnia. Chest. 2015;147(4):1179–92. https://doi.org/10.1378/chest.14-1617.
44. Ursin R. Serotonin and sleep. Sleep Med Rev. 2002;6(1):57–69.
45. Sanlier N, Sabuncular G. Relationship between nutrition and sleep quality, focusing on the melatonin biosynthesis. Sleep Biol Rhythms. 2020;18:89–99.
46. Dinges D, Rogers N, Baynard. Chronic sleep deprivation. In: Kryger MH, Roth T, Dement WC, editors. Principles and practice of sleep medicine. 4th ed. Philadelphia: Elsevier/Saunders; 2005. p. 67–76.
47. Kruger PM, Friedman EM. Sleep duration in the United States: a cross-sectional population-based study. Am J Epidemiol. 2009;169(9):1052–63.
48. Magee CA, Iverson DC, Caputi P. Factors associated with short and long sleep. Prev Med. 2009;49(6):461–7.
49. Cappuccio FP, Cooper D, D'Elia L, et al. Sleep duration predicts cardiovascular outcomes: a systematic review and meta-analysis of prospective studies. Eur Heart J. 2011;32(12):1484–92.
50. Rutters F, Besson H, Walker M, et al. The association between sleep duration, insulin sensitivity and β-cell function: the EGIR-RUISC study. J Clin Endocrinol Metab. 2016;101(9):3237–80.
51. American Psychiatric Association. Diagnosis and statistical manual of mental disorders. 5th ed. Arlington: American Psychiatric Publishing; 2013.
52. CDC (Centers for Disease Control and Prevention). Key sleep disorders. Centers for Disease Control and Prevention, 2014. Available at: https://www.cdc.gov/sleep/about_sleep/key_disorders.html. Accessed 14 Sept 2020.
53. Morin CM, Belanger L, LeBlanc M, et al. The natural history of insomnia: a population-based 3-year longitudinal study. Arch Intern Med. 2009;169:447–53.
54. Riemann D, Nissen C, Palagini L, Otte A, Perlis ML, Spiegelhalder K. The neurobiology, investigation, and treatment of chronic insomnia. Lancet. 2015;14:547558.
55. National Alliance on Mental Illness. Sleep disorders. 2020. Available at: https://nami.org/About-Mental-Illness/Common-with-Mental-Illness/Sleep-Disorders#. Accessed 14 Sept 2020.
56. Ohayon MM. Epidemiology of insomnia: what we know and what we still need to learn. Sleep Med Rev. 2002;6:97–111.
57. Morphy H, Dunn KM, Lewis M, et al. Epidemiology of insomnia: a longitudinal study in a UK population. Sleep. 2007;30(3):274–80.
58. Abad VC, Guilleminault C. Insomnia in elderly patients: recommendations for pharmacological management. Drugs Aging. 2018;35(9):791–817.
59. Johnson EO, Roth T, Breslau N. The association of insomnia with anxiety orders and depression: exploration of the direction of risk. J Psychiatry Res. 2006a;40(8):700–8.
60. Johnson EO, Roth T, Schulz L, Breslau N. Epidemiology of DSM-IV insomnia in adolescence: lifetime prevalence, chronicity, and an emergent gender difference. Pediatrics. 2006b;117(2):247–56.
61. Russo EB, Guy GW, Robson PJ. Cannabis, pain and sleep: lessons from therapeutic clinical trials of Sativex, a cannabis-based medicine. Chem Biodivers. 2007;4:1729–43.
62. Baglioni C, Battagliese G, Feige B, et al. Insomnia as a predictor of depression: a meta-analytic evaluation of longitudinal epidemiological studies. J Affect Disord. 2011;135:10–9.
63. Taylor DJ, Lichstein KL, Durrence HH, Reidel BW, Bush AJ. Epidemiology of insomnia, depression and anxiety. Sleep. 2005;28(11):1457–64.
64. Carley DW, Pavlovic S, Janelidze M, Radulovacki M. Functional role for cannabinoids in respiratory stability during sleep. Sleep. 2002;25(4):388–95.
65. Heslop P, Smith GD, Metcalfe C, et al. Sleep duration and mortality: the effect of short or long sleep duration on cardiovascular and all-cause mortality in working men and women. Sleep Med. 2002;3(4):305–14.

66. Hublin C, Partinen M, Koskenvuo M, Kaprio J. Sleep and mortality: a population-based 22-year follow-up study. Sleep. 2007;30(10):1245–53.
67. Laugsand LE, Vatten LJ, Platou C, Jansky I. Insomnia and the risk of acute myocardial infarction: a population study. Circulation. 2011;124:2073–81.
68. Bonnet MH, Arand DL. Hyperarousal and insomnia: state of the science. Sleep Med Rev. 2010;14:9–15.
69. Gangwisch JE, Heymsfield SB, Boden-Albala B, et al. Short sleep duration as a risk factor for hypertension. Hypertension. 2006;47:833–9.
70. Vozoris NT. The relationship between insomnia symptoms and hypertension using United States population-level data. J Hypertens. 2013;31:663–71.
71. Gangwisch JE, Heymsfield SB, Boden-Albala B, et al. Sleep duration as a risk factor for diabetes incidence in a large U.S. sample. Sleep. 2007;30(12):1667–73.
72. Gangwisch JE, Malaspina D, Boden-Albala B, et al. Inadequate sleep as a risk factor for obesity: analyses of the NHANES I. Sleep. 2005;28(10):1289–96.
73. Kohatsu ND, Tsai R, Young T, et al. Sleep duration and body mass index in a rural population. Arch Intern Med. 2006;166(6):1701–5.
74. Beccuti G, Pannain S. Sleep and obesity. Curr Opin Clin Nutr Metab Care. 2011;14(4):402–12.
75. Taheri S, Lin L, Austin D, et al. Short sleep duration is associated with reduced leptin, elevated ghrelin and increased body mass index. PLoS Med. 2004;1(3):e62.
76. Knutson KL, Van Cauter E. Associations between sleep loss and increased risk of obesity and diabetes. Ann N Y Acad Sci. 2008;1129:287–304.
77. Ayas NT, White DP, Al-Delaimy WK, et al. A prospective study of self-reported sleep duration and incident diabetes in women. Diabetes Care. 2003;26(2):380–4.
78. Touma C, Pannain S. Does lack of sleep cause diabetes? Cleve Clin J Med. 2011;78(8):549–58.
79. Gottlieb DJ, Punjabi NM, Newman AB, et al. Association of sleep time with diabetes mellitus and impaired glucose tolerance. Arch Intern Med. 2005;165:863–7.
80. Chaput JP, Després JP, Bouchard C, Tremblay A. Association of sleep duration with type 2 diabetes and impaired glucose tolerance. Diabetologia. 2007;50(11):2298–304.
81. Kawakami N, Takatsuka N, Shimizu H. Sleep disturbance and onset of type 2 diabetes. Diabetes Care. 2004;27(1):282–3.
82. Cappuccio FP, Taggart FM, Kandala NB, et al. Meta-analysis of short sleep duration and obesity in children and adults. Sleep. 2008;31(5):619–26.
83. Shigeta H, Shigeta M, Nakazawa A, et al. Lifestyle, obesity, and insulin resistance. Diabetes Care. 2001;24(3):608.
84. Singh M, Drake CL, Roehrs T, et al. The association between obesity and short sleep duration: a population-based study. J Clin Sleep Med. 2005;1(4):357–63.
85. Vioque J, Torres A, Quiles J. Time spent watching television, sleep duration and obesity in adults living in Valencia, Spain. Int J Obes Relat Metab Disord. 2000;24(12):1683–8.
86. Chaput JP, Brunet M, Tremblay A. Relationship between short sleeping hours and childhood overweight/obesity: results from the "Québec en Forme" project. Int J Obes. 2006;30(7):1080–5.
87. Seicean A, Redline S, Seicean S, et al. Association between short sleeping hours and overweight in adolescents: results from a US suburban high school survey. Sleep Breath. 2007;11(4):285–93.
88. Van Cauter E. Brief communication: sleep curtailment in healthy young men is associated with decreased leptin levels, elevated ghrelin levels, and increased hunger and appetite. Ann Intern Med. 2004;141(11):846–50.
89. Hogenkamp PS, Nilsson E, Nilsson VC, et al. Acute sleep deprivation increases portion size and affects food choice in young men. Psychoneuroendocrinology. 2013;38(9):1668–74.
90. St-Onge MP, Roberts AL, Chen J, et al. Short sleep duration increases energy intakes but does not change energy expenditure in normal-weight individuals. Am J Clin Nutr. 2011;94(2):410–6.
91. Benedict C, Brooks SJ, O'Daly OG, et al. Acute sleep deprivation enhances the brain's response to hedonic food stimuli: an fMRI study. J Clin Endocrinol Metab. 2012;97(3):E443–7.

92. Cedernaes J, Schiöth HB, Benedict C, et al. Determinants of shortened, disrupted, and mistimed sleep and associated metabolic health consequences in healthy humans. Diabetes. 2015;64(4):1073–80.
93. Cedernaes J, Fanelli F, Fazzini A, et al. Sleep restriction alters plasma endocannabinoids concentrations before but not after exercise in humans. Psychoneuroendocrinology. 2016;74:258–68.
94. Yaffe K, Falvey CM, Hoang T. Connections between sleep and cognition in older adults. Lancet Neurol. 2014;10:1017–28.
95. Sexton C, Storsve AB, Walhovd KB, Johansen-Berg H, Fjell A. Poor sleep quality is associated with increased cortical atrophy in community-dwelling adults. Neurology. 2014;83(11):967–73.
96. Savard J, Laroche L, Simard S, Ivers H, Morin C. Chronic insomnia and immune functioning. Psychosom Med. 2003;65(2):211–21.
97. Finan PH, Smith MT. The comorbidity of insomnia, chronic pain, and depression: dopamine as a putative mechanism. Sleep Med Rev. 2013;17(3):173–83.
98. Asnis GM, Caneva E, Henderson MA. Treatment of insomnia in anxiety disorders. Psychiatr Times. 2012; 29(1).
99. van Mill JG, Hoogendijk WJ, Vogelzangs N, et al. Insomnia and sleep duration in a large cohort of patients with major depressive disorder and anxiety disorders. J Clin Psychiatry. 2010;71:239–46.
100. Backes M. Cannabis pharmacy. New York: Black Dog & Leventhal Publishers; 2014.
101. Sørensen L, Jensen MSA, Rathleff MS. Comorbid insomnia, psychological symptoms and widespread pain among patients suffering from musculoskeletal pain in general practice: a cross-sectional study. BMJ Open. 2019;9:e031971.
102. Parker KP, et al. 2005 ASCO Annual Meeting Proceedings. J Clin Oncol. 2005;23:8020.
103. Parker KP, et al. 2005 ASCO Annual Meeting Proceedings. J Clin Oncol. 2006;24:8526.
104. Heinzelmann M, Gill J. Epigenetic mechanisms shape the biological response to trauma and risk for PTSD: a critical review. Nurs Res Pract. 2013;2013:417010.
105. Norrholm SD, Jovanovic T, Olin IW, et al. Fear extinction in traumatized civilians with post-traumatic stress disorder: relation to symptom severity. Biol Psychiatry. 2011;69:556–63.
106. Kobayashi I, Boarts JM, Delahanty DL. Polysomnographically measured sleep abnormalities in PTSD: a meta-analytic review. Psychophysiology. 2007;44:660–9.
107. Vandrey R, Babson KA, Herrmann ES, Bonn-Miller MO. Interactions between disordered sleep, post-traumatic stress disorder, and substance use disorders. Int Rev Psychiatry. 2014;26(2):237–47.
108. Kilgore WDS. Effects of sleep deprivation on cognition. Prog Brain Res. 2010;185:105–29.
109. Palesh OG, Roscoe JA, Mustian KM, et al. Prevalence, demographics, and psychological associations of sleep disruption in patients with cancer: University of Rochester cancer center-community clinical oncology program. J Clin Oncol. 2010;28(2):292–8.
110. O'Donnell JF. Insomnia in cancer patients. Clin Cornerstone. 2004;6(1):S6–S14.
111. Robertson ME, McSherry F, Herndon JE, et al. Insomnia and its associations in patients with recurrent glial neoplasms. Springerplus. 2016;5:823.
112. Sigurdardottir L, Valdimarsdottir UA, Mucci L, et al. Insomnia among elderly men and risk of prostate cancer. J Clin Oncol. 2012;30(5):78.
113. Lu Y, Tian N, Yin J, et al. Association between sleep duration and cancer risk: a meta-analysis of prospective cohort studies. PLoS One. 2013;8(9):e74723.
114. Redwine L, Hauger RL, Gillin JC, Irwin M. Effects of sleep and sleep deprivation on interleukin-6, growth hormone, cortisol, and melatonin levels in humans. J Clin Endocrinol Metab. 2000;85(10):3597–603.
115. Vgontzas AN, Papanicolaou DA, Bixler EO, et al. Circadian interleukin-6 secretion and quantity and depth of sleep. J Clin Endocrinol Metab. 1999;84:2603–7.
116. Papanicolaou DA, Wilder RL, Manolagas SC, Chrousos GP. The pathophysiologic roles of interleukin-6 in human disease. Ann Intern Med. 1998;128(2):127–37.

117. Irwin MR, Wang M, Campomayor CO, et al. Sleep deprivation and activation of morning levels of cellular and genomic markers of inflammation. Arch Intern Med. 2006;166:1756–62.
118. Irwin MR, Wang M, Ribeiro D, et al. Sleep loss activates cellular inflammatory signaling. Biol Psychiatry. 2008;64(6):538–40.
119. Vgontzas AN, Zoumakis E, Bixler E, et al. Adverse effects of modest sleep restriction on sleepiness, performance, and inflammatory cytokines. J Clin Endocrinol Metab. 2004;89(5):2119–226.
120. Spiegel K, Leproult R, Van Cauter E. Impact of sleep debt on metabolic and endocrine function. Lancet. 1999;354:1435–9.
121. Irwin MR, Olmstead R, Carroll JE. Sleep disturbance, sleep duration, and inflammation: a systematic review and meta-analysis of cohort studies and experimental sleep deprivation. Biol Psychiatry. 2016;80:40–52.
122. Thompson D, Pepys MB, Wood SP. The physiological structure of human C-reactive protein and its complex with phosphocholine. Structure. 1999;7(2):169–77.
123. Mayo Clinic. Insomnia. 2018. Available at: https://www.mayoclinic.org/diseases-conditions/insomnia/symptoms-causes/syc-20355167. Accessed 10 Oct 2020.
124. Mitchell MD, Gehman P, Perlis M, Unscheid CA. Comparative effectiveness of cognitive behavioural therapy for insomnia: a systematic review. BMC Fam Pract. 2012;13:40.
125. Mayo Clinic. Cognitive behavioral therapy. Available at: https://www.mayoclinic.org/testsprocedures/cognitive-behavioral-therapy/about/pac-20384610.
126. WebMD. Drugs to treat insomnia. WebMD Jan. 2020. Available at: https://www.webmd.com/sleep-disorders/insomnia-medications. Accessed 10 Oct 2020.
127. Hammerschlag AR, Stringer S, de Leeuw CA, et al. Genome-wide association analysis of insomnia complaints identifies risk genes and genetic overlap with psychiatric and metabolic traits. Nat Genet. 2017;49(11):1584–92. https://doi.org/10.1038/ng.3888.
128. Chou K-H, Lee P-L, Liang C-S, et al. Identifying neuroanatomical signatures in insomnia and migraine comorbidity. Sleep. 2021;44(3):zsaa202.
129. Wu Y, Zhuang Y, Qi J. Explore structural and functional brain changes in insomnia disorder: a PRISMA-compliant whole brain ALE meta-analysis for multimodal MRI. Medicine. 2020;99(14):e19151.
130. Babson KA, Sottile J, Morabito D. Cannabis, cannabinoids and sleep: a review of the literature. Curr Psychiatry Rep. 2017;19:23.
131. Kesner AJ, Lovinger DM. Cannabinoids, endocannabinoids and sleep. Front Mol Neurosci. 2020;13:125.
132. Pava MJ, Makriyannis A, Lovinger DM. Endocannabinoid signalling regulates sleep stability. PLoS One. 2016;11(3):e0152473.
133. Martinez-Vargas M, Morales-Gomez J, Gonzalez-Rivera R, et al. Does the neuroprotective role of anandamide display diurnal variations? Int J Mol Sci. 2013;14:23341–55.
134. Martinez-Vargas M, Murillo-Rodriguez E, Gonzalez-Rivera R, et al. Sleep modulates cannabinoid receptor 1 expression in the pons of the rat. Neuroscience. 2003;117:197–201.
135. Yamashita T, Yamanaka A. Lateral hypothalamic circuits for sleep–wake control. Curr Opin Neurobiol. 2017;44:94–100.
136. Perez-Morales M, Alberto K, Mendez-Diaz M, et al. 2-AG into the lateral hypothalamus increased REM sleep and c-Fos expression in melanin concentrating hormone neurons in rats. Pharmacol Biochem Behav. 2013;108:1–7.
137. Sanford AE, Castillo E, Gannon RL. Cannabinoids and hamster circadian activity rhythms. Brain Res. 2008;1222:141–8.
138. Murillo-Rodriguez E, Desarnaud F, Prospero-Garcia O. Diurnal variation of arachidonoylethanolamine, palmitoylethanolamide and oleoylethanolamide in the brain of the rat. Life Sci. 2006a;79:30–7.
139. Valenti M, Vigano D, Casico MG, et al. Differential diurnal variations of anandamide and 2-arachidonoylglycerol levels in rat brains. Cell Mol Life Sci. 2004;61:945–50.
140. Hanlon EC, Tasali E, Leproult R, et al. Circadian rhythm of circulating levels of the endocannabinoid 2-arachidonoylglycerol. J Clin Endocrinol Meta. 2014;100:220–6.

141. Hanlon EC, Tasali E, Leproult R, et al. Sleep restriction enhances the daily rhythm of circulating levels of endocannabinoid 2-Arachidonoylglycerol. Sleep. 2016;39(3):653–64.
142. Basile AS, Hanus L, Mendelson WB. Characterization of the hypnotic properties of oleamide. Neuroreport. 1999;10:947–51.
143. Murillo-Rodriguez E, Blanco-Centurion C, Sanchez C, et al. Anandamide enhances extracellular levels of adenosine and induces sleep: an in vivo microdialysis study. Sleep. 2003;26:943–7.
144. Murillo-Rodriguez E, Sanchez-Alavez M, Navarro D, et al. Anandamide modulates sleep and memory in rats. Brain Res. 1998;812:270–4.
145. Huitron-Resendiz S, Sanchez-Alavez M, Wills DN. Characterization of the sleep-wake patterns in mice lacking fatty acid amide hydrolase. Sleep. 2004;27(5):857–65.
146. Murillo-Rodriguez E, Pastrana-Trejo JC, Salas-Crisostomo M, de-la-Cruz M. The endocannabinoid system modulating levels of consciousness, emotions and likely dream contents. CNS Neurol Disord Drug Targets. 2017;16(4):370–9.
147. Murillo-Rodríguez E, Millan-Aldaco D, Millan-Aldaco D, et al. Effects of the fatty acid amide hydrolase inhibitor URB597 on the sleep-wake cycle, c-Fos expression and dopamine levels of the rat. Eur J Pharmacol. 2007;562(1–2):82–91.
148. Murillo-Rodriguez E, Machado S, Barbosa Rosa N, et al. Revealing the role of the endocannabinoid system modulators, SR141716A, URB597 and VDM-11, in sleep homeostasis. Neurosci. 2016;339:433–49.
149. Prospero-Garcia O, Cravatt BE, Siuzdak G, et al. cis-9,10 Octadecenomamide: a novel natural lipid isolated from cat CSF with potential sleep-modulating properties. Sleep Res. 1995;24:50.
150. Yang J-Y, Wu CF, Wang F, et al. The serotonergic system may be involved in the sleep inducing action of oleamide in rats. Naunyn Schmiedeberg's Arch Pharmacol. 2003;368:457–62.
151. Mechoulam R, Fride E, Hanu L, et al. Anandamide may mediate sleep induction. Nature. 1997;389:25–6.
152. Koethe D, Schreiber D, Giuffrida A, et al. Sleep deprivation increases oleoylethanolamine in human cerebrospinal fluid. J Neural Transm (Vienna). 2009;116:301–5.
153. Bilkci-Gorzo A. The endocannabinoid system in normal and pathological brain ageing. Philos Trans R Soc Lond Ser B Biol Sci. 2012;367(1607):3326–41.
154. Piyanova A, Lomazzo E, Bindila L, et al. Age-related changes in the endocannabinoid system in the mouse hippocampus. Mech Ageing Dev. 2015;150:55–64.
155. Maccarrone M, Attina M, Bari M, et al. Anandamide degradation and N-acylethanolamines level in weld-type and CB1 cannabinoid receptor knockout mice of different ages. J Neurochem. 2001;78(2):339–48.
156. Reyes-Prieto NM, Romano-Lopez A, Perez-Morales CJ, et al. Oleamide restores sleep in adult rats that were subjected to maternal separation. Pharmacol Biochem Behav. 2012;103:308–12.
157. Perez-Morales M, Fajardo-Valez A, Menez-Diaz M, et al. 2-Arachidonoylglycerol into the lateral hypothalamus improves reduced sleep in adult rats subjected to maternal separation. Neuroreport. 2014;25:1437–41.
158. Cousens K, DiMascio A. (−)δ9 THC as an hypnotic. Psychopharmacologia. 1973;33:355–64.
159. Feinberg I, Jones R, Walker JM, et al. Effects of high dosage delta-9-tetrahydrocannabinol on sleep patterns in man. Clin Pharmacol Ther. 1975;17(4):458–66.
160. Feinberg I, Jones R, Walker J, et al. Effects of marijuana extract and tetrahydrocannabinol on electroencephalographic sleep patterns. Clin Pharmacol Ther. 1976;19:782–94.
161. Pivik RT, Zarcone V, Dement WC, Hollister LE. Delta-9-tetrahydrocannabinol and synhexl: effects on human sleep patterns. Clin Pharmacol Ther. 1972;13(3):426–35.
162. Pisanti S, Bifulco M. Medical cannabis: A plurimillennial history of an evergreen. J Cell Physiol. 2019;234(6):8342–51.
163. Lee MA. Smoke Signals. New York: Scribner; 2012.

164. Bachhuber M, Arnsten JH, Wurm G. Use of cannabis to relieve pain and promote sleep by customers at an adult use dispensary. J Psychoactive Drugs. 2018;51(5):400–4.
165. Goodhines PA, Gellis LA, Kim J, et al. Self-medication for sleep in college students: concurrent and prospective associations with sleep and alcohol behaviour. Behav Sleep Med. 2019;17(3):327–41.
166. Haug NA, Padula CB, Sottile JE, et al. Cannabis use patterns and motives: a comparison of younger, middle-aged, and older medical cannabis dispensary patients. Addict Behav. 2017;72:14–20.
167. Lintzeris N, Davis J, Elias N, et al. Medicinal cannabis in Australia 2016: the Cannabis as medicine survey (CAMS-16). Med J Aust. 2018;209(5):211–6.
168. Pedersen W, Sandberg S. The medicalization of revolt: a sociological analysis of medical cannabis users. Soc Health. 2013;35(1):17–32.
169. Bonn-Miller MO, Vujanovic AA, Drescher KD. Cannabis use among military veterans after residential treatment for posttraumatic stress disorder. Psychol Addict Behav. 2011;25(3):485–91.
170. Bonn-Miller MO, Babson KA, Vandrey R. Using cannabis to help you sleep: heightened frequency of medical cannabis use among those with PTSD. Drug Alcohol Depend. 2014;136:162–5.
171. Bremner JD, Southwick SM, Darnell A, Charney DS. Chronic PTSD in Vietnam combat veterans: course of illness and substance abuse. Am J Psychiatr. 1996;153:369–75.
172. Piper BJ, DeKeuster RM, Beals ML, et al. Substitution of medical cannabis for pharmaceutical agents for pain, anxiety and sleep. J Psychopharmacol. 2017;31:569–75.
173. Ogeil RP, Phillips JG, Rajaratnma SMW, Broadbear JH. Risky drug use and effects on sleep quality and daytime sleepiness. Hum Psychopharmacol. 2015;30(5):356–63.
174. Schlienz NJ, Scalsky R, Martin EL, et al. A cross-sectional and prospective comparison of medicinal cannabis users and controls on self-reported health. Cannabis Cannabinoid Res. 2020; https://doi.org/10.1089/can.2019.0096.
175. Winiger EA, Hitchcock LN, Bryan AD, et al. Cannabis use and sleep: expectations, outcomes and the role of age. Addict Behav. 2012;112:106642.
176. Vigil JM, Stith SS, Diviant JP, et al. Effectiveness of raw, natural medical *cannabis* flower for treating insomnia under naturalistic conditions. Medicines (Basel). 2018;5(3):75.
177. National Academies of Sciences, Engineering & Medicine. The health effects of cannabis and cannabinoids. Washington DC: The National Academies Press; 2017.
178. Whiting PF, Wolff RF, Deshpande S, et al. Cannabinoids for medical use: a systematic review and meta-analysis. JAMA. 2015;313(24):2456–73.
179. Gates PJ, Albertella L, Copeland J. The effects of cannabinoid administration on sleep: a systematic review of human studies. Sleep Med Rev. 2014;18(6):477–87.
180. Johnson EO, Breslau N. Sleep problems and substance use in adolescence. Drug Alcohol Depend. 2001;64:1–7.
181. McKnight LR, Eaton DK, Lowry JB, et al. Relationships between hours of sleep and health-risk behaviors in US adolescent students. Prev Med. 2011;53(4–5):271–3.
182. Ogeil RP, Cheetham A, Mooney A, et al. Early adolescent drinking and cannabis use predicts late sleep-quality problems. Psychol Addict Behav. 2019;33(3):266–73.
183. Roane BM, Taylor DJ. Adolescent insomnia as a risk factor for early adult depression and substance abuse. Sleep. 2008;31(10):13511356.
184. Wong MM, Brower KJ, Zucker RA. Childhood sleep problems, early onset of substance abuse and behavioural problems in adolescence. Sleep Med. 2009;10(7):787–96.
185. Conroy DA, Kurth ME, Strong DR, et al. Marijuana use patterns and sleep among community-based young adults. J Addict Dis. 2016;35(2):135–43.
186. Gorelick DA, Goodwin RS, Schwilke E, et al. Around-the-clock oral THC effects on sleep in male chronic daily cannabis smokers. Am J Addict. 2013;22:510–4.
187. Bolla KI, Lesage SR, Gambaldo CE, et al. Sleep disturbance in heavy marijuana users. Sleep. 2008;31(6):901–8.

188. Bolla KI, Lesage SR, Gamaldo CE, et al. Polysomnogram changes in marijuana users who report sleep disturbances during prior abstinence. Sleep Med. 2010;11:882–9.
189. Gates P, Albertella L, Copeland J. Cannabis withdrawal and sleep: a systematic review of human studies. Subst Abus. 2016;37(1):255–69.
190. Vandrey R, Smith MT, McCann UD, et al. Sleep disturbance and the effects of extended-release zolpidem during cannabis withdrawal. Drug Alcohol Depend. 2011;117:38–44.
191. Budney AJ, Moore BA, Vandrey RG, Hughes JR. The time course and significance of cannabis withdrawal. J Abnorm Psychol. 2003;112(3):393–402.
192. Budney AJ, Vandrey RG, Hughes JR, et al. Comparison of cannabis and tobacco withdrawal: severity and contribution to relapse. J Subst Abus Treat. 2008;35:362–8.
193. Vandrey RG, Budney AJ, Hughes JR, Liguori A. A within-subject comparison of withdrawal symptoms during abstinence from cannabis, tobacco, and both substances. Drug Alcohol Depend. 2008;92(1-3):48–54.
194. Karniol IG, Carlini EA. Pharmacological interaction between cannabidiol and delta 9-tetrahydrocannabinol. Psychopharmacologia. 1973;33(1):53–70.
195. Davis WM, Borgen LA. Effects of cannabidiol and delta-9- tetrahydrocannabinol on operant behavior. Res Commun Chem Pathol Pharmacol. 1974;9(3):453–62.
196. Guimaraes VM, et al. Cannabidiol increases Fos expression in the nucleus accumbens but not in the dorsal striatum. Life Sci. 2004;75(5):633–8.
197. Monti JM. Hypnotic like effects of cannabidiol in the rat. Psychopharmacology. 1977;55(3):263–5.
198. Murillo-Rodriguez E, Millan-Aldaco D, Palomero-Rivero M, et al. Cannabidiol, a constituent of Cannabis sativa, modulates sleep in rats. FEBS Lett. 2006b;580:4337–45.
199. Murillo-Rodríguez E, Millan-Aldaco D, Palomero-Rivero M, et al. Constituent cannabidiol is a wake-inducing agent. Behav Neurosci. 2008;122(6):1378–82.
200. Murillo-Rodriguez E, Palomero-Rivero M, Millan-Aldaco D, et al. Effects on sleep and dopamine levels of microdialysis perfusion of cannabidiol into the lateral hypothalamus of rats. Life Sci. 2011;88(11–12):504–11.
201. Carlini EA, Cunha JM. Hypnotic and antiepileptic effects of cannabidiol. J Clin Pharmacol. 1981;21(8–9 Suppl):417S–27S.
202. Chagas MH, et al. Effects of acute systemic administration of cannabidiol on sleep-wake cycle in rats. J Psychopharmacol. 2013;27(3):312–6.
203. Hsiao YT, et al. Effect of cannabidiol on sleep disruption induced by repeated combination tests consisting of open field and elevated plus-maze in rats. Neuropharmacology. 2012;62(1):373–84.
204. Murillo-Rodriguez E, Millan-Aldaco D, Cicconcelli D, et al. Sleep-wake cycle disturbances and NeuN-altered expression in adult rats after cannabidiol treatments during adolescence. Psychopharmacology (Berl). 2021;238(6):1437. https://doi.org/10.1007/s00213-021-05769-z.
205. Watson C, Kirkcaldie M, Paxinos G. Techniques for studying the brain. In: Watson C, Kirkcaldie M, Paxinos G, editors. The brain. An introduction to functional neuroanatomy. Academic Press; 2010. p. 153–65.
206. Shannon S, Opila-Lehman J. Cannabidiol oil for decreasing addictive use of marijuana: a case report. Integr Med. 2015;14(6):31–5.
207. Shannon S, Lewis N, Lee H, Hughes S. Cannabidiol in anxiety and sleep: a large case series. Perm J. 2019;23:18–41.
208. Zuardi AW, Guimarães FS, Moreira AC. Effect of cannabidiol on plasma prolactin, growth hormone and cortisol in human volunteers. Braz J Med Biol Res. 1993;26(2):213–7.
209. Nicholson AN, Turner C, Stone BM, Robson PJ. Effect of Delta-9-tetrahydrocannabinol and cannabidiol on nocturnal sleep and early-morning behavior in young adults. J Clin Psychopharmacol. 2004;v24(3):305–13.
210. Zuardi AW, Shirakawa I, Finkelfarb E, Karniol IG. Action of cannabidiol on the anxiety and other effects produced by delta 9-THC in normal subjects. Psychopharmacology. 1982;76(3):245–50.

211. Spindle TR, Cone EJ, Goffi E, et al. Pharmacodynamic effects of vaporized and oral cannabidiol (CBD) and vaporized CBD-dominant cannabis in infrequent cannabis users. Drug Alcohol Depend. 2020;211:107937.
212. Elms L, Shannon S, Hughes S, Lewis N. Cannabidiol in the treatment of post-traumatic stress disorder: a case series. J Altern Complement Med. 2019;25(4):392–7.
213. Chagas MHN, Eckeli AL, Zuardi AW, et al. Cannabidiol can improve complex sleep-related behaviours associated with rapid eye movement sleep behaviour disorder in Parkinson's disease patients: a case series. J Clin Pharm Ther. 2014;39(5):564–6.
214. Megelin T, Ghorayeb I. Cannabis for restless legs syndrome: a report of six patients. Sleep Med. 2017;36:182–3.
215. Babson KA, Bonn-Miller M. Sleep disturbances: implications for cannabis use, cannabis use cessation, and cannabis use treatment. Curr Addict Rep. 2014;1:109–14.
216. Perron RR, Tyson RL, Sutherland GR. Delta9-tetrahydrocannabinol increases brain temperature and inverts circadian rhythms. Neuroreport. 2001;12:3791–4.
217. Kimura T, Takaya M, Usami N, et al. (9)-Tetrahydrocannabinol, a major marijuana component, enhances the anesthetic effect of pentobarbital through the CB1 receptor. Forensic Toxicol. 2019;37:207–14.
218. Watanabe K, Hamajima K, Yamamoto I, Yoshimura H. Different effects of $\Delta^9$-tetrahydrocannabinol and cannabidiol by three routes of administration on pentobarbital-induced sleeping time in mice. Res Commun Subst Abuse. 1981;2:213–20.
219. Mondino A, Cavellia M, Gonzales J, et al. Acute effect of vaporized Cannabis on sleep and electrocortical activity. Pharmacol Biochem Behav. 2019;179:113–23.
220. Hosko MJ, Kochar MS, Wang RIH. Effects of orally administered delta-9-tetrahydrocannabinol in man. Clin Pharmacol Ther. 1973;14:344–52.
221. Barratt ES, Beaver W, White R. The effects of marijuana on human sleep patterns. Biol Psychiatry. 1974;8:47–54.
222. Freemon FR. The effect of delta 9 tetrahydrocannabinol on sleep. Psychopharmacologica. 1974;35:39–44.
223. Tassarini C, Ambrosetto G, Peraita-Adrado MR, et al. The neuropsychiatric syndrome of delta-9-tetrahydrocannabinol and cannabis intoxication in naïve subjects: a clinical and polygraphic study during wakefulness and sleep. In: Braude MC, Szara S, editors. The Pharmacology of Marijuana. New York: Raven Press; 1976.
224. Freemon FR. The effect of chronically administered delta-9-tetrahydrocannabinol upon the polygraphically monitored sleep of normal volunteers. Drug Alcohol Depend. 1982;10(4):345–53.
225. Chait LD. Subjective and behavioral effects of marijuana the morning after smoking. Psychopharmacology. 1990;100:328–33.
226. Neff GW, O'Brien CB, Feddy KR, et al. Preliminary observation with dronabinol in patients with intractable pruritus secondary to cholestatic liver disease. Am J Gastroenterol. 2002;97:2117–9.
227. Farabi SS, et al. Impact of dronabinol on quantitative electroencephalogram (qEEG) measures of sleep in obstructive sleep apnea syndrome. J Clin Sleep Med. 2014;10(1):49–56.
228. Halikas JA, Weller RA, Morse CL, Hoffmann RG. A longitudinal study of marijuana effects. Subst Use Misuse. 1985;20:701–11.
229. Schierenbeck T, Riemann D, Berger M, Hornyak M. Effect of illicit recreational drugs upon sleep: cocaine, ecstasy, and marijuana. Sleep Med Rev. 2008;12:381–9.
230. Fusar-Poli P, Crippa JA, Bhattacharyya S, et al. Distinct effects of {delta}9-tetrahydrocannabinol and cannabidiol on neural activation during emotional processing. Arch Gen Psychiatry. 2009;66(1):95–105.
231. Russo EB. Cannabidiol claims and misconceptions. Trends Pharmacol Sci. 2017;38(3):198–201.
232. Fraser GA. The use of a synthetic cannabinoid in the management of treatment-resistant nightmares in posttraumatic stress disorder (PTSD). CNS Neurosci Ther. 2009;15:84–8.

233. Shalev A, Roitman P, Mechoulam R. Pilot open label trial on oral absorbable Δ-9 THC for chronic PTSD. Hagoshrim: Israel Soc Biological Psychiatry Abstract Book; 2013.
234. Roitman P, Mechoulam R, Cooper-Kazaz R, Shalev A. Preliminary, open-label pilot study of add-on oral Δ9-tetrahydrocannabinol in chronic post-traumatic stress disorder. Clin Drug Invest. 2014;34:587–91.
235. Cameron C, Watson D, Robinson J. Use of a synthetic cannabinoid in a correctional population for posttraumatic stress disorder-related insomnia and nightmares, chronic pain, harm reduction and other indications: a retrospective evaluation. J Clin Psychopharmacol. 2014;34(5):559–64.
236. Jetly R, Heber A, Fraser G, Boisvert D. The efficacy of nabilone, a synthetic cannabinoid, in the treatment of PTSD-associated nightmares: a preliminary randomized, double blind, placebo-controlled cross-over design. Psychoneuro. 2015;51:585–8.
237. Yoshida H, Usami N, Ohishi Y, et al. Synthesis and pharmacological effects in mice of halogenated cannabinol derivatives. Chem Pharm Bull (Tokyo). 1995;43(2):335–7.
238. Karniol IG, Shirakawa I, Takahashi RN, et al. Effects of $\Delta^9$-Tetrahydrocannabinol and cannabinol in man. Pharmacology. 1975;13:502–12.
239. Baron EP. Medicinal properties of cannabinoids, terpenes, and flavonoids in cannabis, and benefits in migraine, headache, and pain: an update on current evidence and cannabis science. Headache Curr. 2018.; 58;(7):1139–86.
240. Nuutinen T. Medicinal properties of terpenes found in *Cannabis sativa* and *Humulus lupulus*. Eur J Med Chem. 2018;157:198–228.
241. Zhou J, Kim JE, Armstrong CL, Chen N, Campbell WW. Higher-protein diets improve indexes of sleep in energy-restricted overweight and obese adults: results from 2 randomized controlled trials. Am J Clin Nutr. 2016;103(3):766–74.
242. Lindseth G, Lindseth P, Thompson M. Nutritional effects on sleep. West J Nurs Res. 2013;35(4):497–513.
243. Afaghi A, Oconnor H, Chow CM. High-glycemic-index carbohydrate meals shorten sleep onset. Am J Clin Nutr. 2007;85(2):426–30.
244. Peuhkuri K, Sihvola N, Korpela R. Diet promotes sleep duration and quality. Nutr Res. 2012;32(5):309–19.
245. Grandner MA, Kripke DF, Naidoo N, Langer RD. Relationships among dietary nutrients and subjective sleep, objective sleep, and napping in women. Sleep Med. 2010;11(2):180–4.
246. Quick V, Byrd-Bredbenner C, White AA, Brown O, Colby S, Shoff S, et al. Eat, sleep, work, play: associations of weight status and health-related behaviors among young adult college students. Am J Health Promot. 2014;29(2):e64–72.
247. Sato-Mito N, Sasaki S, Murakami K, Okubo H, Takahashi Y, Shibata S. The midpoint of sleep is associated with dietary intake and dietary behavior among young Japanese women. Sleep Med. 2011;12(3):289–94.
248. Kim S, DeRoo LA, Sandler DP. Eating patterns and nutritional characteristics associated with sleep duration. Public Health Nutr. 2011;14(05):889–95.
249. Peppard PE, Young T, Barnet JH, et al. Increased prevalence of sleep-disordered breathing in adults. Am J Epidemiol. 2013;177(9):1006–14.
250. Wheaton AG, Perry GS, Chapman DP, Croft JB. Sleep disordered breathing and depression among U.S. adults: National Health and Nutrition Examination Survey, 2005–2008. Sleep. 2012;35(4):461–7.
251. Jennum P. Quality of life, co-morbidity and obstructive sleep apnoea. Clin Respir J. 2010;4(3):129–30.
252. Jumpertz R, Wiesner T, Bluher M, et al. Circulating endocannabinoids and N-acylethanolamides in patients with sleep apnea- specific role of oleoylethanolamide. Exp Clin Endocrinol Diabetes. 2010;118(9):591–5.

253. Calik MW, Radulovacki M, Carley DW. Intranodose ganglion injections of dronabinol attenuate serotonin-induced apnea in Sprague-Dawley rat. Respir Physiol Neurobiol. 2014;190:20–4.
254. Calik MW, Carley DW. Intracerebroventricular injections of dronabinol, a cannabinoid receptor agonist, does not attenuate serotonin-induced apnea in Sprague-Dawley rats. J Negat Results Biomed. 2016;15:8.
255. Carley DW, Prasad B, Reid KJ, et al. Pharmacotherapy of apnea by cannabimimetic enhancement, the pace clinical trial: effects of dronabinol in obstructive sleep apnea. Sleep. 2018;41(1):zsx184. https://doi.org/10.1093/sleep/zsx184.
256. Stein PK, Pu Y. Heart rate variability, sleep and sleep disorders. Sleep Med Rev. 2012;16(1):47–66.
257. Stein D. The Sacred Plant Masterclass: module 6 lesson 2 depression & sleep disorders. Available at: two.thesacredplant.com.
258. Cherasse Y, Urade Y. Dietary zinc acts as a sleep modulator. Int J Mol Sci. 2017;18(11):2334.
259. Bonaventura P, Benedetti G, Albarède F, Pierre MP. Zinc and its role in immunity and inflammation. Autoimmun Rev. 2015;14(4):277–85.
260. Patton SM, et al. Hypoxia-inducible factor pathway activation in restless legs syndrome. Eur J Neurol. 2011;18(11):1329–35.
261. Solinas M, Massi P, Cinquina V, et al. Cannabidiol, a non-psychoactive cannabinoid compound, inhibits proliferation and invasion in U87-MG and T98G glioma cells through a multitarget effect. PLoS One. 2013;8(10):e76918.
262. Seeman P. Cannabidiol is a partial agonist at dopamine D2High receptors, predicting its antipsychotic clinical dose. Transl Psychiatry. 2016;6(10):e920.

# 9 Dementia: Alzheimer's Disease

## Introduction

Dementia is a term that describes a group of diseases which are characterized by gradual impairment of brain function. Changes can include loss of memory, cognitive decline, and changes in speech, behavior mobility, personality, and functional ability [1]. Health and functional ability decline as the disease state progresses [1]. Dementia is increasingly common with increased age, mainly occurring in those 65 and over; however, it can affect younger people. Dementia is a major cause of disability in older people, and it also substantially impacts on caregivers, given that dementia sufferers become very dependent on their caregivers for most areas of daily life [1].

**This Chapter**
In this chapter, we will explore dementia, with a focus on the main form of dementia, Alzheimer's disease. We will discuss the pathophysiology, including how the endocannabinoid system is involved, and then examine the potential mechanisms of action of CBD and THC in treatment of Alzheimer's disease.

## About Dementia

### Prevalence of Dementia

In 2015, worldwide an estimated 50 million people were living with dementia, and this figure is predicted to double every 20 years [2]. In Australia, an estimated 400,000–459,000 Australians had dementia in 2020 (up to 70% was Alzheimer's disease) [1]. To give some context, the population of Australia is around 25 million people.

Alzheimer's disease, the most common form of dementia, affects around 25 million people worldwide [3]. Countries in North America and western Europe have



K. O'Brien, P. Blair, *Medicinal Cannabis and CBD in Mental Healthcare*,
https://doi.org/10.1007/978-3-030-78559-8_9

the highest rates of Alzheimer's disease (6.4% and 5.4%, respectively, at age 60 years). Latin America and China have rates of 4.9% and 4%, respectively, which could be related to adoption of western diets as these areas develop [4]. Prevalence is much lower for Africans (living in Africa) compared western Europe and the Americas [4].

## Types of Dementia

There are several types of dementia, though boundaries between the different types of dementia are indistinct and a person can have several types of dementia concurrently [1]. The most common type of dementia is Alzheimer's disease (hereafter we use the abbreviation AD) (50–70%) and then vascular dementia (20–30%). The etiology and pathogenesis of these two differ [5]. Other types include paralytic dementia, Lewy body dementia, Parkinson's disease, trauma dementia, carbon monoxide-induced dementia, Huntington's dementia (i.e., dementia associated with Huntington's disease), and frontotemporal lobar degeneration (FTLD) [6, 7].

## Risk Factors for Dementia

There are several risk factors for dementia including age, family history, smoking, hearing loss, depression, diabetes, hypertension, and obesity [1, 8]. A systematic review and meta-analysis of 28 prospective observational studies found that in diabetes, there is a 73% increased risk of all types of dementia, a 56% increase in risk of AD dementia, and a 127% increased risk of vascular dementia [9]. The risk factors for AD will be discussed in the section on Alzheimer's Disease.

## Common Neuropsychiatric Symptoms of Dementia

There are neuropsychiatric symptoms (behavioral and psychological symptoms) common to all dementia types, and these include anxiety, agitation, aggression, psychosis, eating disorders, apathy, and wandering [5]. Most dementia sufferers will experience at least one of these symptoms [5]. Anxiety and depression are more common in early stages, while psychosis and aggression are more common in advanced disease [10]. Olfactory dysfunction is often present as a symptom of a neurodegenerative disease including dementia [11]. Loss of smell or anosmia can be an early sign with sensory and central processing impairments in any of the components of olfaction [12]. Hyposmia may be an early predictive symptom associated with AD [13] and more recently recognized, Parkinson's disease [14]. In one study, 9 of 29 patients with hyposmia and mild cognitive impairment (31%) developed AD, which progressed over 18 months [13].

Specific symptoms and signs of AD will be discussed later in this chapter.

## Treatment of Dementia

Currently, there are no current recognized pharmaceutical solutions that can stop the course of dementia. Treatment is aimed at managing the neuropsychiatric symptoms. Treatment of the symptoms associated with dementia includes non-pharmacological interventions aimed at identifying unmet physical and emotional needs which may be triggering the associated symptoms (first-line treatment) and pharmacological interventions (usually second-line treatment) [5].

The most common medications used to treat the symptoms of dementia are the atypical antipsychotics, despite limited evidence of effectiveness and studies which have found them to be associated with harm including falls, cerebrovascular accidents, and death [5]. Other drugs used include antidepressants and antiepileptics for which there is only limited evidence that these types of drugs decrease agitation and psychosis [15].

Four acetylcholinesterase inhibitors (galantamine, donepezil, tacrine, and rivastigmine) have been approved in the USA to improve memory; however, there is no strong evidence of efficacy [4]. A meta-analysis found that risperidone and olanzapine significantly reduced aggression in AD and risperidone reduced psychosis, but both drugs were associated with serious adverse cerebrovascular events and extrapyramidal symptoms [16].

## Impact of Dementia on Caregivers

Dementia has a significant impact on the caregivers of the patient. Patients with dementia become more heavily reliant on the caregiver as the disease progresses. The neuropsychiatric symptoms have been found to have a more profound (negative) effect on caregivers and be a stronger predictor of caregiver burden in AD than the cognitive decline/impairment, disease stage, or other symptoms such as depression and apathy [5, 17]. Effects on caregivers include decreased quality of life, depression, stress/distress, lower income, and potential for injury if the patient behaves aggressively [5].

## Financial Impacts of Dementia

The costs to society and personal and family financial costs of dementia are substantial. In 2018, the estimated cost of caring for US patients with AD and other forms of dementia was $277 billion, without including costs of unpaid caregiving. Approximately US$ 60 billion was out of pocket costs, and these costs are predicted to increase [18].

Interestingly the financial implications of dementia can start 6 years before diagnosis. A cohort study of 81,364 Medicare beneficiaries living in single-person households in the USA found that those with AD and related dementias were more likely to miss bill payments up to 6 years before diagnosis and began to develop suboptimal credit scores 2.5 years before diagnosis compared to those never diagnosed [19].

## Alzheimer's Disease

Alzheimer's disease (AD) is the most common form of dementia, though it is possible to have more than one form of dementia concurrently. AD is an irreversible and progressive neurodegenerative disease which gets worse with time. It is thought that AD begins 20 or more years before symptoms begin to manifest, with small brain changes occurring that are not noticed by the individual [6]. Impairment of short-term memory is one of the first symptoms experienced [3, 20]. As the disease progresses, patients begin to show other symptoms including loss of long-term memory, confusion, sleep disturbances, language disturbances, mood changes, and loss of body function which are a result of the neuron damage in various brain regions affected [3, 6, 21]. People suffering from AD live with the symptoms for years, and with time, the symptoms increase and interfere with daily living. Eventually, neurons in brain regions responsible for basic bodily functions like walking and swallowing become affected. The outcome of AD is death [6].

### Two Types of Alzheimer's Disease

There are two types of AD, one called familial AD which is inherited as an autosomal dominant pattern and typically develops as early onset and the other is the sporadic type which typically develops later in life and the cause of which is poorly understood [22–24].

### Risk Factors for Alzheimer's Disease

The three greatest risk factors for late-onset AD are age (older age—being 65 years or older—is a risk factor for late-onset AD), carrying the E4 form of the ApoE gene (coding for apolipoprotein), and having a family history of AD [6]. Other risk factors for AD include head trauma, vascular conditions including diabetes, obesity, and trans-fat intake, while the Mediterranean diet (characterized by increased monounsaturated olive oil and omega-3 from fish), higher level of education, and physical activity reduce AD [4, 9, 24].

Those who have the genetic variant apolipoprotein E ε2 (ApoE2) allele are protected from developing AD, while the ApoE4 allele is associated with late-onset AD [25]. Implications of variations in the gene coding for apolipoprotein E will be discussed in a later section on pathophysiology.

## Prevalence of Neuropsychiatric Symptoms in Alzheimer's Disease

While memory loss and cognitive decline are common symptoms of AD, behavioral disorders are also a feature of this disease [7]. Over 90% of AD sufferers will be affected by behavioral and psychological symptoms [26]. Interestingly in one study in Thailand [27], in 61.3% of AD patients, the chief complaint was neuropsychiatric symptoms, while memory problems were the chief complaint in a comparatively lower percentage (38.7%). Olfactory disorders such as hyposmia (decreased sense of smell) can accompany AD even in its early stages, and hyposmia may be an early predictive symptom of AD [13].

The following figures from a couple of studies give us an idea of the prevalence of some of the common neuropsychiatric symptoms (in addition to memory loss) in AD:

- Apathy 49–71%
- Depression 42%
- Aggression/agitation 35–45%
- Anxiety 39%
- Irritability 36%
- Sleep disorder 39–56%
- Appetite or eating disorder 34–51%
- Delusion 31–40%
- Aberrant motor behavior 32–61%
- Disinhibition 17%
- Hallucination 16%
- Euphoria 6.5% [27–29]

As you can see from the figures above, behavioral disturbances such as irritability, agitated behavior, aggressive behavior, and aberrant motor behavior are common [28]. Agitated behavior refers to inappropriate verbal or motor activity that is not explained by needs nor confusion and may be nonaggressive or aggressive. Aggressive behavioral symptoms can occur with or without agitation and include fighting, throwing things, swearing, screaming, restlessness, pacing, wandering, inappropriate disrobing, and others [30]. Agitation occurs in 20–50% of those with moderate-severe AD, is common in those residing in long-term care facilities, and is associated with decreased quality of life, increased caregiver burden, higher rates of institutionalization, and higher mortality rates [31]. It is particularly difficult to treat [31].

Something to bear in mind is that agitation and aggressive behavior can be incredibly stressful and challenging for caregivers including nursing staff and family members. The impact of such neuropsychological symptoms on those around the patient with dementia should not be underestimated. In dealing with patients with dementia, healthcare practitioners would do well to also inquire with family members about how they are coping as they may well need your help too.

## Overview of Pathophysiology of Alzheimer's Disease

AD is characterized by a slow and progressive loss of cognitive function which is associated with neurodegeneration and neuroinflammation and a gradual degeneration and death of cerebral cells [7, 32].

AD, like many other age-related neurological disorders, is characterized by proteinopathies—the aberrant accumulation of disease-specific protein aggregates or misfolded proteins, which accompanies cognitive decline. There are several underlying processes involved in AD, including protein misfolding and disrupted protein homeostasis (or proteostasis), microglial activation, oxidative stress, and neuroinflammation [33] and progressive cerebral atrophy [34]. Neurodegeneration associated with AD is characterized by loss of neurons along with synaptic loss and failure, and this leads to loss of memory, impairment of cognition, and changes in behavior [20, 35]. In fact, synaptic loss is one of the factors most strongly correlating with the cognitive impairment occurring in AD patients [35].

### Triad of Changes

AD is characterized by a triad of the following:

1. Extracellular deposits of aggregated β-amyloid peptide (Aβ)
2. Intracellular neurofibrillary tangles (NFT) made of hyperphosphorylated tau proteins
3. Neuroinflammation (including astrogliosis and microglial cell proliferation) [20, 32, 36]

The presence of amyloid plaques is considered a neuropathological diagnostic criterion for AD and is composed of extracellular aggregated β-amyloid peptide (Aβ). Intracellular neurofibrillary tangles (composed of microtubule-associated protein tau), however, are not specific for AD and can be found in many neurodegenerative diseases (such as progressive supranuclear palsy and subtypes of frontotemporal dementia) [37].

According to Gouras et al. [37], Aβ is a normal peptide generated throughout lives, and is not inherently toxic, perhaps even having a physiological function, as distinct from amyloid plaques which are abnormal lesions composed on highly aggregated Aβ fibrils. One study found that Aβ40, either soluble or aggregated, at nano- and micro-molar concentrations in cell-free oxidative systems acts as a potent antioxidant (and argued that Aβ40-Cu(I)/Fe(II) complexes per se were not responsible for oxidative damage in AD) [38]. The function of β-amyloid peptides has not been fully elucidated [37]. Production and secretion of Aβ is stimulated by synaptic activity [37].

## Aggregated Aβ Peptide and Alzheimer's Disease

It is thought that the misfolded, aggregated Aβ peptide is the initiating trigger for AD [39], with progressive accumulation of Aβ protein caused by an imbalance between its production, aggregation, and removal [22]. The proteostasis network is the protein surveillance system which regulates the cellular proteome, including protein synthesis and clearance of misfolded proteins. This network becomes dysfunctional in many different neurodegenerative diseases including AD. Reactive oxidative species (ROS) due to several factors (including inflammation, aging, disease-associated mutations, polymorphisms) can impair the proteostasis network balance, causing oxidative damage, and neuroinflammation and disrupt proteostasis, leading to cell death [33].

As explained by Dash and colleagues [33], what happens in AD, as in other neurodegenerative proteinopathies, is that there is repeated production of a specific protein which is misfolded and aggregated, and this affects specific neurons. Under healthy conditions, the body corrects this: misfolded proteins are either refolded correctly or degraded by the body's quality control system, for example, by chaperone proteins. However, under conditions of cellular aging and proteotoxic stress or mutation, these misfolded proteins manage to evade this quality control system and become aggregated, forming structures varying from amorphous accretions to highly ordered amyloid fibril plaques (which are very resistant to degradation). Several factors are involved in protein aggregation including mitochondrial dysfunction, calcium-induced protein misfolding, and inflammation [33].

### Amyloid Cascade Hypothesis

In AD, Aβ is formed from amyloid-β protein precursor (APP). The "amyloid cascade hypothesis" is that cleavage of amyloid precursor protein (APP) by β-secretase and γ-secretase complex causes an excessive production of Aβ, and this then causes inflammation that triggers tau hyperphosphorylation [32]. Tau is a highly soluble protein maintaining the stability of microtubules in axons that are abundant in the neurons of the central nervous system (CNS). Aggregated Aβ causes an imbalance of various phosphatases and protein kinases involved in maintaining different cellular signals and promoting tau protein hyperphosphorylation. Tau hyperphosphorylation leads to formation of insoluble intracellular aggregates called neurofibrillary tangles (NFT) [33]. This tau phosphorylation is understood to be essential for neurodegeneration [20]. The neurofibrillary tangles then impair intraneuronal communication and lead to cell death [40].

## Neuroinflammation

Support for the role of inflammation in the pathogenesis of AD comes from epidemiological evidence, including findings that long-term use of NSAIDs lowers prevalence of AD by 30–60% [32, 41–43]. Other studies have found increased levels of proinflammatory cytokines including IL-1, IL-6, TNF-α, or S100β associated with AD [36, 44, 45], and elevated plasma levels of C-reactive protein and IL-6 have been found in AD patients well before clinical onset of AD [32, 46, 47]. Also, gliosis is very evident in AD, and most plaques are surrounded by activated astrocytes and/or invaded by activated microglia [32].

### Pathways of Neuroinflammation

Neuroinflammation is a process that helps maintain homeostasis in the CNS and is triggered in response to exogenous and endogenous pathogens, toxins, infections, and aggregated or modified proteins. Neuroinflammation is mediated by glial cells, in particular microglia, the resident macrophages of the CNS. Microglia have the responsibility of initiating, amplifying, and/or equalizing the inflammatory response. They do this by synthesizing inflammatory mediators including cytokines, prostaglandins, and free radicals [48].

While microglia normally play a role in homeostasis, overactivation of microglia appears to be involved in creating the proinflammatory state characteristic of AD. Normally, microglia scavenge damaged neurons and secrete neurotrophic factors, protecting neurons and supporting their survival. However, in AD microglia are overactivated and release excessive amounts of proinflammatory factors like nitric oxide and reactive oxygen species, and this promotes neuronal death [49].

The pathways of neuroinflammation involved in AD are complex, and what follows is a brief summary of key points (see Bedse et al. [22] for a deeper dive). Essentially, the deposition of Aβ neuritic plaques is believed to trigger neuroinflammation which eventually leads to neurodegeneration [22, 50], and the neuroinflammatory response has been found to parallel the disease course [51, 52].

Formation of complex protein aggregates containing Aβ peptide induces a chronic inflammatory response which leads to activation of microglia (CNS phagocytes) and astrocytes [22], and a process of reactive gliosis. These accumulate at the Aβ plaques, engulf them, and try to clear them through autophagy/phagocytosis [22, 36]. Both produce proinflammatory chemicals that trigger secondary damage, contributing to inflammation [53, 54].

Aβ activates many signaling cascades within microglia including, among others, some that lead to production of reactive oxygen species (ROS) and to the synthesis of neurotoxins and excitotoxins [54]. Other factors appear to be involved too, including blood coagulation and fibrinolysis systems, and altered expression of several intercellular adhesion molecules on microglia and astrocytes [54].

Various kinases are stimulated which activate mitogen-activated protein kinase (MAPK) and nuclear factor κB (NF-κB), and Aβ can also directly activate MAPK and extracellular kinase (ERK) pathways [22]. This leads to release of proinflammatory cytokines of which interleukin-1β (IL-1β) and tissue necrosis factor alpha (TNF-α) are the main ones responsible for the chronic inflammation occurring in this disease [22].

IL-1β from glia can activate MAPK and NF-κB signaling in astrocytes as well as neurons, further increasing inflammation as well as triggering tau phosphorylation

[22]. Increased IL-1 is also related to neurofibrillary tangle development in AD [55], though there is some evidence that it may play a beneficial role by dampening the detrimental effects of amyloid accumulation [36].

Aβ induces neuronal cell apoptosis via several mechanisms including increasing permeabilization of lysosomal membranes, activation of caspase-3, and others [22].

### Oxidative Stress

Oxidative stress is a key part of the pathophysiology of AD. Aβ deposition has been shown to lead to free radical-induced oxidative stress, reflected in formation of ROS, lipid peroxidation, DNA oxidation, and modification of proteins by lipid peroxidation products [56–58].

Oxidative stress and synaptic dysfunction are part of the early events occurring in AD, and it is thought that changes in neuronal activity and signaling promote amyloid precursor protein (APP) processing and increased Aβ formation, creating a positive feedback that speeds up the AD pathogenesis [59]. Thus, oxidative stress, neuroinflammation, and synaptic dysregulation/dysfunction are part of the pathogenesis, not just the end result of Aβ-induced damage [59].

Release of the proinflammatory cytokines ultimately causes ROS/reactive nitrogen species (RNS) generation, mitochondrial dysfunction, and neuronal apoptosis [22, 33]. Other pathways are involved including excessive intracellular calcium accumulation leading to ROS/RNS production which detrimentally affects the quality control mechanisms, and excessive aggregation interacts with membrane systems creating transmembrane pores which lead to greater calcium influx [33]. In addition, activation of particular neuronal signaling pathways can inhibit synaptic plasticity [22]. Thus, a neurotoxic environment is created which contributes to AD progression [36, 60].

## Autophagy and mTOR

Inherent in the pathological process is the accumulation of Aβ without adequate clearance. A major clearance mechanism is the process of autophagy. "Autophagy" (a term literally meaning "self-eating") is the body's process of clearing out damaged or dysfunctional cells, organelles, and proteins and then recycling their parts. It is crucial for maintaining cellular homeostasis, and neurons rely heavily on autophagy to maintain normal function. Protein aggregates and damaged organelles are taken into a vesicle-like structure called an autophagosome and then eventually merge with a lysosome for lysing or destruction. The recycled amino acids, fatty acids, sugars, and other components are released into the cytosol to be reused in various pathways [61].

Autophagy is essential for breakdown and recycling of cellular debris and protein aggregates like tau. But this is not without intelligent controls. Autophagy receptors have been found to recognize phagosome contents and differentiate macrophages for the inflammatory versus adaptive state for healing. The mTOR pathway is the master controller of autophagy and is involved in regulation of macrophage polarization. mTOR, activated by the ERK pathway, programs the microglia to decrease autophagy with a proinflammatory response in conjunction with increased cellular glycolysis. However, in the autophagy cascade, Aβ products may be degraded for cellular recycling or inactivated for elimination. This alternative path relies on oxidative phosphorylation of mitochondria. The mTOR pathway may regulate the macrophage inflammatory pathway, differentiation, metabolism, and function [62]. The question of a possible defect in autophagy in the pathophysiology of neurodegenerative conditions has been raised [62].

#### Two Key Systems Regulating Autophagy

There are actually two key systems that regulate autophagy: the mammalian target of rapamycin complex 1 (mTORC1) and AMP-activated protein kinase (AMPK). They have opposite effects, inhibiting or activating autophagy, respectively. The mTOR system primarily senses cellular nutrition and energy (it senses the availability of nutrients and growth factors). In conditions of low cellular energy, AMPK is activated which triggers autophagy. In conditions of sufficiency, mTOR stimulates growth and proliferation, and in cancer, some tumors actually "hijack" mTOR for their growth. Fasting promotes AMPK which can induce this autophagy switch, as can specific diet regimens including caloric restriction and very low carbohydrate/ketogenic diets [61]. Meanwhile, Aβ has been shown to inhibit AMPK, thereby preventing the elimination of neurotoxic Aβ oligomers [63].

#### Associations Between Autophagy Regulation and AD

Autophagy is important for neuron homeostasis, and there is evidence of associations with neurodegenerative disorders including AD, as well as many others including cancer, cardiovascular disease, and obesity (a risk factor for many diseases) [61, 64]. Research in a mice model of AD has demonstrated that an mTOR inhibitor can reduce Aβ levels and abolish cognitive decline [65] and the polyphenol resveratrol (a known antioxidant present in grapes and red wine) has been found to activate the AMPK pathway and trigger autophagic destruction of Aβ [66]. Berberine, one of the active constituents of the Chinese herb *Huang Lian* (*Coptis chinensis*) as well as other herbs, has also been found to promote autophagy and inhibit production of Aβ in a mouse model of AD [67]. There are many different potential compounds which may be able to activate AMPK or inhibit mTOR and other targets in autophagy (see Meng et al. [61]).

#### Changes in the mTOR Pathway Linked to Cognitive Decline and AD

Multiple studies have linked the changes of mTOR pathway to cognitive decline and AD. This is uniquely the case in Down syndrome with very similar pathophysiology to AD, where between 40 and 50 years of age, Down syndrome persons have AD-like pathology and dementia. The premature neurodegeneration in Down syndrome (as early as mid-40s) implicates dysfunction in mitochondria, neurogenesis, oxidative stress, proteostasis, and autophagy, all related to chromosome 21 trisomy. Specifically, in Down syndrome the mTOR signaling has been shown to induce Aβ generation and senile plaques and neurofibrillary tangles [68]. Successful treatment or prevention of dementia in Down syndrome could have major implications for AD.

## Tau Hyperphosphorylation

As described earlier, amyloid deposition is only one part of the pathogenesis of AD [20]. In addition to the extra-neuronal Aβ plaques, AD is also characterized by neurofibrillary tangles composed mostly of hyperphosphorylated tau protein [69]. These intraneuronal aggregations of microtubule-associated protein tau are in the form of filaments [70].

A study was conducted in humans with AD and dementia where they were followed until death, with postmortems then conducted on their brains. The study found moderate correlations between densities of neocortical neurofibrillary tangles and severity/degree and duration of dementia (as measured when they were alive using two validated dementia scales), but the density of senile plaques was not correlated to degree of dementia [71]. They also concluded that densities of neocortical plaque differentiated very old subjects with dementia from controls (those without dementia) [71].

The interactions between extracellular Aβ plaques and intracellular neurofibrillary tangles are not well understood [69]. Research has found that RCAN1 levels (a gene that responds to oxidative stress), GSK-3β (glycogen synthase kinase 3β) protein levels, and tau phosphorylation are increased when cortical neurons are incubated with Aβ peptide, and this effect is blocked by the antioxidants glutathione and trolox [69]. Such research implicates Aβ peptide as a transcription factor in tau hyperphosphorylation via RCAN1 [69]. Additionally, increases in GSK-3β may also promote further Aβ formation by inhibiting AMPK pathways [72].

## Changes Occurring Prior to Signs and Symptoms of AD

One of the key problems, certainly from the perspective of finding therapeutic strategies to prevent or halt it, is that the activation of microglia and astrocytes and the resultant excessive cytokine production can occur decades prior to the pathological changes that hallmark a diagnosis of AD [60]. Aβ deposition occurs at least 20 years prior to the signs and symptoms of AD [73, 74]. Aβ can be detected using positron-emission tomography (PET) or by a reduction in Aβ levels in cerebrospinal fluid (CSF), but unfortunately these only become detectable when Aβ deposition in the brain is already well underway [75].

Recent research in mice suggests that the preclinical phase of AD (i.e., when there is Aβ deposition without clinical symptoms) may be a relatively late manifestation of a much earlier phase of pathogenic Aβ *seed formation* [75]. Other research indicates that Aβ seeding is strongest in the early stages of cerebral β-amyloidosis and decreases with disease progression and age [75–77].

Mice research has demonstrated that acute administration of an antibody, aducanumab, at the pre-amyloid stage led to a significant decrease in Aβ and downstream pathogenic changes 6 months later [75]. This is promising research. Therapeutic interventions that might be able to address this very early pathogenic stage of pre-amyloid seeding may be where the biggest gains might be had in the future.

## Scientific Debate: Is Aβ the Key Toxic Entity After All?

Yet, despite the fact that amyloid plaques are the classic hallmark of AD, and there is much in the literature that indicates Aβ oligomers are responsible for the neurotoxic effects of Aβ rather than the fibrils [22], there are several lines of evidence that amyloid plaques are not the main toxic Aβ entity [37]. Cognitive decline does not correlate with the levels of these cortical plaques. Loss of synapses is the main correlate of disease progression, and loss of cholinergic neurons is a contributor to deficits in memory and attention [3]. Other studies provide evidence that plaques and change in cognition are unrelated. For example, an active Aβ42 vaccine clinical trial found the vaccine was associated with plaque clearance, but there was continued cognitive decline [78]. In two different mouse models of chronic synaptic inhibition, plaque burden decreased, but there was an increase in Aβ42 immunoreactivity within neurons, and increased synaptophysin and synapse loss [79].

Other research that indicates tau deposition is critical in the pathogenesis of dementia [80]. A case report demonstrated that extensive deposition of amyloid in humans who have genetically inherited AD does not lead to dementia if they have an additional genetic mutation that prevents tau deposition [80].

## Cholinergic Involvement in Alzheimer's Disease

Evidence exists that cholinergic and glutaminergic systems are involved in the etiology and pathogenesis of AD. Levels of acetylcholine (ACh) and its functioning are decreased in AD, and this is relevant to AD since this neurotransmitter is critically involved in processing of memory and learning [81]. Cholinergic neurons are widely distributed in the brain, with almost all parts of the brain innervated by these neurons [3]. Cholinergic neurons are found mostly in the spinal cord, hindbrain, basal forebrain, striatum, medial habenula, mesopontine region, olfactory tubercle, and islands of Cajella complex. The cholinergic system is involved in memory, learning, attention, sleep, wakefulness, the stress response, and processing of sensory information [3]. In fact, acetylcholine (ACh) is involved in modulation of all aspects of memory including acquisition, encoding, consolidation, reconsolidation, and retrieval [3].

### Cholinergic Hypothesis of AD

The basalis of Meynert (also called the nucleus basalis) is a group of neurons located in the basal forebrain that projects neurons throughout the cortex and amygdala. In AD, there is a selective and severe degeneration and loss of neurons in the basalis of Meynert which contributes to memory loss [3, 82, 83].

The "cholinergic hypothesis of AD" is based on findings that ACh levels and functioning are decreased in AD, that there is a severe loss of cholinergic neurons in the basal forebrain including in particular in the basalis of Meynert, and that there is decreased acetylcholinesterase activity [81]. It appears that the neurotoxicity associated with the Aβ oligomers affects cholinergic synapses in particular, with loss of cholinergic synapses correlating strongly with cognitive impairment [3, 84].

Because of the extensive distribution of cholinergic neurons, dysfunction of cholinergic transmission has the potential to influence cognition and behavior extensively, including cortical and hippocampal information processing. Disruption of cholinergic signaling to the cortex can detrimentally affect attention and decision-making processes, and loss of cholinergic neurons can impair dopaminergic transmission which might underpin the psychiatric symptoms associated with AD [3].

Deficits in memory and severity of the neuropathy in AD are correlated with changes in synaptic transmission in the hippocampus, and in particular with changes in the expression of the presynaptic vesicle protein synaptophysin [3, 85]. Synaptophysin makes up part of the pore complex that forms when a vesicle fuses with the presynaptic membrane, and in AD, its levels have been found to be lower in particular brain regions [86].

### Acetylcholinesterase Activity Is Reduced in AD

As mentioned earlier, the main cholinergic neurons affected in AD are those in the basalis of Meynert, and neuron numbers here are severely reduced from around 500,000 in normal brains to under 100,000 in those with advanced AD [3, 87]. In the remaining cholinergic neurons, there is reduction in cortical choline acetyltransferase activity (this enzyme is responsible for synthesis of ACh) which correlates with severity of dementia and number of neurofibrillary tangles [88]. Other studies suggest that acetylcholinesterase may also be involved in AD pathology, and on the basis of this, several cholinesterase inhibitor drugs including rivastigmine have reached the market [3].

## Glutaminergic Involvement in Alzheimer's Disease

Glutamate is the most abundant excitatory neurotransmitter in the central nervous system (CNS), widely distributed and mostly located intracellularly [24]. Most of the excitatory neurotransmission is mediated by glutamate and its receptors, mostly ligand-gated ionotropic glutamate receptors (iGluRs) which are involved in synaptic plasticity (which underpins learning and memory). The level of glutamate exists at a low resting concentration in the synaptic cleft, but during synaptic transmission, this concentration increases significantly. Residual glutamate is removed by a glutamate uptake system [24].

There are several lines of evidence to suggest that glutamate excitotoxicity is involved in the pathogenesis of AD. What follows is a summary from Wang and Reddy [24], recommended reading to understand the intricacies better.

One subgroup of iGluRs are the N-methyl-d-aspartate (NMDA) receptors (abbreviated to NMDARs) which are gated selectively by NMDA. Glutaminergic neurotransmission that occurs via NMDARs is necessary for neuronal survival (as these receptors activate neuronal survival pathways) as well as synaptic plasticity (which underpins learning and memory). There needs to be sufficient NMDAR signaling; otherwise, neuronal cell survival is threatened, but if there is excessive NMDAR activity, it leads to excitotoxicity and cell death [24]. It appears that in AD, this delicate balance has become disrupted and that glutamate-mediated excitotoxicity is favored [24].

Where the NMDARs are located determines its action: activation of *synaptic* NMDARs is believed to trigger plasticity and promote cell survival, whereas activation of *extra-synaptic* NMDARs triggers cell death. It is believed that when these processes get out of balance and become tipped toward activation of *extra-synaptic* NMDARs, this contributes to the neurodegeneration that occurs in several diseases including AD [24, 89].

Toxic Aβ may impair the glutamate reuptake systems and thus lead to excess glutamate availability which then contributes to increased excitotoxicity and neurodegeneration [24]. Deficiencies in reuptake of glutamate by astroglial cells in the synaptic cleft can lead to chronic low-level activation of receptors by glutamate [81]. Toxic Aβ can also directly affect the function of NMDARs. Excess glutamate from presynaptic terminals or astrocytes triggers extra-synaptic NMDAR signaling and tilts the balance away from the (pro-survival) synaptic NDMAR activity, thereby favoring excitotoxicity and eventually neurodegeneration [24].

It is also thought that synaptic NMDARs become detrimentally affected by Aβ, resulting in reduced synaptic glutaminergic transmission and synaptic plasticity. Consistent with the synaptic loss of AD and neurodegenerative processes occurring later in AD, the presynaptic vesicle release mechanisms also become dysfunctional, leading to difficulties in initiating an excitatory event [24].

Again, we see how very finely tuned the human being is, illustrated by this example of the balance in NMDAR signaling required to maintain a healthy nervous system. We also see how different factors can work to disrupt that balance and lead to neurodegeneration.

## Glucose, Brain Metabolism, and Vascular Impairments

Glucose hypometabolism may play a key role in the pathophysiology of dementia [25]. There are several lines of research to support this contention. For example, reduced glucose metabolism has been demonstrated in the brains of patients with AD and other types of dementias. Observational studies have demonstrated that patients with diabetes have a higher risk of developing all types of dementia, as well as AD and vascular dementia [9]. Those with type 2 diabetes are 2–4 times more likely to develop AD [90].

## Is AD the New Type 3 Diabetes?

Brain insulin resistance could be an important factor in cerebral degeneration, cognitive impairment, and increased AD [91]. There is evidence that insulin deficiency and insulin resistance within the brain may mediate neurodegeneration in AD, with some arguing that AD is "type 3 diabetes" or "brain diabetes" [91, 92]. Brain insulin resistance is linked to oxidative stress, and this is associated with ceramides, protein aggregates, proinflammatory cytokines, mitochondrial damage and abnormalities, and neuronal death [91].

Insulin plays a vital role in neuronal survival, neuroplasticity, cognition, and memory. Many of the changes seen in AD such as disturbances to neuronal growth and synaptic plasticity, tau hyperphosphorylation, and alterations in energy metabolism may be due to impaired insulin signaling within the CNS. Hyperglycemia impairs endothelial function and increases permeability of the blood-brain barrier allowing for leakage of peripheral ROS species and short-chain ceramides into the cerebral (and eye) circulation. Ceramides, a waxy lipid component of cell membranes, have neurotoxic effects and have been shown to impair brain cell viability and energy metabolism, mediate insulin resistance, and induce inflammation, mitochondrial dysfunction, and oxidative damage in membranes and tissues, and may mediate cognitive problems found in patients with insulin resistance. Aβ plaques and decreased dendritic spine density have been found to be associated with brain insulin resistance [91].

Redox balance is likely to play a key role in cognitive changes and neurodegenerative changes and increased incidence of Alzheimer's disease seen in patients with insulin resistance. In AD, ceramides enhance the formation of amyloid-β peptides through β-secretase that cleaves APP into Aβ. It has been argued that the neurotoxic effects of ceramide may be mediated by oxidative stress, something that might help explain the relationship between brain insulin resistance and the neurodegenerative changes seen in AD [91].

## Diabetes Treatment and AD

An interesting finding is that brain autopsies of diabetics don't have more Aβ plaques and tau tangles than those without diabetes [25]. Why would this be the case? It might be because diabetes medications are decreasing the risk of AD brain pathology [25]. A study found that untreated diabetics displayed significantly greater p-tau, t-tau, and p-tau/Aβ1–42 than treated diabetics, prediabetics, or euglycemic participants and greater t-tau/Aβ1–42 than the prediabetics or euglycemic participants. The untreated diabetic group progressed to dementia at higher rates than the euglycemic group (hazard ratio 1.602 [95% CI 1.057–2.429]; $P = 0.026$) [93].

Further support for a link between glucose metabolism, diabetes, and AD can be seen in improvements in patients with AD with the use of antidiabetic drugs to improve insulin resistance in the body, as well improvements in the brain's mitochondrial function and insulin responsiveness [91]. Endocannabinoid targets include oxidative stress, blood-brain permeability, glucose and lipid metabolism, and nuclear receptor modulation.

### Genes and Glucose Utilization

As mentioned earlier, those with the ApoE2 allele are protected from developing AD, and those with ApoE4 allele have a higher risk of developing late-onset AD [25]. The brains of mice models of ApoE2, ApoE3, and ApoE4 genotypes were found to differ significantly in facilitated glucose transporter (mediates entry of glucose into neurons) and hexokinase (key gateway enzyme involved in glycolysis) [94]. When they examined uptake and metabolism of ketone bodies, a secondary source of energy for the brain during fasting, it was the ApoE3 brains which showed a deficient profile (not the other genotypes) [94]. Thus, this study found that hexokinase was the key cytosolic point in the glucose metabolism pathway that is differentially modulated by the three different genotypes, and they surmised that the differences in expression and activity of hexokinase in the brains of the three ApoE genotypes may underlie the impact on glucose utilization and further susceptibility to AD [94].

Another study in mice found that glycolysis was more robust in ApoE2 mice than ApoE4 mice and that as the ApoE2 mice aged, they produced more hexokinase, while the ApoE4 mice had less hexokinase activity with age (therefore were less efficient at converting glucose to energy), consistent with the finding that the APOE4 allele is associated with late-onset AD [25, 29]. Essentially if the APOE4 mice brain is not as efficient at utilizing glucose, this starves the energy-hungry brain cells and may lead to cognitive impairment [25]. Other animal studies have found impaired glucose transport in mice AD models [95].

## Genes and Familial Alzheimer's Disease

Familial AD is inherited as an autosomal dominant pattern [22, 23]. It is caused by genetic mutations in presenilin (PS1, PS2) and amyloid precursor protein (APP) genes which affect a common pathway in APP synthesis and proteolysis which then leads to overproduction of amyloid-β peptide/protein.

Mutations in genes coding for amyloid precursor protein (APP), presenilin-1 or presenilin-2, have been implicated in familial forms of AD and associated with production of Aβ oligomeric formations and amyloid plaques in brain areas including the hippocampus, cortex, and amygdala. Support for this theory is robust, especially in relation to familial forms of AD, but these only account under 5% of AD cases, indicating that other factors are at play in sporadic forms of AD [32].

The ApoE gene provides the template for apolipoprotein E which is involved in cholesterol transportation in the blood. Each person inherits one of the three alleles/

isoforms of the Apo E gene, ApoE2, ApoE3, and ApoE4 from each parent, and therefore there are six possible ApoE pairs—E2/E2, E2/E3, E2/E4, E3/E3, E3/E4, AND E4/E4 [6, 94]. According to the Alzheimer's Association report, the ApoE4 form increases an individual's risk of developing AD compared with the E3, but does not guarantee that someone will actually develop AD. Those with the ApoE4 variant are more likely to develop AD at a younger age than those with the E2 or E3 forms of the gene [6]. Inheriting one copy of the E4 form is associated with three times the risk of AD than two copies of the E3 form, and inheriting two copies of the E4 form is associated with an 8- to 12-fold risk [6]. The rare genetic variant ApoE2 allele protects people against developing AD, while another variant, ApoE4, is associated with increased dementia risk [25]. Why this is so may have to do with glucose metabolism which may be altered in AD.

## Poor Sleep, Aβ Plaques, and Tau Tangles in the Pathophysiology of Alzheimer's Disease

Those who have poor sleep are at higher risk of AD, and development of Aβ plaques and tau tangles negatively impacts of sleep. Patients with diabetes often have sleep problems [25]. Sleep disruptions, diabetes, and AD appear to be associated in some way. A study that used two different AD mice models (one was a model of Aβ pathology and the other was a model of tauopathy and neurodegeneration) was set up to investigate whether AD pathology and glycemic fluctuations synergize to cause sleep loss and peripheral glucose intolerance, which would increase risk of type 2 diabetes and AD [90]. The study found that sleep disruptions modulated AD and type 2 diabetes risk by changing the relationship between glucose tolerance, cerebral metabolism, neuronal activity, and levels of β-amyloid/tau. Inducing both low and high blood glucose resulted in less sleep in mice models of AD, and effects were exacerbated in mice with more β-amyloid or tau pathology [25, 90].

## Is Age a Risk Factor for Alzheimer's Disease?

Activated microglia are subcategorized into primed, enlarged, and phagocytic, representing the stages of activation [60]. With aging, there is an increase in activated astrocytes, microglia, and neuronal abnormalities and a progressive upregulation of glial inflammatory cytokines including IL-1, and this may increase risk of AD by favoring neuritic plaque formation as well as altering the threshold for AD development in response to genetic and environmental factors [60, 96].

However, the question remains: are these changes a *normal* part of aging, or are they a result of simply a greater number of years living with environmental factors that may predispose us to systemic and neuroinflammation? As mentioned previously, risk factors for AD include many that would be considered environmental including head trauma, diabetes, obesity, trans-fat intake, and lower levels of physical activity [4]. All of these are associated with increased systemic inflammation.

## Deficits in Current Treatments for AD

The difficulty with current treatments is that AD is typically diagnosed after the disease is well advanced. There are no treatments that reverse the disease process and cure AD, and many of the pharmaceutical interventions used to manage the neuropsychiatric symptoms/signs of AD are associated with several undesirable side effects [5, 20].

While recent pharmacological approaches have focused on reducing the β-amyloid deposits, this is only part of the pathophysiology of AD. Therefore, a better approach may be to modulate AD via the many different pathways involved rather than via just one [20]. The very best approach is primary prevention, since the Aβ deposition begins at least 20 years prior to signs and symptoms appearing [75]. Interventions which can target the very early pathogenic Aβ seed formation are likely to be important in the future. Given the regulatory role of the endocannabinoid system, there is clearly interest in how it might be involved in AD and whether this system might be a useful therapeutic target.

## The Endocannabinoid System in Alzheimer's Disease

There is clear evidence that the endocannabinoid system (ECS) is involved in the pathophysiology of AD. This is not surprising, given the homeostatic regulatory role played by the ECS in nearly every system (if not all systems) within the body, and its wide distribution throughout the central nervous system (CNS). As we have seen in previous chapters, the ECS is involved in regulation of cognition, learning, memory, emotions, inflammation, neurogenesis, neuroplasticity, neuro-immunity, and neuroendocrine processes, as well reducing neuroinflammation and promoting neuroprotection.

As discussed in previous chapters, in the brain, CB1 receptors are widely distributed in areas including the cortex, hippocampus, cerebellum, and basal ganglia. CB1 receptor signaling plays a key role in neuroprotection [97]. For example, in human teratocarcinoma cells, the endocannabinoids AEA and noladin ether (2-arachidonyl glyceryl ether) have been shown to protect against Aβ-induced neurotoxicity by activating CB1 receptors [98]. Meanwhile, CB2 receptors are mainly found in association with microglia (and astrocytes), supporting the neuroprotective and anti-inflammatory role of CB2 receptors in the CNS [20]. When microglial cells are activated, CB2 receptors in the microglial are upregulated and act by way of feedback to inhibit immune responsiveness [20, 99].

### Overview of Changes in the Endocannabinoid System in Alzheimer's Disease

A systematic review of 22 human studies [100] found that the following changes in the ECS appear to occur in AD:

- **2-Arachidonyl glycerol (2-AG)**:
  - Postmortem studies found no difference in 2-AG content in mid-frontal and temporal cortex between AD patients and controls.
  - Higher plasma 2-AG in AD compared with controls.
  - Increased DAGL expression with progression in AD (2-AG synthesis).
  - Increased MAGL with progression in AD (2-AG degradation).
- **Anandamide (AEA)**:
  - Reduced AEA concentration in AD was found in postmortem brains (within temporal and mid-frontal cortex) but no change in serum AEA.
  - Increased FAAH expression and activity (AEA degradation) found in relation to AD.
- **CB1 receptors**:
  - Increased CB1 receptors found in early stages of AD in some studies which may reflect a compensatory mechanism (upregulation) related to reduced AEA
  - Decreased CB1 receptor levels in later stage AD found in other studies, with other studies reporting no difference in CB1 receptor levels in AD cases compared to controls
- **CB2 receptors**:
  - Increased CB2 receptor expression and activity in key brain areas (e.g., hippocampus, para-hippocampus, and prefrontal cortex) found in late AD possibly in response to neuroinflammation.
- **TRPV1 receptors**:
  - No changes in TRPV1 expression in relation to AD

Despite changes in the components of the ECS being identified, less evidence exists to link changes in the ECS with cognitive defects [100].

**Fatty Acid Amide Hydrolase (FAAH)**

In addition to the changes above, postmortem examination of brains of individuals who died with AD showed significant upregulation of fatty acid amide hydrolase (FAAH; the enzyme which breaks down AEA) in astrocytes surrounding neuritic plaques. Since the breakdown products of AEA include arachidonic acid (AA), and AA is generally proinflammatory, this may contribute to inflammation [53].

## Preclinical Research: The Endocannabinoid System and Alzheimer's Disease

Mice models of AD have given insight into the pathological changes in AD, including changes in the ECS as well as potential areas for therapeutic intervention. One popular animal model of AD is the 5xFAD (family Alzheimer's disease) transgenic mice model where the mice display microgliosis and astrogliosis in response to amyloid deposition. In this model which represents aggressive and early-onset amyloid pathology, the mice have significant neuronal loss by 9–12 months and cognitive decline beginning at 4 months, increasing greatly with age [20]. While an exhaustive description of the findings of animal experiments is beyond the scope of this book, we will take a quick look at some of the findings.

In one experiment using the 5xFAD model of AD, pharmacologic inhibition of FAAH (remember, FAAH breaks down AEA) had little impact on cognitive impairment, plaque deposition, and gliosis nor on the expression of key cytokines and enzymes. However, genetic inactivation of FAAH (FAAH-null 5xFAD mice) led to increased expression of inflammatory cytokines, reduced soluble amyloid levels, neuritic plaques, and gliosis as well as behavioral improvement in spatial memory (that was not mediated via CB1 receptors and was independent of anxiety level) [50].

Other studies using animal models of AD suggest 2-AG levels may be increased in AD [20], which is consistent with human studies which have also found increased plasma 2-AG in AD [101]. In a study of 41 patients with probable AD, age-matched with normal controls, AD patients were found to have higher plasma 2-AG levels which was thought be the researchers to possibly be a protective mechanism to hinder neurodegeneration [101]. In an experiment using homozygous and heterozygous 5XFAD mice, there was an increase in diacylglycerol lipase (DAGL; which synthesizes 2-AG) levels and a decrease in monoacylglycerol lipase (MAGL; which degrades 2-AG). This may increase 2-AG levels, thereby leading to desensitization of CB1 receptors (which may explain the reduction in CB1 receptor levels found). The authors of this study proposed that excess production of endocannabinoids might be reflective of an anti-inflammatory response to combat the damage due to the amyloid deposition [20].

#### Protective Role of Endocannabinoids

Several lines of evidence suggest that endocannabinoids play a protective role in AD, and this occurs via several pathways. For example, application of AEA, 2-AG, and noladin ether directly to cell culture or via inhibition of their degradative enzymes results in increased viability of neurons exposed to toxic Aβ species [98, 102–104].

As discussed previously, Aβ induces neuronal cell apoptosis via several mechanisms including increasing permeabilization of lysosomal membranes, activation of caspase-3, and others [22]. Endocannabinoids are neuroprotective and can stabilize lysosomes against Aβ permeabilization (increasing cell survival) and prevent DNA fragmentation and caspase-3 activation induced by Aβ [22, 105, 106]. Levels of 2-AG in the brain were found to increase in response to acute in vivo administration of Aβ which again suggests a neuroprotective role [22, 106].

A study in rats and mice found that injection of beta-amyloid peptide (BAP) into rat cortices was associated with markers of neuronal damage in the hippocampus and increased 2-AG levels (but not AEA). Application of VDM-11, an inhibitor of endocannabinoid cellular reuptake, increased rat hippocampal and mouse brain endocannabinoid levels when administered either 3 or 7 days after BAP injection and until the 12th or 14th day. The endocannabinoid reuptake inhibitor reversed the hippocampal damage caused by BAP in the rat experiment and reduced Aβ-induced memory impairment in mice (but only when it was administered at least 3 days after the BAP injection) [106].

## Cannabinoid Receptor Involvement in Pathology

It is reasonable that CB1 receptors should be involved in AD pathology given their critical involvement in the processes of memory, cognition, and regulation of emotions, all of which are affected in AD [20]. In the same experiment mentioned in the previous section using homozygous and heterozygous 5XFAD mice, anxiety-like behavior and memory were altered, and CB1 receptor expression was reduced in the hippocampus in both homo- and heterozygous groups, suggesting this decrease may be related to memory dysfunction. They also found that the number of Aβ plaques was negatively associated with CB1 receptor expression and positively associated with CB2 receptor levels [20].

Increased GPR55 levels and increased CB2 receptor levels were found in the hippocampi of homozygous mice and associated with anxiety-like responses displayed by the mice, perhaps in compensation [20].

Certainly, there is some evidence that CB1 receptor-dependent effects of cannabinoids may be involved in upstream events that might affect intracellular oxidative pathways, for example, activation of CB1 receptors may be able to inhibit glutamate toxicity by countering its hyperpolarizing activity [107]. If we consider that glutamate excitotoxicity is one of the factors that may be involved in pathophysiology of AD, then the ability to modulate CB1 receptors via phytocannabinoids and related substances may be important therapeutically.

Several studies support the notion that upregulation of CB2 receptors is a protective mechanism to limit inflammation and clear amyloid plaques from the brain [22]. In a mice experiment using the 5XFAD model of AD, increased CB2 receptor levels were found in areas of intense inflammation and amyloid deposits, including in the cortex, hippocampus, brainstem, and thalamus [108]. An in vitro experiment demonstrated that CB2 receptor activation facilitated removal of Aβ from frozen human tissue specimens (of people who had AD), and in an animal model of AD, a CB2 receptor agonist induced Aβ clearance, but how CB2 receptors decrease Aβ plaques is not well understood [22].

## Evidence of ECS Involvement in AD: Experiments with Cannabinoid Receptor Agonists

Evidence for involvement of cannabinoid receptors in AD pathology is also found in animal studies investigating the effects of cannabinoid receptor agonists. For example, a mice study found that chronic infusion of a CB1 agonist was able to protect neurons and reduce the cognitive impairment in a mice model of AD [109]. In another study using a genetic mice model of AD, a CB2 receptor agonist was able to improve cognition, and this was associated with decreased microglial reactivity and reduced levels of proinflammatory cytokines (IL-1β, IL-6, TNF-α, and IFN-γ). The CB2 receptor agonist was also able to reduce the expression of active p38 and SAPK/JNK, increase the expression of inactive GSK-3β, and decrease tau hyperphosphorylation near the amyloid-β plaques [110].

Enhancement of endocannabinoids via cannabinoid receptor agonists has been found to have several effects on Aβ including increasing Aβ clearance across the blood-brain barrier (i.e., from the brain to periphery) by increasing Aβ transport protein levels for cellular expulsion. Endocannabinoids, via the CB1 receptor, may activate PPARγ receptors which stimulate expression of the Aβ transport protein [22].

## Human Studies: Evidence of ECS Involvement in Alzheimer's Disease

There have been several postmortem studies examining the brains of people who had AD in comparison with brains of those without AD (see Berry et al. [100]). In one such study, a reduction in CB1 expression was found in the PFC of AD patient brains (Brodmann 10 area), but these did not correlate with any AD molecular marker or cognitive impairment (though it did correlate with hypophagia) [111]. However, in these AD patient brains, the level of CB2 receptors was significantly (40%) higher than controls, and levels of CB2 receptors correlated with two AD markers, $A\beta_{42}$ and senile plaque score (though not cognitive status). They also found increased expression of the glial marker, glial fibrillar acidic protein, in AD patient brains [111]. Yet not all studies have found changes in CB1 receptors associated with AD. Postmortem examination of brains of AD sufferers conducted by one group did not find changes in CB1 receptor density which was not altered within the vicinity of senile plaques [53].

Other postmortem studies have found CB2 receptors and FAAH are overexpressed in cells associated with Aβ-neuritic plaques and FAAH activity is increased in and around $A\beta_{42}$ plaques [22]. The first study to demonstrate the presence of CB2 receptors in the human CNS, published in 2003, was a study comparing AD brains and normal healthy brains [53]. They found that CB2 receptors were selectively upregulated in microglia associated with neuritic plaques in brains of people with AD (though CB1 receptor density was not altered within the vicinity of these senile plaques) and that FAAH protein and activity were upregulated in reactive astrocytes but not in microglia [53].

### Positron-Emission Tomography Studies in Humans

A study which used positron-emission tomography to assess CB1 receptor density in AD patients did not find any difference in CB1 receptor availability between AD patients and healthy normal people. There was no correlation between CB1 receptor availability and neuropsychological test scores, and CB1 receptor availability was not modulated by ApoE genotype. No correlation was found between Aβ plaque deposition and CB1 receptors in those with AD either [112]. As explained by Bedse and colleagues, despite a lack of change in CB1 receptors, it may be the coupling between the CB1 receptor and Gi protein that might underlie reduced CB1 receptor signaling, and indeed CB1 activity appears to change with the stage of AD, with higher activity in some hippocampal regions and internal layers of the frontal cortex in early AD stages and decreased CB1 activity found in later stages. The increase in CB1 receptor activity in early AD might reflect a neuroprotective action in response to early neuronal damage [22].

## Medicinal Cannabis for Treatment of Alzheimer's Disease

There is evidence to indicate that several of the components of medicinal cannabis such as cannabidiol (CBD) may address the underlying pathophysiology of AD [33]. Medicinal cannabis also has the potential to alleviate many of the neuropsychiatric or behavioral symptoms/signs associated with AD including anxiety, depression, psychosis, agitation, aggressive behavior, insomnia, restlessness, memory decline, and pain.

There is a US patent on cannabinoids (this includes CBD, THC from the plant, and synthetic analogues and metabolites) by researchers in the US Government Department of Health and Human Services in relation to their role as antioxidants and neuroprotectants which lists Alzheimer's disease among many others in relation (*US Patent No. 6630507 B1: Cannabinoids as Antioxidants and Neuroprotectants, 7 October 2003*).

In this section, we will firstly look at evidence of efficacy of synthetic cannabinoid agonists in the treatment of AD, and then look at how various constituents of cannabis might address the neuropsychiatric symptoms/signs of AD. We will explore potential mechanisms of action of CBD and THC in the treatment of AD, and preclinical and clinical evidence of efficacy of key cannabinoids. Finally, we shall discuss the scientific evidence that indicates potential roles for terpenes, oleamide, N-Palmitoylethanolamide and Omega 3 polyunsaturated fatty acids in addressing the pathophysiology of AD.

### Synthetic Cannabinoid Agonists in Treatment of Alzheimer's Disease

It's worth noting that there have been many animal studies investigating the potential neuroprotective properties of synthetic CB1 and CB2 agonists in AD [113]. Studies of synthetic agonists of cannabinoid receptors in animal models of AD are perhaps largely driven by a pharmaceutical model which seeks to find a patentable, efficacious compound. Findings of such studies can only be directly applicable to those studied synthetic compounds, but nonetheless they provide some indirect evidence as to how some of the phytocannabinoids might be working too (given that THC is a partial agonist of cannabinoid receptors).

For example:

- In Aβ-injected rats and mice, CB1 agonists, CB2 agonists, and CB1/CB2 receptor agonists have been found to prevent memory deficits via neuroprotective actions [113–117].
- Chronic treatment with WIN55,212-2 (synthetic CB1/CB2 receptor agonist) in a transgenic mouse model of brain amyloidosis prevented neuroinflammation, lowered β-amyloid levels, reduced COX-2 and TNF-α mRNA expression (both of which were raised), and improved cognitive performance [118].

However, the effect of CB1 agonists is not always positive, and it is possible that CB1 agonists may worsen AD by inhibiting acetylcholine release within the brain [22, 119].

Activation of CB2 receptors has been shown to reduce microglia activity and production of inflammatory cytokines, and in an animal model of AD, a CB2 agonist was found to induce Aβ clearance [22, 104]. In another genetic transgenic mice model of AD, a specific CB2 receptor agonist (JWH-133) improved cognition, and the effect was stronger when administered at the presymptomatic stage compared with early symptomatic stage. Improved cognition was associated with reduced microglial reactivity and reduced levels of proinflammatory cytokines (IL-1β, IL-6, TNF-α, and IFN-γ). CB2 agonist treatment was also associated with reduced expression of active p38 and SAPK/JNK and reduced tau hyperphosphorylation near the amyloid-β plaques. However, chronic treatment did not alter the Aβ production or deposition in the cortex and hippocampus. The authors concluded that their results support the idea that stimulation of CB2 receptors ameliorates several parameters associated with AD including neuroinflammation, oxidative stress damage and responses, tau hyperphosphorylation around plaques, and impairment in memory and learning [110]. This study also indicates that the initiation of earlier treatment may be more efficacious.

For a summary of the research into the efficacy of synthetic CB1 and CB2 receptor agonists in animal models of AD, see Aso and Ferrer [113].

## Cannabis Constituents and Target Symptom Treatment

Table 9.1 sets out potentially beneficial components of cannabis for various target symptoms of AD based on pharmacology [4, 120].

## Mechanisms of Action of CBD in Alzheimer's Disease

There are several potential mechanisms of action by which CBD might address the pathological changes associated with AD, as well as addressing some of the

**Table 9.1** Cannabis constituents and potential target symptoms of Alzheimer's disease[a]

| Neuropsychiatric symptom | Component of cannabis |
|---|---|
| Agitation | CBD, THC, linalool |
| Aggression | CBD, THC, linalool |
| Anxiety | CBD, THC (low dose), linalool |
| Depression | CBD, THC, limonene |
| Psychosis | CBD |
| Insomnia/restlessness | THC, linalool |
| Pain | THC, CBD |
| Memory | Alpha pinene + THC |
| Anorexia | THC |
| Neuroprotection | CBD, THC |
| Reduced Aβ plaque formation | CBD, THC, THCA |

[a]Based on pharmacology [4, 120]

**Table 9.2** Potential mechanisms of action of CBD in Alzheimer's disease

| Action | References |
|---|---|
| Protecting against neuroinflammation and oxidative stress, increasing cell survival, and decreasing ROS production and lipid peroxidation | Mukhopadhyay et al. [121]; Iuvone et al. [97] |
| Regulating microglial cell migration | Walter et al. [122] |
| Decreasing microglial activation and reducing reactive gliosis | Martin-Moreno et al. [116]; Esposito et al. [123] |
| Protecting against calcium-induced protein misfolding; regulating proteostasis | Dash et al. [33] |
| Reducing Aβ production by inducing APP ubiquitination | Scuderi et al. [124] |
| Preventing expression of proteins potentially involved in Aβ production and tau phosphorylation in mesenchymal stem cell; downregulating genes linked to AD including genes coding for kinases responsible of tau phosphorylation and for secretases involved in Aβ generation | Libro et al. [125] |
| Inhibiting tau hyperphosphorylation in neuronal cells | Esposito et al. [126] |
| Protecting against Aβ-mediated neurotoxicity and microglial-activated neurotoxicity | Janefjord et al. [104] |
| Inhibiting cell death, inducing degradation, and removal of preformed Aβ aggregation | Schubert et al. [127] |
| Reducing Aβ-induced neuroinflammatory response by decreasing expression of proinflammatory gene and proinflammatory mediators | Esposito et al. [128] |
| Antioxidant activity (potent lipophilic antioxidant) | Marsicano et al. [107]; Kim et al. [129] |
| Reducing apoptosis and therefore improving cell survival; improving cell viability | Scuderi et al. [124]; Harvey et al. [103] |
| Preventing cortical and hippocampal neurodegeneration | Hamelink et al. [130] |
| Preventing neurite degeneration induced by $A\beta_{1-42}$ in human SH-SY5Y neuronal cells and regulating CB1-pSTAT3 signaling for neurite outgrowth | Wang et al. [131] |
| Promoting neurogenesis and facilitating synaptic plasticity | Campos et al. [132]; Esposito et al. [123]; Campos et al. [133] |
| Improving cognition | Farr et al. [134] |
| Improving memory | Coles [135]; Cheng et al. [136]; Cheng et al. [137] |
| Attenuates ceramide synthesis, stimulates sphingosine-1-phosphate (a major regulator of vascular and immune systems) | Bielawiec et al. [138] |

Watt and Karl [139], Dash et al. [33]

neuropsychiatric symptoms and signs, gleaned from in vitro and in vivo studies. These are set out in Table 9.2 (summarized from Watt and Karl [139] in particular and Dash et al. [33]).

### CBD Is Protective Against Neuroinflammation and Oxidative Stress

CBD has been found to be protective against neuroinflammation in several few ways which may be relevant to AD. There is evidence that CBD can reduce neuroinflammation by reducing oxidative stress and producing anti-inflammatory substances and regulating proinflammatory responses [33, 140, 141]. Oxidative stress is involved in the pathogenesis of many different neurological disorders, not just AD, including Parkinson's disease, Huntington's disease, and amyotrophic lateral sclerosis [129].

In one study in glia, under lipopolysaccharide stimulation, CBD inhibited the release of TNF-α and IL-1β (proinflammatory cytokines) and glutamate (a non-cytokine inflammation mediator), and these effects of CBD were mostly receptor-independent (only slightly blunted by CB2 receptor blockade). CBD inhibited a mechanism involving NADPH oxidase-mediated ROS production and NF-κB-dependent signaling events. CBD was also found to prevent the increased glucose uptake in microglial cells challenged with LPS, and this ability to prevent glucose uptake contributed to its anti-inflammatory actions. CBD reduced glucose-derived NAPDH, which is a cofactor necessary for NADPH oxidase activation and generation of ROS. The authors concluded that these findings suggest CBD's anti-inflammatory actions toward microglia are mediated via an intrinsic antioxidant effect and this effect is increased through inhibition of glucose-dependent NADPH synthesis [141].

Another potential mechanism by which CBD may help reduce neuroinflammation is by its action in blocking the orphan G-protein receptor 55 (GPR55). CBD antagonizes GPR55 [142]. GPR55 is expressed in microglial cells and plays a role in different aspects of neuroinflammation, reported in different models [48]. GPR55 appears to be involved in the arachidonic acid (AA) cascade in activated microglia. A study which used a synthetic GPR55 antagonist found that in rat microglia, it reduced neuroinflammatory parameters by inhibiting the prostaglandin E2 (PGE2)/cyclooxygenase-2 pathway [48]. Although this study was in a novel GPR55 receptor antagonist KIT 10, we do know that CBD can block GPR55. Further research may elucidate whether CBD might act via a similar mechanism of action.

In a very recent study, CBD was shown to have neuroprotective effects in vitro in rat pup hippocampal neurons, protecting them against the oxidative stress of hydrogen peroxide. Hydrogen peroxide is a trigger for oxidative stress-induced apoptosis [129]. This is important research because of the crucial role of hippocampal neurons in regulating cognition, normal behavior, and epilepsy as well as dysfunctional behavior [143]. Previous research has demonstrated its cytoprotective effects against cerebellar granular cells and oligodendrocyte progenitor cells [107, 144], but this study is the first in neurons more relevant to brain functioning and behavioral implications [129].

CBD was demonstrated to have higher neuroprotective efficacy than vitamin E and vitamin C in a glutamate neurotoxicity model [145]. CBD was found to be protective against Aβ-induced neurotoxicity, reducing the death of neuron-like pheochromocytoma PC12 cells (in rats) against Aβ plaques from 39% to 12%, as well as decreasing ROS, lipid peroxidation, intracellular calcium, DNA fragmentation, and caspase-3 levels (caspase-3 is a key enzyme in the apoptosis cell-signaling cascade) [97].

CBD has been found to reduce many different inflammatory cytokines including IL-1β, IFN-β, TNF-α, IFN-γ, IL-6, IL-17, NO, and COX-2 by activating PPAR-γ while increasing IL-4 and IL-10 (anti-inflammatory cytokines [33, 146]. CBD can

**Table 9.3** Neuroprotective mechanisms of action of CBD

| Action | References |
|---|---|
| Activates peroxisome proliferator-activated receptor gamma (PPAR-γ) which represses NF-κB signaling[a] | Necela et al. [148] |
| Reduces several different proinflammatory cytokines (IL-1β, IFN-β, TNF-α, INF-γ, IK-6, IL-17, COX-2) via activation of PPAR-γ as well as increase anti-inflammatory cytokines IL-4 and IL-10 and decrease iNOS expression | Rajan et al. [146]; Kozela et al. [149] |
| Suppresses the immune system response: improves the innate and adaptive immune responses | Lee et al. [147] |
| Suppresses microglial cell activation by regulating Th17 proliferation and STAT1/STAYT3 balance | Juknat et al. [150] |
| Upregulates of CD4+ and CD25- T cells | Kozela et al. [149] |
| Inhibits Aβ-induced tau protein hyperphosphorylation (through Wnt/β--catenin pathway) | Esposito et al. [126] |
| Inhibits p38 phosphorylation which reduces neurotoxic effects associated with uncontrolled immune reactions | Esposito et al. [151] |
| Inhibits inducible nitric oxide synthase protein expression and nitric oxide production in β-amyloid-stimulated PC12 neurons through p38MAP kinase and NF-κB involvement | Esposito et al. [151] |
| Upregulates brain-derived neurotropic factor (BDNF)[b] which has been found to correlate with anti-inflammatory actions of CBD (evidenced by decreased TNF-α and IL-6 levels in the prefrontal cortex and hippocampus) | Campos et al. [152] |
| Has potent lipophilic antioxidant activity | Marsicano et al. [107]; Kim et al. [129] |
| Blocks Aβ-induced neurite degeneration through a CB1-mediated mechanism, regulating the CB1-pSTAT3 signaling for neurite outgrowth | Wang et al. [131] |

[a]NF-κB plays a key role in promoting the inflammatory cascade by upregulating cytokines in activated astrocytes and microglia [153]

[b]BDNF has a key role in neuronal development, neuronal survival, synaptic plasticity, and cognitive function [33]

enhance innate and adaptive immune responses in chronic inflammation, demonstrated in an animal study [147]. CBD can also inhibit the ROS-NF-κB pathway, and thereby lower glucose uptake in microglia (which is required for their activation) [141]. In addition, several GPCRs (e.g., CB1R, CB2R, GPR18, GPR55, and others) are modulated by CBD (see Dash et al. [33]).

CBD's neuroprotective actions against neuroinflammation are many, and several are included in Table 9.3 (summarized in the main from Dash et al. [33]).

### CBD, Regulation of Proteostasis, and Induction of Autophagy

As explained earlier, proteostasis is the homeostasis network that regulates the cellular proteome (the set of proteins expressed by the cell). Clearance systems become activated via signaling pathways which respond to misfolded protein and protein aggregations, and aggregates are degraded proteolytically via the ubiquitin-proteasome system (UPS; a target-specific system within the nucleus and cytoplasm) and autophagy (a nonselective system within the cytoplasm). CBD has been shown to induce autophagy in several studies, via regulating different pathways including inhibiting AKT and mTOR and downregulating the JNK MAPK pathway and promoting neuroprotection by inhibiting JNK and p38 MAP kinases [33]. CBD modulation of mTOR depends on cell type and cell state [154]. In a model of Parkinson's disease, CBD promoted ERK activation with interactions of CB2 receptors and TRPV1 leading to enhanced autophagy [64].

As explained by Dash and colleagues [33], calcium ion balance is important in ensuring correct protein formation. An imbalance of Ca2+ disrupts protein conformation, with excessive intracellular Ca2+ inducing oxidative stress, leading to protein aggregation and ultimately cell death. ROS or reactive nitric species (RNS) can modify misfolded proteins and make them more oxidized and prone to aggregation, and aggregated forms inhibit the proteosomal system, resulting in increased accumulation of aggregated protein. Interaction of protein aggregates with particular receptors can lead to upregulated NMDA receptors (ionotropic glutamate receptors involved in Ca2+, Na + , and K regulation within the cytoplasm) and thereby excess Ca2+ influx and subsequent neuronal apoptosis. In addition, due to ongoing hyperpolarization and activation of NMDA receptors, G-protein-coupled receptors (GPCRs) and voltage-gated calcium channels (VGCC) increase Ca2+ influx (implicated in neurodegeneration), and excess Ca2+ adversely affects calcineurin and CaMKII pathways which have been found to lead to memory deficits and depression in AD [33].

CBD can protect against calcium-induced protein misfolding through several mechanisms that impact calcium dynamics at synapses. These include acting as an antagonist to block excitatory glutamate release, indirectly regulating glutamate secretion by 5-HT1A receptors, inhibiting the interaction between σ1R and NMDAR (opposite effect of NMDAR overactivity), and acting as a TRPV1 agonist and VGCC antagonist to regulate intracellular calcium levels (see Dash et al. [33]).

### CBD Prevents Tau Hyperphosphorylation

CBD was also found to reduce tau hyperphosphorylation in Aβ-stimulated neuronal cells, via the Wnt/β-catenin pathway—Wnt activation inhibits tau protein kinase (GSK-3β) which causes the tau hyperphosphorylation and neurofibrillary tangles in AD [22, 126].

### CBD Prevents Neurite Degeneration Induced by Aβ

In very recent research, CBD was shown to prevent neurite lesions induced by $A\beta_{1-42}$ in human SH-SY5Y cells, and also increase FAAH and CB1 receptor expression. In hippocampal neurons, CBD was found to protect against reduction of dendritic spine density and rescue the activity of synaptic Ca2+/calmodulin-dependent protein kinase II from $A\beta_{1-42}$ toxicity. A substudy in a particular strain of the worm *C. elegans* which is bred to overexpress Aβ, CBD was found to block Aβ-induced neurite degeneration through a CB1-mediated mechanism, regulating the CB1-pSTAT3 signaling for neurite outgrowth, thereby increasing the health and lifespan in these worms [131]. Such research again demonstrates the neuroprotective action of CBD.

## Mechanisms of Action of THC in Alzheimer's Disease

Numerous lines of evidence indicate that THC may be a therapeutic treatment strategy for AD with several functions and acting through several pathways [155]. THC has been found to have several actions relevant to AD pathogenesis including the following, set out in Table 9.4.

It is worth noting a key finding from the last study in Table 9.4 [157]: THC dosing in adult rats, where low doses were used, was associated with *increased* cognitive functioning, contrary to other studies that found THC to be associated with cognitive impairment [157, 159]. It is known that the CB1 receptor is involved in adult neurogenesis as well as cognitive functions and that both CB1 and CB2 receptors modulate brain plasticity [157, 159]. Given that THC is a partial agonist at CB1 and CB2 receptors, and low doses of THC were used, this may help explain this seemingly beneficial action. We know from previous chapters that the effects of THC can differ depending on dose (e.g., anxiolytic at low doses but anxiogenic at higher doses).

If you recall in Chap. 4, we also learned of an experiment in mice in which THC was found to restore hippocampal gene transcription patterns such that the expression profiles of 12-month-old mice treated with THC were similar to mice aged

**Table 9.4** Mechanisms of action of THC on AD pathophysiology

| Action | References |
|---|---|
| Significantly reducing fibril and aggregate formation | Janefjord et al. [104] |
| Lowering Aβ levels in vitro at very low concentrations, directly interacting with Aβ peptide and inhibiting aggregation | Cao et al. [155] |
| Lowering GSK-3β levels (tau protein kinase, responsible for tau hyperphosphorylation) and phosphorylated GSK-3β in a dose-dependent manner at low concentrations | Cao et al. [155] |
| Low doses of THC enhanced mitochondria function and did not inhibit melatonin's enhancement of mitochondrial function. No toxicity was found and CB1 receptors were not upregulated | Cao et al. [155] |
| Competitively inhibiting acetylcholinesterase (AChE) and preventing AChE-induced Aβ peptide aggregation by binding to the peripheral anionic site of AChE (critical region involved in amyloid genesis). THC was found to be superior to current AD drugs in inhibiting Aβ aggregation | Eubanks et al. [156] |
| Low doses of THC administered intraperitoneally induce adult neurogenesis in the hippocampus (evidenced by several markers including nestin), and this was associated with improved cognitive performance in rats. Improvements in learning and memory functions were accompanied by upregulation of plasticity markers, doublecortin (DCX) and BDNF | Suliman et al. [157] |
| Has been shown to be a potent lipophilic antioxidant (and oxidative stress is a major part of the pathogenesis of AD) | Marsicano et al. [107] |
| Chronic low-dose THC reversed age-related decline in cognitive function in mice aged 12 and 18 months | Bilkei-Gorzo et al. [158] |

2 months (not treated with THC). Transcripts which were upregulated included transthyretin (gene believed to be protective against AD), BDNF (enhances synapse formation and cognitive functions), and Klotho (Kl) (which extends lifespan in different species and improves cognition). Transcripts which were downregulated after THC treatment were genes associated with aging: caspase-1 (involved in age-related impairments in cognition) and connective tissue growth factor (Ctgf) (which enhances the pro-apoptotic activity of transforming growth factor-β [158].

## Preclinical Evidence of Efficacy of Cannabinoids in Treating AD

Animal studies indicate that CBD and combinations of CBD and THC may be useful in treatment of some of the symptoms/signs associated with AD.

### Cannabidiol

A small number of animal studies have shown CBD may be useful in addressing some of the neuropsychiatric symptoms associated with AD. For example, mice studies have demonstrated CBD can prevent social recognition memory deficits [136], improve social recognition and object recognition [137], and reduce anxiety [160].

- Long-term (8 months) treatment of transgenic mice bred to express signs and symptoms of AD with CBD at a dose of 20 mg/kg from 2.5 months of age prevented the social recognition deficit that develops in such mice, though there was no impact on anxiety or associative learning. The prevention of social recognition defect by CBD was not associated with any changes in amyloid load or oxidative damage; however, there were some subtle changes in neuroinflammation found [136].
- In a transgenic mouse model of AD, chronic treatment with CBD (20 mg/kg for 3 weeks via intraperitoneal injection) was found to reverse cognitive impairment (deficits in social recognition, novel object recognition) suggesting promise as a therapy for specific cognitive impairments in AD [137].

### Efficacy of CBD and THC Combinations in Treating Alzheimer's Disease

There is a growing body of evidence investigating the combination of CBD and THC for neurodegenerative diseases [161–164], and results look promising.

Research that compares CBD or THC alone with the combination of CBD and THC helps tease out whether there is an added advantage of combining the two. At least one study has done so in a mice model of AD [162]. In this study, using a transgenic AD mice model, several benefits of the combination of CBD and THC above the single cannabinoids were found. All three preserved memory when chronically administered during the early symptomatic stage in this mice AD model, and the combination reduced learning impairment. They also found a significant reduction in soluble Aβ42 peptide levels and changes in plaque composition in the combination (CBD plus THC) treatment mice (Aβ42 peptide is thought to be the most toxic form of the Aβ peptide). The redox protein thioredoxin 2 and the signaling protein Wnt16 were found to be important substrates for the effects associated with the combination of CBD plus THC. Treated mice had reduced microgliosis and astrogliosis and inflammatory molecules, and this effect was greater with the combination of CBD and THC compared with either cannabinoid alone [162]. This led the study authors to conclude that the combination of CBD and THC had a better therapeutic profile than either alone [162].

That previous experiment used a model of early-stage AD [162]. In another experiment, this time in a transgenic mouse model of *late* AD, botanical phytocannabinoid extracts of a combination of CBD and THC were still effective in reducing memory impairment but were not effective in modifying the Aβ processing or reducing the glial reactivity associated with the Aβ deposition (unlike in the previous model of early-stage AD). The study also found that natural phytocannabinoids did not affect cognitive impairment associated in healthy aging in normal (wild-type) mice. The mechanism of action of the combination of CBD and THC in the aged mice involved reductions in GluR2/3 levels and increased GABA-A Rα1 levels [163]. These two experiments suggest that early intervention with phytocannabinoids is going to be better than intervention when the disease process is well underway; however, treatment in this late-stage AD model still showed a positive effect on memory.

Other animal studies in neuroinflammatory disease models of multiple sclerosis have shown that THC combined with CBD could suppress mi-RNA-mediated neuroinflammation, reduce CD4+ T cell proliferation, reduce several proinflammatory cytokines (e.g., IL-6, IL-17, TNF-α, and several others), and enhance several anti-inflammatory chemicals (including IL-4, IL-10, TGF-β, and others) [161, 164]. In a mouse model of MS (experimental autoimmune encephalomyelitis), the combination of THC and CBD reduced neuroinflammation, and led to changes in the gut microbiome and the metabolome, and what was interesting was that fecal transfer of THC plus CBD-altered microbiome reduced the experimental autoimmune encephalomyelitis disease severity [161].

Research into Sativex (almost 1:1 ratio of CBD to THC) tested in a "parkin-null, human tau-overexpressing" mouse model of complex frontotemporal dementia, Parkinsonism, and lower motor neuron disease found that Sativex was able to attenuate the neurological deficits and abnormal behaviors of the mice. In these specially bred mice, compared with a placebo treatment, Sativex reduced abnormal behavior related to stress, reduced aggression, reduced intraneuronal MAO-related free radicals produced during dopamine metabolism in the limbic system, decreased gliosis in the hippocampus and cortex, increased the ratio of reduced to oxidized glutathione in the limbic system, decreased inducible NOS levels, and increased complex IV levels in the cerebral cortex, as well as decreasing deposition of amyloid and tau in the hippocampus and cerebral cortex and increasing autophagy [165].

Thus, you can see that there is a growing bank of evidence that the combination of CBD and THC may be valuable. We would add that it will be important to assess full-spectrum CBD/THC combinations that include other plant nutrients (not just THC isolates plus CBD isolates).

## Clinical Evidence of Efficacy of Cannabinoids in Treatment of Alzheimer's Disease

### Cannabidiol for Treatment of AD

There is a lack of human studies investigating the efficacy of full-spectrum CBD-only (i.e., very low THC) in the treatment of AD, despite all the promising preclinical evidence that it addresses many of the pathways involved in its pathogenesis.

Although only in healthy patients, a recent study demonstrated that CBD may increase cerebral blood flow in the hippocampus. In a randomized crossover, double-blind study, 15 healthy people were administered 600 mg oral CBD (or placebo), and regional cerebral blood flow was measured 3 h after ingestion. The study also assessed working memory and episodic memory. The study found that CBD increased cerebral blood flow in the hippocampus (this was statistically significant). There were no differences between CBD and placebo in terms of memory task performance, but there was a greater CBD-induced increase in orbitofrontal cerebral blood flow which was significantly correlated with reduced reaction time in one of the tasks (two-back working memory task). Overall, the study indicates that CBD increases cerebral blood flow to key brain regions involved in memory, in particular the hippocampus, and this may well be relevant to diseases such as AD [166]. This study needs to be repeated in AD patients in the future.

### Tetrahydrocannabinol for Treatment of Dementia Including AD

The clinical research into THC is much greater than for CBD, and much of this relates to synthetic THC for obvious reasons (money). Several clinical studies support the contention that THC may have a promising role to play in the management of many of the neuropsychiatric symptoms and signs associated with dementia.

Table 9.5 sets out several of the studies that have examined the efficacy of THC, with most of these studies in synthetic forms of THC (e.g., dronabinol, Namisol, nabilone) and only one in a plant-based oil [170]. Many of these studies include patients with Alzheimer's disease as well as vascular dementia or mixed forms of dementia.

From these studies we can see evidence of efficacy in treatment of several symptoms or signs listed below:

- Overall functioning
- Agitation
- Aggressive and disturbed behavior
- Irritability
- Sleep
- Nocturnal motor activity
- Appetite disturbances
- Body weight
- Rigidity
- Delusions
- Apathy
- Caregiver distress

See Table 9.5 for details. Not all studies found positive results, for example, Van den Elsen et al. [168] and Van den Elsen et al. [169].

## Combinations of Cannabidiol and Tetrahydrocannabinol for Treatment of AD

There are a few clinical trials underway investigating combinations of CBD and THC on dementia (e.g., Timler et al. [174]) and one published study to date (Broers et al. [173], set out in Table 9.5). This small study in ten women with severe dementia and behavioral problems found significant improvements in behavior and rigidity (the latter making daily care and transfers much easier for staff), with study results indicating the combination of CBD and THC was well tolerated (over half the patients were able to decrease or stop other psychotropic medications) [173].

Anecdotal evidence comes from observations of experienced cannabis clinician Dr. Jeff Hergenrather MD of dementia patients living in a California nursing home, where patients were treated with several types of cannabis products (THC predominant, CBD predominant, and THCA, mostly as tinctures or confections). The treating doctors found the following benefits: decreased agitation, increased appetite,

**Table 9.5** Clinical studies of efficacy of THC in alleviating neuropsychiatric symptoms of dementia

| Reference | Study type, participants, medication | Outcome variables | Results |
|---|---|---|---|
| Herrmann et al. [31] | **Study type:** 14-week RCT double-blind crossover trial, 6 weeks each with 1-week washout period between<br>**Participants**: *n* = 39 patients with moderate-severe **Alzheimer's disease**, mean age 87 +/− 10 years, 77% male<br>**Study medications**: Nabilone dose 1.6 mg +/− 0.5 mg, placebo<br>No. of concomitant medications 12 +/− 5; no. of concomitant psychotropic medications 1.8 +/− 0.7 | **Primary**: **agitation** (Cohen-Mansfield Agitation Inventory [CMAI])<br>Secondary: NPI-NH total, NPI-NH caregiver distress, cognition (sMMSE & Severe Impairment Battery [SIB] or Alzheimer's Disease Assessment Scale of Cognition [CGIC]) & adverse events | Significant improvement in agitation measured by CMAI<br>Significant improvement in NPI-NH total, NPI-NH caregiver distress, sMMSE<br>But in those who completed the SIB (*n* = 25), treatment differences were significant and favored placebo; no significant difference between nabilone & placebo for CGIC<br>More sedation with nabilone (45%) compared with placebo (16%) phases but treatment-limiting sedation was not statistically significant<br>Occurrence of adverse effects was significantly greater during nabilone phase, with sedation the most common (*n* = 17 compared with *n* = 6 for placebo). Sedation improved in 12 when dose of nabilone was reduced<br>**Conclusion**: nabilone may be effective for agitation, but sedation & cognition should be monitored closely |

(continued)

**Table 9.5** (continued)

| Reference | Study type, participants, medication | Outcome variables | Results |
|---|---|---|---|
| Woodward et al. [30] | **Study type**: Retrospective systematic chart review<br>**Participants**: 40 inpatients diagnosed with **dementia** and treated with dronabinol for behavioral or appetite disturbances; 28 women & 12 men; 13 with Alzheimer's disease, 7 with vascular dementia, 15 with mixed etiology dementia, 1 with frontotemporal dementia, 4 with dementia not otherwise specified. Aggression, agitation, and poor appetite were the most common target symptoms. Mean age: not reported<br>**Study medication**: dronabinol as adjunct to current medication (average 3.25 concurrent psychoactive medications prior to augmentation with dronabinol); mean dose 7.03 mg/day; mean duration of dronabinol treatment 16.88 days (range 4–50 days) | Group of psychiatrists consulted medical records to rate patients' behaviors prior to initiation of dronabinol and following up to 7 days of treatment<br>**Outcome variables**: Pittsburgh Agitation Scale (PAS), Clinical Global Impression (CGI), Global Assessment of Functioning | Significant decreases in all domains of Pittsburgh Agitation Scale (PAS)<br>Significant improvements in CGI scores, trend toward improved sleep duration (mean 6.47 h/night before compared with 6.79 h/night during treatment, $p = 0.0596$, though no change in no. awakenings/ night) and significant increase in % meals consumed during treatment<br>26 adverse events reported during treatment, none of which required discontinuation of dronabinol: sedation ($n = 9$), delirium ($n = 4$), urinary tract infection ($n = 3$), confusion ($n = 2$) though relationship to dronabinol could not be assessed<br>**Conclusion**: dronabinol can serve as an adjunct treatment for neuropsychiatric symptoms in dementia |
| Van den Elsen et al. [167] | **Study type**: randomized, double-blind, crossover study<br>**Study participants**: $n = 18$ community-dwelling patients (mean age 77 years); 15 AD, 1 vascular, 2 mixed type dementia<br>**Study medication**: 1.5 mg dronabinol twice daily versus placebo; each phase 3 days followed by a 4-day washout period; use of concurrent psychotropic and some other medications allowed (but not opioids, tricyclic antidepressants) | Balance and gait assessed using: SwayStar and GAITRite within 2 h of administration under conditions of standing with eyes open and eyes closed, preferred speed walking with and without a cognitive dual task | THC significantly increased sway during eyes closed but not during eyes open. THC significantly increased stride length and trunk sway during preferred speed walking; no effects observed during dual task walking. No differences in no. and type of adverse events and no falls occurred during THC administration<br>**Conclusion**: 3 mg/day THC has a benign adverse event profile regarding mobility and was well tolerated |

**Table 9.5** (continued)

| Reference | Study type, participants, medication | Outcome variables | Results |
|---|---|---|---|
| Van den Elsen [168] | **Study type**: randomized, double-blind, placebo-controlled trial<br>**Study participants**: *n* = 50 patients with AD, vascular dementia, mixed dementia<br>**Study medication**: 1.5 mg Namisol (pure THC) orally or matched placebo 3 times daily for 3 weeks; *n* = 24 THC, *n* = 26 placebo<br>Patients also received 1000 mg acetaminophen 3 times daily in case of pain complaints (or suspected pain in noncommunicative patients); use of concurrent psychotropic medication was allowed | **Primary outcome variable**: Neuropsychiatric Inventory (NPI) assessed at baseline, 14 days, and 21 days<br>**Others**: agitation (Cohen-Mansfield Agitation Inventory), quality of life (Quality of Life-Alzheimer's Disease), activities of daily living (Barthel Index) | NPS score reduced in both treatment groups; no significant difference in reduction from baseline between groups<br>No significant difference between groups in changes in scores for agitation, quality of life, or activities of daily living<br>Similar no. participants experiencing adverse events in each group; no effects on vital signs, weight, or episodic memory observed<br>**Conclusion**: oral THC at 4.5 mg/day showed no benefit in terms of NPS but was well tolerated |
| Van den Elsen [169] | **Study type**: Randomized, double-blind, placebo-controlled, repeated crossover trial, consisting of six treatment blocks of 2 weeks each<br>**Study participants**: 22 patients (15 men, mean age 76.4 +/− 5.3 years with dementia (18 AD, 1 vascular dementia, 3 mixed type)<br>**Study medications**: 0.75 and 1.5 mg THC in tablet form (Namisol) twice daily | **Primary outcome variable**: change in Neuropsychiatric Inventory (NPI) score<br>**Secondary variables**: Cohen-Mansfield Agitation Inventory (CMAI); Zarit Burden Interview (ZBI) (assessment caregiver burden) | No difference in change in NPI associated with THC compared with placebo. THC was well tolerated. No difference between treatment groups in incidence of adverse events. Four non-related serious adverse events occurred<br>**Conclusion**: oral THC up to 1.5 mg twice daily did not reduce behavioral disturbances in patients with dementia<br>Safety assessment (assessed using reports of adverse events, vital signs, and mobility) showed that the intervention was well tolerated by this patient group |

(continued)

**Table 9.5** (continued)

| Reference | Study type, participants, medication | Outcome variables | Results |
|---|---|---|---|
| Shelef et al. [170] | **Study type**: open-label prospective trial<br>**Study participants**: $n = 10$ patients, mean age 73.2 +/− 8.59 years (5 females, 5 males) with moderate-severe AD completed the study (1 dropped out from original 11 after 3 days)<br>**Study medication**: Medicinal cannabis oil containing THC as adjunct to pharmacotherapy, over 4 weeks; 2.5 mg THC twice daily (if no adverse events and no/minor improvement after 2 days then dose increased to 5 mg twice daily and after 2 more days to the max dose of 7.5 mg THC twice daily) Minimal dose of 2.5 mg was given to 7 participants during the study with 3 needing higher dose<br>$N = 8$ of the study participants were taking concurrent antipsychotic medications and 4 were taking anticholinesterase inhibitors.<br>Concurrent medication was allowed and was kept unchanged for at least 1 week pre-study | Neuropsychiatric Inventory Scale (NPI), Mini-Mental State Examination (MMSE) scale, Clinical Global Impression Improvement (CGI-I) scale, Clinician Global Impression Severity (CGI-S) scale | Significant reduction in CGI severity score (6.5–5.7, $p < 0.01$) and NPI score (44.4–12.8, $p < 0.01$). NPI domains which significantly decreased were delusions, agitation/aggression, irritability, apathy, sleep, and caregiver distress<br>One of the original 11 participants discontinued after 3 days due to dysphagia (probably not related to med cannabis oil); 1 participant became more confused with 5 mg/day bid—when dose decreased to 2.5 mg bid, confusion improved; another patient had recurrent falls prior to study admission and fell during the study, breaking his pelvis<br>**Conclusion**: Medicinal cannabis oil is safe to add to AD patients' pharmacotherapy |

**Table 9.5** (continued)

| Reference | Study type, participants, medication | Outcome variables | Results |
|---|---|---|---|
| Volicer et al. [171] | **Study type**: placebo-controlled double-blind, crossover trial, each treatment period lasted 6 weeks<br>**Study participants**: $n = 15$ patients with diagnosis of probable AD; final data analysis completed on $n = 11$; average age 72.7 +/− 4.9 years, 11 males and 1 female<br>**Study medication**: dronabinol 2.5 mg as capsule or identical placebo twice daily<br>Concurrent psychoactive medication was maintained during study | Body weight, BMI; Mini-Mental State Examination (MMSE), Katz Activity of Daily Living scale (Katz ADL), Bedford Alzheimer Nursing Scale-Severity (BANS-S) | Body weight of participants increased more during the dronabinol treatment compared with placebo phase<br>Dronabinol treatment was associated with decreased severity of disturbed behavior, and this effect persisted during the placebo period in those who received dronabinol first<br>Adverse reactions were more common in dronabinol phase and included euphoria, somnolence, and tiredness, but discontinuation was not necessary<br>3 patients discontinued the study (1 had grand mal seizure, 2 developed serious intercurrent infections). Another died of a heart attack during the study |
| Walther et al. [172] | **Study type**: open-label pilot study<br>**Study participants**: $n = 6$ patients, mean age 81.5 years (4 women, 2 men) with late-stage dementia (5 with AD, 1 with vascular dementia)<br>**Study medication**: dronabinol 2.5 mg daily for 2 weeks | **Primary outcome variable**: nocturnal motor activity as measured by actigraphy<br>Secondary variables: Neuropsychiatric Inventory (NPI) and NPI subscores for nighttime behaviors, delusions, hallucinations | Compared to baseline: dronabinol led to a significant reduction in nocturnal motor activity; NPI score improved significantly; NPI subscores for agitation, aberrant motor, and nighttime behaviors significantly improved<br>Appetite disturbances and irritability were significantly reduced, and there was a nonsignificant reduction in anxiety<br>**Conclusion**: dronabinol is able to reduce nocturnal motor activity and agitation in severely demented patients |

(continued)

**Table 9.5** (continued)

| Reference | Study type, participants, medication | Outcome variables | Results |
|---|---|---|---|
| Broers et al. [173] | **Study type**: prospective observational study **Study participants**: $n = 10$ female patients with dementia and severe behavioral problems, average age 79.5 years **Study medication**: oral medication combination **CBD/THC oil**; average 7.6 mg THC/13.2 mg CBD daily after 2 weeks; 8.8 mg THC/ 7.6 mg CBD after 1 month; 9.0 mg THC/18.0 mg CBD after 2 months | Neuropsychiatric Inventory (NPI), Cohen-Mansfield Agitation Inventory (CMAI) score, Unified Parkinson Disease Rating Scale (partic Item 22 degree of rigidity with passive movements), Barthel Index for daily activities, visual analogue scale (0–10) for most invalidating or disturbing behavior (determined by staff), VAS (0–10) for most invalidating daily activity (determined by staff) | Study started with cannabis tincture (containing alcohol), but 3 patients got mouth ulcers so swapped to cannabis oil given with a small piece of chocolate cake No patients stopped study medication due to side effects Average NPI score decreased by 40% (from 71.1 to 38.3) after 2 months; CMAI score decreased from 74.5 to 47.5, rigidity score (UPDRS) decreased from 3.4 to 1.7 (i.e., by 50%); scores for daily activities both decreased, but this was due to a decrease (less good functioning) in 2 patients, whereas 7 patients improved; VAS score for most invalidating behavior (screaming, aggressive behavior, tearing clothes) decreased from 9 to 5. Effects persisted after 2 months for the 4 persons for whom longer follow-up was available Nurses observed in nearly all patients less overall rigidity making washing and transfers easier. Two women with almost persistent screaming almost stopped doing so; one patient stopped frequent vomiting Half of the patients decreased or stopped their psychotropic medications; 2 patients were able to stop all morphine and 1 patient decreased by 2/3 in 2 months with the 3 patients having no more constipation. 1 patient decreased benzodiazepine use after 3 months and 1 patient stopped her antipsychotic medications after 1 month Feedback from family was very positive. **Conclusion**: oral THC/CBD cannabis oil in higher dosages than in other studies greatly improved behavior problems, rigidity, and daily care and was well tolerated in demented patients |

decreased aggression, improved sleep, better moods, less self-mutilation, better pain control, less need for neuroleptic drugs, and reduced nursing care demands [4] (Personal communication, J Hergenrather, December 2020).

## Systematic Reviews

A systematic review of the efficacy of cannabinoids for treatment of dementia [26] included five studies evaluating efficacy of cannabinoids for anorexia [171] and agitation in dementia [31, 168, 169, 175]. The systematic review reported that one study which focused specifically on use of dronabinol in treatment of anorexia in AD [171] found that dronabinol 5 mg/day for anorexia positively impacted on weight but sample size was small. Three studies of THC or dronabinol for treatment of agitation/aggression [168, 169, 175] found no significant differences from placebo, but a trial on nabilone (1–2 mg/day) did find an improvement in agitation compared with placebo [31]. The review noted that no studies were available that investigated use of cannabinoids to address cognitive symptoms associated with dementia. The systematic review also criticized the levels of evidence due to methodological issues and low sample sizes and concluded that nabilone might be useful for treatment of agitation associated with dementia but that there was no convincing evidence for THC [26].

Another systematic review of the efficacy of THC for treatment of neuropsychiatric symptoms of AD [5] included 12 studies, mostly of synthetic THC such as dronabinol and nabilone. The researchers concluded that while the efficacy of cannabinoids was not proven in robust RCTs, nonetheless observational studies were promising, in particular in the case of refractory symptoms associated with AD. Furthermore, the safety profile of cannabinoids was favorable with most adverse drug events reported in studies being mild [5].

## Take-Home Points

There are a few points of clinical interest in these studies. Firstly, the studies in Table 9.5 are mostly in pure, synthetic THC. Given the potential for CBD to mitigate some of the less desirable effects of THC, more studies are required to assess full-spectrum THC-dominant medicinal cannabis products (as well as products that might have different ratios of THC and CBD).

Secondly, most study participants in these studies were taking concurrent medications including psychoactive medications; THC was used concurrently. While some side effects occurred, overall, it seems that these were not particularly serious and that THC was relatively well tolerated.

Thirdly, in one study which began with using a medicinal cannabis tincture, three patients had pain on swallowing which was worse with the medicinal cannabis tincture and had mouth ulcers. They then swapped the study medication to a medicinal cannabis oil, and the ulcers disappeared, suggesting that perhaps the alcohol in the tincture might have caused the problem [173]. The take-home message from this study is that when patients with severe dementia can't speak or communicate, treating doctors need to be careful with the type of medicinal cannabis product used and check carefully for any change of behavior and investigate it.

Lastly, another point of interest in a few of the studies is the improvement in caregiver distress found [31, 170, 173]. As mentioned previously, the negative impact of dementia on those around the patient with dementia is substantial, and it is most important that their experience is taken into account.

It is remarkable that despite the relatively positive studies, very little synthetic THC is generally prescribed or used in skilled nursing facilities. This might be explained by several facts. In the USA these drugs are schedule III controlled substances, and a typical prescription at the current time is listed at $330 USD. The FDA-approved indications are for anorexia and nausea induced by chemotherapy. And, although physicians often prescribe outside of approved indications, the polarized cultural climate about cannabis could make physicians less willing to explore this use. Furthermore, few physicians have been educated about the endocannabinoid system or the application of phyto- or synthetic cannabinoids.

## Terpenes and Dementia

Much of the cannabis research in AD, not surprisingly, has revolved around CBD and THC. However, the role of the terpenes bears further thought, since many terpenes may help reduce some of the neurobehavioral symptoms associated with AD. For example, we know that linalool is calming and may assist with agitation, aggression, anxiety, and insomnia [4, 120].

### Beta-Caryophyllene

Beta-caryophyllene is one of the terpenes (though since it does bind with CB2 receptors, it might be more appropriately called a phytocannabinoid) with strong anti-inflammatory and antioxidant actions that could be therapeutically useful in treatment of AD. Oral beta-caryophyllene was found to prevent cognitive impairment in a particular transgenic APP/PS1 AD mice model, and this was associated with a reduction in β-amyloid in the hippocampus and cerebral cortex. Oral beta-caryophyllene was associated with reduced astrogliosis and microglial activation as well as decreased levels of COX-2 protein and mRNA levels of TNF-α and IL-β1 in the cerebral cortex of the mice. When a CB2 receptor antagonist or a PPARγ antagonist was applied, the protective effects were significantly reversed, demonstrating that the anti-inflammatory effects involve CB2 receptors and PPARγ pathways [176].

## PEA and Dementia

N-Palmitoylethanolamide (PEA) belongs to the class of N-acylethanolamine phospholipids and is part of the extended ECS. It is a lipid mediator synthesized in many plants and in cells and tissues of mammals, and has been isolated from several foods including soy lecithin, egg yolk, and peanut meal. PEA has analgesic and anti-inflammatory properties and shows promise in many different areas including pain, eczema, and neurodegenerative and neuroinflammatory diseases. It also shows promise in the treatment of AD [59].

## PEA and the Extended Endocannabinoid System

There are several mechanisms of action of PEA relevant to neuroinflammation and neurodegeneration and, therefore, potentially AD. In addition to acting as an autacoid local injury agonist downregulating mast cell activation, PEA can directly activate PPAR-α and GPR55, with PPAR-α appearing to be the main target receptor involved in the anti-neuroinflammatory actions of PEA. PEA has a weak affinity for the cannabinoid receptors; however, it may indirectly affect cannabinoid receptors by acting as a false substrate for FAAH, thereby leading to reduced AEA degradation (FAAH degrades AEA) and thus increased AEA levels. GPR55 can form receptor heteromers with either CB1 or CB2 receptors, which suggests that PEA might be able to influence CB1/CB2 signaling via targeting such heteromers. PEA can also indirectly activate the TRPV1 channel via several different mechanisms [59].

## Preclinical Studies of PEA in AD

Several in vitro studies have demonstrated that PEA can attenuate Aβ-induced astrocyte activation and reduce Aβ-induced neuroinflammation by decreasing proinflammatory molecules and cytokines (e.g., COX-2, IL-1B, TNF-α, PGE2, and others), and research suggests involvement of PPAR-α. PEA also appears to have antiangiogenic properties which may also be relevant in AD. PEA can counter some of the effects induced by Aβ in cortical cells and astrocytes (e.g., countering the reduction in cell viability, increase in glutamate levels) and reduce Aβ-induced astrocyte activation and improve neuronal survival [59].

There are other actions of PEA of potential value in dementia. PEA may also contribute to gene transcription, maintaining long-term anti-inflammatory effects, decreasing proinflammatory enzymes, and also increasing the synthesis of neurosteroids [177]. Neurosteroids are signaling molecules synthesized from cholesterol in the brain, converted into pregnenolone and then into all other endogenous steroids. Neurosteroids play a role in neural plasticity, learning and memory processes, stress, anxiety, and depression [178]. PEA may also protect the endothelium from oxidative and inflammatory injury, helping to enhance neurovascular unit perfusion and integrity [177].

Animal models of AD also indicate PEA shows promise in its treatment. Studies have shown PEA can reduce or prevent cognitive impairments induced in injection of a specific Aβ protein into mice; reduce brain lipid peroxidation, protein nitrosylation, iNOS induction, and caspase-3 activation; block the upregulation of inflammatory mediators (including iNOS, COX-2, IL-1β, and TNF-α); reduce astrocyte activation; and increase BDNF levels [59].

For a very good summary of the scientific evidence of PEA in AD, see Beggatio et al. [59].

### Human Studies of PEA in AD

There are no published clinical trials of PEA in the treatment of AD and its symptoms currently. There is one case report [177] which may be relevant, that of a 67-year-old woman with mild short-term memory impairment who was treated with high-dose PEALut (a product containing PEA and luteolin), for 9 months. Luteolin is a flavonoid with anti-inflammatory and antioxidant properties [177]. The patient's son and husband had noticed mild memory problems 2.5 years earlier with slow progression since then. The woman had a family history of AD (uncle, mother). At baseline, a brain MRI was normal; however, a brain single-photon emission computed tomography (SPECT) scan revealed bilateral hypoperfusion in several areas (parietal, inferior-temporal, and temporo-occipital). After 3 months of treatment, there was a nonsignificant improvement in cognitive function, and after 9 months there was a significant improvement in memory, as measured by a battery of validated tests, compared with baseline. Interestingly, at 9 months the brain SPECT was almost normal [177]. This was a case of mild cognitive impairment (MCI) and no diagnosis of AD was made; however, MCI is a risk factor for AD [177].

This case report did not report on any potential confounding factors that might have contributed to the cognitive improvement. All being equal, if there were no other changes to the patient's diet and lifestyle apart from adding the PEALut, this could support a therapeutic effect of the combination of PEA and Luteolin. As case studies tend to, it gives us food for thought—might this be worth pursuing?

In these conditions, it has been demonstrated that the increase of endogenous PEA, either by decreasing its degradation or exogenous administration, is able to keep neuroinflammation within its physiological limits [179]. Phytocannabinoids can influence PEA and other N-acyl-ethanolamides (NAEs) by stimulating the synthesis enzyme N-acyl phosphatidyl ethanolamine-specific phospholipase D (NAPE-PLD). Findings show that CBD increased the levels of NAEs and AEA, while THC increased levels of mostly arachidonic acid products [180].

## Oleamide

Many different compounds from plants have the potential to reduce oxidative stress associated with AD, protecting cells from neuronal toxicity resulting from oxidative stress [57]. In a mice model of AD, an extract from the humble radish (*Raphanus raphanistrum*) has been found to reduce lipid peroxidation and Aβ aggregation in mice brain tissues, increase acetylcholine and catalase activity in the brain, and reduce hydrogen peroxide-induced oxidative stress in cells. In vivo behavioral tests were also conducted in the mice. Results indicated attenuation in $A\beta_{1-42}$-induced learning and memory impairment in the mice in those treated with the radish extract. The active compound in radish was found to be oleamide [57].

You will remember from the earlier chapter on the ECS that oleamide is a member of the extended ECS. Oleamide is made within the body of animals—it is structurally related to AEA and is an endogenous amide of the fatty acid oleic acid [57, 181]. Oleic acid is a major monounsaturated fatty acid found in olive oil and other plants [181]. One of the actions of oleamide in our bodies is to promote sleep—it accumulates in the cerebrospinal fluid during sleeplessness. Its exact mechanisms of action are still being investigated but may involve interactions with neurotransmitters such as choline acetyltransferase [57].

Thus, this radish extract appears to be able to protect brain cells against oxidative stress-induced neuronal toxicity, and this may be due to oleamide's antioxidant activity [57]. Other studies have also found that treatment of microglia with extract of radish protects neuronal cells from neurotoxicity induced by microglial activation [49]. Given the role of oxidative stress in the pathophysiology of AD, it makes sense to ensure that the diets of AD patients are rich in those plant foods that have high antioxidant activity.

## Omega-3 PUFAs and Alzheimer's Disease

Epidemiological studies suggest that reduced levels or intake of omega-3 polyunsaturated fatty acids (PUFAs) or fish consumption is associated with increased risk of dementia, including AD, as well as cognitive decline and that increased dietary intake of docosahexaenoic acid (DHA) is protective for AD and other forms of dementia [182]. DHA's neuroprotective mechanisms of action include production of neuroprotective metabolites and reduction in arachidonic acid metabolites (which are often inflammatory in nature), and in AD, it has been shown to limit the production of Aβ toxin and suppress signaling pathways induced by Aβ [182]. This includes suppressing kinases that promote tau phosphorylation and neurofibrillary tangles. Studies suggest that DHA is likely to be more effective in prevention and treatment of AD if treatment is started early or it is used with antioxidants [182].

A systematic review (seven studies met the criteria for inclusion) concluded that there is evidence that supplementation with omega-3 polyunsaturated fatty acids may be beneficial at the stage of AD onset when there is only slight impairment of brain function. The review also concluded that some while studies did show changes in cognitive function in more severe AD, overall, there was not enough data to support omega-3 PUFA supplementation in the treatment of AD [183]. However, none of the studies controlled for the amount of omega-6 intake. This may be important omega-6 competes with omega-3 in the processes leading to the formation of anti-inflammatory endocannabinoid epoxides versus predominantly inflammatory arachidonic products.

Largely overlooked in the literature is the role of omega-3 as a substrate of the extended endocannabinoid epoxy-eicosanoids as well as a ligand for the noncanonical ECS receptor-like PPAR gamma (PPAR-γ). Omega-3 endocannabinoid epoxides are derived from docosahexaenoic acid (DHA) and eicosapentaenoic acid (EPA) to form epoxyeicosatetraenoic acid-ethanolamide (EEQ-EA) and epoxydocosapentaenoic acid-ethanolamide (EDP-EA). They are produced endogenously by activated BV-2 microglia cells, and production is stimulated in response to inflammation. Both these compounds, by way of CB2 receptors and PPARγ, induce anti-inflammatory cytokines and suppress inflammatory ones. Additionally, the omega-3 epoxides exerted antiangiogenic effects in human microvascular endothelial cells and vasodilatory actions on coronary arteries and regulated platelet aggregation [184]. EDP-EA induces apoptotic and anti-migratory actions partially mediated through increased CB1 receptor binding and avoiding hydrolytic metabolism by FAAH, allowing for increased bioavailability [185].

## Guidelines for Treating Dementia with Medicinal Cannabis

### When to Use Medicinal Cannabis

Medicinal cannabis treatment should be considered after a thorough clinical assessment and implementation of a comprehensive treatment plan including lifestyle modification, diet, and behavioral approaches. Sleep is an important factor in AD as we saw earlier, so it is very important to not forget to ask about sleep.

More than any other medical condition, dementia and cognitive decline can be associated with a broad range of possible causes. A reasonably accurate diagnosis should be confirmed by behavioral testing and imaging. Major metabolic disorders should be considered as well as polypharmacy including commonly used statin drugs that reduce essential brain cholesterol, vitamin D3, vitamin K2, thyroid conversion, estrogen, testosterone, and neurosteroids. Behavioral testing may be particularly valuable in establishing a benchmark and measurable parameter in medicinal cannabis treatment.

Dietary approaches are hotly contested, but evidence does suggest that insulin resistance of the brain is well associated with Alzheimer's such that some researchers have called Alzheimer's "type 3 diabetes" [92]. Brain insulin resistance impairs the brain's use of glucose, no matter how high blood sugar rises, and this might explain increased rates of Alzheimer's among those with type 2 diabetes. In a 2004 study, 81% of people with Alzheimer's on autopsy had either type 2 diabetes or prediabetes [186].

Evidence exists for the use of medium-chain triglycerides (MCT) acting as an alternate energy source through the formation of ketone bodies in the insulin-resistant Alzheimer brain. A Japanese study in 2019 showed that supplementation with an MCT-based ketogenic formula led to significant improvements in cognitive function in 20 patients with mild-moderate AD (11 males, nine females, mean age 73.4 ± 6.0 years). A total of 16 of the 20 patients completed the 12-week regimen in which they took the supplement daily. At week 8, there were significant improvements in immediate and delayed logical memory tests compared with baseline measurements. At week 12, compared with baseline, patients showed significant improvements in digit-symbol coding and in an immediate logical memory test. These results suggest that chronic consumption of this MCT-based supplement had positive effects on verbal memory and processing speed in patients with mild-moderate AD [187].

Activity and exercise are also important lifestyle factors for aging and dementia. A 2020 review found considerable benefits improving vascular flow, diabetes control, neurotrophins (BDNF), enhanced neurogenesis, and brain redox status potentially alleviating Aβ [188].

Therefore, insulin resistance and prediabetes should be clinically addressed and treated perhaps in conjunction with medicinal cannabis treatment.

One common barrier to effective medicinal cannabis treatment may be related to omega-3 deficiency. CBD may not be effective without sufficient omega-3 [189]. Dietary adequacy is essential, and testing should be considered if the history suggests inadequate intake of omega 3 (n-3 PUFA), vegetarian diet, or excessive intake of omega-6 (n-6 PUFA). Studies suggest a proper ratio of n-3 to n-6 omegas in the range of 1:2–1:4 is ideal [190].

The objectives of treatment with medicinal cannabis should be clearly established because benefits will vary based on the duration and severity of dementia due to chronic and irreversible brain changes. Palliative therapy is realistic and can provide enormous relief of suffering and behavioral disturbances. Medicinal cannabis can assist with many of the neurobehavioural aspects of dementia and can improve patient management as well as providing compassionate relief to caregivers. Medicinal cannabis can also assist sleep disturbance that are very common and avoid hypnotics and benzodiazepines associated with significant adverse effects. Stabilization of the cognitive decline is also a reasonable target especially when the disease is identified early. Remission or reversal can be achieved in some cases to the great relief of clients and family. Set your targets low so as not to disappoint but also to provide realistic hope.

## What Formulation Should You Use? (Blends)

Let the chief complaint suggest the best starting formulation while additional side benefits may be seen with the use of a wide range of other products. Behaviour management issues (e.g., agitation, aggression) suggest selection of a medicinal cannabis product with more sedative actions, while if lethargy is a concern, the patient may benefit from a product which is more activating. Responses can be very surprising as I have seen with a number of clients ranging from enhanced cooking activity to hypersexuality and even a few episodes of brief protective incarceration that were quickly resolved as misunderstandings. A low THC, high CBD full-spectrum product has been effective in a wide range of my clients. For product forms, consider what is the patient most comfortable with and willing to ingest? Are there taste or texture issues or issues with swallowing?

More and more providers have the opportunity for compounded formulations that might include selected blend of cannabinoids including CBD, CBDA, THC, THCA, D8THC, CBN, or CBG. In addition, there is good experience with terpenes that can be added to enhance a particular tactical effect like myrcene for pain, linalool for sleep, and pinene for memory. Because of its well-established neuroprotective properties, beta-caryophyllene should be a part of any dementia blend. An expert cannabinoid pharmacist can guide you in creating custom blends ideal for your patients.

Topical application of oral formulations can be highly effective particularly in resistant patients or those in restrictive skilled nursing facilities or hospital. In the latter the facility can take credit for their conventional therapy, while the family can supplement with clandestine cannabinoid massage. In one of my cases, a 76-year-old woman with dementia, this approach helped her survive a respiratory arrest after aspiration.

## When Might You Consider Adding THC?

Sedation and tolerance can be effective clinical guides to formula choice and selection. A past history of cannabis use or tolerance may suggest selection of a product with more THC. Increasing the dose of full-spectrum CBD weighted formulations (e.g., high CBD: low THC formulations) will increase the total THC content, perhaps suggesting consideration of a change in formulation to a product with greater THC. Response resistance can also suggest the need for significant increases in THC concentrations and total dose. You may need to remind the family that medicinal cannabis treatment cannot cause respiratory depression and will not induce toxicity.

## Dosing

Doses in the low range of 15 mg CBD per day have been very effective for the average septuagenarians. Once or twice per day frequency is sufficient with bedtime caution for possible activation effects which may be associated with CBD in some. Split the dose to avoid sedation or evening activation.

Topical doses in the same range can be effective when applied to any skin surface. The caregiver can complement the medicinal cannabis treatment with therapeutic touching or massage.

## Titration and Follow-Up

Start low and go slow for this population. Immediate effects of medicinal cannabis occur at the neurotransmitters and ion channels, while changes in cellular metabolism and neuroinflammation take 1–4 weeks. Follow-up visits to the practitioner are valuable in tweaking adjustments to the regimen by typically very cautious caregivers.

Most cases of dementia make some improvement, but some do not and high doses are rarely effective. Correcting an omega-3/6 imbalance is the best potential for nonresponders.

## Other Tips to Enhance Therapeutic Action

First in consideration as non-cannabis agents is beta-caryophyllene (BCP) as a natural CB2R agonist. Until an approved oral formulation becomes available, topical essential oils can be applied to any skin surface with excellent absorption. Depending on the concentration, 5–10 drops delivers about 150 mg and can be used twice daily or as often as desired. For general purpose I prefer the skin on the back of the hands, but BCP can also do double duty as an analgesic for joint pain, bites, burns, or bruises.

Adjunct therapy may include medium-chain triglycerides 45–60gms per day to induce nutritional ketones as part of a dietary supplementation. And, finally, the endocannabinoid palmitoylethanolamide (PEA) 400–800 per day could be additive for pain and dementia. Research suggests that the combination of PEA and luteolin may be useful.

## Drug-Cannabis Interactions

Several medications commonly used in patients with dementia have potential interactions with medicinal cannabis due to CYP450 competition like donepezil, haloperidol, SSRI, and H2 antagonists. Many of the potential drug-cannabis interactions relevant to such drugs relate to the isoenzymes CYP2D6, CYP3A4, 1A2, and potentially 2C, 2D6, 2E1. Several of these pharmaceutical agents are also associated with increased mortality and worsening of dementia. Nevertheless, due to the low doses of the herbal medical cannabis, drug interference or interactions are very uncommon, and none have been reported in the medical literature in relation to dementia. This contrasts vividly with use of pure CBD (i.e., isolate) as in Epidiolex that requires 10–20 mg per kg (in comparison with less than 1 mg/kg for full-spectrum medical cannabis products) where drug-Epidiolex interactions have been reported, in particular in association with antiepileptic medications. For benzodiazepines CBD can facilitate withdrawal while replacing the calming benefits from the drugs being de-prescribed.

## Case Studies from Dr. Blair's Practice

### Case 1: Down Syndrome and Dementia

A 61-year-old woman with Down syndrome (trisomy 13) with mild cognitive impairment from birth was in generally good health with no significant illness or infections. She lived with her widowed sister in Newfoundland, Canada, and was assisted by the state with weekly aides. She required no medications and was not subject to any known chemicals or trauma.

The patient was interactive, playful, cooperative, and kind.

In 2016 the patient developed dementia over 1.5 years. She stopped talking or eating and became oppositional and angry, showing violence and aggression toward her sister. She had no changes in food, medications, infections, trauma, or chemical exposures. The sister was no longer able to care for her in her rural two-story home.

The sister reported: "My life is very hectic now because Terry has dementia and is very difficult. I still have a respite care worker but only for 35 five hours a week, so the rest of the time I am on my own. Terry has had seizures but is on medication for them, so far it is working. It is so awful, this dementia. Terry loved music now she never wants to hear it at all, never gives anyone a hug anymore never says I love You and does not smile. She was always so very sweet and mannerly now she is nasty and rude. If someone comes to visit Terry tells them to *get out and don't come back*."

Because the patient was not cooperative, a topical approach was created. A standard cream base was compounded with full-spectrum 1:20 THC/CBD and beta-caryophyllene (BCP). This was applied to the back twice daily and gently rubbed into the skin. A typical dose was CBD (10 mg/mL), BCP (75 mg/mL) in Cetaphil cream base, 2 mL per treatment.

After 2 weeks her sister reported the following: *"Dr. Blair, Terry is doing really good. She is sleeping better and is smiling more we did not see smiles for months. One of my workers was off for a week she came to work today and she is seeing a difference in Terry for the better. I am attaching a pic of her that I took yesterday we have not seen smiles like this for about a year. Before the cream when I would go out for a walk Terry would yell and shout and cry. Both Grace and Phyllis have told me there is none of that now while I am gone. That is a blessing for them too. One other thing I have noticed (don't know if the cream got anything to do with it or not). Her bowels are working better at least they are for now."*

After 4 weeks the treatment reversed the signs and symptoms associated with dementia and restored docile behavior and normal eating, and her recall in games and play returned.

Her sister continued: *"Terry is still doing so much better since the cream everything that I told you about that was an improvement is still staying improved. There is also one other thing. Terry had not worn her hearing aid for 7 months, just would not have it in her ear. Now she lets me put it in and does not take it out. She used to take it out and throw it. When I came home today my worker, Phyllis, told me this is the best day of all that she has seen Terry since she has had dementia. She said, 'Terry did not yell at me, not even once.' Have still not had to give her anything for her bowels they have worked fine since the cream. Sleeps great, thank God. Will keep you informed and will be for ever grateful for every good day and night I get. I know it can't cure but it sure is helping."*

Her improved health was maintained with the continued medicinal cannabis cream over the next 2 years before dying of aspiration pneumonia following a tonic-clonic seizure without a prior epilepsy diagnosis.

## My Thoughts

AD occurs with high frequency in Down syndrome. Therapy was initiated late in the course of this patient's illness with the hopes of improving behavior and reducing aggression. An oral approach was not reliable, so an alternate topical method was attempted. Most studies suggest less than 10% skin absorption yet despite the limited bioavailability, the patient responded exceptionally well. Reversal of amyloid plaques and tau tangles is unlikely in the short time between medicinal cannabis initiation and response. The probable mechanism engaged in such brief onset of action may have been CB1R antagonism. CBD is a weak but known reverse agonist on CB1R modulating the activity of this receptor. In 2019 Navarro-Romero et al. in a mouse model of Down syndrome (DS) reported that by blocking CB1R, they restored hippocampal-dependent memory, synaptic plasticity, and adult neurogenesis in the dentate gyrus [191]. They repeated the study in another DS model with dysfunctional tyrosine-phosphorylation-regulated kinase 1A (DYRK1A) with the same positive results. In addition, CB2 receptors and FAAH expression are enhanced in both Alzheimer and DS glial cells consistent with Aβ-induced effects. The BCP used in this topical therapy acted as a CB2 agonist modulating those reactive glial components. CBD as a FAAH inhibitor could have provided the necessary synergy to rapidly reverse several parameters on neuropathology and sustain improvements.

Early treatment of DS could prevent the AD, but could it also improve brain development and performance in young patients? In Down syndrome chromosome 21 is triplicated producing excess gene products that neuropathogenic leading to mTOR activation. Early cannabinoid treatment might compensate for several of the DS dysfunctions including mTOR activation, excessive CB1R activation, enhanced neuroplasticity, synaptic vesicle trafficking, mitochondrial protection, and mitochondrial biogenesis, and reducing Aβ formation through regulation of APP. Perhaps early treatment would allow DS children to reach a higher cognitive performance and delay or prevent neurodegenerative disease.

We should not forget the plight of the dedicated caregiver in dementia who are constantly under stress emotionally, behaviorally, financially, and medically. They are often afflicted with fatigue, lack of sleep, anxiety, and depression with possible musculoskeletal injuries from home care. We have shown that the use of cannabinoids can reduce anxiety, agitation, and stress in dementia patients. And, givers of care could also benefit directly. Cannabinoid use in family caregivers can provide essential support for their stress in attending to their loved one. Nursing staff in residential facilities for mental health disorders are another potential target for cannabinoid therapy de-stressing. A 2021 study reported on 21 health care workers exposed to high levels of physical and emotional overloads seeking clinical help during the COVID-19 pandemic. Staff members were evaluated for anxiety, depression, insomnia, and emotional exhaustion before and after 165 mg of purified cannabidiol twice daily without THC for 4 weeks [192]. All four indices improved rapidly for all subjects, and the effects were sustained without additional dosing until 8 weeks. There were no adverse effects and no dropouts, and all subjects continued to work during the trial.

## Case 2: Vascular Dementia Complicated with Trauma and Infection

Although this case is neither mine nor AD, it has several instructional points to consider. It was published in 2019 [193].

An 81-year-old grandfather from Israel married with six children was first diagnosed with dementia in 2012 7 years after his first cerebrovascular event and immediately following his second. He lived at home with his wife, had 24-h live-in care, and, due to severe spasticity, was wheelchair-bound and required assistance for most daily tasks. He was also diabetic and had hypertension. Since the first two cerebrovascular events in 2005 and 2012, he had also had a series of intracerebral hemorrhage following a road accident. A VP shunt was inserted in 2016 and this was followed by convulsions. He also had recurrent urinary tract infections and pneumonia, for which he had been hospitalized several times. In 2016, he had tracheostomy procedure and required a gastrointestinal feeding tube, and when he presented in 2019, he was fed solely through the feeding tube. The patient took six different medications for his various illnesses and symptoms including carbidopa/levodopa. The patient was drowsy most of the time and unable to speak and to communicate with others, and due to his severe spasticity, transferring him from bed to wheelchair to bed was increasingly difficult.

To relieve his spasticity, a trial CBD therapy was begun (one drop of CBD oil three times daily for approximately 7 days, followed by an increase to four drops in the daily dose). Within a few days, he showed signs of alertness and said a number of words to family. One month later, he continued to be more alert and responsive, saying a few words sporadically and moving his lips and attempting to say more. The patient was also able to maintain eye contact with those around him for more than just a few seconds. His spasticity was significantly decreased.

### My Thoughts

This was a case of long-standing dementia of over 7 years since onset and appeared to be vascular dementia complicated with trauma and infection (from the case history). Severe spasticity made management difficult, so CBD was introduced. Generally, spasticity is considered a target of THC which was available in Israel.

We can estimate the first positive response at about 10 days particularly in cognition, followed by improvements in spasticity. The providers addressed the chief complaint regarding the management issue of bed transfers. From a clinical view, the condition seemed fixed from the point of anatomical pathology, evidenced by scan and vascular events. Note the low doses of four drops only, his advanced age, and extended recovery time of 1 month. Since CBD will not correct lost or damaged tissue, one of the other underlying causes of brain dysfunction which was not obvious was improved, allowing at least limited cognitive and physical improvement. We must be cautious in estimating prognosis in all dementia.

## Case 3: Vascular Dementia

The patient is an 82-year-old living in Florida. He is a disabled, Korean War veteran who suffered a stroke 4 years ago and has been diagnosed with vascular dementia, PTSD, diabetes mellitus with neuropathy, and a familial tremor on 15 medications. In fact, he scheduled for an intracranial procedure to dampen that tremor in a just a few months, but Parkinson's disease was not suspected. For the previous year, he sat in a chair watching TV with little interaction and hardly speaking. He was depressed, stubborn, and unable to recall recent events. He slept poorly at night and was disoriented especially after sundown.

The wife and daughter consulted with me, and a full-spectrum low THC medicinal cannabis product was recommended with a starting dose of 7.5 mg CBD once daily. That night he slept until morning and announced that he wanted more CBD. Three days later he started taking CBD four times a day. Within 3 days he began reacting with pain to his diabetic needle sticks for the first time in years. His strength and energy improved, his tremor calmed, and his cognition cleared. He started making plans for the future and telling his personal Korean War stories, not previously heard, with vivid and accurate detail. At his church revival, he announced his healing to the congregation. The pastor thought him delusional, but looking back the pastor admitted that Joe's revival rantings were in fact lucid and logical.

Not having driven in 4 years, the family was apprehensive when the patient insisted on driving to his Veterans Administration PTSD group meeting. The next day with his wife, he navigated the 60-mile drive over a crowded highway crossing multiple lanes of traffic on a rainy day without incident. He knew exactly where he was going. At home, he talks constantly and is well aware of the date, time, location, and current events. At one point he was emotionally moved by the ravaging weather in New England wanted to drive to Massachusetts to help. Yet, the family had no difficulty dissuading him from the adventure because, when discussed, he fully understood his limitations. Now, he's walking without assistance, independently handling personal business matters with clarity, and maintaining a joyful mood that is in stark contrast to his previous suicide ruminations. Furthermore, despite an increased appetite, his blood sugars have steadily dropped from mid-200s to 130s.

In a follow-up home visit after 1 month, the patient eagerly anticipated my visit and called me by name even though we had never previously met. He was fully oriented and aware of current events and volunteered for public interviews and even the media. Throughout my interview with the family, he was fully cooperative, reasonable, and very discerning. He even admitted to a rising libido with an appropriate, if not embarrassing, description of his feelings. His family carefully controls his use of CBD and he consents.

A month later in a phone interview, the patient thanked me for helping him be "reborn" to awareness and stop living like a "vegetable." He admitted his brain is still not functioning at the "top" floor, but he has high hopes of a complete recovery. Although the family is thrilled with the improvements, his improvement caused a number of changes to their future because he was no longer willing to go to a nursing home.

**My Comments**

This patient may have had multiple causes for dementia with previous cognitive decline followed by a stroke as well as his underlying uncontrolled diabetes. CBD appears to have initiated rapid, broad systemic improvements physically, metabolically, and cognitively with no apparent adverse effects using very low doses. In addition, his lifelong PTSD affliction may be correcting because he is now able to publicly tell the tragic stories of his lost comrades and his unexplained survival. The patient had indicators of vascular-type dementia. Dramatic improvement in the health of an octogenarian is not always well received by the family.

## Conclusion

Dementia, in particular that associated with AD, is all too prevalent. The symptoms and signs are devastating and go beyond just loss of memory. The etiology and pathogenesis of AD are incredibly complex, and much is still unknown. The ECS is involved in the pathogenesis in several ways. Scientific evidence indicates that the earlier AD is treated, the better. Since current pharmaceutical interventions do not prevent the deterioration of the disease and are associated with side effects, there is room for other therapies including medicinal cannabis. Preclinical and clinical research indicates that CBD, THC, and many of the other plant nutrients such as some of the terpenes and PEA may be useful in the treatment of the neurobehavioural aspects of the condition. Medicinal cannabis may be a valuable part of a holistic approach to the treatment of AD that considers a range of factors including diet, exercise, stress reduction, and others. At the end of it all, however, as Chinese medicine and other forms of traditional medicine teach, we must address the root cause of illness. Questions remain: why are so many people now getting dementia, and what factors in our environments are contributing to it? Make no mistake: many (most?) of our chronic illnesses afflicting humanity are of our own doing.

## References


1. Australian Institute of Health and Welfare (AIHW). Dementia. 23 July, 2020. Available at: https://www.aihw.gov.au/reports/australias-health/dementia. Accessed 20 Nov 2020.
2. Prince M, Wimo A, Guerchet M, et al. The World Alzheimer Report 2015. The Global Impact of Dementia. An analysis of prevalence, incidence, costs and trends. London: Alzheimer's Disease International; 2015.
3. Ferreira-Vieira TH, Guimaraes IM, Silva FR, Ribeiro FM. Alzheimer's Disease: targeting the cholinergic system. Curr Neuropharmacol. 2016;14(1):101–15.
4. Russo EB. Cannabis therapeutics and the future of neurology. Front Integr Neurosci. 2018;12:51.
5. Hillen JB, Soulsby N, Alderman C, Caughey GE. Safety and effectiveness of cannabinoids for the treatment of neuropsychiatric symptoms in dementia: a systematic review. Ther Adv Drug Saf. 2019;10:2042098619846993.
6. Alzheimer's Association. 2019 Alzheimer's disease facts and figures. Alzheimers Dement. 2019;15(3):321–87.

7. Kim SH, Yang JW, Kim KH, et al. A review of studies of marijuana for Alzheimer's disease; focusing on CBD, THC. J Pharmacopuncture. 2019;22(4):225–30.
8. Livingston G, Sommerlad A, Orgeta V, et al. Dementia prevention, intervention and care. Lancet. 2017;390:2673–734.
9. Gudala K, Bansal D, Schifano F, Bhansali A. Diabetes mellitus and risk of dementia: a meta-analysis of prospective observational studies. J Diabetes Investig. 2013;4(6):640. https://doi.org/10.1111/jdi.12087.
10. Sawa GM, Zacchi J, Mathews FE, et al. Prevalence, correlates and course of behavioural and psychological symptoms of dementia in the population. Br J Psychiatry. 2009;194:202–19.
11. Alves J, Petrosyan A, Magalhães R. Olfactory dysfunction in dementia. World J Clin Cases. 2014;2(11):661–7.
12. Yamagishi M, Ishizuka Y, Seki K. Pathology of olfactory mucosa in patients with Alzheimer's disease. Ann Otol Rhinol Laryngol. 1994;103:421–7.
13. Fioretti A, Fusetti M, Eibenstein A. The predictive role of hyposmia in Alzheimer's disease. In: The clinical spectrum of Alzheimer's disease- the charge towards comprehensive diagnostic and therapeutic strategies, 2011. Available at: https://www.intechopen.com/books/the-clinical-spectrum-of-alzheimer-s-disease-the-charge-toward-comprehensive-diagnostic-and-therapeutic-strategies/the-predictive-role-of-hyposmia-in-alzheimer-s-disease. Accessed 29 Dec 2020.
14. Oppo V, Melis M, Melis M, et al. "Smelling and tasting" Parkinson's Disease: using senses to improve the knowledge of the disease. Front Aging Neurosc. 2020;12:43. https://doi.org/10.3389/fnagi.2020.00043.
15. Seitz DP, Afuniru N, Gruneir A, et al. Antidepressants for agitation and psychosis in dementia. Cochrane Database Syst Rev. 2011:CD008191.
16. Ballard C, Waite J. The effectiveness of atypical antipsychotics for the treatment of aggression and psychosis in Alzheimer's disease. Cochrane Database Syst Rev. 2006;1:CD003476.
17. Allegri RF, Sarasola D, Serrano CM, et al. Neuropsychiatric symptoms as a predictor of caregiver burden in Alzheimer's Disease. Neuropsychiatr Dis Treat. 2006;2:105–10.
18. Preidt R. The high cost of Alzheimer's. WebMD, 2018. Available at: https://www.webmd.com/alzheimers/news/20180320/the-high-costs-of-alzheimers#1. Accessed 28 Dec 2020.
19. Nicholas LH, Langa KM, Bynum JP, et al. Financial presentation of Alzheimer Disease and related dementias. JAMA Intern Med. 2021;181(2):220–7. https://doi.org/10.1001/jamainternmed.2020.6432.
20. Medina-Vera D, Rosell-Valle C, Lopez-Gambero AJ, et al. Imbalance of endocannabinoid/lysophosphatidylinositol receptors marks the severity of Alzheimer's disease in a preclinical model: a therapeutic opportunity. Biology. 2020;9:377.
21. Waldemar G, Dubois B, Emre M, et al. Recommendations for the diagnosis and management of Alzheimer's disease and other disorders associated with dementia: EFNS guideline. Eur J Neurol. 2007;14(1):e1–26.
22. Bedse G, Romano A, Lavecchia AM, et al. The role of endocannabinoid signaling in the molecular mechanisms of neurodegeneration in Alzheimer's disease. J Alzheimers Dis. 2015;43:1115–36.
23. Cruts M, Van Broekhoven C. Molecular genetics of Alzheimer's disease. Ann Med. 1998;30:560–5.
24. Wang R, Reddy PH. Role of glutamate and NMDA receptors in Alzheimer's Disease. J Alzheimers Dis. 2017;54(4):1041–8.
25. Kuehn B. Alzheimer research, glucose metabolism moves to centre stage. JAMA. 2020;323(4):297–9.
26. Charernboon T, Lerthattaslip T, Supasitthumrong T. Effectiveness of cannabinoids for treatment of dementia: a systematic review of randomized controlled trials. Clin Gerontol. 2020;18:1–9.
27. Charernboon T, Phanasathit M. Prevalence of neuropsychiatric symptoms in Alzheimer's disease: a cross-sectional descriptive study in Thailand. J Med Assoc Thai. 2014;97(5):560–5.
28. Ikeda M. Early diagnosis and memory clinic for Alzheimer's disease. Psychogeriatrics. 2004;4(4):130–2.

29. Zhao Q-F, Lan Tan L, Hui-Fu Wang H-F, et al. The prevalence of neuropsychiatric symptoms in Alzheimer's disease: systematic review and meta-analysis. J Affect Disord. 2016;190:264–71.
30. Woodward MR, Harper DG, Stolya A, et al. Dronabinol for the treatment of agitation and aggressive behavior in acutely hospitalized severely demented patients with noncognitive behavioral symptoms. Am J Geriatr Psychiatry. 2014;22(4):415–9.
31. Herrmann N, et al. Randomized placebo-controlled trial of Nabilone for agitation in Alzheimer's disease. Am J Geriatr Psychiatry. 2019;27(11):1161–73.
32. Bonnet AE, Marchalant Y. Potential therapeutical contributions of the endocannabinoid system towards aging and Alzheimer's disease. Aging Dis. 2015;6(5):400–5.
33. Dash R, Ali C, Jahan I, et al. Emerging potential of cannabidiol in reversing proteinopathies. Ageing Res Rev. 2021;65:101209. https://doi.org/10.1016/j.arr.2020.101209.
34. Fox NC, Schott J. Imaging cerebral atrophy: normal ageing to Alzheimer's disease. Lancet. 2004;363(9406):392–4.
35. Crews L, Masliah E. Molecular mechanisms of neurodegeneration in Alzheimer's disease. Hum Mol Genet. 2010;19(R1):R12–20.
36. Shaftel SS, Griffin WS, O'Banion MK. The role of interleukin-1 in neuroinflammation and Alzheimer disease: an evolving perspective. J Neuroinflammation. 2008;5:7.
37. Gouras GK, Olsson TT, Hansson O. β-Amyloid peptides and amyloid plaques in Alzheimer's disease. Neurotherapeutics. 2015;12(1):3–11.
38. Baruch-Suchodolsky R, Fischer B. Aβ40, either soluble or aggregated, is a remarkably potent antioxidant in cell-free oxidative systems. Biochemistry. 2009;48(20):4354–70.
39. Long JM, Holtzman DM. Alzheimer disease: an update on pathobiology and treatment strategies. Cell. 2019;179(2):312–39.
40. Bennett AE, Marchalant Y. Potential therapeutical contributions of the endocannabinoid system towards aging and Alzheimer's disease. Aging Dis. 2015;6(5):400–5.
41. McGeer PL, Schulzer M, McGeer EG. Arthritis and anti-inflammatory agents as possible protective factors for Alzheimer's disease: a review of 17 epidemiologic studies. Neurology. 1996;47(2):425–32.
42. Stewart WF, Kawas C, Corrada M, Metter EJ. Risk of Alzheimer's disease and duration of NSAID use. Neurology. 1997;48(3):626–32.
43. Vlad SC, Miller DR, Kowall NW, Felson DT. Protective effects of NSAIDs on the development of Alzheimer disease. Neurology. 2008;70(19):1672–7.
44. Akiyama H, Barger S, Barnum S, et al. Inflammation and Alzheimer's disease. Neurobiol Aging. 2000;21(3):383–421.
45. Griffin WS, Sheng JG, Royston MC, et al. Glial-neuronal interactions in Alzheimer's disease: the potential role of a "cytokine cycle" in disease progression. Brain Pathol. 1998;8(1):65–72.
46. Engelhart MJ, Geerlings MI, Meijer J, et al. Inflammatory proteins in plasma and the risk of dementia: the Rotterdam study. Arch Neurol. 2004;61(5):668–72.
47. Schmidt R, Schmidt H, Curb JD, et al. Early inflammation and dementia: a 25- year follow-up of the Honolulu-Asia Aging Study. Ann Neurol. 2002;52(2):168–74.
48. Saliba SW, Glaser F, Denkers A, et al. Effects of a novel GPR55 antagonist on the arachidonic acid cascade in LPS-activated primary microglial cells. Int J Mol Sci. 2021;22:2503.
49. Do MH, Kim M, Sang-Yoon C, et al. Wild radish (*Raphanus sativus* var. *hortensis f. raphanistroides*) root extract protects neuronal cells by inhibiting microglial activation. Appl Biological Chem. 2021;64(1):1–9. https://doi.org/10.1186/s13765-021-00604-7.
50. Vazquez C, Tolon RM, Grande MT, et al. Endocannabinoid regulation of amyloid-induced neuroinflammation. Neurobiol Aging. 2015;36(11):3008–19.
51. Sheng JG, Mrak RE, Griffin WS. Glial-neuronal interactions in Alzheimer disease: progressive association of IL-alpha+ microglia and S100beta+ astrocytes with neurofibrillary tangle stages. J Neuropathol Exp Neurol. 1997a;56(3):285–90.
52. Sheng JG, Mrak RE, Griffin WS. Neuritic plaque evolution in Alzheimer's disease is accompanied by transition of activated microglia from primed to enlarged to phagocytic forms. Acta Neuropathol (Berl). 1997b;94(1):1–5.

53. Benito C, Núñez E, Tolón RM, et al. Cannabinoid CB2 receptors and fatty acid amide hydrolase are selectively overexpressed in neuritic plaque-associated glia in Alzheimer's disease brains. J Neurosci. 2003;23(35):11136–41.
54. Strohmeyer R, Rogers J. Molecular and cellular mediators of Alzheimer's disease inflammation. J Alzheimers Dis. 2001;3(1):131–57.
55. Li Y, Liu L, Barger SE, Griffin WST. Interleukin-1 mediates pathological effects of microglia on tau phosphorylation and on synaptophysin synthesis in cortical neurons through a p38-MAPK pathway. J Neurosci. 2003;23:1605–11.
56. Cheignon C, Tomas M, Bonnefont-Rouselot D, et al. Oxidative stress and the amyloid beta peptide in Alzheimer's disease. Redox Biol. 2018;14:450–64.
57. Choi SJ, Park CK, Shin D-H. Protective effects of radish extract against neurotoxicity in mice and PC12 cells. J Med Food. 2020;23(5):523–34.
58. Rivas-Arancibia S, Rodriguez-Martinez E, Mendez-Barcia A, et al. Oxidative stress, inflammation and formation of beta-amyloid 1-42 in brain. In: Ahmad R, editor. Free Radicals and Diseases. Rijeka: InTechOpen; 2016. p. 113–30.
59. Beggiato S, Tomasini MC, Ferraro L. Palmitoylethanolamide (PEA) as a potential therapeutic agent in Alzheimer's Disease. Front Pharmacol. 2019;10:821. https://doi.org/10.3389/fphar.2019.00821.
60. Mrak RE, Griffin WS. Glia and their cytokines in progression of neurodegeneration. Neurobiol Aging. 2005;26:349–54.
61. Meng T, Lin S, Zhuang H, et al. Recent progress in the role of autophagy in neurological diseases. Cell Stress. 2019;3(5):141–61.
62. Wu MY, Lu JH. Autophagy and macrophage functions: inflammatory response and phagocytosis. Cell. 2019;9(1):70.
63. Seixas da Silva G, Melo HM, Lourenco MV, et al. Amyloid-β oligomers transiently inhibit AMP-activated kinase and cause metabolic defects in hippocampal neurons. J Biol Chem. 2017;292(18):7395–406.
64. Gugliandolo A, Pollastro F, Bramanti P, Mazzon E. Cannabidiol exerts protective effects in an in vitro model of Parkinson's disease activating AKT/mTOR pathway. Fitoterapia. 2020;143:104553.
65. Spilman P, Podlutskaya N, Hart MJ, et al. Inhibition of mTOR by rapamycin abolishes cognitive deficits and reduces amyloid-beta levels in a mouse model of Alzheimer's disease. PLoS One. 2010;5(4):e9979.
66. Vingtdeux V, Giliberto L, Zhao H, et al. AMP-activated protein kinase signaling activation by resveratrol modulates amyloid-beta peptide metabolism. J Biol Chem. 2010;285(12):9100–13.
67. Huang M, Jiang X, Liang Y, et al. Berberine improves cognitive impairment by promoting autophagic clearance and inhibiting production of β-amyloid in APP/tau/PS1 mouse model of Alzheimer's disease. Exp Gerontol. 2017a;91:25–33.
68. Domenico F, Tramutola A, Foppoli C, et al. mTOR in Down Syndrome: role in Aβ and tau neuropathology and transition to Alzheimer disease-like dementia. Free Radic Biol Med. 2018;114:94–101.
69. Loret AL, Badia MC, Giraldo E, et al. Alzheimer's amyloid-β toxicity and tau hyperphosphorylation are linked via RCAN1. J Alzheimers Dis. 2011;27(4):701–9.
70. Simic G, Babic M, Wray S. Tau protein hyperphosphorylation and aggregation in Alzheimer's disease and other tauopathies, and possible neuroprotective strategies. Biomolecules. 2016;6(1):6.
71. Berg L, McKeel DW, Miller JP, et al. Neuropathological indexes of Alzheimer's disease in demented and nondemented persons aged 80 years and older. Arch Neurol. 1993;50(4):349–58.
72. Cai Z, Li B, Zhao B. Down-regulation of amyloid-β through AMPK activation by inhibitors of GSK-3β in SH-SY5Y and SH-SY5Y-AβPP695 cells. J Alzheimers Dis. 2012;29(1):89–98.
73. McDade E, et al. Longitudinal cognitive and biomarker changes in dominantly inherited Alzheimer disease. Neurology. 2018;91:e1295–306.
74. Villemagne VL, Dore V, Burnham SC, et al. Imaging tau and amyloid-β proteinopathies in Alzheimer disease and other conditions. Nat Rev Neurol. 2018;14:225–36.

75. Uhlmann RE, Rother C, Rasmussen J, et al. Acute targeting of pre-amyloid seeds in transgenic mice reduces Alzheimer-like pathology later in life. Nat Neurosci. 2020;23(12):1580–8. https://doi.org/10.1038/s41593-020-00737-w.
76. Aoyagi A, et al. Aβ and tau prion-like activities decline with longevity in the Alzheimer's disease human brain. Sci Trans Med. 2019;11:eaat8462.
77. Ye L, et al. Aβ seeding potency peaks in the early stages of cerebral β-amyloidosis. EMBO Rep. 2017;18:1536–44.
78. Holmes C, Boche D, Wilkinson D, et al. Long term effects of Abeta42 immunisation in Alzheimer's disease: follow-up of a randomised, placebo-controlled phase I trial. Lancet. 2008;372:216–23.
79. Tampellini D, Capetillo-Zarate E, Dumont M, et al. Effects of synaptic modulation on β-Amyloid, synaptophysin, and memory performance in Alzheimer's Disease transgenic mice. J Neurosci. 2010;30(43):14299–304.
80. Arboleda-Velasquez JF, Lopera F, O'Hare M, et al. Resistance to autosomal dominant Alzheimer's disease in an APOE3 Christchurch homozygote: a case report. Nat Med. 2019;25:1680–3.
81. Francis PT. The interplay of neurotransmitters in Alzheimer's disease. CNS Spectr. 2005;10(Suppl 18):6–9.
82. Whitehouse PJ, Price DL, Clark AW, et al. Alzheimer disease: evidence for selective loss of cholinergic neurons in the nucleus basalis. Ann Neurol. 1981;10(2):122–6.
83. Whitehouse PJ, Price DL, Struble RG, et al. Alzheimer's disease and senile dementia: loss of neurons in the basal forebrain. Science. 1982;215(4537):1237–9.
84. Terry RD, Masliah E, Salmon DP, et al. Physical basis of cognitive alterations in Alzheimer's disease: synapse loss is the major correlate of cognitive impairment. Ann Neurol. 1991;30(4):572–80.
85. Selkoe DJ. Alzheimer's disease is a synaptic failure. Science. 2002;298(5594):789–91.
86. Tannenburg RK, Dodd PR. Excitatory and neurodegenerative disease. In: Schwartzkroin PA, editor. Encyclopedia of basic epilepsy research. Academic Press; 2009. p. 114–9.
87. Schliebs R, Arendt T. The significance of the cholinergic system in the brain during aging and in Alzheimer's disease. J Neural Transm (Vienna). 2006;113(11):1625–44.
88. Wilcock GK, Esiri MM, Bowen DM, Smith CC. Alzheimer's disease. Correlation of cortical choline acetyltransferase activity with the severity of dementia and histological abnormalities. J Neurol Sci. 1982;57(2–3):407–17.
89. Hardingham GE, Bading H. Synaptic versus extrasynaptic NMDA receptor signalling: implications for neurodegenerative disorders. Nat Rev Neurosci. 2010;11(10):682–96.
90. Carroll CM, Stanley M, Pait M, et al. Aging and pathology cause sleep disruptions and altered metabolism in mouse models of Alzheimer's disease. Program 651.23. 2019 neuroscience Meeting Planner. Chicago: Society for Neuroscience; 2019.
91. Maciejczyk M, et al. Insulin resistance and oxidative stress in the brain: what's new? Int J Mol Sci. 2019;20:874.
92. de la Monte SM. Type 3 diabetes is sporadic Alzheimer's disease: mini-review. Eur Neuropsychopharmacol. 2014;24(12):1954–60.
93. McIntosh EC, Nation DA. Importance of treatment status in links between diabetes type 2 and Alzheimer's Disease. Diabetes Care. 2019;42(5):972–9.
94. Wu L, Zhang X, Zhao L. Human ApoE isoforms differentially modulate brain glucose and ketone metabolism: implications for Alzheimer's disease risk reduction and early intervention. J Neurosci. 2018;38(30):6665–81.
95. Barger SE, Hendrix RD, Ou Y, et al. Alzheimer-related pathology impairs peripheral glucose tolerance by disrupting glucose transporter 1 localization and cerebral glucose delivery. Program 651.09.2019 Neuroscience Meeting Planner. Chicago: Society for Neuroscience; 2019.
96. Sheng JG, Mrak RE, Griffin WST. Enlarged and phagocytic, but not primed, IL-1α-immunoreactive microglia increase with age in normal human brain. Acta Neuropathol. 1998;95:229–34.

97. Iuvone T, Esposito G, Esposito R, et al. Neuroprotective effect of cannabidiol, a non-psychoactive component from Cannabis sativa, on β-amyloid-induced toxicity in PC12 cells. J Neurochem. 2004;89:134–41.
98. Milton NG. Anandamide and noladin ether prevent neurotoxicity of the human amyloid-beta peptide. Neurosci Lett. 2002;332(2):127–30.
99. Koppel J, Davies P. Targeting the endocannabinoid system in Alzheimer's disease. J Alzheimers Dis. 2008;15:495–504.
100. Berry AJ, Zubko O, Reeves SJ, Howard RJ. Endocannabinoid system alterations in Alzheimer's disease: a systematic review of human studies. Brain Res. 2020;1749:147135.
101. Altamura C, Ventriglia M, Martin MG, et al. Elevation of plasma 2-arachidonylglycerol levels in Alzheimer's disease patients as a potential protective mechanism against neurodegenerative decline. J Alzheimers Dis. 2015;46:497–506.
102. Chen X, Zhang J, Chen C. Endocannabinoid 2-arachidonoylglycerol protects neurons against β-amyloid insults. Neuroscience. 2011;178:159–68.
103. Harvey BS, Ohlsson KS, Mååg JL, et al. Contrasting protective effects of cannabinoids against oxidative stress and amyloid-β evoked neurotoxicity in vitro. Neurotoxicology. 2012;33(1):138–46.
104. Janefjord E, Mååg JL, Harvey BS, Smid SD. Cannabinoid effects on β amyloid fibril and aggregate formation, neuronal and microglial-activated neurotoxicity in vitro. Cell Mol Neurobiol. 2014;34(1):31–42.
105. Noonan J, Tanveer R, Klompas A, et al. Endocannabinoids prevent beta-amyloid-mediated lysosomal destabilization in cultured neurons. J Biol Chem. 2010;285:38543–54.
106. van der Stelt M, Mazzola C, Esposito G, et al. Endocannabinoids and beta-amyloid-induced neurotoxicity in vivo: effect of pharmacological elevation of endocannabinoid levels. Cell Mol Life Sci. 2006;63(12):1410–24.
107. Marsicano G, Moosmann B, Hermann H, et al. Neuroprotective properties of cannabinoids against oxidative stress: role of the cannabinoid receptor CB1. J Neurochem. 2002;80(3):448–56.
108. Lopez A, Aparicio N, Pazos MR, et al. Cannabinoid $CB_2$ receptors in the mouse brain: relevance for Alzheimer's disease. J Neuroinflammation. 2018;15(1):158.
109. Aso E, Palomer E, Juvés S, et al. CB1 agonist ACEA protects neurons and reduces the cognitive impairment of AβPP/PS1 mice. J Alzheimers Dis. 2012;30(2):439–59.
110. Aso E, Juvés S, Maldonado R, Ferrer I. CB2 cannabinoid receptor agonist ameliorates Alzheimer-like phenotype in AβPP/PS1 mice. J Alzheimers Dis. 2013;35(4):847–58.
111. Solas M, Francis PT, Franco R, Ramirez MJ. CB2 receptor and amyloid pathology in frontal cortex of Alzheimer's disease patients. Neurobiol Aging. 2013;34:805–8.
112. Ahmad R, Goffin K, Van den Stock J, et al. In vivo type 1 cannabinoid receptor availability in Alzheimer's disease. Eur Neurpsychopharmacol. 2014;24(2):242–50.
113. Aso E, Ferrer I. Cannabinoids for treatment of Alzheimer's disease: moving toward the clinic. Front Pharmacol. 2014;5:37.
114. Fakhfouri G, Ahmadiani A, Rahimian R, et al. WIN55212-2 attenuates amyloid-beta-induced neuroinflammation in rats through activation of cannabinoid receptors and PPAR-γ pathway. Neuropharmacology. 2012;63(4):653–66.
115. Haghani M, Shabani M, Javan M, et al. CB1 cannabinoid receptor activation rescues amyloid β-induced alterations in behaviour and intrinsic electrophysiological properties of rat hippocampal CA1 pyramidal neurones. Cell Physiol Biochem. 2012;29(3–4):391–406.
116. Martín-Moreno AM, Reigada D, Ramírez BG, et al. Cannabidiol and other cannabinoids reduce microglial activation in vitro and in vivo: relevance to Alzheimer's disease. Mol Pharmacol. 2011;79(6):964–73.
117. Wu J, Bie B, Yang H, Xu JJ, et al. Activation of the CB2 receptor system reverses amyloid-induced memory deficiency. Neurobiol Aging. 2013;34(3):791–804.
118. Martín-Moreno AM, Brera B, Spuch C, et al. Prolonged oral cannabinoid administration prevents neuroinflammation, lowers β-amyloid levels and improves cognitive performance in Tg APP 2576 mice. J Neuroinflammation. 2012;9:8.

119. Bisogno T, Di Marzo V. The role of the endocannabinoid system in Alzheimer's disease: facts and hypotheses. Curr Pharm Des. 2008;14:2299–3305.
120. Russo EB, Marcu J. Cannabis pharmacology: the usual suspects and a few promising leads. Adv Pharmacol. 2017;80:67–134.
121. Mukhopadhyay P, Rajesh M, Horváth B, et al. Cannabidiol protects against hepatic ischemia/reperfusion injury by attenuating inflammatory signaling and response, oxidative/nitrative stress, and cell death. Free Radic Biol Med. 2011;50:1368–81.
122. Walter L, Franklin A, Witting A, et al. Nonpsychotropic cannabinoid receptors regulate microglial cell migration. J Neurosci. 2003;23:1398–405.
123. Esposito G, Scuderi C, Valenza M, et al. Cannabidiol reduces Aβ-induced neuroinflammation and promotes hippocampal neurogenesis through PPARγ involvement. PLoS One. 2011;6:e28668.
124. Scuderi C, Steardo L, Esposito G. Cannabidiol promotes amyloid precursor protein ubiquitination and reduction of beta amyloid expression in SHSY5YAPP+ cells through PPARγ involvement. Phytother Res. 2014;28(7):1007–13.
125. Libro R, Diomede F, Scionti D, et al. Cannabidiol modulates the expression of Alzheimer's disease-related genes in mesenchymal stem cells. Int J Mol Sci. 2017;18:26.
126. Esposito G, De Filippis D, Carnuccio R, et al. The marijuana component cannabidiol inhibits beta-amyloid-induced tau protein hyperphosphorylation through Wnt/beta-catenin pathway rescue in PC12 cells. J Mol Med (Berl). 2006a;84(3):253–8.
127. Schubert D, Kepchia D, Liang Z, et al. Efficacy of cannabinoids in a pre-clinical drug screening platform for Alzheimer's disease. Mol Neurobiol. 2019;56:7719–30.
128. Esposito G, Scuderi C, Savani C, et al. Cannabidiol *in vivo* blunts β-amyloid induced neuroinflammation by suppressing IL-1β and iNOS expression. Br J Pharmacol. 2007;151:1272–9.
129. Kim J, Choi JY, Choi IS. Neuroprotective effect of cannabidiol against hydrogen peroxide in hippocampal neuron culture. Cannabis Cannabinoid Res. 2021;6(1):40–7.
130. Hamelink C, Hampson A, Wink DA, et al. Comparison of cannabidiol, antioxidants, and diuretics in reversing binge ethanol-induced neurotoxicity. J Pharmacol Exp Ther. 2005;314:780–8.
131. Wang Z, Peng Z, Xie Y, et al. Cannabidiol regulates CB1-pSTAT3 signaling for neurite outgrowth, prolongs lifespan, and improves health span in Caenorhabditis elegans of Aβ pathology models. FASEB J. 2021;35(5):e21537.
132. Campos AC, Ortega Z, Palazuelos J, et al. The anxiolytic effect of cannabidiol on chronically stressed mice depends on hippocampal neurogenesis: involvement of the endocannabinoid system. Int J Neuropsychopharmacol. 2013;16(6):1407–19.
133. Campos AC, Fogaca MV, Scarante FF, et al. Plastic and neuroprotective mechanisms involved in the therapeutic effects of cannabidiol in psychiatric disorders. Front Pharmacol. 2017;8:18.
134. Farr SA, Goodland MN, Niehoff ML, Young BJ. Cannabidiol (CBD) improves cognition and decreases anxiety in the SAMP8 mouse model of Alzheimer's. FASEB. 2020;34(S1):1–1.
135. Coles M. Evaluation of the therapeutic potential of low dose chronic cannabidiol (CBD) treatment to reverse deficits of APPSwe/PS1ΔE9 transgenic female mice. PhD thesis, University of Western Sydney, 2019. Available at: https://researchdirect.westernsydney.edu.au/islandora/object/uws%3A57347. Accessed 8 Dec 2020.
136. Cheng D, Spiro AS, Jenner AM, et al. Long-term cannabidiol treatment prevents the development of social recognition memory deficits in Alzheimer's disease transgenic mice. J Alzheimers Dis. 2014a;42:1383–96.
137. Cheng D, Low JK, Logge W, et al. Chronic cannabidiol treatment improves social and object recognition in double transgenic APPswe/PSIΔ E9 mice. Psychopharmacology. 2014b;231:3009–17.
138. Bielawiec P, Harasim-Symbor E, Konstantynowicz-Nowick K, et al. Chronic Cannabidiol administration attenuates skeletal muscle de novo ceramide synthesis pathway and related metabolic effects in a rat model of high-fat diet-induced obesity. Biomol Ther. 2020;10(9):1241.
139. Watt G, Karl T. In vivo evidence for therapeutic properties of cannabidiol (CBD) for Alzheimer's Disease. Front Pharmacol. 2017;8:20.

140. De Ternay J, Naassila M, Nourredine M, et al. Therapeutic prospects of cannabidiol for alcohol use disorder and alcohol-related damages on the liver and the brain. Front Pharmacol. 2019;10:627.
141. Dos-Santos-Pereira M, Guimaraes FS, Del-Bel E, et al. Cannabidiol prevents LPS-induced microglial inflammation by inhibiting ROS/NF-κB-dependent signaling and glucose consumption. Glia. 2020;68(3):561–73.
142. Kaplan J. What is the GPR55 receptor and why is it important in CBD's benefits? April 4, 2018. Leafly. Available at: https://www.leafly.com/news/science-tech/health-benefits-cbd-on-g-protein-coupled-receptor-55. Accessed 3 Dec 2019.
143. Lupia CR, Hu Y, Devinsky O, et al. Cannabinoids as hippocampal network administrators. Neuropharmacology. 2017;124:25–37.
144. Mecha M, Torrao AS, Mestre L, et al. Cannabidiol protects oligodendrocyte progenitor cells from inflammation-induced apoptosis by attenuating endoplasmic reticulum stress. Cell Death Dis. 2012;3:e331.
145. Hampson AJ, Grimaldi M, Axelrod J, Wink D. Cannabidiol and (–) Δ9-tetrahydrocannabinol are neuroprotective antioxidants. Proc Natl Acad Sci U S A. 1998;95:8268–73.
146. Rajan TS, De Nicola GR, Iori R, et al. Anticancer activity of glucomoringin isothiocyanate in human malignant astrocytoma cells. Fitotherapia. 2016;110:1–7.
147. Lee WS, Erdelyi K, Matyas C, et al. Cannabidiol limits T cell-mediated chronic autoimmune myocarditis: implications to autoimmune disorders and organ transplantation. Mol Med. 2016;22:136–46.
148. Necela BM, Su W, Thompson EA. Toll-like receptor 4 mediates cross-talk between peroxisome proliferator-activated receptor γ and nuclear factor-κB in macrophages. Immunology. 2008;125:344–58.
149. Kozela E, Juknat A, Kaushansky N, et al. Cannabidiol, a non-psychoactive cannabinoid, leads to EGR2-dependent anergy in activated encephalitogenic T cells. J Neuroinflammation. 2015;12:52.
150. Juknat A, Pietr M, Kozela E, et al. Differential transcriptional profiles mediated by exposure to the cannabinoids cannabidiol and Δ-9 tetrahydrocannabinol in BV-2 microglial cells. Br J Pharmacol. 2012;165:2512–28.
151. Esposito G, De Filippis D, Maiuri MC, et al. Cannabidiol inhibits inducible nitric oxide synthase protein expression and nitric oxide production in β-amyloid stimulated PC12 neurons through p38MAP kinase and NF-κB involvement. Neurosci Lett. 2006b;399:91–5.
152. Campos A, Brant F, Miranda A, et al. Cannabidiol increases survival and promotes rescue of cognitive function in a murine model of cerebral malaria. Neuroscience. 2015;289:166–80.
153. Campos AC, Fogaça MV, Sonego AB, Guimarães FS. Cannabidiol, neuroprotection and neuropsychiatric disorders. Pharmacol Res. 2016;12:119–27.
154. Damstra-Oddy J, Warren EC, Perry CJ, et al. Phytocannabinoid-dependent mTORC1 regulation is dependent upon IPMK activity. Br J Pharmacol. 2021;178(5):1149–63. https://doi.org/10.1111/bph.15351.
155. Cao C, Li Y, Liu H, et al. The potential therapeutic effects of THC on Alzheimer's Disease. J Alzheimers Dis. 2014;42:973–84.
156. Eubanks LM, Rogers CJ, Beuscher AE, et al. A molecular link between the active component of marijuana and Alzheimer's disease pathology. Mol Pharm. 2006;3:773–7.
157. Suliman NA, Taib CNM, Moklas M, Basir R. Delta-9-Tetrahydrocannabinol (Δ-9THC) induce neurogenesis and improve cognitive performances of male Sprague Dawley rats. Neurotox Res. 2018;33(2):402–11.
158. Bilkei-Gorzo A, Albayram O, Draffehn A, et al. A chronic low dose of Δ9-tetrahydrocannabinol (THC) restores cognitive function in old mice. Nat Med. 2017;23(6):782–7.
159. Wolf SA, Bick-Sander A, Fabel L, et al. Cannabinoid receptor CB1 mediates baseline and activity-induced survival of new neurons in adult hippocampal neurogenesis. Cell Commun Signal. 2010;8(1):12.
160. Zieba J, Sinclair D, Sebree T. Cannabidiol (CBD) reduces anxiety-related behavior in mice via an FMRP-independent mechanism. Pharmacol Biochem Behav. 2019;181:93–100.

161. Al-Ghezi ZZ, Busbee PB, Alghetaa H, et al. Combination of cannabinoids, delta-9-tetrahydrocannabinol (THC) and cannabidiol (CBD), mitigates experimental autoimmune encephalomyelitis (EAE) by altering the gut microbiome. Brain Behav Immun. 2019;82:25–35.
162. Aso E, Alexandre SP, Esteban VL, et al. Cannabis-based medicine reduces multiple pathological processes in AβPP/PSI mice. J Alzheimers Dis. 2015;43(3):977–92.
163. Aso E, Pol Andres B, Isidro F. Delineating the efficacy of a cannabis-based medicine at advanced stages of dementia in a murine model. J Alzheimers Dis. 2016;54(3):903–12.
164. Feliu A, Moreno-Martet M, Mecha M, et al. A Sativex (R) – like combination of phytocannabinoids as a disease=modifying therapy in a viral model of multiple sclerosis. Br J Pharmacol. 2015;172:3579–95.
165. Casarejos MJ, et al. Natural cannabinoids improve dopamine neurotransmission and tau and amyloid pathology in a mouse model of tauopathy. J Alzheimers Dis. 2013;35:525–39.
166. Bloomfield MAP, Green SF, Hindocha C, et al. The effects of acute cannabidiol on cerebral blood flow and its relationship to memory: an arterial spin labelling magnetic resonance imaging study. J Psychopharmacol. 2020;34(9):981–9.
167. van den Elsen GA, et al. Effects of tetrahydrocannabinol on balance and gait in patients with dementia: a randomised controlled crossover trial. J Psychopharmacol. 2017;31(2):184–91.
168. van den Elsen GA. Tetrahydrocannabinol for neuropsychiatric symptoms in dementia: a randomized controlled trial. Neurology. 2015a;84(23):2338–46.
169. van den Elsen GA. Tetrahydrocannabinol in behavioral disturbances in dementia: a crossover randomized controlled trial. Am J Geriatr Psychiatry. 2015b;23(12):1214–24.
170. Shelef A, Barak Y, Berger U, et al. Safety and efficacy of medical cannabis oil for behavioral and psychological symptoms of dementia: an-open label, add-on, pilot study. J Alzheimers Dis. 2016;51(1):15–9.
171. Volicer L, et al. Effects of dronabinol on anorexia and disturbed behavior in patients with Alzheimer's disease. Int J Geriatr Psychiatry. 1997;12(9):913–9.
172. Walther S, Mahlberg R, Eichmann U, Kunz D. Delta-9-tetrahydrocannabinol for nighttime agitation in severe dementia. Psychopharmacology (Berlin). 2006;185:524.
173. Broers B, Pata Z, Mina A, et al. Prescription of a THC/CBD-based medication to patients with dementia: a pilot study in Geneva. Med Cannabis Cannabinoids. 2019;2:56–9.
174. Timler A, Bulsara C, Bulsara M, et al. Use of cannabinoid-based medicine among older residential care recipients diagnosed with dementia: study protocol for a double-blind randomised crossover trial. Trials. 2020;21:188.
175. Walther S, Schupbach B, Seifritz E, et al. Randomized, controlled crossover trial of dronabinol, 2.5 mg, for agitation in 2 patients with dementia. J Clin Psychopharmacol. 2011;31(2):256–8.
176. Cheng Y, Dong Z, Liu S. β-Caryophyllene ameliorates the Alzheimer-like phenotype in APP/PS1 Mice through CB2 receptor activation and the PPARγ pathway. Pharmacology. 2014c;94(1–2):1–12.
177. Calabro S, Naro A, De Luca R, et al. PEALut efficacy in mild cognitive impairment: evidence from a SPECT case study! Aging Clin Exp Res. 2016;28:1279–82.
178. Frye CA. Neurosteroids' effects and mechanisms for social, cognitive, emotional, and physical functions. Psychoneuroendocrinology. 2009;34(Suppl 1):S143–61.
179. Petrosino S, Schiano MA. Palmitoylethanolamide: a nutritional approach to keep neuroinflammation within physiological boundaries-a systematic review. Int J Mol Sci. 2020;21(24):e9526.
180. Leishman E, Manchanda M, Thelen R, et al. Cannabidiol's upregulation of N-acyl ethanolamines in the central nervous system requires N-Acyl Phosphatidyl Ethanolamine-Specific Phospholipase D. Cannabis Cannabinoid Res. 2018;3(1):228–41.
181. Leggett JD, Beckett SRG, D'Antona AM, et al. Oleamide is a selective endogenous agonist of rat and human $CB_1$ cannabinoid receptors. Br J Pharmacol. 2004;141(2):253–62.
182. Cole GM, Ma Q-L, Frautschy SA. Omega-3 fatty acids and dementia. Prostaglandins Leukot Essent Fat Acids. 2009;81(2–3):213–21.
183. Canhada S, Castro K, Schweigert Perry I, Luft VC. Omega-3 fatty acids' supplementation in Alzheimer's disease: a systematic review. Nutr Neurosci. 2018;21(8):529–38.

184. McDougle DR, Watson JE, Abdeen AA, et al. Anti-inflammatory ω-3 endocannabinoid epoxides. Proc Natl Acad Sci U S A. 2017;114(30):E6034–43.
185. Jahnabi Roy, et al. Antitumorigenic properties of omega-3 endocannabinoid epoxides. J Med Chem. 2018;61:5569–79.
186. Janson J, Laedtke T, Parisi JE, et al. Increased risk of type 2 diabetes in Alzheimer disease. Diabetes. 2004;53(2):474–81.
187. Ota M, Matsuo J, Ishida I, et al. Effects of a medium-chain triglyceride-based ketogenic formula on cognitive function in patients with mild-to-moderate Alzheimer's disease. Neurosci Lett. 2019;690:232–6.
188. Valenzuela PL, Castillo-García A, Morales JS, et al. Exercise benefits on Alzheimer's disease: State-of-the-science. Ageing Res Rev. 2020;62:101108.
189. Lafourcade M, et al. Nutritional omega-3 deficiency abolishes endocannabinoid-mediated neuronal functions. Nat Neurosci. 2011;14(3):345–50.
190. Huang CH, et al. Dietary ω-6/ω-3 Polyunsaturated fatty acid ratios affect the homeostasis of Th/Treg cells in mice with dextran sulfate sodium-induced colitis. J Parenter Enter Nutr. 2017b;41(4):647–56.
191. Navarro-Romero A, et al. Cannabinoid type-1 receptor blockade restores neurological phenotypes in two models for Down syndrome. Neurobiol Dis. 2019;125:92–106.
192. Pacheco JC, et al. Cannabidiol as a treatment for mental health outcomes among health care workers during the coronavirus disease pandemic. J Clin Psychopharmacol. 2021;41(3):327–9.
193. Hermush O. An 81-year-old male with advanced dementia and recurrent cerebrovascular events: is there a place for cannabidiol therapy? Isr Med Assoc J. 2019;21(11):759–60.

# 10 Autism Spectrum Disorder

## Introduction

Autism spectrum disorder (ASD) is a complex behavioral condition beginning in early childhood and continuing throughout life [1]. ASD is characterized by deficits in communication and social functioning and interaction, restricted and stereotypic or repetitive behaviors, restricted patterns of interest, sensory issues, and a marked preference for behavioral and environmental consistency [1–5]. It also has several comorbidities which need to be kept in mind. The pathophysiology is complex, multifactorial, and not completely understood, with genetic and environmental factors involved. There is no successful treatment for ASD. However, there is a growing body of research that medicinal cannabis might be useful in the treatment of some of the behavioral aspects of this disorder.

**This Chapter**
In this chapter, we will explore the characteristics of ASD, its prevalence, the various comorbidities, orthodox treatment, and its pathophysiology. We will then look at how the endocannabinoid system is involved in ASD, evidence of efficacy of treatment of ASD with medicinal cannabis, and the mechanisms of action by which cannabidiol in particular might work.

## What Is Autism Spectrum Disorder?

ASD is characterized by deficits in communication and social functioning and interaction (e.g., in social-emotional reciprocity; in developing, maintaining, and understanding relationships; in nonverbal communicative behaviors used in social interactions), restricted and stereotypic or repetitive behaviors, restricted patterns of interest, and sensory issues (e.g., extreme responses to certain sounds/textures, fascination with lights or spinning objects) and a marked preference for behavioral and environmental consistency [1–5].



K. O'Brien, P. Blair, *Medicinal Cannabis and CBD in Mental Healthcare*,
https://doi.org/10.1007/978-3-030-78559-8_10

Various authors describe three main symptom/sign behavior domains where there are deficits in ASD:

- Communication and speech
- Repetitive, compulsive behaviors with restricted interests
- Social impairment [4]

In ASD, deficits in social domain functioning are evidenced by particular behaviors including lack of social/emotional reciprocity, lack of mutual enjoyment of social activities, reduced ability to hold conversations, lack of eye contact, and others [4]. In particular, there is an atypical reward system functioning in those with ASD [1]. Children and adults with ASD look less at social stimuli than non-social stimuli [6–8], and functional MRI studies show lower activity in the ventral striatum area of the brain in response to social stimuli [9]. The autism-like characteristics are considered to exist on a spectrum of features and intensity, hence the name ASD.

The behavioral characteristics typically emerge within the first 4 years of life, and whilst it seems that most of the behavioral abnormalities associated with ASD tend to appear between 12 and 48 months, some have a much earlier onset. For example, sensory problems including extreme responses to sounds may appear as early as 7 months. Other behaviors, like disengagement of visual attention, occur later, appearing around 12–14 months [1].

## Prevalence

ASD has substantial clinical and pathogenetic heterogeneity, with the distribution seen as a dimensional continuum across the general population. Worldwide prevalence is around 1% [10], with a higher prevalence in males compared with females—US surveillance data (2010) indicated an overall prevalence of ASD of 14.7 per 1000 (male/female ratio 4.5:1) [11].

There is a much higher incidence of ASD in siblings of children already diagnosed, ranging from 15% to 25% [1, 12].

## Associated Comorbidities

Of those with ASD, 70% have associated comorbidities [13]. These include:

- Intellectual disability (65%)
- ADHD (40–70%)
- Seizures (30%)
- Sleep disorders (40–80%)
- Motor dysfunctions
- Metabolic and gastrointestinal disturbances (including constipation) (in children: 9–91%)

- Mood disorders, anxiety disorders (42–56%)
- Depression, psychosis, and obsessive-compulsive disorders
- Addictive behaviors (e.g., Internet, video gaming, watching TV)
- Self-injury (35–60%) [1, 10, 14–30]

**Sleep Disorders**

Sleep disorders are common in ASD, and 40–80% of children with ASD will experience sleep problems (this figure is around 25–40% in normally developing children) [16].

As we saw in a previous chapter on insomnia, sleep is very important for the developing child including brain development (including synaptic pruning) and cognition and memory consolidation. Thus, sleep disturbances in a child with ASD are particularly serious, with insufficient sleep shown to exacerbate ASD symptoms including social behaviors (such as communication problems) and maladaptive behaviors such as aggression and tantrums [16]. Reduced amounts of sleep are associated with more severe symptoms in children with ASD [31].

**Gastrointestinal Disorders**

Various reports indicate the prevalence of gastrointestinal (GI) disorders in children with ASD is anywhere between 9% and 91% [17]. GI conditions including constipation, diarrhea, food allergies, and malabsorption or maldigestion problems occur more frequently in children with ASD (than in children without ASD) [23, 32]. A review of studies on this topic concluded that cognitive deficits in ASD are clearly related to GI disturbances, at least in certain groups [23].

**ADHD and ASD**

Interestingly, ASD and ADHD can co-occur and share genetic risk factors, and there is overlap in some of their features, as well as distinctions, including in neuroanatomical findings [14]. Approximately 15–25% of youth with ADHD demonstrate ASD symptoms [33, 34], and 12.4% have an ASD diagnosis [35]. In children with ADHD, higher levels of ASD symptoms are associated with a more severe phenotype including higher levels of oppositional, conduct, and anxiety symptoms, lower IQ, deficits in working memory, and general motor problems [33].

## ASD and Reduced Mortality

People with ASD have higher risk of premature mortality, including all-cause mortality and disease-specific mortality across several International Classification of Diseases (ICD) disease categories [36]. A matched case-cohort study found that premature mortality is significantly increased in ASD (odds ratio 2.56 for all-causes), with average lifespan reduced by around 16 years (compared to the general population). The study found that mortality was increased in both low- and high-functioning ASD and in both males and females. Low-functioning ASD was associated with higher mortality compared with high-functioning ASD for mental and behavioral disorders; diseases of nervous, circulatory, respiratory, and digestive systems; and congenital malformations. Across the whole ASD cohort, females with low-functioning ASD were particularly at risk; mortality risk was nine times higher than the general population [36]. Other studies have also found higher death rates associated with ASD [37] and a higher mortality rate in females with ASD compared with males with ASD [37, 38].

## Prenatal, Perinatal, and Neonatal Risk Factors for ASD

Several risk factors have been identified for ASD; however, no cause-effect relationship has been established. These include gestational diabetes, vaginal bleeding in the first trimester, viral infections, fungal infections, meconium in amniotic fluid, and starting medications during pregnancy [39]. Won et al. [39] divide these up into three subcategories:

- Prenatal risk factors: advanced maternal and paternal ages, primiparous women, bleeding, medication, and diabetes
- Perinatal risk factors: induced labor, preterm birth, breech presentation, caesarean section
- Neonatal factors: low birthweight and size and poor conditions at birth (hypoxia, hyperbilirubinemia, encephalopathy, birth defects)

Several genetic and environmental factors have been identified as possible etiological agents, discussed shortly.

## Treatment

There are no established effective primary treatments available to reverse or prevent ASD. Most treatments address behavioral symptoms and learning deficits. Pharmaceuticals are used mainly to treat aggressive behavior and irritability and include antipsychotics, selective serotonin reuptake inhibitors, and stimulants [10]. Pharmaceuticals, of course, often have undesirable side effects. There is clearly room for other therapeutic options.

### Qualifying Medical Condition in US States

ASD is recognized as a medical condition that qualifies for treatment with medicinal cannabis in 15 states of the USA including the territory of Puerto Rico. It may also be recommended by doctors for the treatment of ASD in the following states: California, Michigan, Massachusetts, Oklahoma, Oregon, and the District of Columbia [40] (http://www.mammausa.org/autism-friendly-states.html).

## Etiology and Pathogenesis of Autism Spectrum Disorder

The etiology and pathomechanism of ASD are complex. It appears that altered neurodevelopment during pregnancy and early childhood occurs and genetic, epigenetic, and environmental factors are also involved in its etiology [41–44]. Various studies support the contention that ASD transmission is polygenic (3–15 alleles per individual), along with gene-gene and/or gene-environment (epigenetic) effects [42].

The pathogenesis involves many disparate mechanisms. Research supports the following factors: involvement of atypical development of neural connectivity, mutations in genes, chronic neuroinflammation, immune system dysregulation, microglial activation, GABAergic imbalance, monoaminergic dysregulation, mitochondrial dysregulation, abnormal endocannabinoid tone, and abnormal endocannabinoid signaling [1, 45–52].

We will look at some of the factors that are thought to be involved in the pathogenesis of ASD in this section. However, Bourgeron [53] points out something important: ASD should not be considered a single entity but as a continuum, and it might be better to give up the idea that there is a single defining dysfunction occurring in the brains of those with ASD and, instead, simply try to understand the many factors involved in this disorder. When we look later at the endocannabinoid system involvement in ASD, and knowing how far-reaching the involvement of the endocannabinoid system is broadly within our brains and bodies more generally as a neuroregulatory system, it makes you wonder if the endocannabinoid system might in some ways be a vital link in connecting up all the pathomechanisms that appear to underlie ASD.

### Neuroanatomical Findings

Research indicates that in ASD, there is an increase in total brain volume or increased intracranial volume [54, 55] (though this does not occur uniformly) and increased head circumference [54, 56] and evidence that increased brain volume occurs early in development of the child [54].

Brain volumetric changes have been found in both gray and white matter, though research findings are inconsistent [56]. Some researchers have found that the early brain growth occurs prior to age 2, others have found cortical enlargement occurring at age 2 and 4–5 years, some have found persistent brain enlargement in adolescence and adulthood, and others have found that white matter development is abnormally slow and there is overgrowth of gray matter during adolescence (see Stigler and McDougle [56] for the studies). Neuroimaging of infants at high risk of familial ASD (in comparison with low-risk infants) revealed hyper-expansion of the cortical surface area between 6 and 12 months which preceded brain volume overgrowth between 12 and 24 months in 15 high-risk infants who were diagnosed with ASD at

24 months. The brain volume overgrowth was associated with emergence as well as severity of the social deficits of ASD [54].

Changes have been found in many brain regions in ASD, many of which are set out in Table 10.1 (summarized from studies in Antshel et al. [14], Stigler and McDougle [56], Doherty et al. [57]). This variation may reinforce our understanding of ASD as a syndrome with multivariate pathophysiology as well as clinical manifestations. From this list, we can see that the functions associated with these brain regions are affected in people with ASD. There have been volumetric changes

**Table 10.1** Brain neuroanatomical changes in ASD

| Brain region | Evidence from various studies: Enlargement (↑), decrease (↓) or no change (–) in volume |
|---|---|
| Total brain volume | ↑ |
| Left middle/superior temporal gyrus (region important for language and social communications) (gray matter) | ↑ |
| Frontal lobe | ↑ |
| Frontal-parietal regions (relevant to motor functions in children, particularly postcentral gyrus) | ↑ |
| Dorsolateral prefrontal cortex | ↑ |
| Medial prefrontal cortex | ↑ |
| Orbitofrontal cortex | –/↓ |
| Hippocampus (integration of information, associative learning) | ↑/↓/– |
| Insula (integrates several neurocognitive systems related to empathetic, affective, and interoceptive processes) | **↓ (gray matter)** |
| Amygdala (plays a role in emotional and social behavior and motivation) | ↑/↓ |
| Striatum | ↑ |
| Caudate nucleus (part of basal ganglia involved in executive function, role in repetitive behaviors) | ↑ |
| Inferior frontal gyrus (involved in memory, sentence comprehension) | ↓ |
| Brainstem (involved in sensory modulation) | ↓/– |
| Thalamus (language and emotional processing, role in executive function) | –/↑ |
| Fusiform gyrus (involved in face processing) | ↑/↓/– |
| Superior temporal gyrus (involved in processing of eye movements) | **↓ (gray matter)** |
| Planum temporale (involved in auditory processing, receptive language) | ↑/↓ |
| Anterior cingulate cortex (integration of cognition and emotion and behavioral expression integration) | ↓ |
| Cerebellum (motor coordination, language, emotion, executive function) | **↑/↓ (total volume)**<br>**↑ or ↓ (vermal region)** |
| Corpus callosum (white matter microstructure) | ↓/– |
| Superior longitudinal fasciculus (white matter microstructure) | ↓ |

Summaries of findings of studies in Antshel et al. [14], Doherty et al. [57], Stigler and McDougle [56]

in both white and gray matter in various brain regions found in ASD [56]. In general, there is an increase in total brain volume and increase in volume/size in several areas of the brain associated with ASD. However, in some brain areas, there are discrepancies between study findings with some finding evidence of an increase and others finding evidence of reduction or no change in volume in ASD compared with healthy controls [14, 56, 57]. Abnormalities in cortical thickness may be age-related, with studies of children with ASD finding evidence of increased cortical thickness and studies in adolescents and adults with ASD finding evidence of cortical thinning in certain brain areas, e.g., temporal, parietal, and frontal lobes (see Stigler and McDougle [56]).

Whilst a complete discussion of the neuroanatomical changes occurring in ASD is beyond the scope of this chapter (readers are referred to Antshel et al. [14], Doherty et al. [57], and Stigler and McDougle [56]), we will just choose a couple of examples to demonstrate how changes in particular brain regions appear to be associated with characteristics of ASD.

**Caudate Nucleus and Repetitive Behavior**

The caudate nucleus is part of the basal ganglia that are involved in executive function and is thought to play a role in the repetitive, stereotypic behaviors associated with ASD [58]. Various studies have found ASD to be associated with an increase in volume of the caudate nucleus in adults and children, with volume positively associated with repetitive behavior [56, 58].

**Alterations in Fronto-striatal Circuitry and Inflexible Behavior**

Changes in fronto-striatal circuitry that supports flexible behavior may underpin the restricted and repetitive behaviors, the clear preference for behavioral and environmental consistency, and rigid adherence to preferred behavioral patterns, characteristics of ASD. As explained by D'Cruz et al. [3], flexible behavior requires decision-making and response planning as well as processing of reinforcement cues. A functional magnetic resonance imaging (fMRI) study in 17 people with ASD and 23 controls (age-, gender-, and IQ-matched) assessed behavioral flexibility on using two- and four-choice reversal learning tasks during fMRI. In controls, activation usually increased in both dorsal and ventromedial frontal systems when the correct choice after reversal was uncertain and when a four-choice reversal learning task was used. What they found in this study was that when the choice outcome after reversal was uncertain, there was *decreased* activation in the frontal cortex and ventral striatum in the ASD group. When the outcomes of new responses were certain, there was no difference between the ASD group and controls. The decreased activation in the frontal cortex suggests problems in decision-making and planning of responses, whilst the decreased activation in the ventral striatum suggests problems in processing reinforcement cues [3].

**Anterior Cingulate-Ventral Striatum-Thalamic Pathway and Dysfunctional Reward System**

In typical adults, social rewards elicit greater saccadic eye movement deviation (saccadic eye movements are the movements from one point to another) and greater gaze duration bias and thus this would seem to indicate that social rewards have greater salience and value in comparison on non-social rewards [59]. In ASD, reduced preference for social rewards has been observed [59]. Alterations in the anterior cingulate-ventral striatum-thalamic pathway are implicated in ASD: abnormalities in sensory stimuli processing and gross motor function and reward system deficits and stereotypies suggest that there is impairment of the caudate, putamen, and thalamus and striatal involvement [60]. Humans preferentially look longer at socially rewarding stimuli, and gaze fixation has been linked to striatal activity [1, 59, 61]. Functional MRI studies have demonstrated lower activity in the ventral striatum in response to social stimuli in those with ASD compared with controls [9]. The dopamine system has been implicated in reward-related functions and primate research has demonstrated that reward-dependent modulation of saccadic eye movements is dependent on dopamine-induced changes in caudate nucleus neuronal activity [62].

For more information on the neuroanatomical changes found in ASD, see Antshel et al. [14] and Stigler and McDougle [56]. For a comparison with changes found in brain regions in ADHD, see Doherty et al. [57].

## Abnormal Connectivity and Signalling of Neuronal Networks

Synaptic plasticity has been defined as "the property of synapses to strengthen or weaken in response to changes in both the amplitude and the temporal dynamics of neuronal activity" [53]. Sensory inputs and intrinsic brain activity can alter number of synapses and increase or decrease neuronal connectivity [53].

Altered connectivity of neuronal networks is thought to underpin ASD. ASD-derived neurons showed abnormal neurogenesis and reduced synaptogenesis, leading to functional deficits in neuronal networks [63].

### Dysgenesis of Dendritic Spines

Dendritic spines are small protrusions from dendrites and are the major postsynaptic sites of excitatory glutaminergic synapses—excitatory synapses form on the head of the spine [64, 65]. Spines have variable shapes, changing size and shape in response to synaptic activity (in other words, they are adaptable and responsive, not static) [65]. Many ASD risk genes alter cellular pathways which intersect at postsynaptic glutaminergic synapses, and this implicates abnormalities in dendritic spines in ASD [66]. This is supported by studies in individuals with autism-related disorders which demonstrate dysgenesis and abnormalities of dendritic spines, including reduced dendritic spine density, and spine dysgenesis has been confirmed in experimental mouse models of these syndromes [65, 67]. Studies in mice models of Fragile X ("fmr1 knockout mice") show immature dendritic spines, and Fragile X patients with intellectual disability have been found to have altered dendritic spine morphology (longer or shorter, thinner and fewer than normally developing individuals) [39]. Fragile X is understood as the most common genetic cause of ASD.

We will discuss dendritic spines again in relation to disturbances of signaling pathways shortly.

**Disturbed Signaling Pathways Involved in ASD Pathology**

Insulin-like growth factor 1 (IGF-1) has been implicated in the pathology of ASD. So too has the mammalian target of rapamycin (mTOR, a central regulator of many cell processes including growth, proliferation, autophagy, translation, and actin polymerization) as well as phosphatidylinositol 3-kinases (PI3K, a downstream target of IGF-1 which regulates many cellular operations including growth, differentiation, motility, survival, intracellular transport) and the serine/threonine kinase AKT (which is a central node in cell signaling downstream of growth factors, cytokines, and other stimuli and plays an important role in various cell functions including survival, growth, proliferation, cell migration, and angiogenesis) [68–70].

Disturbance of the IGF-1/PI3K/AKT/mTOR pathway is likely to be involved in the pathophysiology of ASD [68]. Animal and human research points to the likelihood that decreased IGF-1 signaling is involved, particularly in ASD impairment of myelination, neuron development, and synaptic function [68]. Children with ASD have been found to have decreased IGF-1 levels in cerebrospinal fluid [71]. Children with ASD have been shown to have abnormal myelination which is regulated by IGF-1 (e.g., Steinman and Mankuta [72]). For more information on this pathway's involvement in ASD, see Chen et al. [68].

**Dysfunction of mTOR in ASD**

As discussed previously, the mTOR plays a central role in regulation of many cell processes, including growth, proliferation, autophagy, translation, and actin polymerization [69]. The mTOR signaling pathways are present at synapses and can influence dendritic spine development and synaptic plasticity [69]. Dysregulation of mTOR signaling is a key biological pathway involved in autism-relevant behaviors [69].

Overactivity of mTOR has been found in several autism-related conditions, and in mice models of such diseases, treatment with rapamycin (inhibitor of mTOR) was found to reverse the autism-related disorder phenotypes [65, 73]. mTOR forms two different complexes, mTORC1 (sensitive to rapamycin, believed to regulate mRNA translation rates) and mTORC2 (insensitive to rapamycin and a regulator of embryonic development, actin cytoskeleton activity, synaptic efficacy, and long-term memory consolidation), and dysregulation of both complexes has been implicated in memory disorders and the cognitive deficits of various ASDs [69]. Altered mTORC2 has been found associated with cognitive deficits in other diseases such as Parkinson's disease and Alzheimer's disease [69]. Several ASD syndromes are caused by mutations in genes that inhibit mTOR kinase [66].

Evidence suggests that in ASD, dysfunctional mTOR signaling is associated with synaptic (dendritic) spine abnormalities and abnormal synaptic plasticity [65, 66, 69], and this may be the common denominator in the various autism-related disorders [65]. In ASD there is a loss of balance between synaptic protein synthesis and breakdown (autophagy) which is needed for homeostasis and plasticity, and mTOR signaling is critically involved [66].

Overactive mTOR may result in excessive synaptic protein synthesis and inhibit autophagy. Normal neuronal autophagy is essential for spine pruning during postnatal development plus normal social behavior. Neuronal autophagy-deficient mice demonstrate mTOR overactivity that underlies ASD-like synaptic pathology. Inhibition of autophagy was found to be associated with inhibition of normal spine pruning, and when it was corrected by pharmacological blockade of mTOR, dendritic spine pruning deficits and social behaviors were normalized, mainly via activating neuronal autophagy [66]. Other studies have shown ASD brains to be deficient in autophagic mitochondrial turnover [74]. Postmortem human studies have found significantly higher spine density in adolescents with ASD compared with controls, with significantly less synaptic pruning occurring in ASD brains during childhood and adolescence compared with controls; in addition a negative correlation between spine density and mTOR-dependent autophagy during childhood and adolescence has been demonstrated [66].

In ASD, a dysregulation of mTOR may also underlie the reduced life expectancy in this disorder. Regulation of autophagy exerts a significant effect on lifespan, well studied in the nematode *C. elegans* and in rodents. Since autophagic degradation declines with age, damaged proteins and organelles could accumulate leading to cellular senescence and premature death [75]. Impaired autophagy may be the case for other diseases like diabetes, cardiovascular disease, cancer, and neurodegenerative diseases like Alzheimer Aβ (reviewed in Saha et al. [76]).

For a greater insight into the various pathways involved, see Huber et al. [69], Phillips and Pozzo-Miller [65], and Tang et al. [66].

**Brain-Derived Neurotrophic Factor**

Neurotrophic factors play a critical role in regulating neuronal maturation including synaptic synthesis [77]. Brain-derived neurotrophic factor (BDNF) is of particular importance in ASD. BDNF is a key neurotrophin which regulates synaptic plasticity, neuronal differentiation, and neuronal survival in the brain [67, 77]. BDNF participates in dendritic and axonal differentiation during embryonic neuronal development and in the formation and maturation of dendritic spines postnatally [64]. BDNF inhibits apoptosis and stimulates sprouting and neuronal reorganization [67]. Tyrosine kinase receptor B (TrkB) and p75 neurotrophin receptor (p75NTR, a member of the TNF receptor family) mediate the actions of BDNF [67]. BDNF, its receptor, TrkB, and the proteins involved in their signaling pathways affecting dendritic spine protein synthesis and stability are involved with neuritogenesis and have been implicated in ASD [48]. Neuritogenesis is the process by which new neurites (dendrites and axons) are formed in the brain.

Significantly elevated plasma levels of BDNF have been found in boys with ASD compared with matched controls [77]. A more recent meta-analysis of 19 studies (2896 participants) confirmed this, finding that children with ASD have significantly increased blood levels of BDNF compared with healthy children [78]. However, not all studies have found changes in BDNF: in a study conducted in

India, serum BDNF levels were significantly higher in atypical autistic children (this was a milder phenotype of autism) but not in typical ASD children (the more severe phenotype) compared with healthy normal children [67]. They also found that BDNF levels were significantly lower in Rett syndrome (the most severe, X-linked form of typical autism) compared with controls. They surmised that lower levels of BDNF might indicate impairment of neuroprotective mechanisms and higher levels might imply a manifested protective response [67]. At least one other study, in central Saudi Arabia, also found that serum BDNF levels were significantly lower in ASD children [79].

## Genes

Although several studies indicate that ASD is heritable, ASD heritability plays a relatively minor role [80] and appears to account for 10–20% of ASD cases [81]. Thus, interest has turned to environmental factors and their role in pathogenesis which we will discuss shortly. In this section, we will look at a few ways in which genetic alterations appear to be involved in ASD.

**Fragile X Syndrome (FXS)**

Fragile X syndrome (FXS) is an X-linked dominant disorder understood as the most common genetic cause of ASD, where there is a loss of expression of the fragile mental retardation protein (FMRP) which regulates signal transduction at metabotropic glutamate receptor-5 in the brain [82, 83]. Symptoms and signs associated with FXS include ADS (60%), anxiety (80%), social avoidance (80%), stereotypic behaviors (80%), social avoidance (80%), ADHD (70%), intellectual disability (85% males and 25% females), sleep disorders (40%), aggression (40%), epilepsy (16%) and macro-orchidism (90% adults), prominent ears (60%), long faces (60%), soft skin (50%), and hyperextensible joints (60% children) [83].

FMRP plays a key role in regulation of translation of many messenger RNAs that are involved in synaptic plasticity, and its absence is associated with intellectual deficits [83]. It is the deficiency of this FMRP that is thought to increase neuronal excitability (Jung et al. 2021). Mice studies have shown metabotropic glutamate receptor-5 (mGlu5)-dependent long-term depression at excitatory synapses in the prefrontal cortex and ventral striatum (which is mediated by 2-AG) is absent in FMRP-null mice [82]. Males with FXS are more severely affected than females as the single X chromosome in males is typically fully methylated and not producing FMRP, whereas in females, there is usually some FMRP that is expressed from the FMR1 gene on the other X chromosome (which isn't affected)—this explains why FXS males are more likely to have greater intellectual and developmental disabilities than females [83].

Research has shown that the mRNA levels of several genes were significantly increased in ASD, including members of the glutamate system (excitatory amino acid transporter 1 and glutamate receptor AMPA 1), whilst abnormalities in other molecules in the glutamate system were also found (e.g., glutamate receptor binding proteins). AMPA-type glutamate receptor density was also found to be significantly reduced in the cerebellum in those with ASD [84].

**Genetic Alterations in Glucuronidation Pathway**
Genetic aberrations in the glucuronidation pathway may also compromise individuals toward ASD by preventing metabolism and excretion of drugs or environmental substances. This could be either at the enzyme or substrate level. Some studies have shown decreased glucuronidation function in ASD [85, 86].

**ASD-Risk Genes**
Recent genetic studies in ASD implicate "risk genes" which are key regulators of synaptic plasticity, and many of these encode a variety of different proteins (e.g., synaptic scaffolding proteins, receptors, cell adhesion molecules, and proteins involved in chromatin remodeling and transcription, protein synthesis and degradation, and actin cytoskeleton). Changes in these proteins can alter synaptic strength and/or number of synapses and thereby neuronal connectivity [53]. Animal studies have demonstrated that many ASD-risk genes participate in synaptic plasticity, altering synaptic strength and/or number, and that genetic mutations impact on neuronal networks, causing hyper- or hypo-activity and increased or decreased synaptic density [53].

Bourgeron [53] reports that the majority of ASD-related genetic mutations result in increased gene transcription and mRNA translation, something seen when there is increased neuronal activity. He suggests that such mutations may cause increased synaptic strength or synapse numbers within particular neuronal networks and that this might explain why patients with ASD have a higher risk of epilepsy, as well as findings in ASD sufferers of ectopic synapses [53].

**Genetic Mutations, Synaptic Homeostatic Mechanisms, and ASD**
The body has homeostatic mechanisms to ensure that synaptic strength, number, and size and therefore neuronal firing remain in balance. There are several mechanisms, one of which is synaptic scaling (which involves voltage-gated calcium channels and proteins such as BDNF and tissue necrosis factor), whilst others work via altering neuronal excitability [53]. Bourgeron [53] hypothesizes that in a subset of ASD patients with genetic mutations, the process of synaptic homeostasis cannot counterbalance the effects of genetic mutations on synaptic activity. Consequently, there is either hyper- or hypo-activity of neurons. He also suggests that abnormal sprouting or pruning of synapses due to mutations may lead to abnormal coordination as well as competition between neuronal networks, which may explain why those with ASD have trouble integrating information from different sensory modalities.

**Genetic Alterations in Neurexins and Neuroligins in ASD**
Drilling down even more at the level of synapses, neuroexins and neuroligins are cell adhesion molecules located on presynaptic and postsynaptic neurons, respectively. There are four main isoforms of neuroligans (neuroligans 1–4, abbreviation

NL1, NL4, etc.). Neuroexins and neuroligans bind with each other and interact with intracellular proteins. It is through binding with each other that they essentially facilitate connections between neurons and mediate trans-synaptic signaling.

Alterations in genes coding for neurexins and neuroligins have been implicated in ASD as well as a range of other diseases/disorders including mental retardation and schizophrenia [87]. In a mice experiment using a "knock-in" model in which the mice are bred to express a neuroligin mutation, a point mutation in neuroligin-3 has been found to result in impaired social interaction and enhanced spatial learning and memory. In addition, in these mice there was increased inhibitory synaptic strength in the somatosensory cortex, resulting in an imbalance in excitatory and inhibitory synaptic transmission which is likely to be relevant to the ASD-like behaviors demonstrated by the mice. This same study also demonstrated that the impaired inhibitory transmission occurring at cortical synapses in this mice model is at least partly due to impaired endocannabinoid signaling via CB1 receptors acting at interneurons other than parvalbumin-positive or somatostatin-positive interneurons [88].

## Sleep Dysregulation and ASD

Sleep and circadian disorders occur frequently in ASD [89, 90]. Fragile X syndrome with ASD, resulting from loss of fragile X mental retardation (fmr) gene products, is associated with disturbed sleep and altered circadian rhythms. Several studies suggest that Fragile X-related proteins (FRMP) may be involved in abnormal sleep patterns through altering circadian genes, and these have been shown to modulate the number, function, and maturation of synapses and are involved in synaptic plasticity. FRMP is localized on dendrites and synapses and is involved in regulation of metabotropic glutamate receptor (mGluR) activity [39].

### Parvalbumin Cells and Timing of Plasticity

Circadian rhythms regulate our sleep-wake cycles and disturbances of circadian rhythms are implicated in etiology of ASD. We have circadian clocks within our cells and clock-controlled genes which control the onset of the critical period of neocortical plasticity. Parvalbumin (PV) cells are inhibitory interneurons found within the cortex and synchronize with other brain cells to control the timing of critical periods of increased plasticity. Decreases in PV or density of PV- expressing neurons have been implicated in mice models of ASD [91]. It is possible that in ASD, disturbances to circadian mechanisms can downregulate the maturation of PV cells and impact the timing of the critical period of plasticity [90].

### Dysregulation of Melatonin Synthesis and Circadian Rhythms

Dysregulation of melatonin synthesis and melatonin-dependent signaling pathways can detrimentally affect memory, learning, and vigilance and has been linked to autistic behaviors including anxiety [39]. As we learned in Chap. 8, this hormone plays a key role in regulating our circadian rhythms and sleep-wake patterns.

Sleep-circadian disorders may worsen symptoms of ASD and may also detrimentally affect neurodevelopment. Even slight impairment in circadian or sleep rhythms (and impairment can occur prenatally and postnatally) can increase susceptibility to ASD [90]. Studies have found that around 65% of ASD patients have less than 50% of mean levels of melatonin, and there is a global deficit in melatonin production in ASD [90]. Polymorphisms in ASMT (N-acetylserotonin O-methyltransferase, an enzyme involved in melatonin synthesis) which are paralleled by reduced levels of circulating melatonin have been found in ASD [92].

Whilst a deeper discussion on how sleep disturbances are involved in ASD is beyond the scope of this chapter, an important point is that sleep plays a vital role in neuronal development including synaptic pruning, and therefore sleep disturbances can potentially detrimentally affect the developing brain. In people with ASD, it is therefore vital that clinicians actively address sleep hygiene issues. Sleep has such a profound ability to affect our health in so many ways.

## Environmental Factors Contributing to ASD

It has been estimated that environmental factors may contribute to over half of ASD cases [80]. Several environmental factors have been identified, including heavy metals (lead, mercury, cadmium, arsenic); insecticides; phthalates used in vinyl and cosmetics; household cleaning products (e.g., antibacterial soaps), and bacterial or viral infections [93]. The heterogeneity demonstrated in ASD may partly relate to these diverse environmental factors and exposure period in utero and early postpartum [93].

Prenatal valproate (VPA) exposure in rats showed early deficits in social communication and discrimination, compromised sociability and social play, increased anxiety, and stereotypies in offspring, confirming that ASD-like effects are induced by prenatal valproate. VPA-exposed rats showed altered phosphorylation of CB1 receptors in different brain areas, associated with changes in anandamide (AEA) metabolism from infancy to adulthood. Inhibition of AEA breakdown rescued the behavioral deficits, suggesting that abnormalities in anandamide activity underpin the behavioral effects seen [44]. In a similar way, acetaminophen modulates the ECS to elevate AEA levels [94]. The use of acetaminophen after measles-mumps-rubella vaccination was significantly associated with ASD in young children when considering children 5 years or younger (OR 6.11, 95% CI 1.42–26.3), when cases were limited to children with regression in development (OR 3.97, 95% CI 1.11–14.3), and when limited only to children who had post-vaccination sequelae (OR 8.23. 95% CI 1.56–43.3), and this was after adjusting for age, gender, mother's ethnicity, and presence of concurrent illness at time of vaccination [95]. Use of ibuprofen after MMR vaccination was not associated with ASD [95].

**Vaccine Damage and ASD**

The study just mentioned brings us to another possibility in terms of environmental factors that may be associated with ASD. Whilst no one wants to hear this, not the least pharmaceutical companies who manufacture them and government bodies which might have patents on many of them, childhood vaccines have been associated with the development of ASD. This topic is contentious and tends to inflame emotions in many people, both medical and nonmedical. Medical practitioners are reported to have lost their licenses to practice as a result of speaking publicly about the topic, effectively silencing open and frank discussion about vaccine safety and its relationship to public health. A detailed discussion of vaccine associations with ASD or other disorders is beyond the scope of the book.

## Neuronal Hyperexcitability Hypothesis

A key hypothesis concerning the etiology and pathogenesis of ASD is the neuronal hyperexcitability hypothesis which may help explain the higher incidence of epilepsy in people with ASD as well as sensory hyperactivity [96, 97]. Elevated cortical excitability is proposed as a key neurobiological characteristic of many ASD patients, a model supported by genetic and epigenetic evidence including GABA and glutamate system alterations [97].

Glutamate is an excitatory neurotransmitter, whilst GABA is an inhibitory neurotransmitter. ASD is characterized by an imbalance between excitation and inhibition of glutaminergic and GABAergic signaling in different brain structures [98]. Several different lines of evidence suggest that glutamate and GABA systems may be altered in ASD [99]. Such evidence includes postmortem, genetic and human proton magnetic resonance spectroscopy (MRS) studies indicating abnormalities in prefrontal and basal ganglia glutamate and GABA pathways [13, 99, 100] and differences in excitatory-inhibitory responsivity to pharmacologic challenge [99] in people with ASD. These brain regions have been linked to core symptoms of ASD [13]. The ECS is involved in modulating the balance of GABAergic and glutamatergic transmission [101] and, thus, likely plays a significant role in ASD pathology and management. This will be discussed more shortly.

Further evidence is found in EEG studies where epileptiform EEG activity was recorded in ASD children without epilepsy [102]. A study of 889 ASD patients with no known genetic conditions, brain malformations, or clinical seizures found that 60.7% had abnormal EEG epileptiform activity during sleep [102]. This supports the "intense world theory" that associates symptoms of ASD and excessive neuronal activity and connectivity in the central nervous system (CNS) [97, 103].

Lines of evidence supporting the neuronal excitability theory include the following findings in association with ASD:

- Reduced expression of GABA-related genes in the cerebellum and parietal cortex
- Reduced levels of GABAergic neurons

- Reduced binding at GABA receptors in parts of the brain including the hippocampus and anterior posterior cingulate gyrus
- Increased glutamate receptors and glutamate transfer proteins
- Elevations in mRNA levels of glutamate system-related genes
- Histone modifications associated with a glutamate receptor gene [97]

Magnetic resonance spectroscopy findings also support neuronal hyperexcitability in ASD with lower levels of GABA found in several brain areas including motor, somatosensory, visual, and auditory cortices and increased glutamate levels found in occipital region and auditory cortex (see Takarae and Sweeney [97] for the individual studies).

**Other Neurotransmitter Involvement**
According to Bourgeron [53], although glutaminergic synapses are thought to play a key role in ASD susceptibility, other synapses including GABAergic and glycinergic synapses may also be involved in some ASD patients. Yet other neurotransmitters may also be involved in ASD pathology. For example, neurotransmitters oxytocin and vasopressin are modulators of social behaviors [104], including reward, and social reward is a key aspect of social functioning that is impaired in ASD [51].

## Immune System Activation and Inflammation

There is evidence of early immune activation in individuals with ASD, with chronic peripheral and central alterations in the inflammatory response occurring in ASD. Clinical and postmortem data indicate that ASD patients present an altered neuroinflammatory response throughout their lives which may be an ongoing etiological factor contributing to the condition [93].

There is much interaction between the immune system and the nervous system, and immune dysfunction is commonly present in neurological conditions. Cytokines facilitate communication between these systems [105]. Cytokines are proteins that control the immune response and are produced by immune cells (macrophages, dendritic cells, neutrophils, T cells, B cells) though other types of cells like neurons produce and respond to them. They are structurally similar and share signaling pathways with neurotrophins and neurological growth factors [105].

**Altered Cytokines in ASD**
Cytokines mainly act as mediators of immune activity and have important interactions with the nervous system [105]. Since cytokines participate in normal neural development and function, it is possible that dysregulation of cytokines may contribute to the neural dysfunction seen in ASD [105]. Rodent studies support involvement of elevated cytokines in behavioral symptoms of ASD, during development and adulthood [93]. Dysregulation includes differential monocyte responses,

abnormal T helper cytokine levels, decreased T-cell mitogen response, decreased numbers of lymphocytes, and abnormal serum immunoglobulin levels [106].

ASD patients typically have elevated blood levels of pro-inflammatory cytokines including IL-6, TNF-α, and IL-8 and decreased levels of anti-inflammatory cytokines including TGF-β and IL-10 [48]. IL-6 is an important cytokine required for CNS functioning, homeostasis, cognition, memory, and learning. Increased or decreased levels can both lead to problems. Higher levels of circulating IL-6 have been found in both children and adults with ASD [105, 107, 108]. Increased levels of nuclear factor kappa-B (NF-κB, a transcription factor involved in regulation of cytokines, B cell and T cell expression, and CNS development) have also been found in relation to ASD [52]. Lower levels of immune mediators like TGF-β1 have been found to be associated with worsening of symptoms in children with ASD [48, 105].

IL-4, generally considered neuroprotective, has several roles in the nervous system. Several different studies have found that ASD patients have increased levels of IL-4 and IL-4-producing Th2 cells compared with healthy controls, with this increase in IL-4 in ASD possibly a response by the immune system to regulate other detrimental processes (rather than contributing to the pathogenesis) [105]. For example, the neonatal blood was examined in 214 children with ASD, 62 children with typical development and 27 children with developmental delay who participated in the *Childhood Autism Risks from Genetics and Environmental Study.* The study found that IL-1β and IL-4 were independently associated with ASD (compared to normal development), with increased IL-4 being associated with a 40% increased odds of severe ASD (odds ratio 1.40, 95% CI 1.03–1.91) and IL-1β being associated with a much greater odds of mild/moderate ASD (odds ratio 3.02, 95% CI 1.43–6.38) [109]. IL-1β plays a role in CNS pathology and healing, and a balance between IL-1β and its antagonist IL-1ra is necessary for normal brain development and functioning. Alterations to IL-1β systems may occur due to genetic mechanisms or environmental factors, and this may contribute to ASD [105].

Peripheral cytokines have been shown to affect different behaviors (including sickness behavior and depression) by increasing the expression of brain cytokines. The possibility has been suggested that the high peripheral and/or central cytokine expression and the inflammatory response observed in ASD may be responsible for some of the abnormal behaviors associated with ASD, as suggested by animal models; however, more research is required to clarify this [93].

**Microglial Activation and Increased Brain Cytokines**

Within the brains of ASD patients, there is a significant increase in activation of microglia and astroglia and increased production of pro-inflammatory and anti-inflammatory cytokines [50]. ASD patients show increased astro- and microgliosis in the cortex and the cerebellum, and increased expression of cytokines (IL-6, TNF-α, MCP-1, TGF-β1, IFN-γ, IL-8) and other genes associated with the immune response have been reported in these brain regions and in cerebrospinal fluid [93].

A study that assessed the levels of cytokines in the brains of ASD patients compared with age- and gender-matched normal subjects found significant increases in proinflammatory cytokines (TNF-α, IL-6, and GM-CSF), Th1 cytokine (IFN-γ), and chemokine (IL-8) but not Th2 cytokines (IL-4, IL-5, and IL-10) in the brains of ASD patients compared with controls. The Th1/Th2 ratio was significantly increased in ASD patients, compared with controls. The researchers concluded that there is an increased innate and adaptive immune response operating via the Th1 pathway, suggestive of involvement of localized brain inflammation and autoimmune disorder in the pathogenesis of ASD [110]. The findings of this study contrast with what was found in the *Childhood Autism Risks from Genetics and Environmental Study* mentioned previously which examined neonatal blood and found that increased IL-4 was associated with a greater odds of severe ASD [109]. In that study, the increased IL-4 was explained as possibly reflective of a response by the immune system to regulate other detrimental processes (rather than contributing to the pathogenesis).

**Maternal Immune Activation and Inflammation**

Research indicates support for a role of inflammation and maternal immune activation in ASD and ASD-like behaviors [93, 111–114]. Maternal immune activation can alter the levels of specific cytokines in the maternal serum, the placenta, and fetal brain. During development, cytokines and chemokines are expressed at very low levels in the brain under normal circumstances, where they play a role in neuronal and glial cell migration, differentiation, and synaptic maturation. However increased levels of particular brain cytokines and/or chemokines in the maternal blood due to maternal immune activation could reach the fetal brain, thereby impacting on brain development [93].

Several studies in humans lend support to the notion that maternal inflammation is involved in the pathogenesis of ASD [111–114]. For example:

- A Danish cohort study found elevated levels of tumor necrosis factor-α (TNF-α) and TNF-β in amniotic fluid were associated with increased risk of ASD among offspring [112]. In the amniotic fluid of males, increased levels of IL-4, IL-5, and IL-10 were also found [112].
- A Finish study found that early gestational levels of (inflammatory marker) C-reactive protein (CRP) (prospectively assayed in maternal sera in a large national birth cohort) were significantly associated with autism in children. For maternal CRP levels in the highest quintile, the risk was 43% higher than for maternal CRP levels in the lowest quintile [113].
- The Early Markers of Autism Study examining archived maternal serum samples from mid-pregnancy found that significantly increased levels of interferon-γ (IFN-γ), interleukin-4 (IL-4), and interleukin-5 (IL-5) were all associated with ASD [114].

Animal models of maternal immune activation have also demonstrated that the maternal inflammatory response can affect the normal early programming of different behaviors, including sociability, communication, and the regulation of stereotypic behavior [93]. Since neurological development of the brain continues after birth, postnatal infections and postnatal immune activation may also affect neuronal maturation and survival [93]. However, the literature has been equivocal about the association of early life infections and ASD in humans, with some studies supporting and others not finding an association [93].

#### Chronic Inflammatory Disease in ASD

Chronic inflammatory diseases and abnormal response to infection of different blood cell populations have been found in both children and adults with ASD [93]. For example, ASD patients suffer from chronic gastrointestinal disturbances [115]. In children with ASD, peripheral blood mononuclear cells and lymphoblasts produced excessive proinflammatory cytokines (IL-1β, IL-6, and TNF-α) basally and after LPS stimulation compared with controls [116, 117].

### Microbiota-Gut-Brain Axis

A healthy microbial composition is important to health. An increasing number of studies show that the gut microbiota can modulate important processes during development, including neurogenesis, myelination, glial cell function, synaptic pruning, and blood-brain barrier permeability [118].

#### Gut Dysbiosis and ASD

Dysbiosis, often found in gut-related diseases/conditions such as inflammatory bowel disease and diabetes and obesity, has also been found in ASD [119]. Autistic children show an altered metabolism and absorption of disaccharides in their gut, and increased intestinal permeability has been observed in ASD patients [118].

Frequent gastrointestinal (GI) symptoms appear to be related to behavioral problems in children with ASD, with behavioral issues including social withdrawal, irritability, hyperactivity, stereotypies, and inappropriate speech occurring more often in those children with ASD and frequent GI complaints compared with children with ASD without frequent GI complaints [120].

#### Bacterial and Viral Infections

There is some research to suggest that chronic viral and bacterial infections could underlie the chronic inflammatory status observed in ASD patients. For example, certain viruses and bacteria have been associated with the high incidence of gastrointestinal problems observed in ASD [93]. Individuals with ASD with GI disturbances have significantly higher numbers of potential bacterial pathogens including several *Clostridia* species (*C. bolteae, C. histolyticum, C. perfringens*) and *Sutterella* species and significantly lower levels of *Bifidobacterium* [23, 120]. Toxins produced by bacteria may contribute to gut dysbiosis [120].

In addition, in children with ASD, reduced gut microbial diversity and chronic peripheral low-grade inflammation have been found, along with increased TNF-α, TGF-β, and other immune factors [121].

**Gut Integrity**

The importance of the gut-brain axis in health is now well established. Gut microbes communicate to the CNS through at least three parallel and interacting channels involving nervous, endocrine, and immune signaling mechanisms [122]. In the ASD brain, there is an altered expression of genes associated with blood-brain barrier (BBB) integrity coupled with increased neuroinflammation and possibly impaired gut barrier integrity. Claudins (CLDNs) are a family of proteins which are components of tight junctions (along with occludin). Postmortem cerebral cortex and cerebellum tissues and duodenal biopsies from ASD patients found 75% of the ASD samples analyzed had reduced expression of barrier-forming tight junction components (CLDN-1, OCLN, TRIC), whereas 66% had increased pore-forming CLDNs (CLDN-2, CLDN-10, CLDN-15) compared to controls [123].

**Multimodal Approach to Treatment**

Considerable evidence is accumulating to suggest gastrointestinal symptoms and ASD-related symptoms may be able to be modified with a multimodal approach. An open-label trial in 18 ASD patients of Microbiota Transfer Therapy (MTT), including antibiotics, a bowel cleanse, a stomach-acid suppressant, and fecal microbiota transplant, demonstrated significant improvements in gastrointestinal symptoms, autism-related symptoms, and gut microbiota immediately and for 2 years after, with autism-related symptoms showing even more improvement after the end of treatment [124].

Now that we have examined many of the various possible pathomechanisms underpinning ASD, let us now look at how the endocannabinoid system, a major neuroregulatory system of the body, is involved too.

## The Endocannabinoid System in ASD Pathology

Dysregulation of the endocannabinoid system (ECS) is implicated in the etiology and pathogenesis of ASD. Much of the research is found from animal studies.

Indirect evidence of involvement of the ECS in ASD comes from its role in regulating many of the processes altered in ASD including social interactions, emotions, cognition, learning, memory, circadian rhythms, seizure susceptibility, and nociception [44, 98]. As we have seen in earlier chapters, the ECS plays an important role in neurodevelopment and is a major regulator of synaptic plasticity [45], and we also know that disturbances to neural development appear to underlie ASD. The ECS is involved in the modulation of many cellular functions and molecular pathways altered in ASD, such as imbalanced GABAergic and glutamatergic transmission, oxidative stress, inflammation, altered energy metabolism, and immune dysregulation. Genetic and environmental factors may also impact on the ECS. Evidence from animal and human studies implicates the ECS is implicated in four key features of ASD in particular: neural development, social reward responsivity, anxiety, and circadian rhythm alterations [1].

In this section, we will discuss some of the ways in which the ECS is involved in regulation of some of the behavioral aspects characteristic of ASD and how dysregulation of the ECS may be involved in the pathogenesis of ASD. We have already covered the topics of anxiety and sleep disorders in previous chapters.

## ECS and Regulation of Neurotransmitter Excitation and Inhibition in ASD

According to Zamberletti et al. [98], given the role that CB1 receptor signaling plays in synaptic plasticity at both excitatory and inhibitory synapses and its role in regulation of maturity of excitatory and inhibitory neurons, it is conceivable that ECS dysfunction could contribute to ASD through imbalances between excitatory and inhibitory neurotransmission. Abnormal CB1 receptor signaling in early brain development stages could lead to disruption of the optimal balance of excitation/inhibition and increase susceptibility to ASD [98].

There is some evidence implicating changes in CB1 receptors in the pathogenesis of ASD. For example, postmortem studies have shown decreased levels of CB1 receptors [84]. CB1 receptor blockade has been shown in animal models of Fragile X syndrome to improve cognitive deficits [98].

### Fragile X Model of ASD

As discussed previously, Fragile X is a genetic disorder due to Fmr 1 gene mutations and is a leading monogenetic cause of ASD. Research suggests that FXS abnormalities may be underpinned by dysregulation of ECS pathways in the central nervous system, including decreased stimulation of cannabinoid receptors [83].

Fmr 1 knockout mice are used as an animal model of FXS, and the animals show behaviors mimicking ASD in humans (memory deficits, hyperactivity, repetitive behaviors, altered social behaviors, anxiety, etc.), and they also show abnormal dendritic spines and altered glutaminergic and GABAergic neurotransmission (which supports the idea that FXS involves excitatory and inhibitory neurotransmission defects) [98]. Studies in Fmr 1 knockout mice provide some evidence that changes in the ECS may contribute to symptoms of FXS and that endocannabinoid signaling modulation could potentially address some of the symptoms of FXS. For example, experiments have shown that endocannabinoid-mediated long-term depression occurs at excitatory synapses in the forebrain of Fmr1 knockout mice and that administration of a MAGL inhibitor (which enhances 2-AG signaling) could correct this depression and improve hyperlocomotion and anxiety-like responses in these mice. Other experiments in Fmr 1 knockout mice demonstrated that enhancement of AEA signaling by blocking

FAAH reversed social impairment and improved aversive memory and anxiety-like behavior. See Zamberletti et al. [98] for a discussion of the individual studies. Such studies demonstrate the potential for manipulation of endocannabinoid signalling to positively impact on ASD-like behaviors.

## Abnormal Endocannabinoid Signaling in ASD

There is evidence of abnormal endocannabinoid signaling in ASD. This may relate to lower endocannabinoid tone, as well as oxytocin-driven AEA signaling.

### Lower Endocannabinoid Tone in ASD

Several animal models support the contention that reduced endocannabinoid tone is involved in the pathogenesis of ASD, and activation of the ECS was found to reverse autistic symptoms (see Aran et al. [125]). Rodent ASD models suggest that altered AEA signaling may contribute to the communication and social deficits that characterize ASD and support the contention that fatty acid amide hydrolase (FAAH, the enzyme that breaks down AEA) is involved in regulation of social behavioral deficits [98]. In various animal ASD models, enhancing AEA signaling by inhibiting its degradation appears to promote prosocial effects [98].

In children, analysis of blood samples has demonstrated that those with lower AEA levels were significantly more likely to have ASD and that AEA concentrations were significantly lower in ASD compared with control children [126]. In another study, lower plasma levels of AEA and two ECS-related compounds N-palmitoylethanolamide (PEA) and N-oleoylethanolamide (OEA) were found in children with ASD compared to normal children [45]. Plasma levels of polyunsaturated fatty acids, components of endocannabinoids, and endocannabinoid-like substances have also been found to be lower in patients with ASD [127]. A systematic review found that compared with normally developed, ASD was associated with significantly lower levels of docosahexaenoic acid (DHA), eicosapentaenoic acid, and arachidonic acid and higher levels of n-6 long-chain PUFA/n-3 long-chain PUFA ratio [127].

A study in women who had already had a child with ASD and were pregnant or planning a pregnancy followed the children born to these women longitudinally for 36 months. The study found that mothers consuming more total omega-3 in the second half of the pregnancy had a substantially reduced likelihood (40% less likely) to have a child with ASD (RR 0.6, 95% CI 0.3–0.98). There were no significant associations found between maternal trimester 3 plasma PUFA subtype concentrations and risk of ASD, but higher plasma eicosapentaenoic acid and docosahexaenoic acid concentrations were found to be associated with lower risk of non-typical development (RR 0.47–0.88) [128].

This is an important point that we continue to come back to: diet is very important in any disease, and we know that the typical western diet has a ratio that is very skewed toward higher omega 6 polyunsaturated fatty acids (PUFAs) compared with omega 3 PUFAs.

There are other lines of evidence suggesting that secondary abnormal endocannabinoid signaling may contribute to ASD [51]. For example, we met neuroligan-3 earlier, and we know that neuroligans bind with neuroexins to facilitate synapse formation. Neuroligan-3 is needed for tonic secretion of AEA and 2-AG, and we also know from mice experiments that mutations in neuroligan-3 are implicated in ASD [129]. This all supports involvement of impaired endocannabinoid signaling in ASD.

### AEA and Oxytocin Signaling

The neuropeptide oxytocin and the peptide arginine vasopressin are believed to play a role in ASD etiology, in particular in relation to the social impairment found in ASD [4]. Oxytocin promotes social bonding, and social reward is regulated by oxytocin-dependent activation of the ECS in the nucleus accumbens (which we know is a key reward center of the brain) [51]. Oxytocin stimulates AEA release in the nucleus accumbens, and AEA-mediated signaling is required for the prosocial effects of oxytocin [130]. Research implicates defective oxytocin-driven AEA signaling in ASD [51, 98, 130].

Increased AEA levels (via FAAH blockade) acting at CB1 receptors reversed ASD-related social impairment in two different mouse models of ASD, and this was independent of any anxiolytic effect [51]. The researchers concluded that FAAH might be a novel target for ASD [51]. Administration of oxytocin to ASD patients can improve processing of social behaviors, improve emotional recognition, strengthen social interaction, decrease repetitive behaviors, and increase eye gaze [4, 131].

Research in rats also shows that oleoylethanolamide (OEA), one of the endocannabinoid-like substances in our bodies, restored normal oxytocin receptor density in the striatum, induced an increase in oxytocin mRNA levels in the paraventricular nucleus, and decreased corticotropin-releasing factor (CRF) mRNA levels in the central amygdala [132].

## ECS and Regulation of Social Behavior

Observations of human behavior support the notion that the ECS affects social behavior—for example, acute intoxication with cannabis often leads to less hostile feelings and feeling more connected and empathetic and interacting more with others [133, 134] . However, it is animal research which provides evidence of involvement of the ECS in regulation of many of the behavioral aspects of ASD like social behavior and that dysfunction of the ECS may underpin many of the behavioral aspects of ASD.

Endocannabinoids are key modulators of socio-emotional responses which we know to be disturbed in ASD [44]. Rodent studies indicate that the ECS controls emotional responses, behavioral reactivity to context, and social interaction, and it appears that AEA is particularly relevant [1, 135–137]. For example, in one rat study, adolescent rats were allowed to interact with another rat under two different conditions—one in which the other rat was a familiar social partner and the other in which the other rat was a non-familiar social partner. The non-familiar social encounter significantly increased AEA levels in the striatal region (but not other brain regions) of rats compared with non-social controls and rats which were exposed to a familiar partner. No changes were found in FAAH or 2-AG. They concluded that striatal AEA levels were important in emotional arousal resulting from a non-familiar social encounter and are likely to be important in coping to new social contexts [135].

Another study in rats demonstrated that FAAH is involved in regulation of social deficits and that FAAH inhibition could attenuate the social behavioral deficits in male rats prenatally exposed to valproate, but this effect was not duplicated in female rats [138]. Prenatal valproate exposure has previously been shown to be associated with changes in the rat brain ECS, and in an earlier experiment, tissue levels of AEA, palmitoylethanolamide (PEA), and oleoylethanolamide (OEA) were found to be higher in the hippocampus of prenatal VPA-exposed rats immediately after social exposure [139] (see later section on Environmental Toxins, the Endocannabinoid System, and ASD).

As pointed out by Aran et al. [45], research has demonstrated that CB1 receptors and their ligands AEA and 2-AG regulate social play and anxiety in animals [140–142] and in humans [143, 144]. Studies in rats have elucidated key brain regions that are sites of action of cannabinoids in modulation of reward and social behavior. For example, a rat study found that social play increased AEA levels in the amygdala and nucleus accumbens, however, no change was found in the prefrontal cortex or hippocampus. Blockade of AEA hydrolysis increased social play behavior. The AEA hydrolysis inhibitor was injected into various parts of the brain, and effect on social behavior is observed. They found that increased AEA signaling in the amygdala and nucleus accumbens increases social play and that the basolateral amygdala was a key site of action for endocannabinoid modulation of the reward component of social interactions [142].

Another study used a particular mouse model of autism in which the mice have an imbalance in excitatory and inhibitory synaptic activity in the hippocampus and somatosensory cortex and display heightened aggression. Knowing that the amygdala plays a role in modulating aggressive behavior, they investigated the activity in the basolateral amygdala and found that these mice also had increased amplitude of excitatory currents and reduced amplitude of postsynaptic inhibitory currents. Mice administered a CB1 receptor agonist demonstrated reduced aggressive behavior, suggesting that CB1 receptor agonists might be promising therapeutic targets for reducing aggression [145].

These studies in rodent models of ASD provide evidence of involvement of the ECS in various key brain regions associated with social behavioral aspects of ASD, as well as alterations in synaptic activity.

There may be a genetic basis for some of the social behavioral anomalies found in ASD. We will now explore the evidence for this.

## Genetic Changes, the Endocannabinoid System, and ASD

There may be a genetic basis for some of the social behavioral anomalies found in ASD that involves the ECS. The striatum is a key region of the brain involved in reward processing and in directing gaze. The ECS is involved in the functioning of the striatal circuit, working alongside the mesolimbic dopaminergic system. Animal and human studies indicate high levels of CNR1 expression in the striatum as well as in the caudate, putamen, internal globus pallidus, and substantia nigra and shell of the nucleus accumbens, and this gene is believed to modulate striatal dopamine release via mechanisms involving GABAergic and glutaminergic synapses. The main mechanism encoding for reward is phasic dopamine release from the striatum [146].

Variations in the CNR1 gene may underlie atypical social reward responsivity in ASD [1]. Humans generally look longer at rewarding stimuli like happy faces, but ASD is characterized by atypical gaze fixation patterns where this is not the case. Human neuroimaging studies [147, 148] and eye movement studies [146] revealed associations between polymorphisms in CNR1 and social gaze and social reward responsivity, providing some evidence that alterations of CB1 receptors may contribute to deficits in social reward processing in ASD [98]. One study measured gaze patterns of 30 individuals from the general population who observed dynamic emotional expressions on a screen. They found that specific SNPs in the CNR1 gene in ASD were associated with differences in gaze duration for happy faces but not for disgust faces. Functional MRIs conducted showed that the allelic groups associated with a greater striatal response to happy faces were associated with longer gaze duration also. Such studies provide evidence that the CNR1 gene is involved in social reward processing, something that is impaired in ASD [146].

**Mutations in Neuroligans and Endocannabinoid Signaling in Autism**
Research indicates that several genes, including those coding for neuroligins and neurexins (which, to recap from an earlier section, are involved in brokering synapses), are associated with ASD [1, 87]. More than 30 neuroligin gene mutations have been found to be associated with ASD in humans [129]. This includes a neuroligan-3 (NL3) point mutation (the R451 substitution) and a NL3 deletion [129]. Mice studies indicate that these two autism-related mutations in neuroligin-3 are associated with deficits in social behavior and disrupted tonic endocannabinoid signaling [129, 149]. Mice studies have demonstrated that neuroligan-3 is essential for tonic endocannabinoid signaling and that both mutations (R451C substitution and neuroligin-3 deletion) impaired tonic but not phasic endocannabinoid signaling [129]. Given that both the R451C substitution and neuroligan-3 deletion are associated with ASD, this provides support for the involvement of endocannabinoid signaling in ASD [129].

## ECS, Regulation of the Immune System, and Inflammation and ASD

The ECS is a key regulator of the immune system via CB2 receptors which are highly expressed on macrophages and microglial cells [49]. It is known that changes in the immune system associated with ASD involve alterations in macrophage and monocyte responses, as well as increased levels of pro-inflammatory cytokines, and that these changes are mediated by dysfunction of the ECS [150]. Thus, the ECS is a potential therapeutic target for treatment of ASD [150].

The ECS may modulate ASD symptoms by interacting with immune system cells. For example, CB2 receptors (but not CB1 receptors) have been found to be upregulated in peripheral blood mononuclear cells in children with ASD [151] and blood monocyte-derived macrophage cells in patients with ASD [49]. The simultaneous upregulation of CB2 receptors and downregulation of NAPE-PLD in this type of immune cells provides some evidence of ECS mediation of immune-mediated changes in ASD [152] and supports the theory that the ECS may play a role in the immunological dysfunctions associated with ASD [98]. Given the potential role of inflammation in ASD (discussed in detail earlier), the increase in CB2 expression may actually be compensatory, counteracting the pro-inflammatory responses implicated in ASD [1].

## Environmental Toxins, the Endocannabinoid System, and ASD

Prenatal valproate (VPA) exposure is associated with alterations in the brain's ECS and supports the hypothesis that endocannabinoid dysfunction may underlie behavioral abnormalities observed in ASD. Studies in rats help us understand some of the changes occurring. Prenatal VPA exposure in rats was found to be associated with ASD-like behavior during adolescence. It was also associated with a reduction in DAGLα and MAGL expression in the hippocampus and cerebellum, reduced PPAR-α and GPR55 mRNA expression in the frontal cortex, and reduced PPARϒ and GPR55 mRNA expression in the hippocampus. There were no changes in CB1 or CB2 receptor gene expression found in the frontal cortex, hippocampus, or cerebellum in VPA-exposed mice compared with control mice.

Following exposure of VPA-exposed rats to a sociability test, 2-AG levels were not altered, but AEA, OEA, and PEA levels were found to be increased in the hippocampus [139]. PPAR-α, PPAR-γ, and GPR55 are considered part of the endocannabinoidome [153]. Such findings suggest that in adolescent rats prenatally exposed to VPA, alterations in the ECS might underpin some of the ASD-like behaviors demonstrated [139].

There are many other environmental toxins that have been implicated in the etiology and pathogenesis of ASD, and one might surmise that these are likely also to impact the ECS, in particular if such toxins are known to be neurotoxins.

## ECS, the Gut, and Gastrointestinal Conditions in ASD

The gut clearly is intimately involved with our brain. In fact, it is often referred to as a second brain. It would therefore not be at all surprising to think that the involvement of the ECS in ASD may therefore also include mechanisms involving the gut (as well as direct effects on the brain and elsewhere).

As we saw earlier, the gut microbiota can modulate important neurodevelopmental processes such as neurogenesis, myelination, glial cell function, synaptic pruning, and blood-brain barrier permeability [118]. We also know that in ASD, there is a higher prevalence of gut-related conditions, that children with ASD have altered metabolism and absorption of disaccharides in their gut, and that in ASD patients, increased intestinal permeability has been found [118].

The ECS is involved in gut physiology through modulation of gastric emptying, gastrointestinal motility, and inflammation. Chronic activation of the ECS was found to induce severe metabolic disturbances such as glucose intolerance, infiltration of macrophages, and lipid accumulation in muscle. Gut microbiota has also been proposed to control levels of endocannabinoids in the gut and adipose tissue. In addition, microbiota and endocannabinoids have been linked with intestinal integrity. Changing the gut microbiota via high-fat diet, prebiotics, probiotics, or antibiotics affects CNR1 expression (the gene encoding the CB1 receptor) in the intestine. The ECS has also been proposed to control gut-barrier function, gut permeability, and metabolic endotoxemia in obese and diabetic conditions through a CB1-dependent mechanism, as antagonists of CB1 decrease gut permeability and act as "gate keepers" [154].

## Endocannabinoid System and Comorbidities of ASD

Finally, support for the involvement of the ECS in ASD comes from the fact that the ECS is involved in many of the comorbidities of ASD including epilepsy/seizures, anxiety, and sleep disorders [1]. The ECS is involved in regulating circadian rhythms [155], and ASD is associated with atypical sleep patterns and circadian rhythms [156]. The ECS regulates our stress response and emotions including anxiety, as discussed in Chap. 5.

## How CBD May Work in Autism Spectrum Disorder

CBD has multiple potential targets which may be relevant in its use in treating ASD:

- Actions on glutamate and GABA
- Neurogenic effects
- Anti-inflammatory actions
- Enhancing mitochondrial functioning
- Regulating mTOR

- Actions on ECS including increasing endocannabinoid tone
- Recovering gastrointestinal function
- Actions in reducing comorbidities of ASD including anxiety

## Actions of CBD on Glutamate and GABA

The actions of CBD on glutamate and GABA may be important in ASD, given that an imbalance between excitation and inhibition of glutamatergic and GABAergic signaling in different brain structures has been demonstrated in ASD [13, 98]. Animal research indicates that CBD helps regulate brain excitatory glutamate and inhibitory gamma-aminobutyric acid (GABA) levels, including in regions of the brain such as basal ganglia and the dorsomedial prefrontal cortex (DMPFC) which are regions linked to ASD, thereby influencing signaling pathways [13]. CBD can facilitate glutamate and GABA neurotransmission across the brain through agonism at transient receptor potential villanoid type 1 (TRPV1) receptor and may increase GABAergic transmission via antagonism at GPR55, in particular in the basal ganglia [13]. CBD is also believed to act as an agonist at prefrontal 5-HT1A receptors, suppressing glutamate and GABA transmission [13].

A study was conducted using magnetic resonance spectroscopy in 34 adults (17 with ASD, 17 neurotypicals) after a single dose of CBD (600mg) or placebo. CBD increased subcortical but decreased cortical (excitatory) glutamate in both groups. CBD increased (inhibitory) GABA levels in the basal ganglia and DMPFC in neurotypicals but decreased GABA levels in these areas in autistic adults. Thus, it appears that CBD modulates glutamate-GABA systems, and prefrontal-GABA systems respond differently in ASD [13].

## Possible Neurogenic Effects of CBD

Research has shown that increasing AEA levels can increase neurogenesis in the brain and replace dysfunctional neurons [150, 157]. In a mice study, CBD was shown to increase AEA levels in the hippocampus and increase neurogenesis in chronically stressed mice [158]. It has been hypothesized that given that new neurons migrate the from hippocampus to cortex, providing they follow the appropriate endocannabinoid gradients, they might gradually improve the symptoms of ASD [150].

We also know that ASD is related to altered BDNF levels, with some studies finding higher levels and some lower, with one study suggesting that lower levels of BDNF might indicate impairment of neuroprotective mechanisms and higher levels might imply a manifested protective response [67]. A study in animals showed that CBD can induce rapid, sustained antidepressant effects, and this was associated with increased BDNF levels in the mPFC and hippocampus. The antidepressant effect appeared to be associated with rapid changes in synaptic plasticity in the mPFC and mediated via activation of the BDNF-Trk signaling pathway [159].

Whether or not this is relevant to ASD is unknown; however, since depression is a comorbidity of ASD, at the very least, we can see a mechanism by which CBD might address one of the pathomechanisms underpinning depression.

## Anti-inflammatory Action of CBD

CBD's anti-inflammatory actions are likely to be relevant in the treatment of ASD given evidence of involvement of inflammation. Several studies have demonstrated the anti-inflammatory and antioxidant effects of CBD in neuroinflammatory models. For example, short-term CBD treatment in mice after bilateral carotid artery occlusion prevented the cognitive and emotional impairments, attenuated hippocampal neurodegeneration and white matter (WM) injury, and reduced glial response that were induced by the injury [160]. In another mouse study, CBD decreased LPS-induced cell margination, compromised BBB integrity, and reduced expression of inflammatory cytokines COX-2, TNF-a, and iNOS [161]. CBD also protects oligodendrocyte progenitor cells from inflammation-induced apoptosis by attenuating endoplasmic reticulum stress through the decrease of caspase-3 induction via mechanisms that do not involve CB1, CB2, TRPV1, or PPAR-$\gamma$ receptors. The pro-survival effects of CBD in oligodendrocyte progenitor cells were accompanied by decreases in the expression of apoptotic effectors and increased expression of the anti-apoptotic Bcl-2 [162].

## CBD and Mitochondrial Functioning

Whilst there is only a little research about the role of mitochondria in ASD per se, it is known that two fundamental determinants of neuronal survival as well as viability under pathological conditions are calcium homeostasis and metabolic activity, and these both rely on mitochondrial function [163]. In a study investigating mechanisms by which CBD exerts neuroprotective effects, an oxygen-glucose deprivation/reperfusion model in a mouse hippocampal neuronal cell line was used [164]. The study found that mechanisms of action of CBD included attenuating oxidative stress, enhancing mitochondrial bioenergetics, and modulating glucose metabolism via the pentose-phosphate pathway, thus preserving both energy and the redox balance [164].

More studies are needed to understand the potential role of mitochondria, in neuroprotection and in reducing oxidative stress and inflammation as it pertains to ASD.

## Actions on mTOR Pathway

Hyperactive mTOR-mediated signaling has been proven in some forms of ASD and may be a target for pharmacological therapy [165]. CBD may potentially regulate mTOR as one of the pathways to improvement in ASD. At the current time, we have found no studies that discuss CBD effects on ASD through the mTOR mechanism. However, there are a number of studies that have shown that CBD modulates the mTOR system in other medical conditions. The effects of CBD are often contextual as to tissue state of function (e.g., normal or cancerous) or tissue type (e.g., neuronal versus glial) or region in the brain. In preclinical studies CBD has been shown to differentially regulate mTORC1, reducing its activity in epilepsy and cancer while increasing mTORC1 in models of multiple sclerosis (MS) and psychosis [166]. In depression activation of the hippocampal BDNF-TrkB-mTOR pathway is essential for cannabidiol effects [167]. In schizophrenia studies CBD was antipsychotic through selective phosphorylation of the mTOR [168]. Interestingly, in neurons CBD stimulates autophagy by facilitating cross-talk by activating ERK1/2 and suppressing AKT independent of mTORC1 [169]. Thus, CBD may benefit ASD by modulating mTOR/autophagy toward more normal function and resolving this monogenic error.

## Actions of CBD on the Endocannabinoid System

Different animal models of ASD indicate that enhancing anandamide signaling through inhibition of its degradation leads to prosocial effects [51, 98]. CBD is known to be able to inhibit degradation of anandamide by fatty acid amide hydrolase (FAAH). Fatty acid-binding proteins (FABPs) are intracellular carriers that transport anandamide to FAAH. CBD can bind FABPs and thereby block anandamide breakdown—this is believed to be one mechanism by which CBD works in childhood epilepsy, that is, by increasing anandamide levels [170].

In a mouse model of Dravet syndrome epilepsy, the beneficial effects of CBD on inhibitory neurotransmission were mimicked and occluded by an antagonist of GPR55, supporting treatment of epilepsy and autistic-like behaviors linked to Dravet syndrome with CBD [171]. CBD was shown to prevent permeability changes at the blood-brain barrier in an ischemic stroke model mediated by activation of PPAR-$\gamma$ and 5-$HT_{1A}$ receptors [172].

Research in mice has found that CBD attenuates the anxiogenic effects caused by chronic unpredictable stress, via effects on the ECS. Whilst the mechanism is not completely understood, it seems that the way in which CBD prevents the behavioral effects caused by chronic unpredictable stress is probably due to facilitation of endocannabinoid neurotransmission and consequent $CB_1$/$CB_2$ receptors activation, recruiting intracellular/synaptic proteins involved in neurogenesis and dendritic remodeling [173]. Other studies conducted with hippocampal progenitor cells in culture showed that the anxiolytic effect of chronic CBD administration in stressed mice depends on its pro-neurogenic action in the adult hippocampus by facilitating endocannabinoid-mediated signalling [158].

## CBD's Potential Role in Recovering the Gastrointestinal System

As we learned previously, gastrointestinal disorders are a common comorbidity of ASD. Although there are no human studies of CBD action on the gut in ASD patients as yet, there is substantial preclinical information to suggest a potentially significant benefit of CBD on gut function through multiple mechanisms.

Research indicates that increased intestinal permeability, so-called leaky gut, is associated with inflammatory bowel diseases (IBD) [174] and irritable bowel syndrome (IBS) [175]. In IBD, there is impairment of the mucosal barrier, increased intestinal permeability, and an immunological response promoting inflammation [174]. In IBS, increased gut/intestinal permeability has also been linked to low-grade intestinal inflammation [176]. Several preclinical studies indicate that CBD is protective in intestinal inflammation and inhibits GI inflammation by controlling the inflammatory response and the activation of enteric glial cells and maintaining a healthy intestinal barrier [177]. For example, in a CaCo-2 cell model, CBD recovered the intestinal barrier in a concentration- and CB1-dependent manner [178]. Specifically, CBD and THC were protective against excessive intestinal permeability, suggesting that cannabinoids could play an important role in treating inflammatory gastrointestinal diseases such as IBD [178]. Both CBD and PEA were found to prevent increased cytokine production in human colon tissue (explants), with CBD's effect blocked by a CB2 receptor antagonist and PEA's effects blocked by a PPAR-α antagonist. Both were found to be anti-inflammatory in IDB and appendicitis explants [179], demonstrating promise in the treatment of inflammatory gut conditions.

In animal models and in patients with ulcerative colitis, colon inflammation is associated with increased AEA levels (but not 2-AG), and this elevation is a physiologic attempt to control inflammation. When an AEA reuptake inhibitor was administered in a rat model of colon inflammation, it increased AEA levels and simultaneously abolished inflammation [180]. Since CBD has the potential to inhibit the degradation of AEA, one might surmise it could also be useful in reducing colonic inflammation as demonstrated in this study when a AEA reuptake inhibitor was used.

In addition, CBD has significant antibacterial effects on Gram-positive strep and staph bacteria including antibiotic-resistant strains as well as hepatitis C (HCV) and herpes simplex virus (HSV) as well as some types of malaria parasites [181]. Furthermore, CBD is a strong inhibitor of microvesicle release from Gram-negative bacteria (microvesicles are a means by which bacteria protect themselves from host defense and antibiotics and advance their dominance in the gut) [182].

## CBD May Help Treat Other Comorbidities of ASD

Research in humans indicates the CBD may be effective in treating many of the comorbidities of ASD including anxiety [183], sleep disorders [184], epilepsy [185,

186], addictive behavior [185], and ADHD and hyperactivity [187, 188]. We have already discussed in detail how CBD may assist in alleviation of anxiety (Chap. 5) and sleep disorders (Chap. 8).

A study in ADHD adults found that a cannabinoid spray (1:1 ratio of THC:CBD) significantly improved hyperactivity, impulsivity, and inhibition measures, though there was no significant change in cognitive performance [188].

Research has demonstrated the effectiveness of a CBD-enriched oil in children with intractable epilepsy, which reduced seizure frequency in 89% of patients [186]. Other studies support its efficacy in treating Dravet syndrome and Lennox-Gastaut syndrome, severe refractory epilepsy syndromes with onset in early childhood [189–194]. A systematic review of four RCTs with 550 patients with Lennox-Gastaut syndrome and Dravet syndrome concluded that adjunctive treatment with CBD was associated with a significant reduction in seizures. A decrease of at least 50% of all-type seizure frequency occurred in 37% of patients in the 20 mg/kg group compared with 21% of placebo-treated patients (risk ratio 1.76, 95% CI 1.07–2.88). Adverse events occurred in 88% of patients treated with CBD compared with 72% of patients taking placebo (RR 1.22, 95% CI 1.11–1.33) [192].

### Combining CBD, Oxytocin, and Melatonin

Recognizing the convergence of neuroendocrine abnormalities in melatonin, oxytocin, and the endocannabinoid system, one study examined the effect of combinations of these in ASD. Thirty autistic patients were assigned to therapy with either melatonin alone, melatonin plus CBD, or oxytocin plus melatonin plus CBD and evaluated for sleep, anxiety, and social affective improvement. In the 12 patients with melatonin alone, anxiety was reduced by 25%. When all three agents were combined, 83% of subjects had anxiety reduction although this was not statistically significant because of the small numbers involved in the study. However, the social affective improvement was significant at 67% for the combined approach [195]. This approach is a paradigm shift in the collaborative use of exogenous neurochemicals to modulate the common root causes of autism that may have great potential.

## Scientific Evidence of Efficacy: Medicinal Cannabis in the Treatment of Autism Spectrum Disorder

In this section, we will examine the evidence for efficacy of medicinal cannabis and, in particular, cannabidiol (CBD) in the treatment of ASD. We will also look at potential mechanisms of action of CBD in treating ASD. Much of what we understand about mechanisms of action comes from preclinical research using animal models. However, ASD is a condition peculiar to humans and so animal models have limitations.

CBD has multiple potential targets which include: modulation of the endocannabinoid system including inhibition of FAAH, reverse agonism of CB1R and modulation of CB2R, as well as independent actions on glutamate and GABA, anti-inflammatory actions, and actions in reducing comorbidities of ASD including anxiety.

It has been hypothesized that CBD provides therapeutic benefit in ASD treatment by increasing endocannabinoid tone after inhibiting FAAH activity (and thus increasing AEA levels) and that it may also have promoting effects on the number of CB2 receptors in peripheral blood mononuclear cells and decrease pro-inflammatory cytokines [150].

## Preclinical Research into CBD

Animal studies suggest that CBD may have a positive influence on social behavior, which is relevant to ASD. CBD treatment in a mouse model of Dravet syndrome effectively reduced seizures and ASD-like behaviors [171]. In one rat model of schizophrenia, CBD showed an ability to inhibit MK-801-induced social withdrawal [196], whilst in another, chronic CBD administration attenuated the deficits in social interaction and cognition induced by prenatal infection [197]. In a third study, a low dose (1 mg/kg) of CBD increased passive and total social interaction of rats, although social interaction in the rats was not improved by CBD at any dose [198].

CBD is agonistic at the 5-HT1A receptor and shares similar mechanisms with lithium, which indicate a potential role in the treatment of mood disorders [199]. Research in mice has shown that CBD has properties common to classic antidepressants [200], and rodent studies have established the anxiolytic effects of CBD, similar to anxiolytic drugs in various experiments [201–205].

### Fragile X Syndrome

As we learned earlier, several abnormalities characteristic of Fragile X syndrome (FXS) appear to have as their basis a dysregulation of the ECS in the CNS, with a reduction in endocannabinoid signaling [83]. CBD appears to be able to attenuate the reduction in endocannabinoid signaling in animal models of FXS. For example, in one mouse model of FXS, deletion of FRMP (fragile X mental retardation protein, regulator of translation of messenger RNAs involved in synaptic plasticity) led to reduced 2-AG and thereby reduced CB1 receptor activation in the CNS [82]. However, since CBD has been found to be able to increase 2-AG availability [206], CBD has the potential to attenuate one of the abnormal pathways associated with FXS [83]. Other animal studies have found that increasing AEA-mediated signaling at CB1 receptors can improve social deficits associated with FXS, and CBD is known to be able to increase AEA levels (through binding to fatty acid-binding proteins and thus inhibiting AEA catabolism)—this is another potential way in which CBD might be able to address some of the ECS dysfunction occurring in FXS [83]. In addition, it has been hypothesized that CBD may increase synaptic plasticity in FXS which has been found to be altered in FXS [83, 207]. CBD may also have other mechanisms of action in FXS, including enhancing binding affinity for GABA (GABA receptors are downregulated in FXS mice models) and exerting anxiolytic effects via the serotonin 1A receptor [83].

## Human Research

There are only small number of studies published in the literature investigating the treatment of ASD with medicinal cannabis [45, 96, 101, 101, 187, 208, 209]. These studies all suggest medicinal cannabis may be effective in treating some of the symptoms and signs associated with ASD. These studies also indicate that in general, medicinal cannabis appears to be well tolerated with only mild side effects. In three of the studies, many of the children were able to lower the dose of current medications or, in some cases, cease medication [96, 101, 125].

### Retrospective Study: CBD-Rich Cannabis Oil as Adjuvant Treatment

The efficacy and tolerability of CBD-rich medicinal cannabis as adjuvant treatment were assessed in a retrospective study of 60 children with ASD and severe behavioral problems (5–18 years). The medicinal cannabis was a 20:1 ratio of CBD:THC dissolved in olive oil, sublingual dosage two to three times per day with doses up-titrated over 2–4 weeks to effect and tolerability. Mean starting dose was 1mg/kg per day, with maximum dose 10 mg/kg per day. Forty-nine children (82% of participants) were treated with cannabis and medications concomitantly (including antipsychotics, mood stabilizers, benzodiazepines, SSRIs, and stimulants).

Mean total daily dose was 3.8 ± 2.6 mg/kg/day CBD and 0.29 ± 0.22 mg/kg/day THC for children who received three daily doses ($n = 44$) and 1.8 ± 1.6 mg/kg/day CBD and 0.22 ± 0.14 mg/kg/day THC for children who received two daily doses ($n = 16$). Mean treatment duration was 10.9 ± 2.3 months [125].

The results of 57 patients (3 excluded from analysis) showed improvements in behavioral outbreaks (61% of the children), communication problems (47%), anxiety (in 39% of children), stress (in 33% of children), and disruptive behavior (in 33% of children) [125].

Medication usage changed over the study: of the 49 on pharmaceuticals, 16 children (33%) received less medications or lower dosage and 12 (24%) stopped taking medications (all received at least 1 antipsychotic), while four children (8%) received more medications or higher dose [125].

Most prevalent side effects included hypervigilance leading to aggravation of sleep problems (14%) (which was usually resolved by omitting or adjusting the evening dose), restlessness, loss of appetite, and nervousness (9% each). Three children (5%) stopped the treatment due to side effects that included marked irritability after treatment onset in two cases and a psychotic event in one adolescent girl [125].

### Prospective Study in Children with ASD Treated with CBD-Rich Oil

A prospective study was conducted in 188 ASD children (mean age 12.9 ± 7.0 years, 82% males) treated with medicinal cannabis (the majority cannabis oil containing 30% CBD and 1.5% THC) between 2015 and 2017. Most patients consumed oil with 30% CBD and 1.5% THC, on average 79.5 ± 61.5 mg CBD and 4.0 ± 3.0 mg THC, three times a day.

The study found that after 6 months of treatment, of the 93 responding to the questionnaire, 28 patients (30.1%) reported a significant improvement, 50 (53.7%) moderate, 6 (6.4%) slight, and 8 (8.6%) no change in their condition. More than 80% of the parents reported a significant or moderate improvement in child global assessment.

Quality of life was improved. Prior to treatment, good QoL was reported by 31.3% of patients and, after 6 months of treatment, reported by 66.8% of patients. Prior to treatment, positive mood was reported by the parents in 42% of cases, whilst after 6 months, this percentage rose to 63.5% ($p < 0.001$). Good sleep and concentration were reported by 3.3% and 0.0%, respectively, prior to treatment, and this rose to 24.7% and 14.0%, respectively, during treatment (both statistically significant improvements).

Other improvements after 6 months included in relation to seizures as follows: of 13 patients with seizures still on treatment at 6 months, 11 reported disappearance of symptoms and 2 reported improvement. Restlessness and rage attacks improved in 72 patients (91%) and 66 patients (90.3%), respectively.

Regarding medication use from the same 93 patients, 67 reported use of chronic medications at the study baseline. At 6 months, six patients (8.9%) reported an increase in their drug consumption, 38 patients (56.7%) reported their drug consumption remained the same, and 23 patients (34.3%) reported a decrease in drugs used, mainly of the following families: antipsychotics, antiepileptics, antidepressants, and hypnotics and sedatives [101].

Adverse effects were found to be mild. Most common adverse events were somnolence ($n$ = 12 children) and change in appetite (six experienced a decrease in appetite, four an increase in appetite). Of the 93 patients reporting following 6-month treatment, 23 patients (25.2%) experienced at least one side effect. The most common side effects were restlessness (6 patients, 6.6%), sleepiness (3, 3.2%), psychoactive effect (3, 3.2%), increased appetite (3, 3.2%), digestion problems (3, 3.2%), dry mouth (2, 2.2%), and lack of appetite (2, 2.2%). The study authors concluded that cannabis in ASD patients appears to be well tolerated, safe, and effective [101].

After 6–9 months of treatment, most patients showed some level of improvement in more than one of the eight symptom categories measured. The greatest improvements were for seizures, ADHD, sleep disorders, and communication and social interaction deficits. Of the ten non-epileptic patients, nine had a 30% or better improvement in at least one of eight symptom categories, whilst six had an improvement of 30% or better in at least two categories and four had improvement of 30% or more in at least four symptom categories. Of the ten using concurrent medications, nine kept their improvements after reducing or withdrawing from their medications [96].

### Brazilian CBD-Enriched *Cannabis sativa* Extract Observational Study

In a compassionate-use, observational study, a cohort of 18 autistic patients (ten without and five with epilepsy) underwent treatment with a standardized CBD-enriched CE (with a CBD to THC ratio of 75/1) and an average ending dose of 4.55 mg/kg/day. Three dropped out after 1 month due to adverse events. After 6–9 months of treatment, most patients, including epileptic and non-epileptic, showed some level of improvement in more than one of the eight symptom categories but with very infrequent and mild adverse effects. Among the 15 patients who adhered to the treatment (ten non-epileptic and five epileptic), only 1 patient showed lack of improvement in autistic symptoms. The greatest improvements were for seizures, ADHD, sleep disorders, and communication and social interaction deficits. Of the ten non-epileptic patients, nine had a 30% or better improvement in at least one of eight symptom categories, whilst six had an improvement of 30% or better in at least two categories and four had improvement of 30% or more in at least four symptom categories. Of the ten using concurrent medications, nine were able to maintain their improvements after reducing or withdrawing from their medications [96].

### Chilean Study: Whole Plant Cannabis Extract

In a Chilean study, 20 children and 1 adult were treated daily with a sublingual dose of cannabis extract (whole plant, typically 1:1 CBD:THC) for at least 3 months. Results indicated that CBD was more effective than conventional autism medicines. Most patients treated with cannabis (71%) had improved at least one core symptom of ASD including social interaction, communication, or repetitive behaviors, and 67% patients showed significant overall improvements [209].

### Open-Label Study of Children with ASD with 20:1 Ratio CBD:THC Oil

In an open-label study, 53 children with ASD (median age of 11 (4–22)) received cannabidiol for a median duration of 66 days (range 30–588 days). The cannabinoid oil supplied had a concentration of 30% with a 20:1 ratio of CBD:THC. Recommended daily dose of CBD was 16 mg/kg (maximal daily dose of 600 mg) and for THC, daily dose of 0.8mg/kg (maximal daily dose of 40 mg) for the study. Analysis of study data indicated that the THC median interquartile range (IQR) daily dose was 7 (4–11) mg and CBD median (IQR) daily dose was 90 (45–143) mg [187].

The following results were found, set out in Table 10.2.

**Table 10.2** Results of Barchel et al.'s study [187]—changes in associated comorbidities of ASD

| Associated comorbid symptom or sign | Improved (%) | No change (%) | Worse (%) |
|---|---|---|---|
| Self-injury and rage attacks ($n = 34$ children) | 67.6 | 28.9 | 8.8 |
| Hyperactivity symptoms ($n = 38$ children) | 68.4 | 28.9 | 2.6 |
| Sleep problems ($n = 21$ children) | 71.4 | 23.8 | 4.7 |
| Anxiety ($n = 17$ children) | 47.1 | 29.4 | 23.5 |

There was no statistically significant difference compared with conventional treatment as published in the literature for all of these variables, except for self-injury where there was a borderline significance in improvement of symptoms compared to the conventional treatment ($p = 0.063$). There was no statistical difference in worsening of symptoms ($p = 0.307$). Adverse effects, mostly somnolence and change in appetite, were mild [187].

## Case Reports of CBD Treatment in Fragile X Syndrome Patients

There are three case reports of patients diagnosed with FXS syndrome documented by Tartaglia et al. [83], all of which were treated with CBD oil and reported improvements. One of the cases is of a toddler who was diagnosed with FXS and was given an oral paste (18–23.5% CBD) with trace amounts of THC (0.03%) at a dose of 50 mg/day (in coconut oil). Behavioral improvements were noticed by the family within the first month of treatment, and continual improvements over the next 3 months were also noted including better motor coordination, more frequent and longer eye contact, increased positive interactions with other children, and others. Interestingly, when the child was 30 months of age, the parents discontinued the CBD treatment and began the child on minocycline, and the child displayed increased anxiety and poorer sleep (difficult falling asleep and staying asleep) and meltdowns occurred more often. At 3 years of age, the child was on sertraline and minocycline and was making slow progress, but there were problems with attention span, anxiety, sleep, and continued frequent meltdowns. The child was restarted on CBD treatment (50 mg/day), and there was a reduction in anxiety, meltdowns, and sleep. The child continues on CBD [83].

Two other case studies of FXS patients, one of a male and another of a female in their early to mid-20s, were reported which demonstrated benefits of CBD oil including less anxiety, cessation of panic attacks, improved work performance, less social avoidance, better sleep, and improved linguistic skills [83].

## Randomized Controlled Trial of Oral Cannabinoids in ASD

A double-blind, placebo-controlled study was conducted in 150 patients (age 5–21 years) with ASD. Two medicinal cannabis products were compared with placebo: a CBD-dominant product whole plant cannabis extract (with 20:1 ratio of CBD and THC) and a purified product (with 20:1 ratio of CBD and THC). Participants received the treatment medication or placebo for 12 weeks, followed by a 4-week washout period. The groups were then crossed over to receive one of the other study medications for a further 12 weeks (those in the placebo group initially received the whole plant extract; those who initially received the purified extract received the placebo; those who initially received the whole plant extract received the purified extract). The primary outcome variables were change in behavioral problems as measured by the Home Situation Questionnaire-ASD (HSQ-ASD) and the Clinical Global Impression-Improvement scale (CGI-I, with disruptive behavior anchor points). Secondary outcome variables were the Social Responsiveness Scale (SRS-2) and Autism Parenting Stress Index (APSI) [208].

For each treatment period, the starting dose was 1 mg/kg CBD (0.05 mg/kg THC) daily. Dose was increased by 1 mg/kg CBD (and therefore 0.05 mg/kg/day

THC) per day every second day up to 10 mg/kg body weight per day CBD (and 0.5 mg/kg/day THC) for children 20–40 kg in weight, or up to 7.5 mg/kg/day CBD (and 0.375 mg/kg/day THC) for children over 40 kg (to a maximum of 420 mg/kg CBD and 21 mg THC per day) divided as three daily doses. Treatments were oral (sublingual where possible) as an adjunct to any ongoing stable medication (72% took concomitant medications). At the end of the treatment period (4 weeks), the study treatment was gradually decreased over 2 weeks.

There was no difference between the total scores of the HSQ-ASD and APSI scores between groups. Disruptive behavior as measured on the CGI-I was much or very much improved in 49% of the whole plant extract group compared with 21% on placebo (this was statistically significant at $p = 0.005$), but there was no significant difference between the pure cannabinoid and placebo groups. There was also no significant difference between the whole plant and pure cannabinoid groups on the HSQ-ASD, APSI, and CGI-I scores. With respect to the secondary outcome variables, median SRS total score improved significantly more in the whole plant group compared with placebo (improvement of 14.9 points in whole plant group and 3.6 points in the placebo group, $p = 0.009$), and there was no significant difference between the pure cannabinoid and placebo groups. Notably, there were no serious adverse events. Common adverse events included somnolence (28% of whole plant group, 23% of pure cannabinoid group, and 8% of placebo group) and decreased appetite (25% of whole plant group, 21% of pure cannabinoid group, and 15% of placebo group) [208].

#### Systematic Review

A recent systematic review which included ten studies concluded that cannabinoids appear to improve some ASD-associated symptoms including problematic behaviors, sleep problems, and hyperactivity and that there were limited cardiac and metabolic side effects. The review also found that cannabinoids generally allowed reduction of number of prescription medicines and, in patients with comorbid epilepsy, decreased frequency of seizures. It suggested the mechanisms of action may be linked to an imbalance in excitation and inhibition found in ASD. It also concluded that knowledge of the effects on ASD core symptoms was very little [210].

## Guidelines for Treating ASD with Medicinal Cannabis

### When to Use Medicinal Cannabis

Most ASD responds well to medicinal cannabis for either primary abnormalities or comorbidities. Those ASD patients who do not respond may have one of the variants that cannot be modulated by the ECS or associated targets, or it is possible that they may need a particular blend of cannabinoids or terpenes as yet unknown. There is hope that early use of medicinal cannabis could modulate physiologic, cognitive, and emotional development to optimize health and performance without maintenance dosing.

## Type of Product (Blends)

Ideal blends are high in CBD and low in THC. Several terpenes like caryophyllene may be a significant part of the product blend and combine well with hemp phytocannabinoids to complement the effects in both anxiety behavior and neuroinflammatory aspects of ASD.

## What Form of Product Should You Use?

It is particularly challenging to find the best medicinal cannabis formulations for ASD patients because of taste and texture sensitivities. The patient or family may best be able to guide the selection based on taste or texture and the ability to swallow capsules.

- **Oral tinctures and liposomal products**: are fast acting when held in the mouth or under the tongue (sublingual) but not well tolerated in ASD.
- **Capsules**: are fixed in dose and seem to have longer duration of effects, but onset is delayed by 60–90 min.

Masking flavors in another food or drink is occasionally successful, but generally a formulation change is needed. Alternatively, capsules (vegetable glycerin type) can be used as suppositories, and almost all medicinal cannabis liquids are absorbed through the skin.

The clinical response for topically applied CBD has been good for urgent conditions like behavior meltdowns.

## Dosing Guidelines

Start dosing with the recommended product serving size for patients seven (7) years or older. For patients under 7 years of age or those known to be dose sensitive, use half a serving or smaller. Physiologic changes with a responsive dose can occur within minutes of oral-mucosal servings and topical use. Topical use of oral formulas can be effective during "melt-down" crisis management or for calming effect if touching or massage is tolerated.

### Target Dose

Studies suggest 1–2 mg/kg CBD as a common steady dosage, and this is consistent with my experience. Increase the dose by half (½) serving with stress like upper respiratory or febrile illness.

### Frequency

Twice daily of the same dose is the usual but not required. And not all of the doses need to be the same so that if extra coverage is needed at certain times of the day or night, then a larger amount can be used. Alternatively, an extra dose can be added. Medicinal cannabis works primarily by signaling within the body system not by maintaining blood levels like antiepileptic drugs.

### Duration

Over time the amount of medicinal cannabis needed may increase or decrease. Medicinal cannabis does not induce tolerance, but because medicinal cannabis induces epigenetic and metabolic changes, some patients may see their dose change. Stopping or skipping medicinal cannabis is not an issue except if the patient is dependent on its use for controlling certain disruptive behaviors.

### Stopping Other Medications

Many patients have been able to reduce or decrease other drugs that they have been relying on. This should be done with physician guidance. Generally a taper is used, reducing by 25% per week for 4 weeks for most substances. In some cases the drug should be maintained to optimize performance albeit at a lesser dose.

## Titration and Follow-Up

This is a prime condition for following the adage "start low and go slow." Adjust the dose every 2–3 days by about half a single dose depending on behavior changes. Keep a log of several characteristic parameters so that you can track progress or digressions. Since there are usually several causes that could disrupt the patient's progress, those should be tracked as well. Over time patterns may emerge to allow the caregivers to anticipate situations and adjust the dose accordingly.

Improvements often are slow but progressive so that monthly follow-ups are very appropriate as medicinal cannabinoids make subtle metabolic, membrane (as in gastrointestinal, blood-brain barriers), and epigenetic changes.

## Other Tips to Enhance Therapeutic Action

Diets of high fat, particularly saturated fats, work well with cannabinoids. In fact, very-high-fat diets induce ketones that have some of the same anti-inflammatory targets as cannabinoids (e.g., PPAR-$\alpha$) [211]. Sulforaphane, a natural substance found in cruciferous vegetables, targets the nuclear factor-erythroid 2 (NRF2) cellular antioxidant system and improves cases of ASD [212]. CBD also activates this pathway which might explain some clinical synergy [213]. Caryophyllene may also play a role in the same Nrf2 pathway in the brain and is a superb terpene supplement targeting CB2R for controlling inflammation throughout the body [214].

## Adverse Effects and Interactions

The most common side effect from medicinal cannabis is fatigue that indicates too high a dose. In rare patients even the smallest dose may induce anxiety. The literature suggests that lower doses can be activating while higher doses are sedating. Too little medicinal cannabis will not show any appreciable effect. Again in rare patients, medicinal cannabis at even small doses may induce psychoactive effects. All is not lost, however. Some patients have reported very small and careful titrations have allowed them to continue medicinal cannabis, and this may possibly be rebalancing the body endocannabinoid system.

Interactions with other medications are rare at usual doses. Interactions have been reported with pharmaceutical dose levels well over 5 mg/kg when patients were also using the antiepileptic drugs valproate and clobazam. However, because of shared neurotransmitter targets, medicinal cannabis can amplify some drugs. Look for side effects of those pharmaceutical drugs used concurrently in assessing the situation. Become very familiar with the other drug side effects.

From a positive side, medicinal cannabis works well with lifestyle changes including diet, exercise, tranquility, other natural agents, and supplements. This also includes other therapy modalities about which we continue to learn more and more.

## Case Studies from Dr. Blair's Practice

### Case 1, ASD Level 3

Erin 10, Australia, first presentation April 2015.

***Presenting Problem:*** Autism spectrum disorder with onset at 3 years of age, manifesting with social withdrawal, no eye contact, five words or less in speech, attention-deficit hyperactive, self-stimulating to the point of self-injury. He has been enrolled in a number of rehabilitation programs with minimal progress. A history of multiple unsuccessful medications.

***Other Details:*** Bowel habits irregular, sleep limited to a few hours per day. Diet limited by taste and texture sensitivities to a narrow range of processed foods. No known allergies but chronic eczematous rash in atopic pattern of skin fold on arms.

No current medications or food supplements.

***Past History:*** Recurrent minor infections and respiratory illnesses, no operations or procedures, standard immunizations up to 15 months.

***Family History:*** Mother and father with two older sisters in good health.

***Examination and Observation:*** Normal appearing 10-year-old, small for age: weight and height were 25 kg and 50 cm respectively (5th percentile height and weight for age). Videos demonstrate a thin male child poorly responsive to parental direction, jumping and running from place to place in household and climbing onto counters. At each location he would engage in self-stimulation with hand-finger tapping, putting foreign objects into his mouth and spitting them out.

***Assessment:*** ASD level 3 requiring very substantial support: Inflexibility of behavior, extreme difficulty coping with change, or other restricted/repetitive behaviors markedly interfere with functioning in all spheres. Great distress/difficulty changing focus or action.

**Treatment**

After thorough consultation and informed consent, the family agreed to medicinal cannabis therapy using a full-spectrum hemp-derived CBD tincture with a ratio of CBD:THC of 20:1. Starting dose was 10 mg twice per day. Parents were advised to adjust the dose and frequency to control his symptoms and behaviors. During the next 6 weeks, the dose increased to 15 mg three times per day and as needed for stressful situations or infections.

**Follow-Up**

Parents reported Erin was now speaking some words and asking for objects or foods that he wanted as well as being generally more verbal. His teachers reported improved performance in swimming classes including following instructions. No specific measurements were provided, but parents felt he was significantly larger in height and weight.

Sleep significantly improved to 6–8 h per night. Appetite has improved, he is eating more, and he is happy to try new foods. Constipation is resolved with daily bowel movement. His chronic skin rash is completely resolved.

Behavior is relaxed and calm. He listens intently, shows interest in activities around him, and eats at the table with his family. Signs of anxiety or compulsive behavior are indicators for another MC dose. Currently functioning at ASD level 1.

Video clips show Erin sitting quietly in bed listening to a vocabulary picture game on a computer tablet, responding carefully and appropriately to the game and making eye contact with the videographer. Other videos show close sibling contact while viewing television and evidence that Erin is allowing physical affection towards himself.

## Case 2, ASD Level 2

Nate, 15 year-old boy, Massachusetts, USA, first presentation August 2017

***Presenting Problem:*** Anxiety and anger control in 15-year-old boy with ASD level 2 requiring special school environment. Diagnosed with bipolar syndrome. Taking

SSRI antidepressants for several years, no lithium. Average intelligence but socially limited interaction with occasional outbursts requiring supportive environment in special school. He easily becomes anxious with loud noises or new environments. He experiences wide swings in mood and behavior and supervision.

***Other Details:*** Sleep and bowel function normal. Height and weight are average (170 cm, 65 kg).

***Past History:*** No remarkable illnesses or infections or chronic physical disorders. Normal blood pressure and pulse. History of normal regular physical examination and immunizations.

***Family History:*** Lives with father, stepmother, and their daughter. Birth mother has history of bipolar behavioral disorder.

***Diet:*** Balanced omnivore diet.

### Treatment

Initial therapy started with a liposomal water-soluble full-spectrum hemp-derived medicinal cannabis with CBD:THC ratio of 20:1. This product was shown to have improved bioavailability on the order of 5:1 compared with tincture. He began with standard serving size of 5 mg in water or juice twice per day or as needed for anxiety. After showing an immediate response, the dose was increased to 15 mg per day. The broccoli extract sulforaphane was introduced as a food supplement.

### Follow-Up

Within 4 weeks the parents reported improvements in compassion, social skills, cooperation, maturity, mood, and sleep. He was noticeably less anxious—tornado warnings, thunderstorms, and power outages that had bother him and caused him to perseverate. After starting medicinal cannabis, he handled them as if they were no big deal. A close lightning strike and extremely loud thunderclap made him jump, but then he laughed it off and went back to doing what he was doing. "In the past, he might have shown increased anxiety and talked about it excessively. He did not seem to be phased at all!"

At this point the father also started therapy with medicinal cannabis for his stress management and well-being.

Medicinal cannabis capsules of 15 mg were added to Nate's program before school for their sustained effects over the course of the school day. Liposome product was used at home and as needed for stressful or anxious episodes.

Over the course of the next 2 months, Nate was able to re-integrate to regular high school and enroll in carpentry program with great enjoyment. His medications remained unchanged during this time except for the addition of CoQ10 and magnesium citrate providing some additional mood stability.

Over the next 9 months, Nate's condition continued, but medicinal cannabis was no longer providing any specific benefit and at times was felt to worsen his mood and behaviors. This was also a time for some major hormonal changes. At this point the medicinal cannabis and sulforaphane were discontinued in regular use. However, the family was confident that medicinal cannabis was instrumental in Nate's recovery and transition to greater independence and ASD level 1.

## Conclusion

ASD is a complex behavioral condition associated with several comorbidities (including anxiety, depression, sleep disorders, learning difficulties). It begins in early childhood and extends throughout life. The etiology and pathogenesis of ASD are complex and involve altered neurodevelopment and neural connectivity, genetic and environmental factors, inflammation, immune system dysregulation, and abnormal endocannabinoid tone and signaling. The endocannabinoid system is involved in the modulation of many cellular functions and molecular pathways altered in ASD. Several lines of research indicate that CBD may have a role to play in alleviating many of the neurobehavioral aspects of ASD, operating via multiple potential targets relevant to ASD.

There are many other potential factors that might feed into the neurobehavioral problems associated with ASD. Although we have not addressed them in this chapter, it bears repeating that it is important to look carefully at nutritional and environmental factors. Toxins in the environment of a child or indeed adult with ASD may add to the toxic load on the body and brain. Remember that the child with ASD has a neurological system that is still critically developing. Environmental toxins can be chemicals in water used to drink and bathe in, chemicals in personal care products, cleaning products, and others. It is vital that nutrition and diet are optimal. Pro-inflammatory diets will not help any chronic condition, including neurological conditions like ASD. Chemicals in food packaging (in plastics in particular, which can leach into foods), foods sprayed with pesticides, and chemicals used as flavorings, coloring, and preservatives, for example, can all add to a toxicity overload on a sensitive neurological system. Electromagnetic frequencies emitted from cell phones and tablets may have detrimental effects on our brains. An integrative approach which takes into account many factors that may contribute to poor health is going to be the best way to help patients and empower them with knowledge, in particular about things they can personally change.

## References

1. Chakrabarti B, Persico A, Battistia N, Maccarrone M. Endocannabinoid signaling in autism. Neurotherapeutics. 2015;12:837–47.
2. American Psychiatric Association, editor. Diagnostic and statistical manual of mental disorders. 5th ed. Arlington: American Psychiatric Association; 2013.

3. D'Cruz AM, Mosconi MW, Ragozzino ME, et al. Alterations in the functional neural circuitry supporting flexible choice behavior in autism spectrum disorders. Transl Psychiatry. 2016;6(10):e916.
4. Green JJ, Hollander E. Autism and oxytocin: new developments in translational approaches to therapeutics. Neurotherapeutics. 2010;7:250–7.
5. Lord C, Cook EH, Leventhal BL, et al. Autism spectrum disorders. Neuron. 2000;28:355–63.
6. Fletcher-Watson S, Leekam SR, Benson V, et al. Eye-movements reveal attention to social information in autism spectrum disorder. Neuropsychologia. 2009;47:248–57.
7. Klin A, Ones W, Schultz R, et al. Visual fixation patterns during viewing of naturalistic social situations as predictors of social competence in individuals with autism. Arch Gen Psychiatry. 2002;59:809–16.
8. Sasson NJ, Dichter GS, Bodfish JW. Affective responses by adults with autism are reduced to social images but elevated to images related to circumscribed interests. PLoS One. 2012;7:e42457.
9. Richey JA, Rittenberg A, Hughes L, et al. Common and distinct neural features of social and non-social reward processing in autism and social anxiety disorder. Soc Cogn Affect Neurosci. 2014;9:367–77.
10. Lai MC, Lombardo MV, Baron-Cohen S. Autism. Lancet. 2014;383:896–910.
11. Centers for Disease Control and Prevention (CDC). Developmental Disabilities Monitoring Network Surveillance Year 2010 Principal Investigators. Prevalence of autism spectrum disorder among children aged 8 years – autism and developmental disabilities monitoring network, 11 sites, United States, 2010. MMWR Surveill Summ. 2014;63:1–21.
12. Ozonoff S, Young GS, Carter A, et al. Recurrence risk for autism spectrum disorders: a Baby Siblings Research Consortium study. Pediatrics. 2011;128:e488–95.
13. Pretzche CM, Freyberg J, Voinescu B, et al. Effects of cannabidiol on brain excitation and inhibition systems; a randomised placebo-controlled single dose trial during magnetic resonance spectroscopy in adults with and without autism spectrum disorder. Neuropsychopharmacology. 2019;44:1398–405.
14. Antshel KM, Zhang-James Y, Wagner K, et al. An update on the comorbidity of ASD and ADHD: a focus on clinical management. Expert Rev Neurother. 2016;16:1744–8360. https://doi.org/10.1586/14737175.2016.1146591.
15. Chen YL, Chen SH, Gau SSF. ADHD and autistic traits, family function, parenting style, and social adjustment for internet addiction among children and adolescents in Taiwan: a longitudinal study. Res Dev Disabil. 2015;39:20–31.
16. Cohen S, Conduit R, Lockley SW, et al. The relationship between sleep and behavior in autism spectrum disorder (ASD): a review. J Neurodev Disord. 2014;6:44.
17. Coury DL, Ashwood P, Fasano A, et al. Gastrointestinal conditions in children with autism spectrum disorder: developing a research agenda. Pediatrics. 2012;130(Suppl 2):S160–8.
18. De Bruin EI, Ferdinand RF, Meester S, et al. High rates of psychiatric co-morbidity in PDD-NOS. J Autism Dev Disord. 2007;37:877–86.
19. Fombonne E. Epidemiology of autistic disorder and other pervasive developmental disorders. J Clin Psychiatry. 2005;66:3–8.
20. Ghaziddin M, Zafar S. Psychiatric comorbidity of adults with ASD. Clin Neuropsychiatry. 2008;5:9–12.
21. Gillott A, Standen PJ. Levels of anxiety and sources of stress in adults with autism. J Intellect Disabil. 2007;11:359–70.
22. Lalanne L, Weiner L, Bertschy G. Treatment of addiction in adults with autism spectrum disorder. Cham: Springer; 2017. p. 377–95.
23. Lefter R, Ciobica A, Timofte D, et al. A descriptive review on the prevalence of gastrointestinal disturbances and their multiple associations in autism spectrum disorder. Medicina (Kaunas). 2019;56(1):11.
24. Richards C, Moss J, Nelson L, et al. Persistence of self-injurious behaviour in autism spectrum disorder over 3 years: a prospective cohort study of risk markers. J Neurodev Disord. 2016;8:21. https://doi.org/10.1186/s11689-016-9153-x.

25. Richdale AL, Schreck KA. Sleep problems in autism spectrum disorders: prevalence, nature, & possible biopsychosocial aetiologies. Sleep Med Rev. 2009;13(6):403–11.
26. Romano M, Truzoli R, Osborne LA, Reed P. The relationship between autism quotient, anxiety, and internet addiction. Res Autism Spectr Disord. 2014;8:1521–6.
27. Simonoff E, Pickles A, Charman T, et al. Psychiatric disorders in children with autism spectrum disorders: prevalence, comorbidity, and associated factors in a population-derived sample. J Am Acad Child Adolesc Psychiatry. 2008;47:921–9.
28. Souders MC, Mason TB, Valladares O, et al. Sleep behaviors and sleep quality in children with autism spectrum disorders. Sleep. 2009;32:1566–78.
29. Tarazi F, Sahli Z, Pleskow J, Mousa S. Asperger's syndrome: diagnosis, comorbidity and therapy. Expert Rev Neurother. 2015;15:281–93.
30. Tuchman R, Rapin I. Epilepsy in autism. Lancet Neurol. 2002;1:352–8.
31. Veatch OJ, Stucliffe JS, Warren ZE, et al. Shorter sleep duration is associated with social impairment and comorbidities in ASD. Autism Res. 2017;10(7):1221–38.
32. Horvath K, Papadimitriou JC, Rabsztyn A, et al. Gastrointestinal abnormalities in children with autistic disorder. J Pediatr. 1999;135(5):559–63.
33. Cooper M, et al. Autistic traits in children with ADHD index clinical and cognitive problems. Eur Child Adolesc Psychiatry. 2014;23(1):23–34.
34. Kotte A, et al. Autistic traits in children with and without ADHD. Pediatrics. 2013;132(3):e612–22.
35. Jensen CM, Steinhausen HC. Comorbid mental disorders in children and adolescents with attention-deficit/hyperactivity disorder in a large nationwide study. Atten Defic Hyperact Disord. 2015;7(1):27–38.
36. Hirvikovski T, Mittendorfer-Rutz E, Boman M, et al. Premature mortality in autism spectrum disorder. Br J Psychiatry. 2016;208:232–8.
37. Gillberg C, Billstedt E, Sundh V, Gillberg IC. Mortality in autism: a prospective longitudinal community-based study. J Autism Dev Disord. 2010;40:352–7.
38. Isager T, Mouridsen SE, Rich B. Mortality and causes of death in pervasive developmental disorders. Autism. 1999;3:7–16.
39. Won J, Jin Y, Choi J, et al. Melatonin as a novel interventional candidate for fragile x syndrome with autism spectrum disorder in humans. Int J Mol Sci. 2017;18:1314.
40. Romano T. Autism and cannabis: here's what the science says. Leafly.com, 20 June 2018. Available at: https://www.leafly.com/news/health/autism-and-cannabis-heres-what-the-science-says. Accessed 1 Dec 2019.
41. Amaral DG, Schumann CM, Nordahl CW. Neuroanatomy of autism. Trends Neurosci. 2008;31:137–45.
42. Di Cicco-Bloom E, Lord C, Zwaigenbaum L, et al. The developmental neurobiology of autism spectrum disorder. J Neurosci. 2006;26:6897–906.
43. Dietert RR, Dietert JM, Dewitt JC. Environmental risk factors for autism. Emerg Health Threats J. 2011;4:7111.
44. Sevadio M, Melancia F, Manduca A, et al. Targeting anandamide metabolism rescues core and associated autistic-like symptoms in rats prenatally exposed to valproic acid. Transl Psychiatry. 2016;6:e902. https://doi.org/10.1038/tp.2016.182.
45. Aran A, Eylon M, Harel M, et al. Lower circulating endocannabinoid levels in children with autism spectrum disorder. Mol Autism. 2019a;10:2.
46. Belmonte MK, Allen G, Beckel-Mitchener A, et al. Autism and abnormal development of brain connectivity. J Neurosci. 2004;24(42):9228–31.
47. Morgan JT, Chana G, Pardo CA, et al. Microglial activation and increased microglial density observed in the dorsolateral prefrontal cortex in autism. Biol Psychiatry. 2010;68:368–76.
48. Ohja K, Gozal E, Fahnestock M, et al. Neuroimmunologic and neurotrophic interactions in autism spectrum disorders: relationship to neuroinflammation. Neuromolecular Med. 2018;20(2):161–73.

49. Siniscalco D, Bradstreet JJ, Cirillo A, Antonucci N. The in vitro GcMAF effects on endocannabinoid system transcriptionomics, receptor formation, and cell activity of autism-derived macrophages. J Neuroinflammation. 2014;11:78.
50. Vargas DK, Nascimbene C, Krishnan C, et al. Neuroglial activation and neuroinflammation in the brain of patients with autism. Ann Neurol. 2005;7(1):67–81.
51. Wei D, Dinh D, Lee DY, et al. Enhancement of anandamide-mediated endocannabinoid signaling corrects autism-related social impairment. Cannabis Cannabinoid Res. 2016;1:1. https://doi.org/10.1089/can.2015.0008.
52. Young AM, Campbell E, Lynch S, et al. Aberrant NF-kappa B expression in autism spectrum condition: a mechanism for neuroinflammation. Front Psychiatry. 2011;2:27.
53. Bourgeron T. From the genetic architecture to synaptic plasticity in autism spectrum disorder. Nat Rev Neurosci. 2015;16(9):551–63.
54. Hazlett H, Gu H, Munsell B, et al. Early brain development in infants at high risk for autism spectrum disorder. Nature. 2017;542:348–51.
55. Kucharsky Hiess R, Alter R, Sojoudi S et al. Corpus Callosum Area and Brain Volume in Autism Spectrum Disorder: Quantitative Analysis of Structural MRI from the ABIDE Database. Journal of Autism and Developmental Disorders. 2015;45(10):3107–14.
56. Stigler KA, McDougle CJ. Chapter 3.1 - Structural and functional MRI studies of autism spectrum disorders. In: Buxbaum JD, Hof PR, editors. The neuroscience of autism spectrum disorders. Academic Press; 2013. p. 251–66.
57. Doherty CC, Evans DW, Myers SM, et al. A comparison of structural brain imaging findings in autism spectrum disorder and attention-deficit hyperactivity disorder. Neuropsychol Rev. 2015;26:25–43.
58. Qiu T, Chang C, Li Y, et al. Two years changes in the development of caudate nucleus are involved in restricted repetitive behaviors in 2–5-year-old children with autism spectrum disorder. Dev Cogn Neurosci. 2016;19:137–43.
59. Chakrabarti B, Haffey A, Canzano L et al. Individual differences in responsivity to social rewards: Insights from two eye-tracking tasks. PLoS ONE. 2017;12(10):e0185146.
60. Haznedar M, Buchsbaum MS, Hazlett EA, et al. Volumetric analysis and three-dimensional glucose metabolic mapping of the striatum and thalamus in patients with autism spectrum disorders. Am J Psychiatry. 2006;163:1252–63.
61. Hikosaka O. Basal ganglia mechanisms of reward-oriented eye movement. Ann N Y Acad Sci. 2007;1104:229–49.
62. Nakamura K, Hikosaka O. Role of dopamine in the primate caudate nucleus in reward modulation of saccades. J Neurosci. 2006;26(20):5360–69.
63. Piven J, Elison JT, Zylka MJ. Toward a conceptual framework for early brain and behavior development in autism. Mol Psychiatry. 2017 Oct;22(10):1385–94.
64. Chapleau CA, Larimore JL, Theivert A, et al. Modulation of dendritic spine development and plasticity by BDNF and vesicular trafficking: fundamental roles in neurodevelopmental disorders associated with mental retardation and autism. J Neurodev Disord. 2009;1:185–96.
65. Phillips M, Pozzo-Miller L. Dendritic spine dysgenesis in autism related disorders. Neurosci Lett. 2015;601:30–40.
66. Tang G, Gudsnuk K, Kuo SH, et al. Loss of mTOR-dependent macroautophagy causes autistic-like synaptic pruning deficits. Neuron. 2014;83(5):1131–43.
67. Kasarpalkar NJ, Kothari ST, Dave UP. Brain-Derived Neurotrophic Factor in children with Autism Spectrum Disorder. Ann Neurosci. 2014;21(4):129–33.
68. Chen J, Alberts I, Li X. Dysregulation of the IGF-I/PI3K/AKT/mTOR signaling pathway in autism spectrum disorders. Int J Dev Neurosci. 2014;35(1):35–41.
69. Huber M, Klann E, Costa-Mattioli M, Zukin RS. Dysregulation of mammalian target of rapamycin signaling in mouse models of autism. J Neurosci. 2015;35:13836–42.
70. Manning BD, Cantley LC. AKT/PKB Signaling: navigating downstream. Cell. 2007;129(7):1261–74.
71. Riikonen R, Makkonen I, et al. Cerebrospinal fluid insulin-like growth factors IGF-1 and IGF-2 in infantile autism. Dev Med Child Neurol. 2006;48(9):751–5.

72. Steinman G, Mankuta D. Insulin-like growth factor and the etiology of autism. Med Hypotheses. 2013;80(4):475–80.
73. Ehninger D, Li W, Fox K, Stryker MP, Silva AJ. Reversing neurodevelopmental disorders in adults. Neuron. 2008;60(6):950–60.
74. Tang G, Gutierrez Rios P, Kuo SH, et al. Mitochondrial abnormalities in temporal lobe of autistic brain. Neurobiol Dis. 2013;54:349–61.
75. Schmeisser K, Parker JA. Pleiotropic effects of mTor and autophagy during development and aging. Front Cell Dev Biol. 2019;7:192. https://doi.org/10.3389/fcell.2019.00192.
76. Saha S, Panigrahi DP, Patil S, Bhutia SK. Autophagy in health and disease: a comprehensive review. Biomed Pharmacother. 2018;104:485–95.
77. Bryn V, Halvorsen B, Ueland T, et al. Brain derived neurotrophic factor (BDNF) and autism spectrum disorders (ASD) in childhood. Eur J Paediatr Neurol. 2015;19(4):411–4.
78. Qin X-Y, Feng J-C, Cao C, et al. Association of peripheral blood levels of brain-derived neurotrophic factor with autism spectrum disorder in children. A systematic review and meta-analysis. JAMA Pediatr. 2016;170(11):1079–86.
79. AL-Ayadhi L. Serum levels of brain-derived neurotrophic factor (BDNF) in autistic children in central Saudi Arabia. Open Conf Proc J. 2011;2(1):36–40.
80. Hallmayer J, Cleveland S, Torres A, et al. Genetic heritability and shared environmental factors among twin pairs with autism. Arch Gen Psychiatry. 2011;68:1095–102.
81. Abrahams BS, Geschwind DH. Advances in autism genetics: on the threshold of a new neurobiology. Nat Rev Genet. 2008;9:341–55.
82. Jung KW, Sepers M, Henstridge CM, et al. Uncoupling of the endocannabinoid signalling complex in a mouse model of fragile X syndrome. Nat Commun. 2012;3:1080.
83. Tartaglia N, Bonn-Miller M, Hagerman R. Treatment of Fragile X Syndrome with cannabidiol: a case series study and brief review of the literature. Cannabis Cannabinoid Res. 2019;4(1):3–9. https://doi.org/10.1089/can.2018.0053.
84. Purcell AE, Jeon OH, Zimmerman AW, et al. Postmortem brain abnormalities of the glutamate neurotransmitter system in autism. Neurology. 2001;57:1618–28.
85. Santocchi E, Guiducci L, Fulceri F, et al. Gut to brain interaction in Autism Spectrum Disorders: a randomized controlled trial on the role of probiotics on clinical, biochemical and neurophysiological parameters. BMC Psychiatry. 2016;16:183.
86. Stein TP, Schluter MD, Steer RA, Ming X. Autism and phthalate metabolite glucuronidation. J Autism Dev Disord. 2013;43:2677–85.
87. Sudhof TC. Neuroligins and neurexins link synaptic function to cognitive disease. Nature. 2008;455(7215):903–11.
88. Speed HE, Masiulis I, Gibson JR, Powell CM. Increased cortical inhibition in autism-linked neuroligin-3R451C mice is due in part to loss of endocannabinoid signaling. PLoS One. 2015;10:e0140638.
89. Corbett BA, Mendoza S, WEgelin JA, et al. Variable cortisol circadian rhythms in children with autism and anticipatory stress. J Psychiatry Neurosci. 2008;33(3):227–34.
90. Geoffray MM, Nicholas A, Speranza M, Georgieff N. Are circadian rhythms new pathways to understand Autism Spectrum Disorder? J Physiol Paris. 2016;110(4, Part B):434–8.
91. Wohr M, Srduz D, Gregory P, et al. Lack of parvalbumin in mice leads to behavioral deficits relevant to all human core symptoms and related neural morphofunctional abnormalities. Trans Psych. 2015;5:e525.
92. Melke J, Goubran Botros H, Chaste P. Abnormal melatonin synthesis in autism spectrum disorders. Mol Psychiatry. 2008;13:90–8.
93. Depino AM. Peripheral and central inflammation in autism spectrum disorders. Mol Cell Neurosci. 2013;53:69–76.
94. Högestätt ED, Jönsson BA, Ermund A, et al. Conversion of acetaminophen to the bioactive N-acylphenolamine AM404 via fatty acid amide hydro- lase-dependent arachidonic acid conjugation in the nervous system. J Biol Chem. 2005;280:31405–12.

95. Schultz ST, Klonoff-Cohen HS, Wingard DL, et al. Acetaminophen (paracetamol) use, measles-mumps-rubella vaccination, and autistic disorder: the results of a parent survey. Autism. 2008;12(3):293–307.
96. Fleury-Teixeira P, Caixeta FV, Ramires da Silva LC, et al. Effects of CBD-enriched cannabis sativa extract on autism spectrum disorder symptoms: an observational study of 18 participants undergoing compassionate use. Front Neurol. 2019;10:1145.
97. Takarae Y, Sweeney J. Neural hyperexcitability in autism spectrum disorders. Brain Sci. 2017;7:129.
98. Zamberletti E, Gabaglio M, Parolaro D. The endocannabinoid system and autism spectrum disorders: insights from animal models. Int J Mol Sci. 2017;18:1916.
99. Ajram LA, Horder J, Mendez MA, et al. Shifting brain inhibitory balance and connectivity of the prefrontal cortex of adults with autism spectrum disorder. Transl Psychiatry. 2017;7(5):e1137.
100. Horder J, Lavender T, Mendez MA, et al. Reduced subcortical glutamate/glutamine in adults with autism spectrum disorders: a [$^{1}$H]MRS study. Transl Psychiatry. 2013;3:e279.
101. Bar-Lev Schleiber L, Mechoulam R, Saban N, et al. Real life experience of medical cannabis treatment in autism: analysis of safety and efficacy. Sci Rep. 2019;9(1):1–7.
102. Chez MG, Chang M, Krasne V, et al. Frequency of epileptiform EEG abnormalities in a sequential screening of autistic patients with no known clinical epilepsy from 1996-2005. Epilepsy Behav. 2006;8:267–71.
103. Markam K, Markam H. The intense world theory- a unifying theory of the neurobiology of autism. Front Hum Neurosci. 2010;4:224.
104. Meyer-Lindenberg A, Domes G, Kirsch P, Heinrichs M. Oxytocin and vasopressin in the human brain: social neuropeptides for translational medicine. Nat Rev Neurosci. 2011;12:524.
105. Goines PE, Ashwood P. Cytokine dysregulation in autism spectrum disorders (ASD): possible role of the environment. Neurotoxicol Teratol. 2013;36:67–81.
106. Schultz ST. Can autism be triggered by acetaminophen activation of the endocannabinoid system? Acta Neurobiol Exp. 2010;70:227–31.
107. Ashwood P, Krakowiak P, Hertz-Picciotto I, et al. Elevated plasma cytokines in autism spectrum disorders provide evidence of immune dysfunction and are associated with impaired behavioral outcome. Brain Behav Immun. 2011;25(1):40–5.
108. Emanuele E, Orsi P, Bosco M, et al. Low-grade endotoxemia in patients with severe autism. Neurosci Lett. 2010;471(3):162–5.
109. Krakowiak P, Goines PE, Tancredi DJ, et al. Neonatal cytokine profiles associated with Autism Spectrum Disorder. Biol Psychiatry. 2017;81(5):442–51.
110. Li X, Chauhn A, Shiekh AM, et al. Elevated immune response in the brain of autistic patients. J Neuroimmunol. 2009;207(1-2):111–6.
111. Abdallah MW, Larsen N, Grove J. Amniotic fluid chemokines and autism spectrum disorders: an exploratory study utilizing a Danish Historic Birth Cohort. Brain Behav Immun. 2012;26(1):170–6.
112. Abdallah MW, Larsen N, Grove J, et al. Amniotic fluid inflammatory cytokines: potential markers of immunologic dysfunction in autism spectrum disorders. World J Biol Psychiatry. 2013;14(7):528–38.
113. Brown AS, Sourander A, Hinkka-Yli-Salomaki S, et al. Elevated maternal C-Reactive Protein and autism in a national birth cohort. Mol Psychiatry. 2014;19(2):259–64.
114. Goines PE, Croen LA, Braunschweig D, et al. Increased midgestational IFN-$\gamma$, IL-4 and IL-5 in women bearing a child with autism: a case-control study. Mol Autism. 2011;2:13.
115. Hornig M, Briese T, Buie T, et al. Lack of association between measles virus vaccine and autism with enteropathy: a case–control study. PLoS One. 2008;3:e3140.
116. Jyonouchi H, Sun S, Le H. Proinflammatory and regulatory cytokine production associated with innate and adaptive immune responses in children with autism spectrum disorders and developmental regression. J Neuroimmunol. 2001;120:170–9.

117. Malik M, Sheikh AM, Wen G, et al. Expression of inflammatory cytokines, Bcl2 and cathepsin D are altered in lymphoblasts of autistic subjects. Immunobiology. 2011;216:80–5.
118. Heiss CN, Olofsson LE. The role of the gut microbiota in development, function and disorders of the central nervous system and the enteric nervous system. J Neuroendocrinol. 2019;31(5):e12684.
119. Srikantha P, Mohajeri MH. The possible role of the microbiota-gut-brain-axis in autism spectrum disorder. Int J Mol Sci. 2019;20(9):2115.
120. Parracho HM, Bingham MO, Gibson GR, et al. Differences between the gut microflora of children with autistic spectrum disorders and that of healthy children. J Med Microbiol. 2005;54:987–91.
121. Carissimi C, Laudadio I, Palone F, et al. Functional analysis of gut microbiota and immunoinflammation in children with autism spectrum disorders. Dig Liver Dis. 2019;51(10):1366–74.
122. Martin CR, Osadchiy V, Kalani A, Mayer EA. The brain-gut-microbiome axis. Cell Mol Gastroenterol Hepatol. 2018;6(2):133–48.
123. Fiorentino M, Sapone A, Senger S, et al. Blood-brain barrier and intestinal epithelial barrier alterations in autism spectrum disorders. Mol Autism. 2016;7:49.
124. Kang DW, Adams JB, Coleman DM, et al. Long-term benefit of microbiota transfer therapy on autism symptoms and gut microbiota. Sci Rep. 2019;9(1):5821.
125. Aran A, Cassuto H, Lubotzky A, et al. Brief report: Cannabidiol-rich cannabis in children with autism spectrum disorder and severe behavioral problems-a retrospective feasibility study. J Autism Dev Disord. 2019b;49(3):1284–8.
126. Karhson DS, Krasinska KM, Ahloy Dallaire J, et al. Plasma anandamide concentrations are lower in children with autism spectrum disorder. Mol Autism. 2018;9:18.
127. Mazahery H, Stonehouse W, Delshad M, et al. Relationship between Long Chain n-3 Polyunsaturated fatty acids and Autism Spectrum Disorder: systematic review and meta-analysis of case-control and randomised controlled trials. Nutrients. 2017;9:155.
128. Huang Y, Iosif A-M, Hansen RL, Schmidt RJ. Maternal polyunsaturated fatty acids and risk for autism spectrum disorder in the MARBLES high-risk study. Autism. 2020;24(5):1191–200.
129. Földy C, Malenka RC, Südhof TC. Autism-associated neuroligin-3 mutations commonly disrupt tonic endocannabinoid signaling. Neuron. 2013;78(3):498–509.
130. Wei D, et al. Endocannabinoid signaling mediates oxytocin-driven social reward. Proc Natl Acad Sci. 2015;112:14084–9.
131. Lin IF, et al. The effect of intranasal oxytocin versus placebo treatment on the autonomic responses to human sounds in autism: a single-blind, randomized, placebo-controlled, cross-over design study. Mol Autism. 2014;5:20.
132. Romano A, Micioni Di Bonaventura MV, Gallelli CA, et al. Oleoylethanolamide decreases frustration stress-induced binge-like eating in female rats. Neuropsychopharmacology. 2020;45:1931–41.
133. Salzman C, van der Kolk BA, Shader R. Marijuana and hostility in a small group setting. Am J Psychiatry. 1976;133(9):1029–33.
134. Tart CT. Marijuana intoxication common experiences. Nature 1970; 226(5247): 701–04.
135. Marco EM, Rapino C, Caprioli A, et al. Social encounter with a novel partner in adolescent rats: activation of the central endocannabinoid system. Behav Brain Res. 2011;220:4314–22.
136. Marco EM, Scattoni ML, Rapino C, et al. Emotional, endocrine and brain anandamide response to social challenge in infant male rats. Psychoneuroimmunology. 2013;38:2152–62.
137. Sciolino NR, Bortolato M, Einstein SA, et al. Social isolation and chronic handling alter endocannabinoid signaling and behavioural reactivity to context in adult rats. Neuroscience. 2010;168:371–86.
138. Kerr DM, Gilmartin A, Roche M. Pharmacological inhibition of fatty acid amide hydrolase attenuates social behavioural deficits in male rats prenatally exposed to valproic acid. Pharm Res. 2016;113:228–35.

139. Kerr DM, Downey L, Conboy M, et al. Alterations in the endocannabinoid system in the rat valproic acid model of autism. Behav Brain Res. 2013;249:124–32.
140. Moreira FA, Kaiser N, Monory K, Lutz B. Reduced anxiety-like behaviour induced by genetic and pharmacological inhibition of the endocannabinoid-degrading enzyme fatty acid amide hydrolase (FAAH) is mediated by CB1 receptors. Neuropharmacology. 2008;54(1):141–50.
141. Seillier A, Martinez AA, Giuffrida A. Phencyclidine-induced social withdrawal results from deficient stimulation of cannabinoid CB (1) receptors: implications for schizophrenia. Neuropsychopharmacology. 2013;38(9):1816–24.
142. Trezza V, Damsteegt R, Manduca A, et al. Endocannabinoids in amygdala and nucleus accumbens mediate social play reward in adolescent rats. J Neurosci. 2012;32(43):14899–908.
143. Gunduz-Cinar O, MacPherson KP, Cinar R, et al. Convergent translational evidence of a role for anandamide in amygdala-mediated fear extinction, threat processing and stress-reactivity. Mol Psychiatry. 2013;18(7):813–23.
144. Phan KL, Angstadt M, Golden J, et al. Cannabinoid modulation of amygdala reactivity to social signals of threat in humans. J Neurosci. 2008;28(10):2313–9.
145. Hosie S, Malone DT, Liu S, et al. Altered amygdala excitation and CB1 receptor modulation of aggressive behavior in the neuroligin-3R451C mouse model of autism. Front Cell Neurosci. 2018;12:234.
146. Chakrabarti B, Baron-Cohen S. Variation in the human cannabinoid receptor CNR1 gene modulates gaze duration for happy faces. Mol Autism. 2011;2:10.
147. Chakrabarti B, Kent L, Suckling J, et al. Variations in the human cannabinoid receptor (CNR1) gene modulate striatal responses to happy faces. Eur J Neurosci. 2006;23: 1944–8.
148. Domschke K, Dannlowski U, Ohrmann P, et al. Cannabinoid receptor 1 (CNR1) gene: Impact on antidepressant treatment response and emotion processing in major depression. Eur Neuropsychopharmacol. 2008;18:751–9.
149. Jaramillo TC, Liu S, Pettersen A, et al. Autism-related neuroligin-3 mutation alters social behavior and spatial learning. Autism Res. 2014;7(2):264–72.
150. Schultz S, Siniscalco D. Endocannabinoid system involvement in autism spectrum disorder: an overview with potential therapeutic applications. AIMS Mol Sci. 2019;6:27–37.
151. Siniscalco D, Sapone A, Giordano C, et al. Cannabinoid receptor type 2, but not type 1, is up-regulated in peripheral blood mononuclear cells of children affected by autistic disorders. J Autism Dev Disord. 2013;43:2686–95.
152. Brigida AL, Schultz S, Cascone M, et al. Endocannabinoid signal dysregulation in autism spectrum disorders: a correlation link between inflammatory state and neuro-immune alterations. Int J Mol Sci. 2017;18(7):1425.
153. Veilleux A, Di Marzo V, Silvestri C. The expanded endocannabinoid system/endocannabinoidome as a potential target for treating diabetes mellitus. Curr Diab Rep. 2019;19(11):117.
154. Cani PD, Plovier H, Van Hul M, et al. Endocannabinoids — at the crossroads between the gut microbiota and host metabolism. Nat Rev Endocrinol. 2016;12(3):133–43.
155. Vaughn LK, Denning G, Stuhr KL, et al. Endocannabinoid signalling: has it got rhythm? Br J Pharmacol. 2010;160(3):530–43.
156. Glickman G. Circadian rhythms and sleep in children with autism. Neurosci Biobehav Rev. 2010;34:755–68.
157. Soltys J, Yushak M, Mao-Draayer Y. Regulation of neural progenitor cell fate by anandamide. Biochem Biophys Res Commun. 2010;400:21–6.
158. Campos AC, Ortega Z, Palazuelos J, et al. The anxiolytic effect of cannabidiol on chronically stressed mice depends on hippocampal neurogenesis: involvement of the endocannabinoid system. Int J Neuropsychopharmacol. 2013;16(6):1407–19.
159. Sales AJ, Fogaca MV, Sartim AG, et al. Cannabidiol induces rapid and sustained antidepressant-like effects through increased BDNF signaling and synaptogenesis in the prefrontal cortex. Mol Neurobiol. 2019;56(2):1070–81.

160. Mori MA, Meyer E, Soares LM, et al. Cannabidiol reduces neuroinflammation and promotes neuroplasticity and functional recovery after brain ischemia. Prog Neuro-Psychopharmacol Biol Psychiatry. 2017;75:94–105.
161. Ruiz-Valdpenas L, Martinez-Orgado JA, Benito C, et al. Cannabidiol reduces lipopolysaccharide-induced vascular changes and inflammation in the mouse brain: an intravital microscopy study. J Neuroinflammation. 2011;8(1):5.
162. Mecha M, Torrao AS, Mestre L, et al. Cannabidiol protects oligodendrocyte progenitor cells from inflammation-induced apoptosis by attenuating endoplasmic reticulum stress. Cell Death Dis. 2012;3:e331.
163. Ryan D, Drysdale AJ, Lafourcade C, et al. Cannabidiol targets mitochondria to regulate intracellular Ca 2+ levels. J Neurosci. 2009;29(7):2053–63.
164. Sun S, Hu F, Wu J, Zhang S. Cannabidiol attenuates OGD/R-induced damage by enhancing mitochondrial bioenergetics and modulating glucose metabolism via pentose-phosphate pathway in hippocampal neurons. Redox Biol. 2017;11:577–85.
165. Sato A. mTOR, a Potential Target to Treat Autism Spectrum Disorder. CNS Neurol Disord Drug Targets. 2016;15(5):533–43.
166. Damstra-Oddy JL, et al. Phytocannabinoid-dependent mTORC1 regulation is dependent upon inositol polyphosphate multikinase activity. Br J Pharmacol. 2021;178(5):1149–63.
167. Sartim AG, Sales AJ, Guimarães FS, Joca SR. Hippocampal mammalian target of rapamycin is implicated in stress-coping behavior induced by cannabidiol in the forced swim test. J Psychopharmacol. 2018;32(8):922–31.
168. Hudson R, Rushlow W, Laviolette SR. Phytocannabinoids modulate emotional memory processing through interactions with the ventral hippocampus and mesolimbic dopamine system: implications for neuropsychiatric pathology. Psychopharmacology. 2018;235(2):447–58.
169. Vrechi T, et al. Cannabidiol induces autophagy via ERK1/2 activation in neural cells. Sci Rep. 2021;11(1):5434.
170. Deutsch DG. A personal retrospective: elevating anandamide (AEA) by targeting fatty acid amide hydrolase (FAAH) and the fatty acid binding proteins (FABPs). Front Pharmacol. 2016;7:370.
171. Kaplan JS, Stella N, Catterall WA, Westenbroek RE. Cannabidiol attenuates seizures and social deficits in a mouse model of Dravet Syndrome. Proc Natl Acad Sci. 2017;114:11229–34.
172. Hind WH, England TJ, O'Sullivan SE. Cannabidiol protects an in vitro model of the blood–brain barrier from oxygen-glucose deprivation via PPARγ and 5- HT1A receptors. Br J Pharmacol. 2016;173:815–25.
173. Fogaca MV, Campos AC, Coelho LD, et al. The anxiolytic effects of cannabidiol in chronically stressed mice are mediated by the endocannabinoid system: Role of neurogenesis and dendritic remodeling. Neuropharmacology. 2018;135:22–33.
174. Michielan A, D'Inca R. Intestinal permeability in inflammatory bowel disease: pathogenesis, clinical evaluation, and therapy of leaky gut. Mediat Inflamm. 2015;2015:628157.
175. Camilleri M, Lasch K, Zhou W. Irritable bowel syndrome: methods, mechanisms, and pathophysiology. The confluence of increased permeability, inflammation, and pain in irritable bowel syndrome. Am J Physiol Gastrointest Liver Physiol. 2012;303(7):G775–85.
176. Bertiaux-Vandaële N, Youmba SB, Belmonte L, et al. The expression and the cellular distribution of the tight junction proteins are altered in irritable bowel syndrome patients with differences according to the disease subtype. Am J Gastroenterol. 2011;106(12):2165–73.
177. Hasenoehrl C, Storr M, Schicho R. Cannabinoids for treating inflammatory bowel diseases: where are we and where do we go? Expert Rev Gastroenterol Hepatol. 2017;11(4):329–37.
178. Alhamoruni A, Lee AC, Wright KL, et al. Pharmacological effects of cannabinoids on the Caco-2 cell culture model of intestinal permeability. J Pharmacol Exp Ther. 2010;335(1):92–102.
179. Couch DG, Tasker C, Theophilidou E, et al. Cannabidiol and palmitoylethanolamide are anti-inflammatory in the acutely inflamed human colon. Clin Sci (Lond). 2017;131:2611–26.

180. D'Argenio G, Valenti M, Scaglione G, et al. Up-regulation of anandamide levels as an endogenous mechanism and a pharmacological strategy to limit colon inflammation. FASEB J. 2006;20:568–70.
181. Hernández-Cervantes R, Méndez-Díaz M, Prospéro-García Ó, Morales-Montor J. Immunoregulatory role of cannabinoids during infectious disease. Neuroimmunomodulation. 2017;24:183–99.
182. Kosgodage US, Matewele P, Awamaria B, et al. Cannabidiol is a novel modulator of bacterial membrane vesicles. Front Cell Infect Microbiol. 2019;9:324.
183. Bergamaschi MM, Queiroz RH, Chagas MH, et al. Cannabidiol reduces the anxiety induced by simulated public speaking in treatment-naïve social phobia patients. Neuropsychopharmacology. 2011;36(6):1219–26.
184. Shannon S, Lewis N, Lee H, Hughes S. Cannabidiol in anxiety and sleep: a large case series. Perm J. 2019;23:18–41.
185. Devnisky O, Cilio MR, Fernandez-Ruiz J, et al. Cannabidiol: pharmacology and potential therapeutic role in epilepsy and other neuropsychiatric disorders. Epilepsia. 2014;55:791–802.
186. Tzadok M, Uliel-Siboni S, Linder I, et al. CBD-enriched medical cannabis for intractable pediatric epilepsy – the current Israeli experience. Seizure. 2016;35:41–4.
187. Barchel D, Stolar O, De-Haan T, et al. Oral cannabidiol use in children with autism spectrum disorder to treat related symptoms and co-morbidities. Front Pharmacol. 2019;9:1521.
188. Cooper RE, Williams E, Seegobin S, et al. Cannabinoids in attention-deficit/hyperactivity disorder: a randomised-controlled trial. Eur Neuropsychopharmacol. 2017;27:795–808.
189. Devinsky O, Cross JH, Laux L, Marsh E, Miller I, Nabbout R, et al.; Cannabidiol in Dravet Syndrome Study Group. Trial of cannabidiol for drug-resistant seizures in the Dravet syndrome. N Engl J Med. 2017;376:2011–20.
190. Devinsky O, Patel AD, Cross JH, Villanueva V, Wirrell EC, Privitera M, et al. GWPCARE3 Study Group. Efect of cannabidiol on drop seizures in the Lennox–Gastaut syndrome. N Engl J Med. 2018;378:1888–97.
191. FDA. FDA Briefing Document Peripheral and Central Nervous System Drugs Advisory Committee Meeting April 19, 2018. NDA 210365 Cannabidiol. Available at: https://www.fda.gov/media/112565/download. Accessed 2 Nov 2019.
192. Lattanzi S, Brigo F, Trinka E, et al. Efficacy and safety of cannabidiol in epilepsy: a systematic review and meta-analysis. Drugs. 2018;78(17):1791–804.
193. Lattanzi S, Trinka E, Russo E, et al. Cannabidiol as adjunctive treatment of seizures associated with Lennox-Gastaut syndrome and Dravet syndrome. Drugs Today (Barc). 2019;55(3):177–96.
194. Thiele EA, Marsh ED, French JA, et al. GWPCARE4 Study Group. Cannabidiol in patients with seizures associated with Lennox–Gastaut syndrome (GWPCARE4): a randomised, double-blind, placebo controlled phase 3 trial. Lancet. 2018;391:1085–96.
195. Caddeo A, Trampetti R, Messina G, Porta E, Di Fede E, Tartarelli R, et al. A neuroendocrine therapeutic approach with the Pineal Hormone Melatonin, Cannabidiol and Oxytocin (mco regimen) in the treatment of the autism spectrum disorders. J Immun Allergy. 2020;1(2):1–7.
196. Gururajan A, Taylor DA, Malone DT. Effect of cannabidiol in a MK-801-rodent model of aspects of schizophrenia. Behav Brain Res. 2011;222(2):299–308.
197. Osborne AL, Solowij N, Babic I, Weston-Green K. Improved social interaction recognition and working memory with cannabidiol treatment in a prenatal infection (poly I:C) rat model. Neuropsychopharmacology. 2017;42:1447–57.
198. Almeida V, Levin R, Fiel F, et al. Cannabidiol exhibits anxiolytic but not antipsychotic property evaluated in the social interaction test. Prog Neuro-Psychopharmacol Biol Psychiatry. 2013;41:30–5.
199. Rong C, Lee Y, Carmona DS, et al. Cannabidiol in medical marijuana: research vistas and potential opportunities. Pharmacol Res. 2017;121:213–8.
200. Pupin A, Mendes J, Milani H, et al. Influence of single and repeated cannabidiol administration on emotional behaviour and markers of cell proliferation and neurogenesis in non-stressed mice. Prog Neuro-Psychopharmacol Biol Psychiatry. 2016;64:27–34.

201. Guimarães FS, Graeff FG, Chiaretti TM, Zuardi A. Antianxiety effect of cannabidiol in the elevated plus-maze. Psychopharmacology. 1990;100:558–9.
202. Lemos JI, Restell LB, Guimaraes FS. Involvement of the prelimbic prefrontal cortex on cannabidiol-induced attenuation of contextual conditioned fear in rats. Behav Brain Res. 2010;207(1):105–11.
203. Moreira FA, Aguiar DC, Guimaraes FS. Anxiolytic-like effect of cannabidiol in the rat Vogel conflict test. Prog Neuro-Psychopharmacol Biol Psychiatry. 2006;30(8):1466–71.
204. Resstel LB, Joca SR, Moreira FA, et al. Effects of cannabidiol and diazepam on behavioural and cardiovascular responses induced by contextual conditioned fear in rats. Behav Brain Res. 2006;172:294–8.
205. Resstel LB, Tavares RF, Lisboa SF, et al. 5-HT1A receptors are involved in the cannabidiol-induced attenuation of behavioural and cardiovascular responses to acute restraint stress in rats. Br J Pharmacol. 2009;156(1):181–8.
206. Maione S, Piscitelli F, Gatta L. Non-psychoactive cannabinoids modulate the descending pathway of antinociception in anaesthetized rats through several mechanisms of action. Br J Pharmacol. 2011 Feb;162(3):584–96.
207. Huber KM, Gallagher SM, Warren ST, Bear MF. Altered synaptic plasticity in a mouse model of fragile X mental retardation. Proc Natl Acad Sci U S A. 2002;99(11):7746–50.
208. Aran A, Harel M, Cassuto H, et al. Cannabinoid treatment for autism: a proof-of-concept randomized trial. Mol Autism. 2021;12:6.
209. Kuester G. XXIII world congress in neurology. 2017, Sept 16–21, Kyoto, Japan.
210. Fusar-Poli L, Cavone V, Tinacci S, et al. Cannabinoids for people with ASD: a systematic review of published and ongoing studies. Brain Sci. 2020;10(9):572.
211. Grabacka M, Pierzchalska M, Dean M, Reiss K. Regulation of ketone body metabolism and the role of PPARα. Int J Mol Sci. 2016;17:2093.
212. Liu H, Talalay P, Fahey JW. Biomarker-guided strategy for treatment of autism spectrum disorder. CNS Neurol Disord Drug Targets. 2016;15:602–13.
213. Casares L, García V, Garrido-Rodríguez M et al. Cannabidiol induces antioxidant pathways in keratinocytes by targeting BACH1. Redox Biol. 2020;28:101321.
214. Galán-Ganga M, Del Rio R, Jimenez-Moreno N, et al. Cannabinoid CB2 receptor modulation by the transcription factor NRF2 is specific in microglial cells. Cell Mol Neurobiol. 2020;40:167.

# Routes of Administration, Pharmacokinetics and Safety of Medicinal Cannabis

# 11

## Introduction

As we learned earlier in this book, 'oils ain't oils', and there are many different cannabis strains/cultivars that may have different effects on the mind-body depending on the chemical profile of that particular strain. It is not just about the ratio of cannabidiol (CBD) to tetrahydrocannabinol (THC). Similarly, there are different routes of administration of cannabis, and different countries might favour different delivery methods. This is likely to be a product of local regulations, time that medicinal cannabis has been legalised and other factors. It takes time for some things to change. In Australia, for example, within the legal medicinal market, the majority of medicinal cannabis products on the legal medical market were mostly oils for oral use when medical use first became legalized (in 2016). Increasingly, more doctors are beginning to prescribe flower for vaporisation, but vaporising of oils as a route of delivery of medicinal cannabis is not common in Australia. In the USA, vaping of oils is popular, as is smoking cannabis for medicinal purposes. Safety of any form of medicine is important, and so it is with medicinal cannabis. Whilst we will not talk about quality assurance in this book, suffice to say that it is much safer to use a cannabis product that has been manufactured under Good Manufacturing Practice (GMP) conditions.

**This Chapter**
In this chapter, we discuss four main delivery methods, the pharmacokinetics associated with these different routes of delivery, and safety aspects of cannabis, THC and CBD.



K. O'Brien, P. Blair, *Medicinal Cannabis and CBD in Mental Healthcare*,
https://doi.org/10.1007/978-3-030-78559-8_11

## Routes of Administration (Delivery Methods)

The pharmacokinetics and pharmacodynamics of medicinal cannabis and cannabinoids will vary with individuals and with the route of administration and formulation [1, 2]. The plant chemistry of cannabinoid is far more complex than that of pure THC [1], or pure CBD or synthetic cannabinoids. Therefore, different effects may be expected due to the presence of additional cannabinoids and the other active constituents/chemicals in the plant [1].

### Types of Delivery Methods

The various forms of delivery include the following:

1. **Inhaled:** smoking, vaporising
2. **Oral:** liquid, edibles, tablets, capsules, sprays, fresh juice
3. **Topical:** creams, balms, patches
4. **Other routes:** intranasal, suppositories (rectal, vaginal)

Each of these delivery methods has particular advantages, depending on the clinical condition involved and the patient's preference. For patients with chronic illness, the oral route may be beneficial as the duration of action is longer than that of the inhaled route. However, for dealing with acute exacerbations, for example, pain or anxiety, the inhaled route may be better as the effect is much quicker. For this reason, in conditions in which there can be exacerbations, a combination of oral and inhalation routes may be useful.

Smoking of cannabis is not recommended due to the potential for cannabis leaves to be mixed with tobacco. Vaping of flowers (buds) or oils is preferable over smoking cannabis for this reason. Topical use is good for localised symptoms and systemically has a lesser effect.

Dr. Blair often prescribes terpenes for use in addition to CBD- dominant products, and these can be taken internally or can be rubbed onto the back of the hand or other skin surfaces to be absorbed that way.

We will first talk about each of the routes of delivery before looking at the pharmacokinetics of the inhaled route in comparison with the oral route.

### Inhalation: Smoking Cannabis

Smoking cannabis can include the use of 'joints', pipes and bongs. Smoking of cannabis has been found to be the most common form of delivery of cannabis in several surveys of persons who are self-medicating with cannabis (e.g [3, 4]). An estimated 30–50% of cannabis is lost to 'side-stream' smoke [5].

Smoking heats cannabis to high temperatures, 600–900 °C. Smoking cannabis is associated with toxic by-products, including tar, PAH (polycyclic aromatic hydrocarbons), carbon monoxide (CO) and ammonia (NH3). Chronic use has been found to be associated with respiratory symptoms, including cough, bronchitis and increased phlegm, but there is no evidence that it causes lung cancer or chronic obstructive airway disease (COPD) [5, 6]. The National Academies of Sciences, Engineering and Medicine report *The Health Effects of Cannabis and Cannabinoids*, published in 2017, concluded that 'There is moderate evidence of no statistical association between cannabis smoking and the incidence of lung cancer' ([6], p. 143). However, patients may mix cannabis with tobacco, thereby increasing the risk of respiratory diseases, including cancer [5].

It is common practice amongst recreational cannabis users (less so for medicinal users) to mix cannabis with commercially available tobacco when smoking it. The reason for this is that cannabis-only cigarettes tend to stop burning as soon as the user stops to puff, requiring the user to keep having to relight the cigarette. Adding tobacco increases the burning efficiency of the cannabis cigarette; depending on how much is added, the combination will burn similarly to a normal tobacco cigarette. Adding tobacco also reduces the cost of the cannabis cigarette [7]. A study found that adding tobacco to cannabis led to more efficient release of THC per gram of cannabis, increasing the vaporisation efficiency of THC by up to 45%, which may be due to greater burning efficiency and differences in combustion temperatures between the two [7].

**Systematic Review**

A systematic review of 2159 lung cancer cases and 2985 controls from six case-control studies concluded that there was no statistically significant difference in the risk of lung cancer for habitual cannabis smokers compared with non-habitual cannabis smokers (defined as those with cumulative cannabis consumption of less than 1 joint-year, including never-users). For a subgroup of participants who did not smoke tobacco, the risk of lung cancer was not significantly different for habitual cannabis smokers compared with non-habitual cannabis smokers [8].

## Inhalation: Vaporising

Vaporising or vaping (these terms are often used interchangeably) heats cannabis at a lower temperature (160–230 °C) than smoking. Both cannabis flower and oil may be vaporised. It has some advantages over smoking in that there is no side-stream smoke (and thus fewer concerns about passive smoking), it has fewer toxins (CO is reduced, though PAHs are not completely eliminated), it produces much less harmful biproducts and fewer pulmonary symptoms are reported [5].

The advantages of smoking and vaporising are that the active constituents pass quickly into the bloodstream via the highly vascularised lung tissue, bypassing the 'first-pass mechanism' of the liver. Thus, the onset of action is faster than with the oral route. As peak effects are faster than the oral route, this may be useful for the treatment of acute conditions, such as pain or chemotherapy-induced nausea and vomiting, in which fast action is desirable. For chronic conditions in which a longer effect duration is required, the oral route may be better.

Another advantage of vaporising is the delivery of cannabinoids to the full range of respiratory endothelium. This would include inflamed nasal and sinus tissue depending on the expiratory method used and the pharynx. There is also some suggestion that the antibacterial and antiviral properties of the cannabinoids could reduce pathogen populations and even entry into the body. For example, SARS-CoV-2 uses receptor-mediated entry into humans via the angiotensin-converting enzyme 2 (ACE2). ACE2 is expressed in the lung tissue, nasal and oral mucosa, kidney, gastrointestinal tract and testes. Recent research has demonstrated that various high CBD cannabis extracts could downregulate the ACE2 gene expression and decrease the ACE2 protein levels, with some also downregulating serine protease TMPRSS2 (both proteins are critical for SARS-CoV-2 entry into the host cells) in artificial 3D human models of oral, airway and intestinal tissues. This suggests promise for treatment of respiratory viruses that use the ACE receptor as a molecular gateway, such as SARS-CoV-2 [9].

Vaping is not without risks. In 2019 the safety of vaping cannabis oils was called into question with the occurrence of several hospitalisations and deaths associated with it in the USA. A syndrome named e-cigarette or vaping-associated lung injury (EVALI) was coined. As of January 2020, over 2600 people became sick, most requiring hospitalisation (at least one requiring a lung transplant), and over 50 people died [10]. The illness was finally determined to be due to a synthetic form of vitamin E acetate (α-tocopheryl acetate), used in e-cigarettes to thicken marijuana oil in order to disguise its dilution with other substances, confirmed in various investigations, which was detected in THC-containing products and samples of lung fluid from EVALI patients [10]. For example twenty-four products obtained from victims in 2019 contained vitamin E acetate [11] and in August 2019, the Utah Public Health Laboratory (UPHL) showed evidence of vitamin E acetate in 17 of 20 (89%) THC-containing cartridges in the review of 79 lung injury cases for that US state [12]. In 48 of 51 bronchioalveolar lavage samples taken from patients, vitamin E acetate was detected, along with THC or metabolites in most of the samples [13].

This brings home the important point of quality control of any type of cannabis product, including oils used in vaporising devices and the vaporising/vaping devices themselves in ensuring that health is not harmed. We might add that cannabis that is not organically grown, like other herbs, can be contaminated with adulterants, heavy metals and pesticides.

## Oral Routes

Oral routes of delivery technically include oral ingestion, oro-mucosal and sublingual routes. When we speak of the oral route of delivery, we are referring in general to oral ingestion. Cannabis products that may be consumed by mouth include oils, capsules, tinctures, lozenges, edibles, juicing fresh plants and cannabis teas. The oral route has the advantage of convenience, and duration of action is much longer than that of smoking/vaporising. Thus, these may be more advantageous for the treatment of chronic illnesses. Oils and capsules have the advantage of more accuracy with respect to dosing, unlike edibles (brownies, cookies and gummies), which may be more difficult to dose. Gummies are usually made with some kind of sweetener and may affect the blood sugar levels in vulnerable people, such as those with diabetes. Disadvantages of the oral route of delivery are the low bioavailability of cannabinoids, due to low water solubility (limiting absorption), gastric instability and the hepatic first pass effect [14]. Another potential disadvantage may be dosage-related side effects, given fluctuations in plasma drug levels associated with first order kinetics have been seen in oral and other systemic delivery systems [14]. Related oral routes of delivery include the oro-mucosal route (e.g. buccal route) and sublingual route. There are several products on the market including oromucosal sprays (e.g. nabiximols, which delivers a standardised dose of CBD and THC [5]) and sublingual wafers which are absorbed via the sublingual blood vessels. An advantage of these delivery routes is that the active constituents are absorbed via the blood vessels within the oral cavity, and so the cannabinoids rapidly enter the systemic circulation [14]. This route of delivery is reasonably fast acting (not as fast as inhalation but faster than when oils are swallowed) and has a longer duration of action compared to the inhalation route (see Table 11.1).

The raw plant contains the acid forms of the main phytocannabinoids, THCA and CBDA, which have been found to have therapeutic properties. Juicing and cannabis teas do not allow for adequate decarboxylation of the raw plant [5], which may be considered an advantage or disadvantage, depending on whether you want the acid forms of THC and CBD or whether you want the decarboxylated THC and CBD.

## Topical Route

Topicals (for external use) are ideal for localised symptoms, including skin conditions and arthritis, though there is less research available with respect to their efficacy [5]. Advantages of the trans-dermal route of delivery are that it is more user-friendly (and therefore may increase compliance), and it avoids the hepatic first pass effect and degradation of cannabinoids by gut enzymes [14]. Transdermal patches are a promising route of delivery since they may be able to achieve a constant therapeutic drug level which may be useful for treating conditions like chronic pain [15].

## Other Delivery Routes

Suppositories may be indicated for the treatment of specific conditions (e.g. rectal cancer). They may also be useful for specific subpopulations, such as the elderly or young. However, there is variable absorption [5]. The bioavailability of rectal routes

**Table 11.1** THC routes of administration, bioavailability, onset and duration of action

| Route of administration | Bioavailability of THC | First-pass mechanism | Onset of action | Duration of action | Advantages of route of delivery |
|---|---|---|---|---|---|
| Inhalation | 2–56% [1, 16]<br>Average 30% [24]<br>18 +/– 6% [25]<br>27 +/- 10% for the heavy users and 14 +/- 1% for the light users [26]; 10–35% [27])<br>30% [28]<br>18% [29]<br>10–25% [30] | Avoids first-pass metabolism | 5–10 min [5]<br>3–10 min; peak concentration 2–10 min [30] | 2–4 hours [5]<br>Peak 'psychoactive' effects (euphoria, depersonalisation and sensory perceptions): 15 minutes [30]<br>Peak cognitive effects (short-term memory, attention and concentration): 15 minutes [30] | Rapid action, useful for episodic or acute symptom treatment (e.g. pain, chemotherapy-induced nauseas and vomiting) [5] |
| Oral Ingestion | 4–12% [19, 24]<br>10–20% [31]<br>THC in chocolate cookie: 6 +/– 3% [25]<br>4–20% [1]<br>3–14% [32]<br>6% [33, 34]<br>10% (variable: 6–20%) [30] | First-pass mechanism involved | 60–180 min [5]<br>First onset of effects: 60–90 min; peak concentration 1–3 hours [30]; Maximum Δ9 THC plasma concentration within 1–2 hours (could be delayed by few hours in certain cases) [35] | 6–8 hours [5]<br>Peak psychoactive effects (euphoria, depersonalisation and sensory perceptions): 3 hours; peak cognitive effects (short-term memory, attention and concentration): 5 hours [30] | Advantage for chronic illnesses; less odour compared with smoking, more discrete [5] |
| Oro-Mucosal | 5 and 15 mg oral THC bioavailability was 13.1% and 11.0% for low- and high-dose nabiximols (Sativex), respectively [33] | Largely avoids first-pass metabolism | 15–45 min [5] | 6–8 hours [5] | Pharmaceutical forms available, e.g. nabiximols (efficacy and safety documents) [5] |

| | | | | | |
|---|---|---|---|---|---|
| Rectal suppositories | Uncertain. Evaluation in monkeys showed that THC-hemisuccinate provided bioavailability of 13.5% [1]. Human study: total systemic exposure to THC was much higher for rectal administration of THC-hemisuccinate compared with oral administration of dronabinol capsules (THC area under the plasma concentration versus time curve (AUC(0–∞)) for rectal administration of THC-hemisuccinate was 2.44-fold higher than oral administration of dronabinol capsules [36] | Avoids first-pass metabolism | Little information available. In a small experiment with 2 subjects, after rectal doses of 2.5–5 mg THC, peak plasma levels from 1.1 to 4.1 ng/ml THC and 6.1 to 42.0 ng/ml THC-COOH were measured within 2–8 h and 1–8 h, respectively [37]. | | May be suitable for particular diseases; bypasses first pass mechanism; absorption into bloodstream. |
| Topical | Little data at this time | Avoids first-pass metabolism | Variable [5] | Variable [5] | Local effects; less systemic effect; good for localised symptoms [5] |

is uncertain – evaluation in monkeys showed that a THC-hemisuccinate provided bioavailability of 13.5% [1]. The intranasal route of delivery is an alternative route of systemic delivery. It is non-invasive and rapid acting, delivering cannabinoids into the systemic circulation quickly, and avoids the first-pass mechanism of the liver and enzymatic degradation in the gut [14]. Bioavailability of THC via the intranasal route is approximately 27% [14]. Because of its rapid action, it may be useful for treatment of acute conditions and potential uses include treatment of breakthrough pain or nausea [15]. However, there are disadvantages of the intranasal route which include the fact that most cannabinoids are lipophilic, so crossing the aqueous media of the nasal tissue is problematic. Rapid absorption of cannabinoids such as THC into the central nervous system could result in increased side effects associated with THC. A further disadvantage is the potential to irritate the nasal mucosa. Thus it may not be so suitable for chronic administration [14].

## Pharmacokinetics

The pharmacokinetics of cannabis depends on the route of delivery. Most human clinical trials have measured pharmacokinetic activity after inhalation or ingestion (oral route). The onset, rate of absorption and bioavailability of THC and CBD are much higher with inhalation compared with oral administration [16].

The factors that determine the onset and duration of action of different delivery routes are absorption, distribution and metabolism. Absorption has a wide variability, ranging from 20% to 30% orally and from 10 to 60% for inhalation [1]. The sublingual route of administration has a rate of absorption in between that of inhalation and oral (swallowed) route [17]. Factors that affect absorption include product lipophilicity, bioavailability and the inherent organ tissue differences (e.g. alveolar, dermal, gastric) [5]. Several factors can affect cannabis absorption including recent meals, depth of inhalation, duration of breath holding and temperature of vaporiser [5].

Cannabinoids are lipophilic and have low water solubility. In general, the bioavailability of cannabinoids delivered via the oral (ingestion) route is low, due to low water solubility (that limits absorption), hepatic degradation and gastric instability [14, 15]. Over 95% of ingested cannabinoids are degraded by the first pass mechanisms of the liver [14, 17]. For topical and oral routes of administration, absorption is enhanced in the presence of fat, oils or polar solvents (e.g. ethanol). Nano- or ionised particles and the use of omega fats in carrier oil may enhance absorption. For topical products, ingredients that mildly disrupt the skin barrier may allow greater absorption of active ingredient [5].

It is important to understand the impact that the variability of bioavailability between individuals participating in randomised controlled trials (RCTs) may have on the outcome variables measured. Individualisation of dosage for participants in the RCT could optimise therapeutic efficacy (compared with a standard dose).

## Cannabidiol

### Bioavailability of CBD

The onset, rate of absorption and bioavailability of CBD are much higher with inhalation compared with oral administration [16]. The bioavailability of CBD via inhalation is 11–45% [18, 19].

CBD has a low and highly variable oral bioavailability, estimated at 6–10%, due to the first-pass mechanism of the liver [16], though some studies have reported figures of 13–19% [20]. In a study of the intranasal delivery of CBD in rats, the bioavailability was 34–46% [15].

### Metabolism and Half-Life of CBD

CBD is extensively metabolised by the cytochrome P450 (CYP) enzymes of the liver. The major isoforms that contribute to the metabolism of CBD are CYP3A4, CYP2C19, CYP2C9, CYP1A2, 2C8, 2B6 and 2E1, with CYP3A4 and CYP2C19 being the dominant contributors to the breakdown of CBD to its active metabolite [21, 22].

CBD is highly lipid-soluble and is rapidly distributed in the brain, adipose tissue and other organs [18]. The primary route of CBD metabolisation is hydroxylation to 7-OH-CBD and then further metabolism into several (inactive) metabolites (e.g. CBD-COOH) by the liver cytochrome P450 enzymes, with excretion mainly via faeces and less in urine [18].

The half-life of CBD depends on the route of administration. For example, the half-life (humans) was found to be 18–33 hours for intravenous administration, 27–35 hours after smoking and 2–5 days after oral administration [23].

## Tetrahydrocannabinol

### Bioavailability of THC

The bioavailability of THC is variable and depends on the route of administration (see Table 11.1). For inhalation, the bioavailability is variable, and various studies suggest it is somewhere between 10 and 35% [24, 25, 27–30] (see Table 11.1). Factors that could affect the bioavailability via the inhalation route include frequency of smoking and smoking technique. In one study, a bioavailability of 23–27% was found for frequent users compared with 10–14% for occasional users [35]. Differences may be due to variations in smoking technique, e.g. puff duration, intake volume and holding time. Up to 30% of THC is lost due to pyrolysis, with additional loss in side-stream smoke and incomplete absorption in the lungs [16].

The bioavailability of orally ingested THC is between 4% and 20%, which is lower compared with that of inhalation (see Table 11.1), due to the fact that the cannabinoids undergo extensive first-pass metabolism by the CYP450 genes in the liver, prior to entering the systemic circulation [16]. Oxidation of THC into 11-OH-THC and other metabolites reduces the amount of THC reaching the bloodstream, reducing the oral bioavailability [16].

**Onset and Duration of Action of THC**

The onset of action of inhaled THC (5–10 minutes) is much quicker than that of the oral route (between 60–180 minutes) [5].

- **Inhaled route:** peak plasma concentration of THC is reached in 5–10 minutes [1, 28, 35, 38]
- **Oral route**: peak plasma concentrations of THC may be reached as early as 1–2 hours or as late as 4–6 hours after ingestion [1, 35].

This longer onset of action for the oral ingestion route can be a trap, in particular, for naïve users who consume cannabis edibles like cookies or gummies – a lack of effect soon after consumption can cause the individual to eat more of the cookie or more gummies, with the increased likelihood of having too much and experiencing unpleasant side effects when the THC kicks in.

The duration of effects is longer for oral administration (6–8 hours) compared with inhalation (2–4 hours) [5, 39], and this can be an advantage in treating more chronic conditions.

**Metabolism of THC**

THC is rapidly absorbed through the lungs after inhalation and quickly reaches a high concentration in the blood. Around 90% of THC in the blood is circulated in plasma, with the remaining 10% in the red blood cells [35]. THC is detectable in plasma in below 1 minute after inhalation [1, 16, 27], with peak plasma concentration being reached in 5–10 minutes [1, 28, 35, 38].

In contrast, after oral ingestion, systemic absorption is comparatively slow since it must travel to the gut and be processed by the liver. Peak plasma concentrations may be reached as early as 1–2 hours or as late as 4–6 hours after ingestion, and there can be more than one plasma peak [1, 35]. A much higher concentration of 11-OH-THC occurs after ingestion compared with inhalation [35, 40].

**Liver Metabolism**

THC is highly lipophilic. After assimilation via the blood, THC rapidly penetrates fat tissues and highly vascularised tissues (e.g. brain, muscle, liver, lung and spleen), resulting in a rapid decrease in plasma concentration [35, 41]. Following this, there is a slow redistribution of THC from the deep fat deposits back into the blood stream [35].

THC is metabolised in the liver by enzymes of the cytochrome P450 complex. Hydroxylation of THC generates the psychoactive compound 11-OH-THC, which is the main active metabolite of THC. Further oxidation produces THC-COOH, an inactive secondary metabolite [42]. It is thought that 11-OH-THC and THC-COOH are at least or even more pharmacologically active as THC and that THC-COOH modulates the actions of THC [42]. In one study, the maximum concentration of THC was observed around 8 minutes after the onset of smoking, 11-OH-THC peaked at 15 minutes and THC-COOH peaked at 81 minutes. The THC concentration decreased quickly to 1–4 ng/mL within 3–4 hours [35, 38].

**Excretion of THC**

More than 65% of cannabis is excreted in the faeces, and around 20% is excreted in urine [40]. Most of the cannabis (80–90%) is excreted within 5 days as hydroxylated and carboxylated metabolites [28]. Amongst the major metabolites (THC, 11-OH-THC and THC-COOH), THC-COOH is the primary glucuronide conjugate in urine, with 11-OH-THC being the main form in faeces [43, 44]. Because THC is lipophilic, this results in tubular reabsorption in the kidneys, leading to low renal excretion of unchanged drug.

**Half-Life of THC**

THC and its metabolites can stay around in the body for quite some time, longer for chronic users than an infrequent user [35]. In one study, the half-life of THC for an infrequent user was 1.3 days compared with 5–13 days for a frequent user [45], and after smoking a cigarette that contains 16–34 mg of THC, THC-COOH was detectable in plasma for 2–7 days [35].

THC-COOH is the compound of interest for diagnostic purposes, and it is excreted in urine mainly as a glucuronic acid conjugate [35]. Studies have shown a urinary excretion half-life for THC-COOH of around 30 hours (after 7 days of monitoring) and 44–60 hours (after 12 days monitoring) [35, 43, 46]. It also appears that the time THC metabolites stay in the body depends on whether the individual is an infrequent or frequent cannabis user. Here are some of the various studies' results:

- A study of 6 healthy males with histories of cannabis smoking was conducted, in which the subjects smoked a single cannabis cigarette (placebo 1.75% or 3.55% THC) each week. Urine specimens were then analysed (blinded) for THC-COOH. The mean half-lives were 31.5+/−1.0 hours (range 28.4–35.3 hours) for the low-dose cannabis cigarette and 28.6 +/−1.5 hours (24.9–34.5 hours) for the high-dose cigarette when a 7-day monitoring time period was used [43].
- In a study of prisoners, based on the measurements of THC-COOH/C during the first five days following the last use of cannabis, the mean urinary excretion half-life was 1.3 days in infrequent users, whilst in frequent users, the *median* was 1.4 days with terminal urinary half-lives of up to 10.3 days found. In the infrequent users, the last positive urine specimens for THC-COOH were found at 4 days using a cut-off of 15.0 ng/ml, 5 days using a cut-off of 10.3 ng/ml and 12 days for cannabinoids. But these figures were longer for frequent users, 17, 22 and 27 days, respectively, which demonstrates that THC and its metabolites can

stay in the body for some time, and it seems to stay longer in the bodies of those who use it frequently [45].

- A study of volunteers in a low-step detoxification program found the maximum elimination times of THC-COOH to be 433.5 hours in urine and 74.3 hours in serum (using a cut-off value of 20 ng/ml) [47].

**Passive Smoking and Breastfeeding**

Note that cannabis can be detected in the body fluids of individuals who have been exposed through passive inhalation and through breastfeeding [35].

**Does Intoxication ('High') from Cannabis Coincide with Plasma Concentration?**

An early study investigated the relationship between the plasma concentrations of THC and self-rated perceptions of being intoxicated in 11 men with prior histories of using cannabis. Three forms of THC were administered to each participant in three separate experiments: smoking a cannabis cigarette containing 19% THC, eating a chocolate cookie containing 20 mg THC and intravenous injection of 5% THC. They found that the injected THC and smoked THC followed a similar pattern, rapidly reaching a peak plasma concentration. Then, because THC is very lipophilic, it was quickly distributed to the brain and other fat storage depots in the body. Consequently, the degree of intoxication increased as the plasma concentrations decreased. In contrast, for the orally ingested THC, the degree of intoxication paralleled the peak plasma concentrations, and the degree of intoxication was attained at a much lower concentrations compared with the inhaled or injected routes of administration. The study authors postulated that oral administration might allow a greater amount of THC to enter the liver and allow it to be metabolised to its more potent metabolite (11-OH-THC). They concluded that unlike alcohol, one cannot make neat correlations between the degree of intoxication and plasma concentrations of THC [48].

**Random Drug Testing**

The fact that THC metabolites can remain for days in the body makes it problematic for cannabis users (medicinal or recreational) in countries where it is illegal to have any amount of THC in the body whilst driving, such as in Australia. In Australia, this applies regardless of whether the person is intoxicated or not and regardless of whether he/she has a prescription. Thus, even those prescribed medicinal cannabis products containing THC by a doctor run the risk of testing positive in a random roadside drug test and breaking the law. Clearly this is not a sensible legislation and something that needs to change.

From Dr. Blair's personal experience, even medicinal cannabis with low THC (<0.3%) and high CBD can test positive for THC by urinalysis. Some suggestion has speculated on CBD conversion to THC that occurs in vitro with acid preparations simulating the gut, but this has not been validated in vivo.

Another concern for testing occurs in employees of transportation companies that require a urine drug screen (USD) for employment and accident investigation.

Despite legitimate therapeutic use of medicinal cannabis, positive testing could lead to extreme administrative action impacting on livelihood as well as possible criminal action in unique cases because the standards used are absolute detection values unrelated to impairment.

In one small series that characterises a typical clinical environment, a group six participants sampled two products both orally and by vaporisation for urine drug testing: pure CBD and a full-spectrum medicinal cannabis. The full spectrum contained 10.5% CBD and 0.39% THC (a 27:1 ratio of CBD/THC). This blend is very similar to many legal hemp/CBD products. Two subjects who inhaled the low THC blend confirmed positive test results, whereas none of the group that inhaled pure CBD produced positive urine specimens (for THC). Interestingly, one UDS was positive for oral 100-mg pure CBD but was not confirmed at 15 ng/mL. The implications are that even vaporised low THC products run the risk of positive drug screening [49].

## Safety of Cannabis

Recreational use of cannabis is not the same as its medicinal use, in which the dose is typically individualised to the patient, titrating upwards from a low dose slowly until a therapeutic effect is experienced. This point is very important to understand, as much of the published literature around safety, in particular, around adverse effects and driving safety, is in relation to recreational use, typically of strains of cannabis with high amounts of THC.

### Adverse Events Associated with Cannabis

Observational, population-based studies provide most of the evidence of potential toxicity associated with cannabis use. There are several limitations of such studies, including many confounding factors, and it is not possible to derive evidence of unequivocal causality. Of particular importance is that most of the available evidence of adverse effects associated with cannabis is related recreational use, where it is primarily smoked and self-administered at an unknown quality [2].

**Mortality and Cannabis**

Cannabis has a superior safety profile in comparison with many pharmaceuticals [5]. The World Health Organization 2018 report on THC states that the absence of mortality with THC may reflect the low density of CB1 receptors in the brainstem regions controlling vital cardiovascular and respiratory functions. It also states that a lethal dose in a 70-kg human is approximately 4000 mg (4g) (this amount is the median amount and refers to the quantity of THC alone; it does not include other materials [50]) and that this could not be realistically achieved following oral consumption or smoking or vaporising as THC has a large safety margin

[51]. Experiments in animals indicates that the LD50 of THC is 800 mg/kg in rats, 3000 mg/kg in dogs, and up to 9000 mg/kg in monkeys [52].

However, there are reports in the literature challenging the popular idea that no one has ever died of cannabis, as deaths due to acute myocardial infarction associated with cannabis use have been reported [53]. See section below for more on cardiovascular risk.

In one study, patients who have used cannabis had a greater all-cause mortality and greater morbidity than those who denied cannabis use [54] and another study found that the mortality rate was 29% higher in patients reporting cannabis use [55]. However, the 1999 Institute of Medicine (IOM) report Marijuana and Medicine: Assessing the Science Base states that 'epidemiological data indicate that in the general population marijuana use is not associated with increased mortality' ([56], p. 109). The US National Academies of Sciences, Engineering and Medicine report The Health Effects of Cannabis and Cannabinoids concluded: 'There is no or insufficient evidence to support or refute a statistical association between self-reported cannabis use and all-cause mortality (self-reported cannabis use); occupational accidents or injuries (general, non-medical cannabis use); death due to overdose' ([6], p. 17).

Whilst much of the safety issues around cannabis is associated with its recreational use, some reports suggest that a more measured approach might need to be taken with such statements about its safety and lack of association with mortality (see [53, 57] for further information).

**Cardiovascular Risk and Cannabis**

Smoking cannabis has been found to be associated with a significant increase in the risk of acute myocardial infarction. There have been reports of atrial fibrillation, ventricular tachycardia, acute coronary syndromes, cardiac arrest and stroke associated with smoking cannabis, often in younger people with no significant risk factors [57]. Deaths due to acute myocardial infarction associated with cannabis use have been reported [53]. A retrospective evaluation of the Personality and Total Health Through Life study also found a 3.3-fold risk of stroke/transient ischemic attack in cannabis users within the past year in participants who used cannabis weekly or more often (but not those who used cannabis less often) [58]. Yet a recent large retrospective study of 56,742 subjects found that cannabis use was not associated with increased prevalence of cardiovascular disease – in fact, it showed a trend of reduced odds for cardiovascular disease, adjusted for possible confounding variables, of 0.74 (95% CI 0.54–1.01) [59]. However, because the confidence interval includes 1.0, we see that this figure did not reach statistical significance. Although the results, statistically speaking, could still have occurred by chance, the study fails to confirm the previous positive associations of cannabis and cardiovascular disease.

According to Page and colleagues, evidence of whether cannabis causes adverse cardiovascular events is still inconclusive as most of the available research evidence is short term, observational, and retrospective in nature and there are methodological issues including lack of exposure determination and recall bias [60]. It is important to consider all kinds of evidence. Epidemiological evidence gives broad data from larger populations. Case studies speak about what happened to individuals. We can see that there have been reports of cardiovascular harm related to smoking cannabis. However, evidence of association does not equate with causality. It is also important to note that cannabis strains bred for the recreational market is often much higher in THC content. Nonetheless, THC is generally contraindicated in people with pre-existing heart disease [21].

In summary, whilst much of the safety issues around cannabis is associated with recreational use of cannabis, such reports suggest a more measured approach might need to be taken with statements about its safety and purported lack of association with mortality (see [53, 57] for further information). MacCallum and Russo state that cannabis should be used with caution in those with unstable cardiac conditions including angina, because of tachycardia and possible hypotension due to the THC (though they report that it produces no QTc issues) [5]. Brown and Winterstein state that THC is generally contraindicated in people with pre-existing heart disease [21]. See the section on ***Safety of THC*** for more information about cardiovascular effects, including effects on blood pressure and heart rate (HR).

### Side Effects of Cannabis

Warnings about cannabis and THC often focus on neuropsychiatric side effects and these are dose-limiting and a major cause of discontinuation. In clinical studies, synthetic THC (dronabinol) was shown to exacerbate mania, depression, and schizophrenia [61]. Cannabis consumption is associated with the following effects: euphoria; laughter; talkativeness; increased appetite; increasing visual, olfactory and auditory perceptions; and dry mouth and red eyes (it dilates the conjunctival blood vessels) [2]. It may also cause balance problems, confusion, dizziness, disorientation, diarrhoea, drowsiness, fatigue, hallucination, nausea, somnolence, vomiting [62] and anxiety [63]. Cannabis intoxication can impair attention and short-term memory function, and in some vulnerable persons, it may trigger psychotic reactions [2]. The effects are subject to tolerance following repeated exposure. Thus, many of the more marked reactions in naive users are reduced in frequent users [2].

Young children are at risk of the side effects of cannabis, with case reports of young children experiencing respiratory depression, tachycardia and temporary coma following accidental ingestion [2, 64, 65].

## Drug-Cannabis Interactions

The potential for interactions between pharmaceuticals and THC and CBD will be discussed shortly. However, it is worth noting that according to the World Health Organization (WHO) report, data from randomised controlled trials has not reported significantly increased incidences of severe adverse effects associated with the combination of cannabis/cannabinoids and other medications [2].

## Cannabis Dependence, Abuse and Cannabis Use Disorder

Cannabis use disorder (cannabis addiction) is defined in the Diagnostic and Statistical Manual of Mental Disorders (DSM-5) as the continued use of cannabis despite clinically significant impairment. There has been some debate in the literature as to whether cannabis abuse and cannabis dependence constitute different entities. Abuse has been seen as being associated with less severe social consequences and dependence being associated with more severe cognitive, physiological and psychosocial consequences; however it has been argued that the distinction has limited validity in adolescents [66].

In a systematic review and meta-analysis of epidemiological studies on prevalence risk, in people who used cannabis, 22% had a cannabis use disorder, 13% had cannabis abuse and 13% had cannabis dependence, with risks higher in people who used it daily or weekly and in young people [67].

However, as contrary as it might sound, research suggests that medicinal cannabis may be able to assist people with cannabis dependence. In an Australian study, a 12-week, randomised controlled trial involving 128 patients with cannabis dependence found that the use of nabiximols (1:1 ratio of THC/CBD) reduced the number of days that patients with cannabis dependence consumed cannabis by approximately 40% compared with those in the placebo group [68]. The study allowed flexible dosing (up to 32 sprays daily; THC, 86.4 mg; CBD, 80 mg) with a mean dose of nabiximols of 17.6 [9.5] sprays daily (equivalent to a mean [SD] of 47.5 [25.7]-mg THC and 44.0 [23.8]-mg CBD). The medication was well tolerated with few side effects [68].

## Pregnancy and Cannabis Use

According to a very practical paper by MacCallum and Russo, cannabis is generally contraindicated in pregnancy and lactation and the effect on the foetus and neonate is controversial [5]. Knowing what we do about the involvement of the ECS in the beginning of life, as well as in growth and development, it is perhaps not surprising that cannabis could potentially impact on the developing foetus. The ECS is involved in pre-implantation development, embryo transport to the uterus and uterine receptivity, and in post-implantation, where it is involved in many pathways, including folic acid, BDNF, VEGF and MAPK/ERK. The disruption of any of these pathways can lead to altered in utero processes, including neural development, cellular replication, angiogenesis and tissue differentiation [69].

There is a lack of information about the potential effect of maternal cannabis use on the developing foetus. We do know that preclinical research indicates that THC readily crosses the placenta, though foetal exposures appear lower than maternal [70]. Neurodevelopmental research suggests that prenatal THC exposure may lead to subtle changes in some aspects of higher-level cognition and psychological well-being [70]. In utero cannabis exposure has been associated with miscarriage, birth defects and developmental delay, though the pathomechanisms are not understood. The ability of cannabinoids to inhibit cancer cell growth and apoptosis suggests potential pathomechanisms [70].

**Association of Prenatal Cannabis Exposure with Sleep Disorders in Offspring**
A study comparing 18 children with prenatal cannabis exposure and 20 control children analysed sleep variables from polysomnographic recordings at the age of 3 years. They found that those with prenatal cannabis exposure showed more nocturnal arousals (8.2+/−5.3 cf. 3.2+/−4.6, $p < 0.003$) and lower sleep efficiency than the controls [71].

A study analysed baseline data from the Adolescent Brain and Cognitive Development (ABCD) study to determine whether maternal reports of prenatal cannabis use was associated with sleep disorders in 11,875 children aged 9–10 years. The data indicates that any cannabis use in mothers prenatally was associated with a variety of sleep problems, including disorders associated with initiating and maintaining sleep, disorders of arousal, sleep-wake disorders, disorders of excessive somnolence and a summed sleep disorder score (all $p < 0.03$). More frequent prenatal daily cannabis use was significantly associated with disorders of excessive somnolence ($p = 0.03$) [72]. Whilst this study does not prove causality, it does add to a bank of evidence suggesting that prenatal cannabis use can be detrimental to offspring.

**Association of Prenatal Maternal Cannabis Use and Autism Spectrum Disorder in Offspring**
A recent study in Ontario, Canada, retrospectively analysed information on all live births between 1 April 2007 and 31 March 2012. They found a statistically significant association between prenatal maternal cannabis use and incidence of autism spectrum disorder (ASD) in offspring: the incidence of ASD was 4.00 per 1000 person-years in children with exposure compared with 2.42 in unexposed children, with an adjusted hazard ratio of 1.51 (95% confidence interval: 1.17–1.96) in the matched cohort. They also found that the incidence of intellectual disability and learning disorders was higher amongst offspring of mothers who used cannabis during pregnancy, although this association was less statistically robust [73]. Although evidence of an association is not evidence of causality, and there could be other confounding factors involved, it nonetheless indicates a need for caution.

**Jamaican Study: Women Who Smoked During Pregnancy**
However, results of a 1991 observational study found no detrimental effects on the development of Jamaican children born of mothers who smoked cannabis during pregnancy [74]. Children were divided into two groups (one group comprises children whose mothers smoked cannabis during pregnancy and the control group comprises children whose mothers did not smoke cannabis during pregnancy). Children's development was assessed at 1, 3 and 30 days of age using the Brazelton Neonatal Behavioural Assessment Scale and at 4 and 5 years of age using the McCarthy Scales of Children's Abilities. There were no significant differences between the

two groups, except at 30 days when the children of mothers who heavily smoked cannabis actually had more favourable scores for autonomic stabilities and reflexes as well as improved behaviours. Developmental scores at ages 4 and five were correlated with aspects of the home environment and regularity of basic preschool attendance [74]. Part of the discrepancy with other studies of babies exposed to cannabis may be due to the culturally accepted use, but not abuse, of cannabis. Furthermore, unlike in comparable studies in developed countries, the use of other drugs of abuse were not typically available to or used by this rural Jamaican cohort [74].

**Side Effects of Cannabis-Based Medicines**

The following side effects may be associated with cannabis-based medicines [5]:

- **Most common:** drowsiness/fatigue, dizziness, dry mouth, cough/phlegm/bronchitis (smoking only), anxiety, nausea and cognitive effects
- **Common:** euphoria, blurred vision, headache
- **Rare:** orthostatic hypotension, toxic psychosis/paranoia, depression, ataxia/discoordination, tachycardia (after titration), cannabis hyperemesis, diarrhoea

## Alcohol and Cannabis

Research indicates that the combination of alcohol and THC has been associated with impairment of on-road driving performance and increased driving fatalities [75]. The effect on driving of alcohol and cannabis together appears greater than either alone, with research suggesting an additive or synergistic effect [75]. This topic will be discussed in greater detail in the section on THC.

## Workplace Injuries and Recreational Cannabis Use

A natural concern about cannabis use is whether it could cause accidents in the workplace, in particular, in those industries associated with a higher risk of physical injury. Several studies have examined the potential association between cannabis use and work-related injury. One study was a case-control study that compared the proportion of cannabis-positive urine specimens in post-accident samples compared with random samples. Any urine samples testing positive for substances other than cannabis were excluded from the study. The study failed to find a statistically significant association between the numbers of cannabis-positive urine tests for a group of random drug tests compared with a group of post-accident drug tests [76].

Another study was a cross-sectional analysis of the Canadian Community Health Survey (2013–2016). They found that amongst the 136,536 working individuals, 2% ($n$ = 2577) had had a work-related injury in the past 12 months. Of these individuals who had had a work-related injury, 4% reported cannabis use during the past 12 months. The study found no statistically significant association between past-year cannabis use and work-related injury (odds ratio (OR) for work-related injury, 0.81; 95% CI 0.66–0.99), and this association did not change when they conducted a sub-analysis of occupational groups with a high risk of injury [77].

In another study researchers examined the relationship between three temporal-based cannabis measures and five different types of workplace performance using data of 281 employees and their direct supervisors. This study found that cannabis use before and during work was negatively related to task performance, organisation-aimed citizenship behaviours and two types of counterproductive work behaviours; however after-work cannabis use was not related to any form of performance of employees, positively or negatively, as judged by their supervisors [78].

A systematic review that analysed information from 16 studies found that seven (7) studies supported a positive association between cannabis use and occupational injury, one study showed evidence that supported a negative association, and eight (8) studies found no evidence of a statistically significant association between cannabis use and occupational injury. This review also stated that only three (3) of these studies showed clear evidence that cannabis use preceded the occupational injury event. The conclusion of this systematic review was that the current body of evidence does not provide sufficient evidence that cannabis use increases the risk of occupational injury. They also noted that the quality of the studies suggests significant biases in the literature due to potential confounding variables, participant selection and measurement of exposures and outcomes and that future high-quality studies are necessary to better elucidate the relationship between cannabis use and occupational injury [79]. The National Academies of Sciences, Engineering and Medicine report on cannabis and cannabinoids, which used only evidence from systematic reviews and randomised controlled trials, stated that 'There is no or insufficient evidence to support….a statistical association between cannabis use and…. occupational accidents or injuries' [6].

## Cannabis Use, Psychosis and Schizophrenia

Whilst a discussion of this topic is beyond the scope of this book, we believe that there is evidence to suggest an association between cannabis use (recreational) and psychosis and schizophrenia in susceptible individuals. Whether or not this is a causative association is still unclear. A review paper [80] provides a comprehensive discussion of scientific evidence from a variety of studies, with a focus on adolescents.

Early reports that cannabis might induce psychotic symptoms were published 40–50 years ago [81–83] however there has been debate as to whether cannabis use causes schizophrenia or not for decades [80]. Research indicates that in those with a predisposition for schizophrenia, using cannabis exacerbates symptoms and worsens the prognosis [80, 84]. Some epidemiological studies suggest that cannabis use is a risk factor for the onset of schizophrenia [80], however it is important to note that such studies typically are in relation to recreational use of cannabis and the risk appears to be particularly related to high consumption of cannabis (e.g. [85, 86]). For example, a comprehensive 15-year follow-up study of more than 45, 000 Swedish conscripts found a relative risk for schizophrenia amongst high consumers of cannabis (having used cannabis on more than 50 occasions) compared with non-users, and this study did factor in other potentially confounding factors like other psychiatric illnesses and social background [85]. Another study of more than 50,000 Swedes found an odds ratio of 6.7 for heavy cannabis users [86]. Other studies described in a review paper by Malone et al. [80] also indicate that lifetime cannabis use increases the risk of development of psychosis.

Whether cannabis use actually *causes* schizophrenia as opposed to precipitating it in vulnerable individuals has not been definitively proven either way. A recent study analysed genome-wide data, specifically single nucleotide polymorphisms (SNPs) associated with cannabis initiation and schizophrenia. This study found some evidence consistent with a causal effect of cannabis initiation on the risk of developing schizophrenia (odds ratio OR 1.04 per doubling odds of cannabis initiation, 95% CI 1.01–1.07, $p = 0.019$), but the evidence was much stronger in the other direction – there was strong evidence consistent with a causal effect that those individuals with high risk of schizophrenia were significantly more likely to use cannabis (OR 1.10 per doubling of the odds of schizophrenia, 95% CI 1.05–1.14, $p = 2.64 \times 10^{-5}$, which is highly statistically significant and very unlikely to be due to chance) [87]. There other evidence of a disturbance of the endocannabinoid system associated with psychosis. For example, a meta-analysis published recently Minichino et al. [88] indicated that patients with psychosis have an elevated endocannabinoid tone, with significantly higher levels of AEA in their blood and cerebrospinal fluid along with a higher expression of CB1 receptors in peripheral immune cells than in the brain [89]. A neuroimaging study using positron emission tomography in humans found that the normal inverse relationship between peripheral endocannabinoids and CB1 receptor availability was not maintained in first episode psychosis patients providing further evidence of endocannabinoid system dysregulation in schizophrenia [90].

Adolescents may be particularly vulnerable to the effects of cannabis and THC, and when one considers the developmental changes occurring in the adolescent brain, this is biologically plausible. As we saw in the chapter on the endocannabinoid system, the brain is undergoing robust development and maturation during adolescence, in particular in certain areas of the brain, such as the corticolimbic region relevant to emotions and our stress response. Adolescence, in addition to early life, is also a period of high neural plasticity and during this time the endocannabinoid system is also undergoing changes. Research indicates endocannabinoid system involvement in the early post-natal and adolescent development on stress reactivity of the HPA axis, the corticolimbic system and behaviour. Adolescence therefore represents a critical stage in development and a period of susceptibility to disturbance [91].

According to Malone et al. [80], exposure to cannabis and THC in adolescence may disturb the normal developmental processes occurring in the central nervous system and could possibly lead to a predisposition to develop schizophrenia. This might involve GABAergic and dopaminergic dysfunction. Genetic predispositions including polymorphism in the COMT gene might also be involved [80]. However, whether or not cannabis use in adolescence causes schizophrenia is still undecided [80].

It is worth noting, however, that it is the THC in cannabis that appears to be of concern in relation to psychosis and schizophrenia. CBD, on the other hand, appears to have antipsychotic effects with potential as a non-dopaminergic treatment for psychosis [89]. There appears to be several potential mechanisms of action underpinning its antipsychotic effects, including being able to antagonise CB1 agonists, upregulating AEA, modulating the function of neural substrates involved in various cognitive processes that are impaired in patients with psychosis and modulating brain function in those regions believed to be altered in patients with psychosis and involved in the onset of psychosis and psychotic symptoms (e.g. hippocampus, striatum and midbrain) [89]. Since there is evidence that inflammation and immune reactivity is also involved in the pathomechanism of schizophrenia [92], one can also hypothesise that this might be another way in which CBD might potentially be of therapeutic value. In general, MacCallum and Russo caution that cannabis is contraindicated as a medicine in patients with psychosis, except CBD-predominant preparations [5].

## Safety of THC

Adverse events due to medicinal cannabis products containing THC, in particular, proprietary forms where dosage can be controlled, are usually dose-dependent. With low doses of THC, there may be none or only slight effects as described below. Any adverse effects will depend on the individual including, in particular, their metabolism.

According to McPartland & Russo, more psychological side effects occur with synthetic THC than whole cannabis (e.g. symptoms such as dysphoria, depersonalization, anxiety, panic reactions, and paranoia) [93, 94]. Other constituents in cannabis may mitigate the side effects as well as improve the therapeutic activity of THC [95]. Brown states that medicinal cannabis containing THC should be used with caution in individuals with pre-existing depression, schizophrenia or anxiety as THC has been shown to exacerbate these conditions, and recommends avoiding the concurrent use of THC and drugs which are known to increase the risk of such conditions [61]. He also recommends taking care in patients taking immunosuppressant medications due to the possibility of increased infection risk associated with THC found in animal studies [61].

### Possible Side Effects of THC

THC has very similar pharmacological and subjective effects to cannabis. The following may be experienced: euphoria; laughter and increased loquacity; increased appetite; dry mouth and occasional dizziness; enhanced visual, olfactory and auditory perceptions; drowsiness; slowed reaction time; headache; subtle cognitive deficits (e.g. impaired attention and short-term memory impairment); blurred vision, depression, paranoia and impaired verbal recall [30, 51, 96]. With higher doses, side effects can include anxiety, panic, confusion and disorientation in some users [51].

THC can also cause nausea and vomiting in some users [51, 97]. Cannabinoid hyperemesis syndrome, characterised by uncontrolled vomiting (with some relief by taking warm showers), is a rare side effect, with roughly 80 reported cases, occurring mostly in chronic cannabis users [98].

THC can provoke transient psychosis-like psychological phenomena in some healthy people [51, 99, 100]. In a study of 22 healthy individuals (who had been previously exposed to cannabis but did not meet the lifetime criteria for cannabis use disorder), it was found that administration of *intravenous* THC (99.6% purity) was associated with several transient phenomena, including positive symptoms, negative symptoms, perceptual alterations, euphoria, anxiety and deficits in working memory, recall and executive control of attention without altering general orientation. Positive symptoms included suspiciousness, paranoid and grandiose delusions, conceptual disorganisation, illusions, depersonalisation, derealisation, distorted sensory perceptions, altered body perception, feelings of unreality and extreme slowing of time. Negative effects included blunted affect, reduced rapport, lack of spontaneity, psychomotor retardation and emotional withdrawal [99].

In contrast, in a study of cannabis-dependent subjects who were smoking an average of four cannabis joints per day for several years, minimal effects of THC on cognitive test performance were found [101].

**World Health Organization Report on THC**
According to the World Health Organization:

- The effects of THC are mostly subject to tolerance with repeated exposure [102].
- Randomised controlled trials (RCTs) in which THC has been given daily for years generally report low to moderate toxicity and a low incidence of serious adverse events [51].

**Meta-analysis of Medicinal Cannabis for Mental Health: Safety Findings**
A recent meta-analysis of medicinal cannabis products for mental health conditions also looked at safety data. It found the following for pharmaceutical-grade medicinal cannabis products containing THC and CBD, set out in Table 11.2. In five of the seven studies, there is no evidence that there were more adverse events associated with medicinal cannabis compared with placebo.

## Toxicity of THC

According to the WHO report on THC, the toxicity of THC is very low compared with most other recreational and pharmaceutical drugs. The report states that: 'It has been calculated that a lethal dose in a 70 kg human would be approximately 4 g and

**Table 11.2** Adverse events for pharmaceutical-grade THC-CBD medicinal cannabis products for mental health conditions (adapted from [103] meta-analysis)

| Adverse Events THC-CBD | Comparison | No. of studies (No. of participants) | Odds Ratio (OR), 95% Confidence Interval (CI) | Statistical Interpretation |
|---|---|---|---|---|
| Adverse events, all-cause | Active | 1 (60) | 1·59 (0·57 to 4·45) | Not significant, i.e. could have occurred by chance |
| Adverse events, all-cause | Placebo | 10 (1495) | 1·99 (1·20 to 3·29) THC-CBD > Placebo | Significant |
| Serious adverse events, all-cause | Placebo | 4 (954) | 1·29 (0·94 to 1·77) | Not significant, i.e. could have occurred by chance |
| Treatment-emergent adverse events, all-cause | Placebo | 2 (385) | 1·32 (0·79 to 2·20) | Not significant, i.e. could have occurred by chance |
| Withdrawals, all-cause | Placebo | 15 (2299) | 1·51 (0·96 to 2·36) | Not significant, i.e. could have occurred by chance |
| Withdrawals due to adverse events* | Active | 2 (252) | 0·54 (0·17 to 1·68) | Not significant, i.e. could have occurred by chance |
| Withdrawals due to adverse events* | Placebo | 11 (1621) | 2·78 (1·59 to 4·86) THC-CBD > Placebo | Significant |

that such a dose could not be realistically achieved in a human following oral consumption, smoking or vaporising the substance, as Δ9-THC has a large margin of safety' [51]. It also states that the absence of mortality with THC may reflect the low density of CB1 receptors in the brainstem regions controlling cardiovascular and respiratory functions [51]. However, as mentioned previously in the section "Safety of Cannabis", there is evidence that challenges this idea that no one has died from cannabis (see this section as this is relevant to THC).

## Cardiovascular Effects of THC

THC is generally contraindicated in people with pre-existing heart disease [21]. As previously discussed, MacCallum and Russo state that cannabis should be used with caution in those with unstable cardiac conditions including angina, because of tachycardia and possible hypotension due to the THC (though they report that it produces no QTc issues) [5]. THC has sympathomimetic properties, and dronabinol (synthetic THC) has been associated with increased risk of hypertension, hypotension, syncope and tachycardia [21]. Therefore, there can be additive side effects (e.g. hypotension, hypertension, syncope and tachycardia) due to the concurrent use of cannabinoids and medications with similar cardiovascular adverse events [104].

A meta-analysis found that acute THC exposure in humans induces tachycardia with an average increase in HR of 8.16 beats per minute (bpm), which is highly statistically significant ($p < 0.00001$) [105]. The effects of THC on cardiovascular function are generally dose-dependent, such as the dose-dependent tachycardia [105]. However, research indicates that the haemodynamic effects of THC may vary with exposure over time and that tolerance to these effects may occur [51]. For example, as stated in the WHO report on THC [51], in a study where oral THC was administered to 12 healthy male participants with an escalating dosing regimen over 20 days (up to 210-mg THC per day; 7 × 30 mg oral doses), they found that THC promoted tachycardia early in the treatment period; however at later stages it decreased supine systolic and diastolic blood pressure (DBP) and decreased HR [106].

Animal studies are not considered particularly relevant to understanding the cardiovascular effects in humans since THC generally promotes bradycardia and hypotension in laboratory animal species (opposite to what is observed in humans) [51].

Warning labels for Sativex (combination of THC and CBD in a 1:1 ratio) state that it is contraindicated in people with pre-existing cardiovascular disease, which is likely to be due to the sympathomimetic properties of THC [61]. Studies in dronabinol (synthetic THC) have found that it can cause hypotension, hypertension, syncope and tachycardia [61].

**Blood Pressure and THC**

There is a difference in the findings of studies in the literature in relation to the effect of medicinal cannabis and THC on blood pressure, and this could be due to the differences in acute dosing compared with chronic dosing. A few studies have found that cannabis and THC is associated with increased systolic blood pressure (SBP), for example, one which investigated the effect of a single smoked cannabis cigarette on people with OCD [107]. In another acute dosing study, nine cannabis smokers (most in their 20s, age range of 19–43 years) were randomised to receive (over five experimental sessions) placebo, oral synthetic THC (5 and 15 mg) and low (5.4-mg THC, 5.0-mg CBD) and high (16.2-mg THC and 15.0-mg CBD) doses of nabiximols. This study found no differences in SBP between groups, but it did find significant decreases in DBP in the high THC group (mean change of 2.71+/−1.01 mmHg), low nabiximols group (mean change of 4.52+/−1.00 mmHg) and high nabiximols group (mean change 4.27 ± 1.01 mmHg) compared with the placebo group [33, 34]. In both the 15-mg oral THC and high-dose nabiximols group, the HR was significantly increased (mean change of 5.86 ± 1.09 and 6.93 ± 1.09, respectively) compared with that in placebo [33, 34]. Many of the acute dosing studies have been conducted on younger people [108].

A few studies of older adults focused on an oral drug containing pure THC yielded mixed results. A study of dementia patients found a small increase (2.6 mmHg) in SBP with a higher dose (1.5 mg twice daily) of THC (Namisol) compared with placebo (this effect occurred within 4 hours of the first tablet intake), but no effects on HR or DBP were observed [109]. Another RCT in dementia patients (mean age of 78 years) used a dosage of 1.5 mg three times daily over three weeks and found no differences between the treatment and control (placebo) groups in terms of blood pressure, HR and weight [110]. In a small study ($n$ = 12) of healthy older adults (mean age of 72.1 years, range 65–80 years) which assessed three doses of pure THC (Namisol, 3 mg, 5 mg and 6.5 mg) and placebo found no 'clinically relevant changes in systolic or diastolic blood pressure' defined as a difference of 20 mmHg and 15 mmHg at rest, respectively) nor HR (defined as a difference of 20 bpm) compared with placebo [111].

A recent study assessed change in blood pressure with more chronic dosing, which is more reflective of real life, and in an older population. A prospective study of 26 patients aged 60 years or older (mean age of 70.42+/−5.37 years) with hypertension and a new prescription for cannabis (20 used oil orally, 4 smoked cannabis and 2 used a combination of oil and smoking) found that at the end of three months, the mean 24-hour systolic and DBP were decreased by 5.0 mmHg and 4.5 mmHg, respectively ($p < 0.001$ for both), and the percentage of dippers increased from 27.3% before treatment to 45.5% at the end of 3 months. In addition, fasting blood glucose was significantly decreased in men (not women), with a mean decrease of 15.58 ± 24.36 mg/dL in males. There were no significant changes in other parameters, including lipids, HbA1C, fasting insulin, C-reactive protein, kidney function tests, electrolytes, ECG parameters and anthropometric measurements [108].

Some of the changes in blood pressure are related to different activities after dosing. One caution is orthostatic hypotension that can occur with THC or CBD because of reduced vascular resistance. Thus, patients, especially the elderly, should be cautioned about rapid postural changes in the early use of medicinal cannabis to avoid falls and unnecessary emergency visits [112]. Brown cautions that there may be the potential for THC to adversely reduce blood pressure in older people, in particular in those taking antihypertensives or other drugs that cause hypotension or syncope (e.g. medications with anticholinergic effects), potentially leading to falls [61].

Since there seems to be a potential for THC to lower blood pressure, it is prudent to monitor blood pressure in patients taking medicinal cannabis products containing THC.

## THC, Alcohol and Driving

Research indicates that the effect of the combination of cannabis and alcohol is greater than that when either is taken alone, and the effect is either additive or possibly synergistic [75].

A low dose of alcohol (i.e., blood alcohol concentrations around 0.04%) was found to impair driving performance in all tests, and the effects of smoking cannabis on driving performance were small (100 μg/ kg THC) or moderate (200 and 300 μg/ kg THC) when taken alone. However, when combined with a low dose of alcohol (alcohol sufficient for attaining a BAC of about 0.04%), low to moderate doses of THC (100 and 200 μg/kg) severely impaired driving performance [113]. This was supported by a case-control study that found that drivers positive for both have greater odds of making an error in driving than for either substance alone [75]. Other research supports the content that the risk associated with a combination of alcohol and cannabis is greater than from either alone or placebo [114–116].

In a study of the potential effect of alcohol, cannabis and combined alcohol and cannabis use on driving, current occasional (≥1×/last 3 months, ≤3 days per week) cannabis smokers were given either placebo or low-dose alcohol and inhaled 500-mg placebo, low (2.9%) or high (6.7%) THC vaporised cannabis over 10 min ad libitum in separate sessions (within-subject, six conditions). They then participated in simulated driving 0.5–1.3 h post-inhalation (6 sessions). Cannabis use was associated with slower driving, an increased tendency to drive below the speed limit and increased following distance. In comparison, alcohol was associated with increased standard deviation of speed and time spent above the speed limit, but it had no effect on following distance. THC concentration-dependent associations were found with decreased speed, increased time below the speed limit and increased following distance. This seems to indicate drivers may have been aware of their potential impairment and were trying to compensate [117]. This study did not find interactions between cannabis and alcohol for most of the driving behaviors investigated, except for a less than additive interaction between THC and breath alcohol concentration for % 'speed high'. Whilst the researchers explained this could suggest a possible mitigation of alcohol effects by THC on time spent above the speed limit, it does not necessarily mean that the combination of THC and alcohol results in safer driving and that certainly other studies suggest the combination is likely to be less safe [117].

The take-home message to patients should be to not combine THC-containing medicines and alcohol.

## Drug-THC Interactions

See Section on "Drug-Cannabinoid Interactions" after the section on CBD.

## THC in Individuals with Substance Use Disorders

Whilst much of the literature on cannabis use disorder and cannabis dependency or addiction relates to smoking of cannabis, typically for recreational purposes, there nonetheless remains the potential for development of dependency for THC with medicinal forms of cannabis. For this reason it should be used with caution in individuals with previous or current substance use disorders, such as opioids, nicotine, alcohol and illicit drugs [21].

However, there are studies indicating that medicinal cannabis may be an 'exit drug' for other addictive medicines. As mentioned previously, an Australian study of patients with cannabis dependence found that nabiximols use reduced the number of days patients consumed cannabis by approximately 40% [68]. Additionally, evidence suggests medicinal cannabis may be able to reduce opioid use [118]. For example, a cohort study in New Mexico followed 37 habitual chronic pain sufferers taking opioids who were enrolled in the Mexico Cannabis Program (MCP) and compared them with 29 patients with chronic back pain not enrolled in the MCP. At the end of 21 months, enrolment in the MCP was associated with a 17.27 higher odds of ceasing opioid use (CI 1.89–157.36, $p = 0.012$), a 5.12 higher odds of reducing daily opioid dosage and a 47% reduction in daily opioid dosage compared with 10.4% change in the control group. The MCP group had significant improvements in pain reduction, quality of life, social life and activity levels and few side effects one year after enrolling in the MCP [118].

## Safety of CBD

CBD is regarded as having a good safety profile, with a relatively low toxicity [102]. A WHO Expert Committee on Drug Dependence Report on CBD published in 2018 concluded that: 'Across a number of controlled and open label trials of the potential therapeutic effects of CBD it is generally well tolerated, with a good safety profile' [102].

A recent meta-analysis conducted at the University of NSW in Australia found that the few RCTs that examined adverse events and withdrawals due to pharmaceutical-grade CBD products or 'medicinal cannabis' (which they defined as cannabis buds/leaves or whole plant extracts) found no significant increases in the numbers of people having adverse events or withdrawing from the RCTs in comparison with active or placebo comparators [103]. CBD is not associated with the typical effects caused by cannabis or THC, e.g. psychological effects, impairment of psychomotor and cognitive performance and increased HR [119]. CBD has actually been found to cause the opposite effects to THC [119].

## CBD Adverse Effects

CBD adverse effects appear to be generally mild. An audit of 397 patients prescribed CBD at Cannabis Care in New Zealand (medicinal cannabis has been available since 2017 in New Zealand) assessed indications for use, patient-reported satisfaction, incidence of side effects and patient titrated dosage levels of CBD. CBD was found to be well tolerated with mild adverse events, most commonly related to sedation (this occurred in 2% of the sample who completed follow-up) [120]. Of the 253 patients who were followed up and provided data on adverse effects, adverse effects were experienced in 25 (9.9%) of the patients. Adverse effects included sedation (2.0%), vivid dreams (2.0%), emotional disturbances (e.g. irritable, depressed and anxious) (2.0%), disorientation (1.2%), sleeplessness (0.4%), nausea (0.4%), constipation (0.4%), diarrhoea (0.4%), headaches (0.4%), oral mucosa irritation (0.4%) and hallucinations (0.4%). Positive side effects found were improved appetite (2.8%) and improved sleep (12.3%) [120].

## CBD Is Not Addictive

CBD is not addictive. The WHO Report states: 'In humans, CBD exhibits no effects indicative of any abuse or dependence potential'. It also states: 'To date, there is no evidence of recreational use of CBD or any public health related problems associated with the use of pure CBD [102].

## CBD Does Not Convert to THC

There has been some contention in the literature, with some animal studies suggesting that CBD might convert to THC and other studies refuting this [121]. However, the evidence seems very clear that in humans, this does not occur [102, 121, 122].

## What Does the Preclinical Research on CBD Show in Relation to Safety?

The World Health Organization 2018 report on CBD reveals some preclinical research findings:

- 'CBD affects growth of tumoral cell lines, but has no effect in most non tumour cells. However, a pro-apoptotic effect has been observed in lymphocytes.
- It has no effect on embryonic development (limited research)
- Evidence on potential hormonal changes is mixed, with some evidence of possible effects and other studies suggesting no effect, depending on the method used and the particular hormone
- It has no effect on a wide range of physiological and biochemical parameters or significant effects on animal behaviour unless extremely high doses are administered (eg. in excess of 150 mg/kg iv as an acute dose or in excess of 30 mg/kg orally daily for 90 days in monkeys)
- Effects on the immune system are unclear; there is evidence of immune suppression at higher concentrations, but immune stimulation may occur at lower concentrations' [102].

## Toxicity of CBD

The LD50 for CBD in rhesus monkeys was found to be 212 mg/kg with intravenous administration [123], which indicates very low toxicity [124]. Whilst the oral LD50 has not been reported in the literature yet, an oral dose of CBD 20–50 times higher than the intravenous dose used in rhesus monkeys was found to cause severe toxicity [123, 124]. Several studies have been conducted and have not found any mutagenic or teratogenic effects induced by CBD [124, 125].

A recent hepato-toxicology study in mice found that for acute toxicity testing, no significant changes in liver enzymes were found for a dose of 246 mg/kg CBD (equivalent to MED of 20 mg/kg, analogous to those used in clinical trials). At 3 times this dose, there were significant increases in ALT and AST. Ten times the initial dose was associated with increased liver-to-body weight ratio, ALT, AST and total bilirubin. In the sub-acute toxicity testing using a starting dose of 61.5 mg/kg (equivalent to a MED of 5 mg/kg, analogous to starting target doses used in clinical trials in treatment-resistant epilepsy), no changes were observed at the base dose or 3X starting dose. Mice receiving 10X starting dose developed a moribund condition around days 3 and 4 and had increased liver-body weight ratios and raised liver enzymes [126].

In clinical studies of Epidiolex®, a plant derived CBD isolate, high doses were associated with elevated liver transaminases. However, it is important to put this in perspective of total dose and other drugs in use. In Epidiolex epilepsy trials, elevations in liver function tests for alanine aminotransferase (ALT) were reported in 1% of patients taking CBD 10 mg/kg/day compared with 17% of patients taking CBD 20 mg/kg/day. However, all but one case occurred in patients taking valproate and/or clobazam [127]. Most elevations resolved whilst the patient continued on treatment either with the same treatment regimen or with reduced medications, such as reduced CBD or AED doses [128].

In full spectrum medicinal cannabis products, the average doses are considerably lower than those used for the highly purified CBD (Epidiolex) associated with liver stress. In one typical clinical study, the starting dose for CBD in an open-labelled study of PTSD was 25 mg per day (which represents 0.35 mg/kg/day based on 70 kg body weight), and the mean daily dose at the end of the 8-week study was 48.64 mg (i.e. 0.69 mg/kg/day) [129]. In another study clinicians in a community psychiatric facility found that 12 mg to 25 mg of once-daily CBD herbal extract appears to provide relief of key symptoms in anxiety and sleep disorders with minimal side effects [130]. Thus, there appears to be a wide margin of safety between the low doses of CBD herbal extracts (less than 0.5 mg/kg) and high doses of purified CBD (20 mg/kg/day) seen in toxicity reports.

In a study of individuals with mild, moderate and severe impaired liver function, ingesting a single 200-mg dose of isolate CBD achieved higher total corresponding levels of CBD 1.48, 2.45 and 5.15 times that of controls (area under the curve exposure), but there were no acute changes in liver function studies from baseline, nor were there any significant adverse events [131].

## CBD-Drug Interactions

See Section on "Cannabinoid-Drug Interactions" at the end of the CBD section.

## Studies of CBD in Epilepsy: Side Effects

Several studies conducted on epilepsy, including severe forms of epilepsy, such as Dravet syndrome and Lennox-Gastaut syndrome, have assessed side effects associated with concomitant anti-epilepsy medication and CBD. These have included popular rashes, diarrhoea, somnolence, pyrexia, decreased appetite, vomiting, fatigue, pyrexia, convulsion and abnormal results on liver-function tests [132–113]. Interactions with the drugs clobazam, valproate and n-desmethylclobazam were implicated in several of the studies [133, 134, 137]. In general, the adverse reactions have been mild-moderate in severity and have resolved upon reduction of the dosage or discontinuation of the pharmaceutical or CBD. Transient elevations of liver enzymes were noted in some studies [134, 138].

The difficulty of extrapolating these findings to other conditions is that the dosages of CBD used to treat epilepsy tend to be of the order of 20 mg/kg per day (i.e. a 30-kg child would take 600 mg per day), which is typically a much greater dosage than is required to treat many other conditions. In addition, these patients tend to be taking several anti-epileptic medications. Thus, the CBD-drug interactions may be dose-related, that is, they may be due to the high doses of CBD used (as well as polypharmacy).

## CBD and Alcohol

The question of whether CBD may also interact adversely with alcohol has been investigated. This is important given the fact that beer containing CBD is now being manufactured in some countries. It should be noted that even high doses of oral CBD have not been found to cause THC- or cannabis-like effects [119].

A small double-blind, randomised cross-over study published in 1979 in 10 healthy volunteers (6 men, 4 women) compared placebo (glucose capsule and orange juice), CBD (200-mg capsule and orange juice), alcohol (1 g/kg in orange juice and glucose capsule) and CBD (200-mg capsule) plus alcohol (1 g/kg in orange juice). The combination of alcohol plus CBD resulted in significantly lower blood alcohol levels compared with alcohol alone. However, alcohol alone and alcohol plus CBD (but not CBD alone) both induced significant impairments in motor and psychomotor performances, and there were few differences between the pharmacological effects of alcohol and alcohol plus CBD [139].

In fact, the use of CBD as a potential therapy for alcoholism is being investigated. Transdermal and intraperitoneal delivery of CBD has been found to prevent alcohol-induced neurodegeneration in a rodent model of alcohol use disorder [140].

## CBD and Blood Pressure

It is known from preclinical studies that CBD causes vasorelaxation of isolated arteries as well as reduces vascular inflammation [141]. A systematic review and meta-analysis of in vivo haemodynamic effects of CBD found that under non-stress conditions, CBD had no significant effects on haemodynamics but that in response to stress, it reduced the increase in blood pressure and HR; it also increased cerebral blood flow in mice stroke models [142].

There have been a limited number of studies assessing the effect of CBD on blood pressure and other haemodynamic indices in humans.

A small randomised, double-blind, cross-over study was conducted on 9 healthy men who were given 600 mg of CBD or placebo [143]. The study found that CBD reduced resting SBP with a mean decrease of 6 mmHg (95% CI −12 to −1 mmHg, $p < 0.05$). There was no difference in DBP and mean arterial pressure (MAP) between the two groups.

Volunteers were then exposed to a mental stress test and a physical exercise stress test, with results as follows:

- <u>Mental stress test</u>: CBD was associated with a significantly lower resting SBP (mean −6 mmHg, 95% CI −12 to −1 mmHg, $p < 0.05$) compared with the placebo group, but there was no difference between groups in DBP or MAP.
- <u>Physical exercise stress test</u>: CBD was associated with significantly lower SBP (mean −5 mmHg, 95% CI −10 to −1 mmHg, $P < 0.05$) and significantly lower MAP (mean −5 mmHg, 95% CI −9 to −2 mmHg, $p < 0.05$). They found that those who had taken CBD had increased HR during the physical stress test (mean increase of 10 bpm, 95% CI +5–14 bpm, $p < 0.01$) [143].

In a later randomised, placebo-controlled, double-blind, parallel study design, the effects of acute and seven days of repeated dosing of CBD on haemodynamics, including SBP, DBP, HR and MAP, were assessed. Twenty-six healthy males were given either CBD (600 mg, $n = 13$) or placebo ($n = 13$) orally for seven days. Cardiovascular parameters were assessed at rest and under stress (in response to isometric exercise) after acute and repeated dosing [141]. The results were as follows:

- <u>Acute CBD dosing at rest:</u> no significant difference between groups in the SBP or DBP or HR, but there was a significantly reduced MAP of −2 mmHg (95% CI −3.6 to −0.3)
- <u>Repeated dosing (7 days) at rest:</u> no difference between the two groups in the SBP, DBP, HR or MAP (suggesting tolerance)
- <u>Acute CBD dosing under physical stress:</u> those in the CBD group had significantly lower SBP than the placebo group (mean decrease of 6 mmHg, 95% CI −0 to −1 mmHg, $p = 0.001$)
- <u>Repeated CBD dosing (7 days) under physical stress</u>: those in the CBD group had significantly lower SBP than the placebo group (mean decrease of 5.7 mmHg, 95% CI −10 to −1 mmHg, $p = 0.02$) and CBD was associated with a significant increase in internal carotid artery diameter (mean increase of +0.55 mm, $p = 0.01$) [141]

Thus, acute or repeated dosing over 7 days of CBD did not affect blood pressure in the resting state, but it did lower SBP under conditions of physical stress.

Within the CBD group, repeated dosing significantly reduced arterial stiffness by day 7 compared with day 1, suggesting that CBD may benefit vascular function, in particular under stress [141].

Like the previous study by Jadoon et al. [143], this study found a blunting effect of CBD on blood pressure changes in response to stress, but unlike the previous study, this later study did not find a significant increase in HR in association with CBD [141]. CBD was relatively well tolerated. The following side effects were reported post-CBD administration: lack of appetite on day 4 ($n = 1$), headache on day 3 ($n = 1$), insomnia on days 2 and 3 ($n = 1$), hyperactivity on days 2 and 3 ($n = 1$) and dysuria on days 5 and 6 ($n = 1$). Those in the placebo group reported migraine ($n = 1$) and light headedness on day 6 ($n = 1$) [141].

## Whole Spectrum CBD Versus Pure Isolate: Any Difference in Side Effects (and Efficacy)?

A meta-analysis of observational studies of treatment of refractory epilepsy was conducted to investigate whether there was any difference between CBD-rich extracts compared with purified CBD products in terms of safety and efficacy. The analysis included 11 studies (670 participants) [144]. The results indicate that higher efficacy, fewer adverse events and lower mean daily doses were achieved with the CBD-rich extracts compared with purified CBD:

- A greater percentage of patient reports of improvement was found in those treated with CBD-rich extracts compared with those treated with purified CBD (71% compared with 46%, $p < 0.0001$), though when the standard clinical threshold of a '50% reduction or more in the frequency of seizures' was applied, there was no statistically significant difference between the two groups (39% compared with 37% in the pure CBD group, $p = 0.52$).
- Those treated with CBD-enriched products had fewer mild (33% compared with 76%, $p < 0.001$) and severe (7% compared with 26%, $p < 0.0001$) adverse events compared with those treated with purified CBD [144].
- Those treated with CBD-rich extracts used a lower mean dose per day (6.0 mg/kg/day) compared with those treated with purified CBD (25.3 mg/kg/day) [144].

This meta-analysis was conducted on epilepsy only. Comparisons within other clinical conditions would be very interesting.

## What Doses of CBD Are Considered Safe?

CBD has been found to have a large therapeutic window. Chronic use and high doses of up to 1500 mg per day were repeatedly shown to be well tolerated by humans [145]. In the New Zealand study on CBD mentioned earlier [120], amongst those who completed the course of CBD, dosage information was available for 110 of the 253 followed-up patients. Dose varied widely between patients, ranging from 40 mg/day to 300 mg/day. Statistical analysis did not find any significant association between dosage and patient-reported benefit from CBD ($p = 0.145$). The study found that 9.9% of the followed-up patients reported adverse effects, the most common being sedation (2%), vivid dreams (2%) and emotional disturbances (2%).

Very high doses of CBD are typically prescribed for epilepsy. Product information on the tolerability of Epidiolex, a pharmaceutical-grade, plant-derived CBD product registered for use in the treatment of severe forms of epilepsy, states: 'Based on individual clinical response and tolerability, EPIDIOLEX can be increased up to a maximum recommended maintenance dose of 10 mg/kg twice daily (20 mg/kg/day)' [127]. A 12-week study conducted on children and young adults with epilepsy (who were taking a median of three anti-epileptic drugs) found that the mean CBD dose of 22.9 mg/kg (SD 9.1) at the end of 12 weeks was not correlated with the number of adverse events [132].

## Drug-Cannabinoid Interactions

It is important to be careful of the potential interactions between pharmaceuticals and cannabinoids, but it is also important to keep it in perspective.

According to a review of the potential for phytocannabinoids to act as substrates, inhibitors or inducers of human drug-metabolising enzymes, 'Studies of THC, CBD and CBN inhibition and induction of major CYP-450 isoforms generally reflect a low risk of clinically significant drug interactions with most use, but specific human data are lacking' [146].

CBD is implicated more in drug-phytocannabinoid interactions than THC [21]. According to the WHO, there is potential for CBD to be associated with drug interactions through the inhibition of some cytochrome P450 enzymes, but it is not yet clear whether these effects occur at physiological concentrations [102].

### Metabolism and Drug-Drug Interactions

To recap, most xenobiotic medicines are metabolised by the phase I hepatic cytochrome P450 enzyme system followed by phase II conjugation reaction, which is catalysed by the hepatic UDP-glucuronosyltransferase (UGT) enzymes. These two systems together metabolise over 90% of pharmaceuticals dependent on metabolism in the liver [104]. Most drugs are metabolised by a small number of the CYP enzymes [147].

In general, interactions between drugs are explained by alterations in the hepatic (and extra-hepatic tissue) metabolic enzymes, with many of the pharmacokinetic interactions due to the liver CYP enzymes being affected in some way by the administration of other drugs. Following co-administration, some drugs act as enzyme inducers, and others can act as enzyme inhibitors, with the latter being much more common [147], whilst some compete as substrates for an enzyme.

However, there can also be pharmacodynamic effects associated with drug-cannabinoid interactions. For example, cannabis can have sedative effects, which can be potentiated by concomitant use of medications with similar effects, such as benzodiazepines and opioids [21].

Interactions between phytocannabinoids and drugs can arise if the cannabinoid inhibits, induces or competes as a substrate for a metabolic enzyme that metabolises a drug (or another herb or food) [104].

Overall, cannabinoid metabolism is mainly by the CYP3A4, CYP2C9 and CYP2C19 enzymes and the UGT1A9 and UGT2B7 [104]. Around 60% of clinically prescribed drugs are metabolised by CYP3A4 [145].

## Main P450 Enzymes Metabolising CBD

CYP3A4 and CYP2C19 are the main contributors to CBD metabolism [21, 146], with others being CYP2C9, CYP1A2, 2C8, 2B6 and 2E1 [21, 22].

CBD has mixed effects on the CYP enzymes. CBD inactivates some CYP enzymes in the short term but then, like anticonvulsants, induces them with chronic dosing [145]. Upregulation of the CYP3A4, CYP2C and CYP2B10 messenger RNA has occurred in mice, and induction of CYP1A1 occurred in vivo. In contrast, CBD seems to be the inhibitor of the CYP2C8, CYP2C9, CYP2C19, UGT1A9 and UGT2B7 (uridine glucuronyl transferase) metabolism [148]. Drugs such as rifampin and ketoconazole that act as inducers or inhibitors of CYP pathways can reduce or increase CBD levels by 59% downward or 165% upward, respectively [148].

## Main CYP Enzymes in the Metabolism of THC

THC is less implicated in drug-phytocannabinoid interactions than CBD [61]. However, it can have effects at clinically relevant doses.

It is understood that CYP2C9 and CYP3A4 are the main enzymes involved in the primary metabolism of THC [146], with secondary metabolism occurring through several pathways: THC-COOH by several UGT isoforms, 7-OH $\Delta^8$-THC by CYP-450 isoforms (mostly CYP3A4), 11-OH-$\Delta^9$-THC by several UGT isoforms, 11-oxo-$\Delta^8$-THC by CYP450 isoforms (mainly CYP2C9) and some of the $\Delta^8$-THC epoxide metabolites by epoxide hydrolase (see [146]).

Potential interactions between THC and drugs are mainly due to THC conversion/metabolism by CYP3A4 and CYP2C9, which can be impacted by common pharmaceuticals [61].

However, THC has broad inhibitory effects on several P450 enzymes and also on carboxylesterase 1 (important in the metabolism of many drugs) [61, 149]. This can obviously then impact on metabolism and the bioavailability of other drugs metabolised by these enzymes.

A meta-analysis [149] found the following:

- CYP2D6, CYP2C19, CYP2B6 and CYP2J2 are inhibited by THC (and CBD).
- CYP2C9*, CYP1A1/2** and CYP1B1 are likely to be inhibited by THC (and CBD and cannabinol, CBN).
- THC also activates CYP2C9* and induces CYP1A1**.
- Carboxylesterase 1 (CES1) is potentially inhibited by THC and CBD (another study by [150] concluded that there is potential for clinically significant inhibition of CES1 by both CBD and THC).
- UGT1A9 is inhibited by CBD and CBN, whereas UGT2B7 is inhibited by CBD but activated by CBN [149].

* Separate studies found that THC can induce or inhibit CYP2C9: one research group found that THC and its metabolites (11-hydroxy-THC and 11-nor-9-carboxy-THC) induced CYP2C9 as demonstrated by increased phenytoin hydroxylation in human liver microsomes and recombinant enzyme systems [151], whilst another group found an inhibitory effect of THC (and CBD and CBN) on CYP substrates warfarin and diclofenac in human liver microsomes and recombinant enzyme systems [152]. A possible explanation for the opposite findings of these two groups, though not confirmed, is the different substrates and concentrations used between the studies, as well as the potential existence of an allosteric interaction between THC and CYP2C9 [149].

**For CYP1A1, studies indicate that phytocannabinoids may inhibit or induce this enzyme: two studies [153, 154] found that THC inhibits CYP1A1 (reference [154] also found that CBD and CBN inhibit CYPA1A); however [153] also found that THC was able to *induce* CYP1A1 mRNA levels in a mouse hepatoma cell line after 24 hours of incubation with THC [149].

**Genetic Variations in the P450 Enzymes in Individuals and THC Metabolism**
Research suggests that where individuals have diminished CYP29C or 3A4 function, there is potential for clinically meaningful elevations in THC exposure, and for those who have decreased CYP3A4 function, there is potential for clinically relevant elevations in CBD exposure [146].

CYP2C9 polymorphisms that affect up to 35% of Caucasians (but are not so prevalent in other racial groups) reduce the CYP2C9 metabolic activity and thus increase the bioavailability of THC, in some studies increasing the THC exposure two to three times [61, 155, 156].

## Effect of Co-administration of Drugs and Cannabinoids: Looking in Both Directions

When we look at the potential interactions between cannabinoids and pharmaceuticals, we must consider it from both directions, that is, what the effect of one will be on the other and vice versa.

Brown and Winterstein [21] describe these effects in relation to CBD and provide advice on what clinical action should be taken below. The same logic can be applied to THC.

- Effect on CBD of drugs that are P450 inhibitors: drugs that inhibit P450 enzymes involved in the CBD metabolism will potentially increase the CBD bioavailability and possibly increase the risk of adverse events. Action: start with a low dose of CBD initially and titrate up slowly to therapeutic effect, monitoring for any adverse effects [21].
- Effect on CBD of drugs that are P450 inducers: drugs that induce various P450 enzymes involved in the CBD metabolism will decrease the CBD bioavailability and therefore reduce its effectiveness. Action: higher doses of CBD may be needed when inducers are also being used [21].
- Drugs that are enzyme substrates (for CYP enzymes): The potential effect of concurrent use of CBD is the increase in the bioavailability of the substrate and thereby increase in the risk of adverse effects since CBD competes with the enzyme substrate (drug) for the metabolising enzyme. Action: avoid concurrent use, reduce substrate dose, and monitor for adverse effects/toxicity.

The same argument can be made for the impact of drugs that are CYP inducers or inhibitors on the THC bioavailability (for those P450 enzymes relevant to the THC metabolism, including CYP3A4 inducers or inhibitors or CYP2C9 inducers or inhibitors). Inducers can decrease the bioavailability and therefore effectiveness of THC, and inhibitors can increase the bioavailability of THC and therefore the potential for THC adverse events [61].

For example, a case study of an interaction between warfarin and CBD (Epidiolex®) found increased INR at 10 mg/kg/d and therefore risk of bleeding [157]. Warfarin is a CYP2C19 substrate. However, in most cases, warfarin doses can be adjusted and accommodated, as in this report, allowing for a plateau effect of INR with stable doses of warfarin despite increasing CBD doses up to 35 mg/kg [157].

## CBD Interactions with Liver UGT Enzymes in the Liver

UGT enzymes catalyse the glucuronidation of xenobiotics, a main pathway of phase II metabolism, creating a more readily excreted product. Inhibition of UGTs will therefore decrease excretion of the substrate. CBD has inhibitory effects on UGT1A9 and UGT2B7 enzymes [21]. Moreover, CBD is itself metabolised by UGT1A9 and UGT2B7 in the liver and UGT1A7 in the gastrointestinal tract [104].

Concurrent use of CBD with a range of pharmaceuticals that are UGT1A9 and UGT2B7 substrates can cause increased risk of side effects associated with the substrate [21].

- UGT1A9 substrates: include regorafenib, acetaminophen, ibuprofen and others
- UGT2B7 substrates: include ibuprofen, naproxen, lovastatin, valproate and others [21]

As you can see, some of these are very commonly used medications, such as acetaminophen, ibuprofen and naproxen. Brown and Winterstein [21] recommend CBD to be used with caution in patients who are newly prescribed these medicines or stabilised on them, since UGT inhibition will decrease their excretion and increase bioavailability. This is particularly important with drugs with narrow therapeutic windows and high potential toxicities.

## CBD and Other Enzymes: Breast Cancer Resistance Protein and Bile Salt Export Pump

The inactive hydroxylated metabolite of CBD, 7-COOH-CBD, is a substrate for P-glycoprotein and an inhibitor of the breast cancer resistance protein (BCRP) and bile salt export pump (BSEP). These are involved in the efflux of xenobiotics from tissues and transport into excretion pathways [21]. Here are some potential issues associated with concurrent use of CBD and BCRP and BSEP substrates:

- **BCRP Substrates:** Increased side effects of BCRP substrates with concurrent use of CBD are possible, with increased distribution into the tissues and decreased efflux into excretory organs. BCRP substrates include statins, prazosin, imatinib and others [21].
- **BSEP Substrates:** Increased side effects associated with BSEP substrates can occur with concurrent use of CBD. BESP substrates include paclitaxel, digoxin, statins, celecoxib and others [21].

Brown and Winterstein [21] recommend to avoid co-administration, monitor for adverse events and reduce substrate dosage when possible.

## Pharmacodynamic Interactions: Use of Sedating Medications and Antidepressants

THC alters cognitive functioning and could cause excessive sedation as well as impair motor skills. Thus, concurrent use with medications such as opioids and benzodiazepines, which have similar effects, could exacerbate such symptoms [] [61]. As mentioned previously, Brown states that THC has been known to exacerbate depression, schizophrenia and anxiety and the combination of THC and other drugs which are known to increase the risk of such conditions should be avoided [61]. As previously earlier, there may be the potential for THC to adversely reduce blood pressure in older people, in particular in those taking antihypertensives or other drugs that cause hypotension or syncope (e.g. medications with anticholinergic effects), that could potentially lead to falls [61].

## Safety of Terpenes

Generally, terpenes have low toxicity and high bioavailability and readily cross the skin and blood-brain barrier. Terpenes show very low acute toxicity; terpenes such as β-caryophyllene, myrcene, limonene, pinenes (α, β) and others have oral LD50 values of around 5000 mg/kg or higher [158]. Terpenes have been found to be toxic to particular cancer cell lines, but not to normal cells and tissue. In fact, they have been found to be nephron-, neuro- and hepato-protective [158].

## Conclusion

The four main routes of administration of medicinal cannabis, inhalation, oral route, topical/external application and other routes (suppositories, intranasal delivery) all have their place in healthcare practice. Much more is known about the pharmacokinetics of inhaled and oral routes of administration, in particular, in relation to THC, compared with the other routes of delivery. Having different routes of delivery allows tailoring of medicinal cannabis products to the patient's condition.

Safety of any kind of medicine is an important consideration, and there are possible drug-cannabis/THC/CBD interactions that may occur, though how prevalent any adverse interactions are in clinical practice is not definitively known. It is known that, in particular, high doses of CBD can interact with some anti-epileptic medications. Australia legalised the prescribing of medicinal cannabis in 2016, and at the time of writing, there were no reports of adverse events in relation to CBD recorded by the government, which suggests that either reporting rates are sub-optimal or these are not common. It is Dr. Blair's experience that with whole-spectrum high CBD-low THC medicinal cannabis, significant adverse side effects or interactions with pharmaceuticals are very uncommon at low-moderate doses (<200 mg/day for CBD products). What will be needed in the future is better capture and publishing of data in relation to safety in clinical practice, to reassure doctors and patients that medicinal cannabis prescribed properly is relatively safe.

## References

1. Huestis MA. Human cannabinoid pharmacokinetics. Chem Biodivers. 2007;4:1770–804.
2. World Health Organization (WHO). World Health Organization Expert Committee on Drug Dependence Pre-Review. Cannabis Plant and Cannabis Resin. Geneva: World Health Organization, 2018a. Available at: https://www.who.int/medicines/access/controlled-substances/ecdd_40_meeting/en/. Accessed 20 Jan 2021.
3. Lintzeris N, Davis J, Elias N, et al. Medicinal cannabis in Australia 2016: the Cannabis as medicine survey (CAMS-16). Med J Aust. 2018;209(5):211–6.
4. Sexton M, Cuttler C, Finnell J, Mischley L. A cross-sectional survey of medical cannabis users: patterns of use and perceived efficacy. Cannabis Cannabinoid Res. 2016;1:131–8.
5. MacCallum CA, Russo EB. Practical considerations in medical cannabis administration and dosing. Eur J Internal Med. 2018;49:12–9.

6. National Academies of Sciences, Engineering and Medicine. Report. The health effects of Cannabis and cannabinoids. Washington DC: The National Academies Press; 2017.
7. Van Der Kooy F, Pomahacova B, Verpoorte R. Cannabis smoke condensate II: influence of tobacco on tetrahydrocannabinol levels. Inhal Toxicol. 2009;21(2):87–90.
8. Zhang LR, Morgenstern H, Greenland S, et al. Cannabis smoking and lung cancer risk: pooled analysis in the international lung cancer consortium. J Cancer. 2015;136(4):894–903.
9. Wang B, Kovalchuk A, Li D, et al. In search of preventive strategies: novel high-CBD Cannabis sativa extracts modulate ACE2 expression in COVID-19 gateway tissues. Aging (Albany NY). 2020;12(22):22425–4444.
10. Cobb, Solanki. E-cigarettes, vaping devices, and acute lung injury. Respiratory Care. 2020;65(5):713–8.
11. Taylor J, Wiens T, Peterson J, et al. Characteristics of e-cigarette, or vaping, products used by patients with associated lung injury and products seized by law enforcement — Minnesota, 2018 and 2019. MMWR Morb Mortal Wkly Rep. 2019a;68:1096–100.
12. Lewis N. E-cigarette use, or vaping, practices and characteristics among persons with associated lung injury - Utah, April-October 2019. MMWR Morb Mortal Wkly Rep. 2019;68(42):953–6.
13. Blount BC, Karwowski MP, Morel-Espinosa M, et al. Evaluation of bronchoalveolar lavage fluid from patients in an outbreak of e-cigarette, or vaping, product useassociated lung injury - 10 states, August-October 2019. MMWR Morb Mortal Wkly Rep. 2019;68(45):1040–1.
14. Tijani AO, Thakur D, Mishra D, et al. Delivering therapeutic cannabinoids via skin: Current state and future perspectives. J Control Release. 2021;334:427–51.
15. Paudel KS, Hammell DC, Agu RU, et al. Cannabidiol bioavailability after nasal and transdermal application: effect of permeation enhancers. Drug Dev Ind Pharm. 2010;36(9):1088–97.
16. Nahtigal I, Blake A, Hand A, et al. The pharmacological properties of Cannabis. J Pain Manag. 2016;9(4):481–91.
17. Whittle BA, Guy GW, Robson P. Prospects for new cannabis-based prescription medicines. Cannabis Therap HIV/AID. 2012;67:183–206.
18. Chayasirisobhon S. Mechanisms of action and Pharmacokinetics of Cannabis. Perm J. 2020;25:1–3.
19. Grotenhermen F. Pharmacokinetics and pharmacodynamics of cannabinoids. Anesthesiology. 1997;86:24–33.
20. Mechoulam R, Gallily R. Cannabidiol: an overview of some pharmacological aspects. J Clin Pharmacol. 2002;42:11–9.
21. Brown JD, Winterstein AG. Potential adverse drug events and drug–drug interactions with medical and consumer cannabidiol (CBD) use. J Clin Med. 2019;8:989.
22. Jiang R, Yamouri S, Takeda S, et al. Identification of cytochrome P450 enzymes responsible for metabolism of cannabidiol by human liver microsomes. Life Sci. 2011;89(5–6):165–70.
23. Zhornitsky S, Potvin S. Cannabidiol in humans—the quest for therapeutic targets. Pharmaceuticals. 2012;5:529–52.
24. McGilveray IJ. Pharmacokinetics of cannabinoids. Pain Res Manag. 2005;10(Suppl A):15A–22A.
25. Ohlsson A, Lindgren JE, Wahlen A, et al. Plasma delta-9 tetrahydrocannabinol concentrations and clinical effects after oral and intravenous administration and smoking. Clin Pharmacol Ther. 1980;28(3):409–16.
26. Ohlsson A, Lindgren JE, Wahlén A, et al. Single dose kinetics of deuterium labelled delta 1-tetrahydrocannabinol in heavy and light cannabis users. Biomed Mass Spectrom. 1982;9(1):6–10.
27. Grotenhermen F. Pharmacokinetics and pharmacodynamics of cannabinoids. Clin Pharmacokinetics. 2003;42:327–60.
28. Goulle J, Saussereau E, Lacroix C. Delta-9tetrahydrocannabinol pharmacokinetics. Ann Pharm Françaises. 2008;66:232–4.
29. McPartland JM, Russo EB. Cannabis and cannabis extracts: greater than the sum of their parts? J Cannabis Therap. 2001;14:103–32.

30. Cyr C, Arboleda MF, Aggarwal SK, et al. Cannabis in palliative care: current challenges and practical recommendations. Ann Palliat Med. 2018; https://doi.org/10.21037/apm.2018.06.04.
31. Wall ME, Sadler BM, Brine D, et al. Metabolism, disposition, and kinetics of delta-9-tetrahydrocannabinol in men and women. Clin Pharmacol Ther. 1983;34(3):352–63.
32. Nadulski T, Pragst F, Weinberg G, et al. Randomized, double-blind, placebo controlled study about the effects of cannabidiol (CBD) on the pharmacokinetics of delta9-tetrahydrocannabinol (THC) after oral application of THC verses standardized cannabis extract. Ther Drug Monit. 2005;27:799–810.
33. Karschner EL, Darwin WD, Goodwin RS, Wright S, Huestis MA. Plasma cannabinoid pharmacokinetics following controlled oral a 9-tetrahydrocannabinol and oromucosal cannabis extract administration. Clin Chem. 2011a;57:66–75.
34. Karschner EL, Darwin WD, McMahon RP, Liu F, Wright S, Goodwin RS, et al. Subjective and physiological effects after controlled Sativex and oral THC administration. Clin Pharmacol Ther. 2011b;89:400–7.
35. Sharma P, Murthy P, Bharath MMS. Chemistry, metabolism, and toxicology of cannabis: clinical implications. Iran J Psychiatry. 2012;7:149–56.
36. ElSohly MA, Gula W, Walkera LA. Pharmacokinetics and tolerability of Δ9-THC-hemisuccinate in a suppository formulation as an alternative to capsules for the systemic delivery of Δ9-THC. Med Cannabis Cannabinoids. 2018;1:44–53.
37. Brenneisen R, Egli A, Elsohly MA et al. The effect of orally and rectally administered delta 9-tetrahydrocannabinol on spasticity: a pilot study with 2 patients. Int J Clin Pharmacol Ther. 1996;34(10):446–52.
38. Huestis MA, Henningfield JE, Cone EJ. Blood cannabinoids. I. Absorption of THC and formation of 11-OH-THC and THCCOOH during and after smoking marijuana. J Anal Toxicol. 1992;16:276–82.
39. Abramovici H. Information for health care professionals: cannabis (marihuana, marijuana) and the cannabinoids. Health Canada 2013. http://www.hc-sc.gc.ca/dhp-mps/alt_formats/pdf/marihuana/med/infoprof-eng.pdf.
40. Lemberger L, Axelrod J, Kopin IJ. Metabolism and disposition of delta-9-tetrahydrocannabinol in man. Pharmacol Rev. 1971;23:371–80.
41. Huestis MA. Pharmacokinetics and metabolism of the plant cannabinoids, delta9- tetrahydrocannabinol, cannabidiol and cannabinol. Handb Exp Pharmacol. 2005:657–90.
42. Lemberger L, Martz R, Rodda B, et al. Comparative pharmacology of Delta9-tetrahydrocannabinol and its metabolite, 11-OH-Delta9-tetrahydrocannabinol. J Clin Investig. 1973;52:2411–7.
43. Huestis MA, Cone EJ. Urinary excretion half-life of 11-nor-9-carboxy-delta9-tetrahydrocannabinol in humans. Ther Drug Monit. 1998;20:570–6.
44. Vandevenne M, Vandenbussche H, Verstraete A. Detection time of drugs of abuse in urine. Acta Clin Belg. 2000;55:323–33.
45. Smith-Kielland A, Skuterud B, Morland J. Urinary excretion of 11-nor-9-carboxy-delta9- tetrahydrocannabinol and cannabinoids in frequent and infrequent drug users. J Anal Toxicol. 1999;23:323–32.
46. Kelly P, Jones RT. Metabolism of tetrahydrocannabinol in frequent and infrequent marijuana users. J Anal Toxicol. 1992;16:228–35.
47. Reiter A, Hake J, Meissner C, et al. Time of drug elimination in chronic drug abusers. Case study of 52 patients in a "low-step" detoxification ward. Forensic Sci Int. 2001;119(2):248–53.
48. Hollister LE, Gillespie HK, Ohlsson A, et al. Do plasma concentrations of Δ-9 tetrahydrocannabinol reflect the degree of intoxication? J Clin Pharmacol. 1981;21:171S–7S.
49. Spindle TR, Cone EJ, Kuntz D, et al. Urinary Pharmacokinetic profile of cannabinoids following administration of vaporized and oral cannabidiol and vaporized CBD-dominant Cannabis. J Anal Toxicol. 2020;44(2):109–25.
50. Gable RS. Toward a comparative overview of dependence potential and acute toxicity of psychoactive substances used nonmedically. Am J Drug Alcohol Abuse. 1993;19(3):263–81.

51. World Health Organization (WHO). World Health Organization Expert Committee on Drug Dependence Pre-Review. Delta-9-Tetrahydrocannabinol. Geneva: World Health Organization, 2018c. Available at: https://www.who.int/medicines/access/controlled-substances/ecdd_40_meeting/en/
52. Bhaskar A, Bell A, Boivin M et al. Consensus recommendations on dosing and administration of medical cannabis to treat chronic pain: results of a modified Delphi process. J Cannabis Research. 2021;3:22.
53. Patel RS, Kamil SH, Bachu R, et al. Marijuana use and acute myocardial infarction: a systematic review of published cases in the literature. Trends Cardiovac Med. 2019;S1050-1738(19):30112–4.
54. De Filippas EM, Sing A, Divakaran S, et al. Cocaine and marijuana use among young adults with myocardial infarction. J Am Coll Cardiol. 2018;71:2540–51.
55. Frost L, Mostofsky E, Rosenbloom JI, et al. Marijuana use and long-term mortality among survivors of acute myocardial infarction. Am Heart J. 2013;165:170–5.
56. IOM (Institute of Medicine). Marijuana and medicine: assessing the science base. Washington, DC: National Academy Press; 1999.
57. Rezkalla S, Kloner RA. Cardiovascular effects of Marijuana. Trends Cardiovasc Med. 2019;29(7):403–7.
58. Hemachandra D, McKetin R, Cherbuin N, Anstey KJ. Heavy cannabis users at elevated risk of stroke: evidence from a general population survey. Aust N Z J Public Health. 2016;40:226–30.
59. Jivanji D, Mangosing M, Mahoney SP, et al. Association between Marijuana use and cardiovascular disease in US adults. Cureus. 2020;12(12):e11868. https://doi.org/10.7759/cureus.11868.
60. Page RL, Allen LA, Kloner RA, et al. Medical Marijuana, recreational cannabis, and cardiovascular health: a scientific statement From the American Heart Association. Circulation. 2020;142:e131–52.
61. Brown JD. Potential adverse drug events with tetrahydrocannabinol (THC) due to drug–drug interactions. J Clin Med. 2020;9(4):919.
62. Lim K, See YM, Lee J. A systematic review of the effectiveness of medical cannabis for psychiatric, movement and neurodegenerative disorders. Clin Psychopharmacol Neurosci. 2017;15(4):301–12.
63. Whiting PF, Wolff RF, Deshepande S, et al. Cannabinoids for medical use: a systematic review and meta-analysis. JAMA. 2015;313:2456–73.
64. Appelboam A, Oades PJ. Coma due to cannabis toxicity in an infant. Eur J Emerg Med. 2006;13(3):177–9.
65. Carstairs SD, Fujinaka MK, Keeney GE, Ly BT. Prolonged coma in a child due to hashish ingestion with quantitation of thc metabolites in urine. J Emerg Med. 2011;41(3):e69–71.
66. Piontek D, Kraus L, Legleye S, Buhringer G. The validity of DSM-IV cannabis abuse and dependence criteria in adolescents and the value of additional cannabis use indicators. Addiction. 2011;106(6):1137–45.
67. Leung J, Chan GCK, Hide L, Hall WD. What is the prevalence and risk of cannabis use disorders among people who use cannabis? a systematic review and meta-analysis. Addict Behav. 2020;109:106479.
68. Lintzeris N, Bhardwaj A, Mills L, et al. Nabiximols for the treatment of cannabis dependence: a randomized clinical trial. JAMA. 2019;179(9):1242–53.
69. Friedrich J, Khatib D, Parsa K, et al. The grass isn't always greener: the effects of cannabis on embryological development. BMC Pharmacol Toxicol. 2016;17:45.
70. Grant KS, Petroff R, Isoherranen N, et al. Cannabis use during pregnancy: pharmacokinetics and effects on child development. Pharmacol Ther. 2018;182:133–51.
71. Dahl RE, Scher MS, Williamson DE, et al. A longitudinal study of prenatal marijuana use: effects on sleep and arousal at age 3 years. Arch Pediatr Adolesc Med. 1995; https://doi.org/10.1001/archpedi.1995.02170140027004.

72. Winiger EA, Hewitt JK. Prenatal cannabis exposure and sleep outcomes in children 9-10 years of age in the adolescent brain cognitive development SM study. Sleep Health. 2020; https://doi.org/10.1016/j.sleh.2020.05.006. Accessed 20 Jan 2021.
73. Corsi DJ, Donelle J, Sucha E, et al. Maternal cannabis use in pregnancy and child neurodevelopmental outcomes. Nat Med. 2020; https://doi.org/10.1038/s41591-020-1002-5.
74. Hayes JS, Lampart R, Dreher MC, Morgan L. Five year follow up of rural Jamaican children whose mothers used marijuana during pregnancy. West Indian Med J. 1991;40(3):120–3.
75. Dubois S, Mullen N, Weaver B, Bedard M. The combined effects of alcohol and cannabis on driving: impact on crash risk. Forensic Sci Int. 2015;248:94–100.
76. Price JW. Marijuana and workplace safety: an examination of urine drug tests. J Addict Dis. 2014;33(1):24–7.
77. Zhang JC, Carnide N, Holness L, Cram P. Cannabis use and work-related injuries: a cross-sectional analysis. Occup Med (Lond). 2020;70(8):570–7.
78. Bernerth JB, Walker HJ. Altered states or much to do about nothing? A study of when Cannabis is used in relation to the impact it has on performance. Business Manag INK. 2020;45(4):459–78.
79. Biasutti WR, Leffers KSH, Callaghan RC. Systematic review of Cannabis use and risk of occupational injury. Subst Use Misuse. 2020;55(11):1733–45.
80. Malone DDT, Hill MN, Rubino T. Adolescent cannabis use and psychosis: epidemiology and neurodevelopmental models. 2010;160(3):511–22.
81. Ames F. A clinical and metabolic study of acute intoxication with Cannabis sativa and its role in the model psychoses. J Ment Sci. 1958;104:972–99.
82. Chopra GS, Smith JW. Psychotic reactions following cannabis use in East Indians. Arch Gen Psychiatry. 1974;30:24–7.
83. Spencer DJ. Cannabis induced psychosis. Br J Addiction. 1970;65:369–72.
84. Hall W, Degenhardt L, Teesson M. Cannabis use and psychotic disorders: an update. Drug Alcohol Rev. 2004;23:433–43.
85. Andreasson S, Allebeck P, Engstrom A, Rydberg U. Cannabis and schizophrenia. A longitudinal study of Swedish conscripts. Lancet. 1987;2:1483–6.
86. Zammit S, Allebeck P, Andreasson S, et al. Self reported cannabis use as a risk factor for schizophrenia in Swedish conscripts of 1969: historical cohort study. BMJ. 2002;325:1199.
87. Gage SH, Jones HJ, Burgess S, et al. Assessing causality in associations between cannabis use and schizophrenia risk: a two-sample Mendelian randomization study. Psychol Med. 2017;47:971–80.
88. Minichino A, Senior M, Brondino N, et al. Measuring disturbance of the endocannabinoid system in psychosis. JAMA Psychiat. 2019; https://doi.org/10.1001/jamapsychiatry.2019.0970.
89. Davis C, Bhattacharyya S. Cannabidiol as a potential treatment for psychosis. Ther Adv Psychopharmacol. 2019;9:1–16.
90. Dickens AM, Borgan F, Laurikainen H, et al. Links between central CB1-receptor availability and peripheral endocannabinoids in patients with first episode psychosis. Schizophrenia. 2020;6:21.
91. Lee TTY, Gorzalka BB. Timing is everything: evidence for a role of corticolimbic endocannabinoids in modulating hypothalamic–pituitary–adrenal axis activity across developmental periods. Neuroscience. 2012;204:17–30.
92. Muller N, WEidinger E, Leitner B, Schwartz MJ. The role of inflammation in schizophrenia. Front Neurosci. 2015;9:372.
93. Grinspoon L, Bakalar JB. Marihuana, the forbidden medicine, revised edition. New Haven, CT: Yale University Press, 1997, in: McPartland JM, Russo E. Cannabis and Cannabis Extracts: Greater Than the Sum of Their Parts? Cannabis Therapeutics. 2001;14:103–32.
94. McPartland JM, Russo E. Cannabis and Cannabis Extracts: Greater Than the Sum of Their Parts? The Haworth Press; 2001. Available at: http://cannabismed.org/data/pdf/2001-03-04-7.pdf

95. McPartland JM, Duncan M, Di Marzo V, Pertwee R. Are cannabidiol and Δ9-tetrahydrocannabivarin negative modulators of the endocannabinoid system? A systematic review. Brit J Pharmacol. 2015;172:737–53.
96. Ranganathan M, D'Souza DC. The acute effects of cannabinoids on memory in humans: a review. Psychopharmacology. 2006;188(4):425–44.
97. Walter C, Oertel BG. Felden Lisa et al. Effects of oral Δ9-tetrahydrocannabinol on the cerebral processing of olfactory input in healthy non-addicted subjects. Eur J Clin Pharmacol. 2017;73(12):1579–87.
98. Sorensen CJ, DeSanto K, Borgelt L, et al. Cannabinoid hyperemesis syndrome: diagnosis, pathophysiology, and treatment- a systematic review. J Med Toxicol. 2017;13:71–87.
99. D'Souza DC, Perry E, MacDougall L, et al. The psychotomimetic effects of intravenous delta-9-tetrahydrocannabinol in healthy individuals: implications for psychosis. Neuropsychopharmacology. 2004;29(8):1558–72.
100. Morrison PD, Zois Z, McKeown DA, et al. The acute effects of synthetic intravenous Delta9-tetrahydrocannabinol on psychosis, mood and cognitive functioning. Psychol Med. 2009;39(10):1607–16.
101. Hart CL, van Gorp W, Haney M, et al. Effects of acute smoked marijuana on complex cognitive performance. Neuropsychopharmacology. 2001;25(5):757–65.
102. World Health Organization (WHO). World Health Organization Expert Committee on Drug Dependence. Cannabidiol (CBD) Critical Review Report. Expert Committee on Drug Dependence Fortieth Meeting Geneva, 4–7 June 2018. World Health Organization (WHO), 2018b. Available at URL: https://www.who.int/medicines/access/controlled-substances/CannabidiolCriticalReview.pdf. Accessed 20 Jan 2021.
103. Black N, Stockings E, Campbell G, et al. Cannabinoids for the treatment of mental disorders and symptoms of mental disorders: a systematic review and meta-analysis. Lancet Psychiatry. 2019; https://doi.org/10.1016/S2215-0366(19)30401-8.
104. Kocis PT, Vrana KE. Delta-9-Tetrahydrocannabinol and cannabidiol drug-drug interactions. Med Cannabis Cannabinoids. 2020;1 https://doi.org/10.1159/000507998.
105. Sultan SR, Millar SA, O'Sullivan SE, England TJ. A systematic review and meta-analysis of the in vivo haemodynamic effects of Δ9-Tetrahydrocannabinol. Pharmaceuticals. 2018;11(1):13.
106. Benowitz NL, Jones RT. Cardiovascular effects of prolonged delta-9-tetrahydrocannabinol ingestion. Clin Pharmacol Ther. 1975;18(3):287–97.
107. Kayser RR, Haney M, Raskin M, Arout C, Simpson HB. Acute effects of cannabinoids on symptoms of obsessive-compulsive disorder: a human laboratory study. Depress Anxiety. 2020; https://doi.org/10.1002/da.23032.da.23032.
108. Abuhasira R, Haviv YS, Leiba M, et al. Cannabis is associated with blood pressure reduction in older adults – a 24-hours ambulatory blood pressure monitoring study. Eur J Internal Med. 2021; https://doi.org/10.1016/j.ejim.2021.01.005.
109. Van Den Elsen GAH, Ahmed AIA, Verkes RJ, et al. Tetrahydrocannabinol in behavioral disturbances in dementia: a crossover randomized controlled trial. Am J Geriatr Psychiatry. 2015a;23:1214–24.
110. Van Den Elsen GAH, Ahmed AIA, Verkes R-J, et al. Tetrahydrocannabinol for neuropsychiatric symptoms in dementia: a randomized controlled trial. Neurology. 2015b;84:2338–46.
111. Ahmed AIA, van den Elsen GAH, Colbers A, et al. Safety and pharmacokinetics of oral delta-9-tetrahydrocannabinol in healthy older subjects: a randomized controlled trial. Eur Neuropsychopharmacol. 2014;24:1475–82.
112. Sidney S. Cardiovascular consequences of Marijuana use. J Clin Pharmacol. 2002;42(11 Suppl):64S–70S.
113. Robbe H. Marijuana's impairing effects on driving are moderate when taken alone but severe when combined with alcohol. Human Psychopharmacol. 1998;13(S2):S70–8.
114. Downey LA, King R, Papafotiou K, Swann P, Ogden E, Boorman M, Stough C. The effects of cannabis and alcohol on simulated driving: Influences of dose and experience. Accid Anal Prev. 2013;50:879–86.

115. Ramaekers JG, Robbe HWJ, O'Hanlon JF. Marijuana, alcohol and actual driving performance. Hum Psychopharmacol. 2000;15:551–8.
116. Ronen A, Chassidim HS, Gershon P, et al. The effect of alcohol, THC and their combination on perceived effects, willingness to drive and performance of driving and non-driving tasks. Accid Anal Prev. 2010;42:1855–65.
117. Hartman RL, Brown TL, Milavetz G, et al. Cannabis effects on driving longitudinal control with and without alcohol. J Appl Toxicol. 2016;36(11):1418–29.
118. Vigil JM, Stith SS, Adams IM, Reeve AP. Associations between medical cannabis and prescription opioid use in chronic pain patients: a preliminary cohort study. PLoS One. 2017;12(11):e0187795.
119. Grotenhermen F, Russo E, Zuardi AW. Even high doses of oral cannabidiol do not cause THC-like effects in humans: comment on Merrick et al. Cannabis Cannabinoid Res. 2016;1(1):102–12.
120. Gulbransen G, Xu W, Arroll B. Cannabidiol prescription in clinical practice: an audit on the first 400 patients in New Zealand. BJGP Open. 2020;4(1):bjgpopen20X101010.
121. Crippa JA, Zuardi AW, Hallak JEC, et al. Oral Cannabidiol does not convert to Δ 8-THC or Δ 9-THC in humans: a pharmacokinetic study in healthy subjects. Cannabis Cannabinoid Res. 2020;5(1):89–98.
122. Consroe P, Kennedy K, Schram K. Assays of plasma cannabidiol by capillary gas chromatography/ion trap mass spectroscopy following high-dose repeated daily oral administration in humans. Pharmacol Biochem Behav. 1991;40:517–22.
123. Rosenkrantz H, Fleischman RW, Grant RJ. Toxicity of short-term administration of cannabinoids to rhesus monkeys. Toxicol Appl Pharmacol. 1981;58(1):118–31.
124. Dash R, Ali C, Jahan I, et al. Emerging potential of cannabidiol in reversing proteinopathies. Ageing Res Rev. 2020; https://doi.org/10.1016/j.arr.2020.101209.
125. Scuderi C, Filippis DD, Iuvone T, et al. Cannabidiol in medicine: a review of its therapeutic potential in CNS disorders. Phytother Res. 2009;23(5):597–602.
126. Ewing LE, Skinner CM, Quick CM, et al. Hepatoxicity of a cannabidiol-rich cannabis extract in the mouse model. Molecules. 2019;24:1694. https://doi.org/10.3390/molecules24091694.
127. EPIDIOLEX® (cannabidiol) oral solution, CV Initial U.S. Approval: 2018. Prescribing Information Revised 12/2018. Available at: https://www.epidiolex.com/sites/default/files/EPIDIOLEX_Full_Prescribing_Information.pdf. Accessed 12 Feb 2019.
128. Thiele E, Marsh E, Mazurkiewicz-Beldzinska M, et al. Cannabidiol in patients with Lennox-Gastaut syndrome: Interim analysis of an open-label extension study. Epilepsia. 2019;60(3):419–28.
129. Elms L, Shannon S, Hughes S, Lewis N. Cannabidiol in the treatment of post-traumatic stress disorder: a case series. J Altern Complement Med. 2019;25(4):392–7.
130. Shannon S, Lewis N, Lee H, Hughes S. Cannabidiol in anxiety and sleep: a large case series. Perm J. 2019;23:18–041.
131. Taylor L, Crockett J, Tayo B, Morrison G. A phase 1, open-label, parallel-group, single-dose trial of the pharmacokinetics and safety of cannabidiol (CBD) in subjects with mild to severe hepatic impairment. J Clin Pharmacol. 2019b;59(8):1110–9.
132. Devinsky O, Marsh E, Friedman D, et al. Cannabidiol in patients with treatment-resistant epilepsy: an open-label interventional trial. Lancet Neurol. 2016;15(3):270–8.
133. Morrison G, Crockett J, Blakey G, Sommerville K. A phase 1, open-label, pharmacokinetic trial to investigate possible drug-drug interactions between clobazam, stiripentol, or valproate and cannabidiol in healthy subjects. ACCP. 2019;8(8):1009–31.
134. Thiele EA, Marsh ED, French JA, et al. Cannabidiol in patients with seizures associated with Lennox-Gastaut syndrome (GWPCARE4): a randomised, double-blind, placebo-controlled phase 3 trial. Lancet. 2018;391(10125):1085–96.
135. Devinsky O, Cross JH, Laux L, et al. Trial of cannabidiol for drug-resistant seizures in the Dravet syndrome. N Engl J Med. 2017;376:2011–20.
136. Devinsky O, Nabbout R, Miller I, et al. Long-term cannabidiol treatment in patients with Dravet syndrome: An open-label extension trial. Epilepsia. 2019;60(2):294–302.

137. Geffrey AL, Pollack SF, Bruno PL, Thiele EA. Drug-drug interaction between clobazam and cannabidiol in children with refractory epilepsy. Epilepsia. 2015;56(8):1246–51.
138. Gaston TE, Bebin EM, Cutter GR, et al. Interactions between cannabidiol and commonly used antiepileptic drugs. Epilepsia. 2017;58(9):1586–92.
139. Consroe P, Carlini EA, Zwicker AP, Lacerda LA. Interaction of cannabidiol and alcohol in humans. Psychopharmacol (Berl). 1979;66(1):45–50.
140. Liput DL, Hammell DC, Stinchcomb AL, Nixon K. Transdermal delivery of cannabidiol attenuates binge alcohol-induced neurodegeneration in a rodent model of an alcohol use disorder. Pharmacol Biochem Behav. 2013;111:120–7.
141. Sultan SR, O'Sullivan SE, England TJ. The effects of acute and sustained cannabidiol dosing for seven days on the haemodynamics in healthy men: a randomised controlled trial. Br J Clin Pharmacol. 2020;86(6):1125–38.
142. Sultan SR, Millar SA, England TJ, O'Sullivan SEA. Systematic review and meta-analysis of the Haemodynamic effects of cannabidiol. Front Pharmacol. 2017;8:81.
143. Jadoon KA, Tan GD, O'Sullivan SE. A single dose of cannabidiol reduces blood pressure in healthy volunteers in a randomized crossover study. JCI Insight. 2017;2(12):e93760.
144. Pamplona FA, da Silva LR, Coan AC, et al. Potential clinical benefits of CBD-rich *cannabis* extracts over purified CBD in treatment-resistant epilepsy: observational data meta-analysis. Front Neurol. 2018;9:759.
145. Bergamaschi MM, Queiroz RH, Zuardi AW, et al. Safety and side effects of cannabidiol, a Cannabis sativa constituent. Curr Drug Saf. 2011;6:237–49.
146. Stout SM, Cimino NM. Exogenous cannabinoids as substrates, inhibitors, and inducers of human drug metabolizing enzymes: a systematic review. Drug Metabol Rev. 2014:46(1). https://doi-org.ezproxy.uws.edu.au/10.3109/03602532.2013.849268.
147. Tanaka E. Clinically important pharmacokinetic drug-drug interactions: role of cytochrome P450 enzymes. J Clin Pharm Therap. 1998;23:403–16.
148. White CM. A review of human studies assessing cannabidiol's (CBD) therapeutic actions and potential. J Clin Pharmacol. 2019;00(0):1–12.
149. Qian Y, Gurley BJ, Markowitz JS. The potential for pharmacokinetic interactions between cannabis products and conventional medications. J Clin Psychopharmacol. 2019a;39(5):462–71.
150. Qian Y, Wang X, Markowitz JS. In vitro inhibition of carboxylesterase 1 by major cannabinoids and selected metabolites. Drug Metab Dispos. 2019b;47:465–72.
151. Bland TM, Haining RL, Tracy TS, et al. CYP2C-catalyzed delta9-tetrahydrocannabinol metabolism: kinetics, pharmacogenetics and interaction with phenytoin. Biochem Pharmacol. 2005;70:1096–103.
152. Yamaori S, Koeda K, Kushihara M, et al. Comparison in the in vitro inhibitory effects of major phytocannabinoids and polycyclic aromatic hydrocarbons contained in marijuana smoke on cytochrome P450 2C9 activity. Drug Metab Pharmacokinet. 2012;27:294–300.
153. Roth MD, Marques-Magallanes JA, Yuan M, et al. Induction and regulation of the carcinogen-metabolizing enzyme CYP1A1 by marijuana smoke and delta (9)-tetrahydrocannabinol. Am J Respir Cell Mol Biol. 2001;24:339–44.
154. Yamaori S, Kushihara M, Yamamoto I, et al. Characterization of major phytocannabinoids, cannabidiol and cannabinol, as isoform-selective and potent inhibitors of human CYP1 enzymes. Biochem Pharmacol. 2010;79:1691–8.
155. Sachse-Seeboth C, Pfeil J, Sehrt D, et al. Interindividual variation in the pharmacokinetics of delta9-tetrahydrocannabinol as related to genetic polymorphisms in CYP2C9. Clin Pharmacol Ther. 2009;85:273–6.
156. Wang B, Wang J, Huang SQ, et al. Genetic polymorphism of the human cytochrome P450 2C9 gene and its clinical significance. Curr Drug Metab. 2009;10(7):781–834.
157. Grayson L, Vines B, Nichol K, et al. An interaction between warfarin and cannabidiol, a case report. Epilepsy Behav Case Rep. 2018;9:10–1.
158. Nuutinen T. Medicinal properties of terpenes found in *Cannabis sativa* and *Humulus lupulus*. Eur J Med Chem. 2018;157:198–228.

# Conclusion 12

In writing this book, we sought to demonstrate that there is already much known about the endocannabinoid system (ECS), its homeostatic role within the body and how it may be involved in regulation of stress and emotions as well as in pathophysiology of various mental health conditions. There is also much that is unknown. We also sought to demonstrate how the plant Cannabis sativa and its key active constituents, in particular cannabidiol (CBD), may be able to assist in the treatment of many conditions associated with mental health. It seems evident that there is much research into mechanisms of action and efficacy of CBD and THC in animals, and there is a growing evidence-base also in relation to efficacy of medicinal cannabis in humans also. Western science and biomedicine, in particular, take a reductionistic approach to understanding how the human body works and what happens in disease, seeking to examine specific biological or neurological pathways and disruptions therein within specific diseases. The pharmaceutical model seeks to find an active constituent that can be isolated, copied, manipulated in some way and then patented and sold. It is very difficult to patent plant medicines. The reductionist approach to understanding the functioning of the human body, therefore, marries up with the pharmaceutical approach quite well.

However, our ranges of experiences as clinicians, educators and researchers (Kylie) and a deep quest to understand the nature of health and illness have shaped a somewhat different understanding of what might be important in helping people achieve wellness.

## Philosophical Thoughts

In examining how the ECS might be involved in various mental health conditions (and in this book, we also included insomnia given its comorbidity with many mental health illnesses and indeed other diseases), it is apparent that within many parts of the brain and body, the ECS is operational. It is a homeostatic regulatory system that seeks to bring the body back into balance. Many researchers strive to find those



K. O'Brien, P. Blair, *Medicinal Cannabis and CBD in Mental Healthcare*,
https://doi.org/10.1007/978-3-030-78559-8_12

parts of the brain, in which the ECS is involved in specific mental illnesses, and understand what is happening with the individual components of the endocannabinoidome (i.e. endocannabinoids, receptors, enzymes and transporters). One can see how pharmaceutical companies might be interested in all endocannabinoid mechanisms, including, for example, those enzymes involved in the degradation of the endocannabinoids such as fatty acid amide hydrolase (FAAH). Synthetic FAAH inhibitors have been developed as patented new drugs. But there is a risk. In 2016 the FAAH inhibitor BIA 10–2474 was undergoing Phase I clinical trials in France when serious adverse effects occurred. BIA 10–2474 was developed 'for the treatment of medical conditions in which there is advantage in enhance the levels of endogenous AEA and tonically increase the drive of the endocannabinoid system' [1]. The unfortunate result was that volunteers on the test drug were adversely affected, with one declared brain-dead and four others reported to have irreversible brain damage [1].

Prior to this tragic episode, rimonabant, an antagonist and inverse agonist for the cannabinoid receptor CB1, was approved by the European Union in 2006 as an anorectic anti-obesity drug. Post-marketing surveillance data revealed that the risk of psychiatric disorders in people taking rimonabant was double that observed in clinical trials. In addition, other side effects were reported, including gastroenteritis, anxiety, irritability, insomnia and other sleep disorders, hot flushes, diarrhoea, dry or itchy skin, tendonitis, muscle cramps and spasms, fatigue, increased risk of falling and flu-like symptoms, by up to 10% of users, whilst nausea and upper respiratory tract infections were reported by more than 10% of users [2]. Rimonabant was subsequently removed from the market due to the very serious mental health side effects and harm caused. Our sense is, if you start to manipulate any unique component of a biological pathway, in this case the CB1 receptors, given the widespread crucial regulatory nature of the ECS, you are going to impact many systems, not just one part of the brain. It is the totality of the human being, the overall state of the ECS, that is going to be important. That brings us to another point.

The potential problems associated with drugs that target specific biological pathways or receptors are in considerable contrast to natural phytocannabinoids that show considerable contextual modulation of neuroendocrine and metabolic physiological effects on different cell types even within the same organ.

At many points in the preceding chapters, we have eluded to a 'dysfunctional' ECS that may not be justified. Most of the 'dysfunction' relates to environmental, behavioural or genetic stresses causing imbalances in our ECS 'chemical-software' for signalling. No doubt there are significant genetic shifts and even defects in our individual endocannabinoidome genes that impact our health and how we individually respond to endocannabinoid-modulating herbs and drugs. There are already several companies attempting to correlate ECS genes with health conditions and ideal cultivar selections for treatment. Confirming evidence in this area may lead us to more personalised cannabinoid treatments in the future.

More importantly, the dysregulated ECS is a key pathomechanism of clinical disease induced by a root cause that comes from a wide range of possible adverse aetiologies. These include toxins from drugs, chemicals or nature as well as infectious sources. Nutritional patterns and deficiencies may be implicated. Dysfunctional behaviours may also play a role as we have seen with chronically stressed animals, sleep deprivation, unnatural light and vibration exposures. And, we cannot leave out trauma or cancer as root causes of ECS imbalances.

Assuming this is the case, a medicinal cannabis consultation can and should be the start of the journey to identify and address the root cause(s) of many of the syndromes our modern society faces. Integrative mental health providers are already doing this through the field of functional medicine [3]. These health professionals routinely perform root-cause investigations using cost-effective investigations into patterns of organic acids in the urine that can indicate deviations in, for example, the Krebs cycle or neurotransmitter metabolites [4]. Test abnormalities can suggest toxins, infections, nutritional deficiencies and genetic metabolic defects and suggest possible holistic therapeutic approaches. These include conventional drugs along with lifestyle modifications, herbs, supplements and biomodulation through, for example, acupuncture, massage or sauna. Unfortunately, no ECS parameters are available at the current time, but future research may reveal specific patterns correlating with mental health disorders providing clinical clues to the use of ECS modulation.

## Mind and Body Are Not Really So Separate

We still have a sense of Cartesian duality permeating our understanding of mental health. We split the mind and the body and treat them as separate. We delve into parts of the brain to understand what is going wrong in various mental health conditions, and indeed we have reported such research findings in this book. Yet we do not really understand what the 'mind' is. Ancient medical systems such as Chinese medicine and ayurvedic medicine see mind and body as a continuum. In Chinese medicine, the heart is seen as the 'seat of consciousness', not the brain, and the emotions are not ascribed to the brain. Instead, each organ system (and the concept of 'organ' in Chinese medicine is quite different from the biomedical one, though it includes this) has a related emotion, and the organ systems are inter-related [5]. Emotions are understood to be potential aetiological factors in illness [5]. These notions would once have seemed somewhat ridiculous to a western mind. However, we now know that there is a neurochemical basis for the impact of emotions on our functioning, and the fields of psychoneuroimmunology, psychoneuroendocrinology and neurocardiology are well established.

Research has also demonstrated that clusters of autonomic nervous system neurons that regulate organs such as the heart, lung, gastrointestinal tract, kidney and bladder lie near the organs and communicate with each other, forming networks that facilitate information exchange [6]. Not only does the heart receive signals from the central nervous system (CNS) neurons, but afferent signals arising from the heart are known to affect neurons in the CNS (as well as ganglia in the thorax and the heart itself) [6]. The heart is understood to have its own 'little brain', and there is a sophisticated two-way communication between the two, with each influencing each other's function [6]. We also now understand much about the gut microbiome and its integral role in our health and in illness. The 'gut-brain axis' is now an established entity, and much is understood about how the gut and brain interact. Perhaps the notion of the organ systems being associated with particular emotional states, as in Chinese medicine, is not such a stretch of the imagination.

## The Notion of Balance

What also underpins traditional medical systems like Chinese medicine is the concept of balance. In Chinese medicine, this was captured in the Theory of Yin and Yang, which describes two complementary but opposite, interdependent forces. In health, yin and yang are in balance, whereas in illness, they are out of balance [5]. This is not so foreign to western medicine, as here we also have a similar concept, called homeostasis. Indeed, the ECS is an important regulator, perhaps the most important regulator, of homeostatic balance.

In Chinese medicine, however, the concept of balance is not only related to the internal workings of the body but also includes how the human interacts with her/his environment. This concept even extends to how the organ systems inter-relate internally. We can therefore see that an individual's environment can play an important role in health. The 'environment' can include levels of stress in the individual's life, her/his home surroundings and work environment and the greater environment, e.g. town, city and country where the person lives. Here again, the ECS may be an impartial and central mediator of these negative signals of stress. If a person is living with a great amount of personal stress, it will not be surprising to find that her/his health is not optimal. A person's personal home environment can detrimentally affect her/his health – toxic personal products used on the body daily, off-gassing of toxic components of paint and contact with toxic cleaning products are only a few ways that we expose ourselves to everyday toxins that can accumulate in the body and eventually cause us harm.

Another important principle that Chinese medicine teaches us is to find and treat the root cause of illness, termed 'ben', and not only treat the signs and symptoms of the illness (the 'biao' or branches) [5].

From traditional medicine systems, then, we learn something important. We do not exist in a vacuum. Rather we are inter-dependent with our environment, and that concept of environment extends from the inside (our inner milieu) to outside: our personal environment, work environment, societal environment and planetary environment. Branches of medicine such as 'environmental medicine' understand the impact of environmental toxins and pathogens on health. Thus, when a person comes into our practice with a health problem, we are going to need to look much more broadly than many practitioners are perhaps used to doing. We need to look at the person in front of us in their totality and try to understand all the potential factors that have brought this person out of balance, because fundamentally, disease is a reflection of a loss of balance.

## The Many Factors that Keep Us Healthy

Medicinal cannabis is not a magic panacea for every condition. It can be very helpful in many conditions; however if we are to help people truly heal, we must look at the many factors that can adversely as well as positively impact health.

Lifestyle factors are increasingly recognised as critical in achieving and maintaining well-being as well as contributors to illness. Lifestyle factors include physical activity, sleep, nutrition and diet, stress levels and environment. These are important pillars of health and can all contribute to poor health, including poor mental health. For example, research clearly shows us that a sedentary lifestyle can take years off our life and contribute to many diseases and disease risk factors, including obesity, diabetes, cardiovascular disease and cancer [7, 8].

## Physical Activity

Physical activity is critical to our well-being and our mental health. For example, tai chi (a form of Chinese exercise therapy) has been shown to cause changes in the Th1 and Th2 immune responses associated with immune modulation of natural killer cells and dendritic cells [9] as well as improve sleep, reduce anxiety and depression, improve stress management, reduce pain, increase strength and flexibility and increase cardiopulmonary function [10, 11]. A meta-analysis demonstrated a significant effect of tai chi on reducing depression [11]. That is only one form of exercise!

Active lifestyles and aerobic exercise have been found to help protect against age-related cognitive declines and have a positive impact on brain structure and function, in particular executive brain functioning [12]. Animal research shows that physical exercise can induce hippocampal neurogenesis, cell proliferation and dendritic branching and increase gene expression of brain-derived neurotrophic factor (BDNF) in the hippocampus [12]. For an in-depth exploration of the benefits of physical exercise on brain health and functioning, see Watson [13].

## Nutrition

The importance of nutrition for health, in general, and mental health, specifically, cannot be understated. There is now so much scientific evidence on the impact of poor and good nutrition on health that it is not debatable – good nutrition underpins health, and this includes mental health. There is much in the literature that links poor nutrition and nutritional factors to depression [14], for example, and indeed to many other diseases, including cancer, cardiovascular disease, diabetes and obesity [7]. As we have stressed in an earlier chapter, the western diet is characterised by a high omega 6/omega 3 ratio, which is essentially pro-inflammatory. We have an epidemic of diseases underpinned by inflammation, and you will note that in our discussions of many of the mental health conditions in this book, there is evidence that inflammation is part of the pathomechanism.

Therefore, it is very important in a holistic approach to helping people regain and/or maintain health, including mental health, that dietary factors are examined. There are many good books that can provide information on the role of nutrition in various mental health conditions, including those conditions in this book.

What is an unfortunate fact is that there is still a paucity of nutritional medicine education in orthodox medical degree training. If you are not trained in nutritional medicine, we suggest that you expand your network and include other healthcare practitioners who are knowledgeable in this area (naturopaths, nutritional medicine practitioners and dieticians) and refer your patients to see them for advice on nutrition. You can also learn more about nutritional and environmental medicine via online courses, such as those provided by the Australasian College of Nutritional and Environmental Medicine (www.acnem.org) – this was set up nearly 40 years ago to provide postgraduate training to medical and allied healthcare practitioners in these important areas.

## Other Factors

A person's environment can play a key role in illness, including mental health. In using the word 'environment', we are taking a broad definition – it includes not only the inner milieu (inner environment, including our gut microbiota and state of our immune system) but also our personal environment, home and office environment and planetary environment. If we are ingesting toxins or are exposed in other ways to environmental toxins (e.g. exposure to electromagnetic frequencies from cell phones and telecommunication towers), damage can be cumulative, and it can cause neurological damage to our brains. We must consider the environment in which the patient is living and existing. Again, if you do not know much about environmental medicine, you can learn through colleges, such as the ACNEM mentioned earlier, or refer to colleagues who are experienced in this field, including building biologists who can inspect homes, offices and other spaces and help identify environmental toxins and solutions.

Stress can be an aetiological factor in many illnesses. If a patient is under personal stress, you might refer them also to see a counsellor or psychologist. If they are stressed because they have lost their home after divorce and are living in their car, medicinal cannabis or any other form of medicine is not likely to suddenly alleviate their extreme stress, anxiety or depression, but referring them to social services where they might obtain some practical help possibly will (in Chinese medicine, this is the 'root cause' of the illness). We need to pull back sometimes and listen to the patient in front of us. If we listen well, they will lead us to what is at the bottom of their health problems.

## Medicinal Cannabis

This brings us back to medicinal cannabis. By understanding the pathomechanisms of various illnesses, including mental health illnesses, and by understanding the various mechanisms of action of cannabis, including its key phytocannabinoids and terpenes, we can start to understand the reasons why cannabis may help alleviate such conditions as well as the signs and symptoms. Whilst we recognise that this is taking a mechanistic approach to the study of the mind-body and cannabis, it is still very useful. Evidence of how medicinal cannabis may work in relation to the underlying pathogenesis of a condition, coupled with evidence of efficacy in animal and human studies, provides a rationale for healthcare practitioners to consider the option of prescribing medicinal cannabis for a particular condition.

When we look at results of human studies including epidemiological and clinical research, we are stepping back from the world of biological and biochemical pathways to see if and how medicinal cannabis impacts humans. You can see from the research described in this book that there is a varying degree of human research investigating the efficacy of medicinal cannabis for various mental health conditions. The same applies more generally to the state of research into medicinal cannabis across the board. Some conditions have a greater bank of evidence than others. This will change in time with the opening up of the world to the potential therapeutic benefits of medicinal cannabis.

If you understand research methodology, you will also understand that randomised controlled trials (RCTs) and meta-analyses are inherently flawed as research approaches, despite being top of the hierarchy of evidence in medicine. RCTs typically have a narrow set of inclusion and exclusion criteria, which is applied to recruit participants to studies. Thus, the study population is relatively homogeneous. This does not reflect the real population. Therefore, it is wise to take all kinds of research into consideration when trying to reach a conclusion of whether medicinal cannabis might be efficacious in particular conditions or not. This includes research such as epidemiological studies, cohort studies and case reports, as well as the clinical experiences of the many healthcare practitioners prescribing it and the many experiences of the patients who are taking it.

## An Herbal Medicine Rediscovered

This is one of the most fascinating herbal medicines on the earth, and it has been rediscovered at a time when it is increasingly needed. We are seeing a resurgence of its use within many countries after decades of being wrongfully outlawed. What will be very important is that access to this plant medicine is not denied or made difficult for those who wish to use it and that the forces that seek to suppress it because of its medicinal value are not allowed to do so. Healthcare practitioners can be an important part of increasing access, but they can also be party to restricting access. Our thoughts are that it is the patient's right to access a medicinal plant that grows on this earth. Healthcare practitioners trained in medicinal cannabis are simply there to provide guidance to patients who wish to seek their advice on how to use it and certainly not to carry out a 'medical takeover' of this herb. People have the right to access this herb for their own self-care too.

We believe that medicinal cannabis has a place in healthcare broadly, including mental healthcare, and hope that reading this book has opened your eyes to the growing scientific evidence that exists. Our heroes are the researchers who have dedicated their efforts to understand this remarkable plant medicine and our endocannabinoid system, the work of many of whom we have captured in these pages, as well as those healthcare practitioners who are guiding patients in its use. We wish you well on your journey of discovery about medicinal cannabis, contextualised as part of a holistic treatment strategy that addresses the varied fundamental factors that have led to imbalance in each of your patients.

## References


1. Kaur R, Sidhu P, Singh S. What failed BIA 10-2474 Phase I clinical trial? Global speculations and recommendations for future Phase I trials. J Pharmacol Pharmacother. 2016;7(3):120–6.
2. Moreira FA, Crippa JA. The psychiatric side-effects of rimonabant. Rev Bras Psiquiatr. 2009;31(2):145–53.
3. Lake J, Helgason C, Sarris J. Integrative Mental Health (IMH): paradigm, research, and clinical practice. Explore (NY). 2012;8(1):50–7.
4. Shaw W, Kassen E, Chaves E. Increased urinary excretion of analogs of krebs cycle metabolites and arabinose in two brothers with autistic features. Clin Chem. 1995;41:1094–104.
5. O'Brien KA, Xue CC. The theoretical framework of Chinese medicine. In: Leung P-C, Xue CC, Cheng Y-C, editors. A Comprehensive Guide to Chinese Medicine. 2nd ed. New Jersey: World Scientific Press; 2016.
6. Armour JA. Neurocardiology. Anatomical and functional principles. California: Institute of HeartMath; 2003.
7. O'Brien K, Sali A. A Clinician's Guide to Integrative Oncology: What You Should Be Talking About with Cancer Patients and Why. US: Springer; 2017.
8. Peterson CB, Bauma A, Gronbaek M, et al. Total sitting time and risk of myocardial infarction, coronary heart disease and all-cause mortality in a prospective cohort of Danish adults. International J Behavioural Nutrition & Physical Activity. 2014;11:13.
9. Liu J, Chen P, Wang R, et al. Effect of tai chi exercise on immune function in middle-aged and elderly women. Sports Med Doping Stud. 2012;2(6):1000119.
10. Li JX, Hong Y, Chan KM. Tai chi: physiological characteristics and beneficial effects on health. Br J Sports Med. 2001;35:148–56.
11. Wang F, Lee EK, Wu T, et al. The effects of tai chi on depression, anxiety, and psychological wellbeing: a systematic review and meta-analysis. Int J Behav Med. 2014;21(4):605–17.
12. Bonavita S, Tedeschi G. Neural structure, connectivity and cognition changes associated with physical activity. In: Watson RR, editor. Physical Activity and the Aging Brain: Effects of Exercise on Neurological Function. London: Elsevier Science & Technology; 2017.
13. Watson RR, editor. Physical Activity and the Aging Brain: Effects of Exercise on Neurological Function. London: Elsevier Science & Technology; 2017.
14. Owens M, Watkins E, Bot M, et al. Habitual Behavior as a Mediator Between Food-Related Behavioral Activation and Change in Symptoms of Depression in the MooDFOOD Trial. Clinical Psychological Science. 2020;9(4):649–65.

# Index





K. O'Brien, P. Blair, *Medicinal Cannabis and CBD in Mental Healthcare*,
https://doi.org/10.1007/978-3-030-78559-8

MIX
Papier aus verantwortungsvollen Quellen
Paper from responsible sources
FSC® C105338

If you have any concerns about our products, you can contact us on
**ProductSafety@springernature.com**

In case Publisher is established outside the EU, the EU authorized representative is:
**Springer Nature Customer Service Center GmbH**
**Europaplatz 3, 69115 Heidelberg, Germany**

Printed by Libri Plureos GmbH
in Hamburg, Germany